AN INTRODUCTION TO

COMMUNITY HEALTH

AN INTRODUCTION TO

COMMUNITY HEALTH

James F. McKenzie
Ball State University

Robert R. Pinger
Ball State University

HarperCollinsCollegePublishers

We would like to dedicate this book to our wives, Bonnie and Harriet, and our children: Anne, Craig, Katherine, Andrew, and Michael.

Editor-in-Chief: Glyn Davies
Executive Editor: Bonnie Roesch
Developmental Editor: Maxine Effenson-Chuck
Project Editor: Janet Frick
Text and Cover Designer: Wendy Ann Fredericks
Cover Photographs: clockwise from top left: Peter Simon/Stock, Boston; Robert Bremer/PhotoEdit; Scott Foresman; Gale Zucker/Stock Boston; Centers for Disease Control; and John Griffin/The Image Works
Art Studio: Academy Artworks, Inc.
Photo Researcher: Rosemary Hunter
Electronic Production Manager: Valerie A. Sawyer
Desktop Administrator and Electronic Page Makeup: Sarah Johnson
Electronic Page Makeup: Interactive Composition Corporation
Manufacturing Manager: Helene G. Landers
Printer and Binder: RR Donnelley & Sons Company
Cover Printer: The Lehigh Press, Inc.

An Introduction to Community Health

Library of Congress Cataloging-in-Publication Data

McKenzie, James F., 1948-
    An introduction to community health / James McKenzie, Robert R. Pinger
        p. cm.
    Includes index.
    ISBN 0-06-500797-2.
    1. Public health. 2. Community health services.
3. Regional medical programs. I. Pinger, R. R.
II. Title.
    [DNLM: 1. Community Health Services—United States. 2. Community Medicine—methods—United States. 3. Delivery of Health Care—United States. 4. Occupational Health. 5. Public Health—United States. WA 546 AA1 M471 1994]
RC425.M238 1995
362.1'2—dc20
DNLM/DLC   94-20883
for Library of Congress   CIP

94 95 96 97   9 8 7 6 5 4 3 2 1

Contents

v

Chapter 11
Community
Mental Health 336

Chapter 12
Abuse of Alcohol
and Other Drugs 368

UNIT III
HEALTH CARE
DELIVERY 405

Chapter 13
Health Care System:
Structure Scenario 406

Chapter 14
Health Care System: Function   434

UNIT IV
ENVIRONMENTAL HEALTH AND SAFETY   469

Chapter 15
Environmental Concerns: Wastes and Pollution   470

Chapter 16
The Impact of Environment on Human Health   529

Chapter 17
Injuries as a Community Health Problem   571

Chapter 18
Safety and Health in the Workplace   609

Preface

As its title implies, *An Introduction to Community Health* was written to introduce students to community health. In comparison with other such textbooks, this text is unique. It incorporates a variety of pedagogical elements that will assist and encourage students to understand complex community health issues.

Each chapter of the book includes: (1) chapter objectives, (2) a scenario, (3) an introduction, (4) content, (5) marginal definitions of key terms, (6) a chapter summary, (7) a scenario analysis and response, (8) review questions, (9) activities, and (10) references. In addition, many figures, tables, boxes, and photos and a glossary have been presented to clarify and illustrate the concepts presented in the text. Selected content in each chapter is related to the *Healthy People 2000* goals and objectives.

Chapter Objectives

The chapter objectives identify the content and skills that should be mastered after reading the chapters, answering the end-of-chapter questions, and completing the activities. To use the objectives effectively, it is suggested that they be reviewed before reading the chapters. This will help focus the reader on the major points in each chapter and facilitate answering the questions and completing the activities at the end.

Scenarios

Short scenarios are presented at the beginning of each chapter. The scenarios pro-vide real-life situations related to the chapter content. The content presented in the chapter will allow the student to offer a solution to the community health problem presented in the scenario.

Introduction

Each chapter begins with a brief introduction that informs the reader of the topics to be presented and discussed and explains how these topics relate to others in the book.

Marginal Definitions

Key terms are introduced in each chapter of the textbook. These terms are important to the understanding of the chapter. Such terms are presented in boldface type within each chapter, and the definitions are presented in the lower margins. Before reading the chapter, it is suggested that the student skim the chapters, paying particular attention to the key terms. This should provide greater understanding of the content. The bold-faced terms, including those defined in the margin, appear in the glossary at the end of the book.

Content

Although each chapter in the textbook could be expanded, and in some situations there are entire books written on topics that are covered here in a chapter or less, it is felt that each chapter contains the necessary information to help the reader understand the issues related to community health. To enhance and facilitate learning, the chapters are organized in four units: Foundations of Community Health, The Nation's Health, Health Care Delivery, and Environmental Health and Safety.

Chapter Summary

At the end of each chapter, the reader will find a two- or three-paragraph review of the major concepts contained in each chapter.

Scenario: Analysis and Response

Following the chapter summary, students are provided an opportunity to respond to the scenario presented earlier in the chapter. The content presented in the chapter will help the students to formulate their responses.

Review Questions

The purpose of the questions at the end of each chapter is to provide the readers with some feedback regarding their mastery of the chapter's content. The questions reinforce the chapter objectives and key terms.

Activities

The final pedagogical element, and one unique to this text, is the activities. These activities will not only allow the readers to apply their new knowledge but also to apply it in a meaningful way. The activities are presented in a variety of formats and should appeal to the different learning styles of the readers.

It is felt that this textbook is one that students will find easy to understand and use. If they read the chapters carefully and make an honest effort to answer the review questions and complete some of the activities, we feel confident that students will gain a good understanding of the realm of community health.

Introduction to Community Health is accompanied by an Instructor's Manual/ Test Bank by James McKenzie. This helpful supplement includes teaching outlines and strategies, and a set of over 900 test questions.

Acknowledgments

A project of this nature could not be completed without the assistance and understanding of a number of individuals. First, we would like to thank all our past and present students, who have inspired us to produce a better community health textbook. Second, we would like to thank several colleagues for their contributions. They include: Dale B. Hahn, Ph.D., for encouraging us to take on this project; Molly S. Wantz, Ed.S., Ball State University, for her review of Chapter 6; Wayne A. Payne, Ed.D., Ball State University, for his review of Chapter 10; Jacquie Rainey, Dr. P.H., Ball State University, for her writing of Chapter 8; Alice K. Thomas, M.S.W., for her review of Chapter 11; Ellen J. Hahn, D.N.S., University of Kentucky, for her review of Chapter 12; Diana Godish, Ph.D., Ball State University, for her review of Chapter 15; Diane L. Calvin, M.L.S., Ball State University, for her help in finding the facts; and Kate Prager, Sc.D., National Center for Health Statistics, for her help in locating the latest government health statistics. Third, we would like to express our thanks to those professionals who took the time and effort to review our manuscript and provide feedback. They include: A. Davanni, California State University—Sacramento; Donald Ensley, East Carolina University; Mary Hawk, Western Washington University; Joseph Hudak, Ohio Eastern University; Marilyn Morton, State University of New York—Plattsburgh; Carol M. Parker, University of Central Oklahoma; Jane Petrillo, Western Kentucky University; Carl Peter, Western Illinois University; Gayle

Schmidt, Texas A & M University; J. L. Sexton, Fort Hays State University; and Bob Walsh, Idaho State University. Fourth, we would like to thank several employees of HarperCollins College Publishers for their work: Bonnie Roesch, Executive Editor and Director of Development, for her initial and continued support of the project; Janet Frick, Project Editor, for her untiring effort to produce a quality book; and Juliana Nocker, Editorial Assistant, for her ability to answer all the questions. Fifth, we would like to thank Maxine "Max" Effenson-Chuck of B. Czar Productions, Inc., for the endless amount of time she spent in her role as Developmental Editor. Sixth, we express our appreciation to Suzanne Ivester for her copy editing skill. Seventh, we are grateful to Billie Kennedy for her assistance in typing the manuscript. And finally, we would like to thank our families for their support, encouragement, and tolerance of the time that writing takes away from family activities.

James F. McKenzie, Ph.D., M.P.H.

Robert R. Pinger, Ph.D.

UNIT I
FOUNDATIONS OF
COMMUNITY HEALTH

AIDS and the Education
of Our Children

A Guide for Parents and Teachers

Chapter 1

COMMUNITY HEALTH— YESTERDAY, TODAY, AND TOMORROW

Chapter Outline

Chapter Objectives

After studying this chapter, you will be able to:

1. Accurately define the terms *health, community, community health,* and *public health.*
2. Explain the difference between personal and community health.
3. Describe the role of community health in our society today.
4. Explain the concept of community.
5. List and discuss the factors that influence a community's health.
6. Briefly relate the history of community/public health, including the recent history of community and public health in the twentieth-century United States.
7. Provide a brief overview of the current health status of Americans and list some of the health goals for the year 2000.
8. Describe the status of efforts to improve world health and list some objectives for the future.

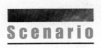

Amy and Todd are a young working couple and have "the world by the tail." They have high-paying jobs, drive new cars, are buying a home in a good neighborhood, and have two healthy preschool children. While reading the newspaper one evening, Amy learns that hepatitis has been reported at three day care centers near the one their two preschoolers attend. As the couple discusses whether or not they should take their children to day care as usual the following day, they discover that they have many unanswered questions. How serious is hepatitis? What is the likelihood that their children will be at serious risk for getting the disease? Is any state or local agency responsible for standardizing health practices at private day care centers in the community? Does the city, county, or state carry out any type of inspection when they license these facilities? If the children do not attend day care, which parent will stay home with them?

INTRODUCTION

As the twentieth century comes to an end, the achievement of good health has become a worldwide goal. Governments, private organizations, and individuals throughout the world are working to improve health. Although individual actions to improve one's own personal health certainly contribute to the overall health of the community, community actions are sometimes needed when health problems exceed the resources of any one individual. When such actions are not taken, the health of the entire community is at risk.

This chapter introduces the concepts and principles of community health, explains how community health differs from personal health, and provides a brief history of community health. Some of the key health problems facing Americans in the 1990s are described, and an outlook for the twenty-first century is given.

Definitions

The word *health* means different things to different people. Similarly there are other words that can be defined in various ways. Some basic terms we will use in this book are defined in the paragraphs that follow.

Health

The word **health** is derived from *hal,* which means "hale, sound, whole." When it comes to the health of people, the word *health* has been defined in a number of different ways—often in its social context, as when a parent describes the health of a child or when an avid fan defines the health of a professional athlete. Until the beginning of the health promotion era, in the mid-1970s, the most widely accepted definition of health was the one published by the World Health Organization in 1947. That definition states that "health is a state of complete physical, mental, and social well-being and not merely the absence of disease and infirmity."[1] However, in more recent times the word has taken on a more holistic approach; Payne and Hahn have defined **health** as the blending of physical, emotional, social, intellectual, and spiritual

---

health The blending of all one's personal resources for the enjoyment of a satisfying, productive life.

resources as they assist in mastering the developmental tasks necessary to enjoy a satisfying and productive life.[2]

Community

A **community** is a group of people with a shared location, shared environment, and shared fate. Our community is the social unit within which we interact. It may be as small as a residence hall floor or as large as the nation or world in which we live.

> Although a community is a difficult thing to define, it is easy to define what is *not* a community. No single person, no nuclear family, no bureaucracy, no government, no corporation, no place, and no process can be considered as a community. Each person *belongs to,* each family *is important to,* each effective bureaucracy *is beholden to,* and many corporations *affect the lives of* communities.[3]

Community Health

Community health includes both private and public efforts of individuals, groups, and organizations to promote, protect, and preserve the health of those in the community.

Public Health

Public health is the sum of all official (governmental) efforts to promote, protect, and preserve the people's health.

Roles of Community Health in Society

The average American spends little time each day thinking or planning for good

community People with a shared location, shared environment, and shared fate.
community health Both private and public efforts to promote, protect, and preserve the health of those in the community.
public health Government efforts to promote, protect, and preserve the people's health.

health. Most think about health only when confronted with illness. Even fewer people worry about community health. When was the last time you got up in the morning worrying about polluted air or water, the homeless, the spread of a communicable disease, or that someone in your town may be denied health care? If you are like most Americans, the last time you worried about a community health problem was when you were directly impacted by it. Actually, all Americans are impacted by community health activities on a daily basis. Let's examine this concept more closely.

Community Health versus Personal Health

To further clarify the definitions presented in this chapter it is important to distinguish between the terms *personal health* and *community health*.

The Domain of Personal Health

Personal health activities are individual actions and decision making that affect the health of an individual or his or her immediate family members. These activities may be preventive or curative in nature but seldom directly affect the behavior of others. Choosing to eat wisely, to wear a safety belt regularly, and to visit the physician are all examples of personal health activities.

The Domain of Community Health

Community health activities are those that are aimed at protecting or improving the health of a population or community. Maintenance of accurate birth and death records, protection of the food and water supply, and participating in fund drives for voluntary health organizations such as the American Cancer Society are examples of community health activities.

In this course, you will be introduced to the many community health activities and to the organizations that have responsibility for carrying them out. Below are some of the key topics covered in this text:

Organizations that contribute to community health.

How communities measure disease, injury, and death.

Control of communicable and noncommunicable diseases.

How communities organize to solve health problems.

Community health in schools.

Health needs of mothers, infants, and children.

Health needs of special populations.

Community mental health.

Abuse of alcohol, tobacco, and other drugs.

The health care delivery system.

Environmental health problems.

Intentional and unintentional injuries.

Occupational safety and health.

The Concept of Community

Traditionally, the community has been thought of as a geographic area with specific boundaries—for example, a neighborhood, city, county, or state. However, as noted earlier, a community is a social unit that shares the same fate. This community could be defined by a political boundary, as the city of San Francisco, for example. But it might also be defined by a physical feature or by social or cultural forces. Therefore, a community could be defined by occupation; for example, we speak of the business community, the banking community, or the industrial community. There are separate communities that include those involved in agriculture, education, or religion. There are communities made up of those on welfare, those with social concerns like homelessness, those with similar ethnic backgrounds, and so on. It is important to remember that communities do not necessarily require a political or governmental boundary.

Factors That Affect the Health of a Community

There are a great many factors that affect the health of a community. As a result, the health status of each community is different. These factors may be physical, social, and/or cultural. They also include the ability of the community to organize and work together as well as the individual behaviors of those in the community (see Figure 1.1).

Physical Factors

Physical factors include the influences of geography, the environment, community size, and industrial development.

Geography

A community's health problems can be directly influenced by its altitude, latitude, and climate. In tropical countries where warm, humid temperatures and rain prevail throughout the year, parasitic and infectious diseases are a leading community

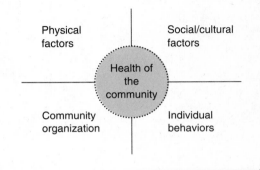

FIGURE 1.1

Factors that affect the health of a community.

health problem (see Figure 1.2). In many tropical countries, survival from these diseases is made more difficult because poor soil conditions result in inadequate food production and malnutrition. In temperate climates with fewer parasitic and infectious diseases and a more than adequate food supply, obesity and heart disease are important community health problems.

Environment

The quality of our environment is directly related to the quality of our stewardship over it. Many experts believe that if we

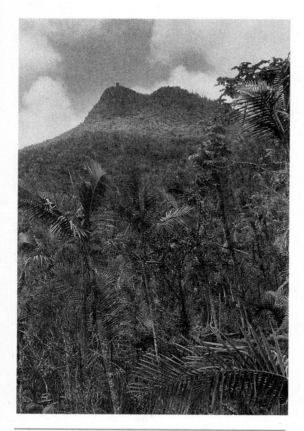

In tropical countries, parasitic and infectious diseases are a leading community health problem.

continue to allow uncontrolled population growth and continue to deplete nonrenewable natural resources, succeeding generations will inhabit communities that are less desirable than ours. Many feel that we must accept responsibility for this stewardship and drastically reduce the rate at which we foul the soil, water, and air.

Community Size

The larger the community, the greater its range of health problems and the greater its health resources. For example, larger communities have more health professionals and better health facilities than smaller communities. These resources are often needed because communicable diseases can spread more quickly and environmental problems are often more severe in densely populated areas. For example, the amount of trash generated by the 7-plus million people in New York City is many times greater than that generated by the entire state of North Dakota, with its population of about 750,000.

It is important to note that a community's size can impact both positively and negatively on that community's health. The ability of a community to effectively plan, organize, and utilize its resources can determine whether size can be used to good advantage.

Industrial Development

Industrial development, like size, has either positive or negative effects on the health status of a community. Industrial development provides a community with added resources for community health programs but may bring with it environmental pollution and occupational illnesses. Communities that experience rapid industrial development must eventually regulate the way in which industries: (1) obtain raw materials, (2) discharge by-products, (3) dispose of wastes, (4) treat and protect their employees, and (5) clean up environmental accidents. Unfortunately, these laws are usually passed only after these communities have suffered significant reductions in the quality of their life and health.

Social and Cultural Factors

Social factors are those that arise from the interaction of individuals or groups within the community. For example, people who live in urban communities, where the life is fast-paced, experience higher rates of stress-related illnesses than those who live in rural communities, where life is more leisurely. On the other hand, those in rural areas may not have access to the same quality or selection of hospitals or medical specialists available to those who live in cities.

Cultural factors arise from guidelines (both explicit and implicit) that individuals "inherit" from being a part of a particular society. These guidelines tell them how to view the world and how to behave in it in relation to other people, to supernatural forces or gods, and to the natural environment.[4] Some of these factors are discussed below.

Beliefs, Traditions, and Prejudices

The beliefs, traditions, and prejudices of community members can affect the health of the community. The beliefs of those in a community about such specific health behaviors as exercise and smoking can influence policy makers on whether or not they will spend money on bike trails and no-smoking legislation. The traditions of specific ethnic groups can influence the types of food, restaurants, and bars in a community. Prejudices in one specific ethnic or racial group against another can result in acts of violence and crime. Racial and ethnic disparities will continue to put certain groups, such as black Americans, at greater risk.

Economy

Both national and local economies can affect the health of a community through reductions in health and social services. An economic downturn means that lower tax revenues (fewer tax dollars) will be available for programs including welfare, food stamps, and community health care. This occurs because revenue shortfalls cause agencies to experience budget cuts. With less money, they often must alter their eligibility guidelines thereby restricting aid to only the neediest individuals. Obviously, many people who had been eligible for assistance before the economic downturn become ineligible.

Employers usually find it increasingly difficult to provide health benefits for their employees as their income drops. The unemployed and underemployed face poverty and deteriorating health. Thus, the cumulative effect of an economic downturn significantly affects the health of the community.

Politics

Those who happen to be in political office, either nationally or locally, can improve or jeopardize the health of their community by the decisions they make. In the most general terms, the argument is over greater or lesser governmental participation in health issues. For example, there has been a long-standing discussion in the United States on the extent to which the government should involve itself in health care. Historically, Democrats have been in favor of such action while Republicans have been against it. However, as the cost of health care has continued to grow, both sides see the need for some kind of increased regulation. Local politicians also influence the health of their communities each time they vote on health-related measures brought before them.

Religion

A number of religions have taken a position on health care. For example, some religious communities limit the type of medical treatment their members may receive. Some do not permit immunizations; others do not permit their members to be treated by physicians. Still others prohibit certain foods.[4] For example, Kosher dietary regulations permit Jews to eat the meat only of animals that chew a cud and the flesh only of fish that have both gills and scales. They are forbidden to eat the meat of animals with cloven hooves.

Some religious communities actively address moral and ethical issues like abortion, premarital intercourse, and homosexuality. Still other religions teach health-promoting codes of living to their members. Obviously, religion can affect a community's health positively or negatively (see Figure 1.3).

Social Norms

The influence of social norms can be positive or negative and can change over time. Cigarette smoking provides a good example. During the 1940s, 1950s, and 1960s it was socially acceptable to smoke in most

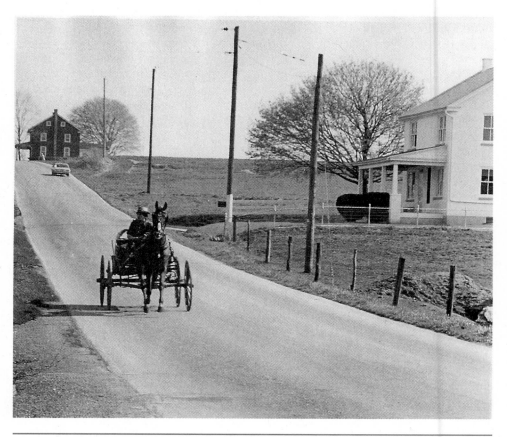

FIGURE 1.3

Religion can affect a community's health either positively or negatively.

settings. As a matter of fact, in 1960, 53% of American men and 32% of American women smoked. Thus, in 1960 it was socially acceptable to be a smoker, especially if you were male. In 1990, those percentages have dropped to 28% (for males) and 23% (for females), and in most public places it has become socially unacceptable to smoke. Thus, there is less social pressure to smoke. Unlike smoking, alcohol consumption represents a continuing negative social norm in America, especially on college campuses. The normal expectation seems to be that drinking is fun (and almost everyone wants to have fun). Despite the fact that most college students are too young to drink legally, 80–90% of college students drink. It seems fairly obvious that the American alcoholic-beverage industry has influenced our social norms.

Socioeconomic Status (SES)

Segments of the community with the lowest socioeconomic status also have the poorest health and the most difficulty in gaining access to the health care. The point of entry into the health care system for most Americans is the family doctor. The economically disadvantaged seldom have a family doctor. For them, the point of entry is the local hospital emergency room—a resource they access usually only when very ill. It is little wonder that people with incomes below the federal poverty level have death rates twice as high as those of people with incomes above the poverty level.[5]

Community Organization

The way in which a community is able to organize its resources directly influences its ability to intervene and solve problems, including health problems. **Community organization** is "the method of intervention whereby individuals, groups and organizations engage in planned action to influence social problems. It is concerned with the enrichment, development, and/or change of social institutions."[6] It is not a science but an art of building consensus within a democratic process.[7] If a community can organize its resources effectively into a unified force, it will be better able to address and resolve a community health problem. For example, many communities in the United States have faced communitywide drug problems. Some have been able to organize their resources to reduce or resolve these problems while others have not. (See Chapter 5 for a full explanation of community organization.)

Individual Behavior

The behavior of the individual members of a community contributes to the health of the entire community. It takes the concerted effort of many—if not most––of the individuals in a community, to make a voluntary program work. For example, if each individual consciously recycles his or her trash each week, community recycling will be successful. Likewise, if each occupant would wear a safety belt, there could be a significant reduction in the number of facial injuries and deaths from car crashes for the entire community. In another example, the more individuals who become immunized against a specific disease, the slower the disease will spread and the fewer people will be exposed. This concept is known as **herd immunity.**

---

community organization Planned action by members of a community to influence social problems.

herd immunity The resistance of a population to the spread of an infectious agent based on the immunity of a high proportion of individuals.

A BRIEF HISTORY OF COMMUNITY AND PUBLIC HEALTH

The history of community and public health is almost as long as the history of civilization. This brief summary provides an account of some of the accomplishments and failures in community and public health. It is hoped that a knowledge of the past will enable us to better prepare for future challenges to our community's health.

Earliest Civilizations

In all likelihood, the earliest community health practices went unrecorded. Perhaps these practices involved taboos against defecation within the tribal communal area or near the source of drinking water. Perhaps they involved rites associated with burial of the dead. Certainly, the use of herbs for the prevention and curing of diseases and communal assistance with child birth are practices that predate archeological records.

Ancient Societies (Before 500 B.C.)

Excavations at sites of some of the earliest known civilizations have uncovered evidence of community health activities (see Figure 1.4). Archeological findings from the Indus Valley of northern India, dating to about 2000 B.C., provide evidence of bathrooms and drains in homes, and sewers below street level. Drainage systems have also been discovered among the ruins of the Middle Kingdom of ancient Egypt (2000–2700 B.C.). The Myceneans, who lived on Crete in 1600 B.C., had toilets, flushing systems, and sewers.[8] Written medical prescriptions for drugs have been deciphered from a Sumarian clay tablet dated at about 2100 B.C. By 1500 B.C. more than 700 drugs were known to the Egyptians.[9]

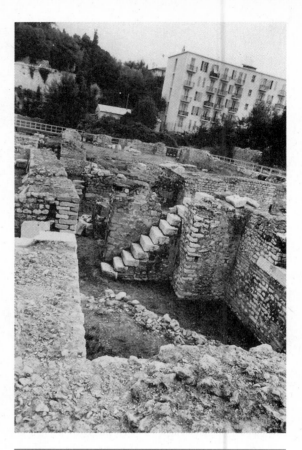

FIGURE 1.4

Archeological findings reveal community health practices of the past.

Perhaps the earliest written record concerning public health is the Code of Hammurabi, the famous king of Babylon, who lived 3900 years ago. Hammurabi's code of conduct included laws pertaining to physicians and health practices (see Figure 1.5). The Bible's Book of Leviticus, written about 1500 B.C., provides guidelines for personal cleanliness, sanitation of campsites, disinfection of wells, isolation of lepers, disposal of refuse, and the hygiene of maternity.[10]

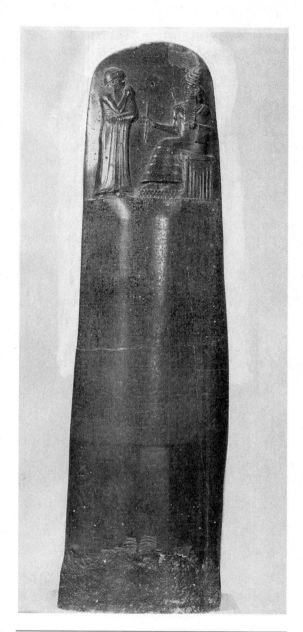

FIGURE 1.5

The Code of Hammurabi included laws pertaining to physicians and health practices.

Classical Cultures (500 B.C.–500 A.D.)

During the thirteenth and twelfth centuries B.C., the Greeks began to travel to Egypt and continued to do so over the next several centuries. Knowledge from the Babylonians, Egyptians, Hebrews, and other peoples of the eastern Mediterranean was included in the Greeks' philosophy of health and medicine.[9] During the "Golden Age" of ancient Greece (in the sixth and fifth centuries B.C.) men participated in physical games of strength and skill and swam in public facilities. There is little evidence that this emphasis on fitness and on success in athletic competition was imparted equally to all members of the community.[11] Participation in these activities was not encouraged or even permitted for women, the poor, or slaves.

The Greeks were also active in the practice of community sanitation. They supplemented local city wells with water supplied from mountains as far as 10 miles away. In at least one city, water from a distant source was stored in a cistern 370 feet above sea level.[8]

The Romans improved upon the Greek engineering and built aqueducts that could transport water for many miles. Evidence of some 200 Roman aqueducts remains today, from Spain to Syria and from northern Europe to North Africa. The Romans also built sewer systems and initiated other community health activities, including the regulation of building construction, refuse removal, and street cleaning and repair.[10]

The Romans were the repository for Greek medical ideas, but with few exceptions, they did little to advance medical thinking. The Romans did make one important contribution to medicine and health care—the hospital. Although the first hospitals were merely infirmaries for slaves, before the end of the Roman era, Christians had established public hospitals as benevolent organs of charity.[9] When the Roman Empire eventually fell in 479 A.D., most public health activities ceased.

Middle Ages (500–1500 A.D.)

The period from the end of the Roman Empire in the West to about 1500 A.D. has become known as the Middle Ages. The Eastern Roman Empire (the Byzantine Empire) with its capital in Constantinople, continued until 1453 A.D. While the Greco-Roman legacy of society was largely preserved in the Eastern Roman Empire, it was lost to most of western Europe. Most of what knowledge remained was preserved only in the churches and monasteries.

The medieval approach to health and disease differed greatly from that of the Roman Empire. There was a growing revulsion of Roman materialism and a growth of spirituality. Health problems were considered to have both spiritual causes and spiritual solutions.[8] This was especially true at the beginning of the Middle Ages, during a period known as the "Dark Ages" (500–1000 A.D.). Both pagan rites and Christian beliefs blamed disease on supernatural causes. St. Augustine, for example, taught that diseases were caused by demons sent to torment the human spirit, and most Christians generally believed that disease was a punishment for sins.[9]

The failure to take into account the role of the physical and biological environment in the causation of communicable diseases resulted in the failure to control the unrelenting epidemics during this **spiritual era of public health.** These epidemics were responsible for the suffering and death of millions. One of the earliest recorded epidemic

diseases was leprosy. It has been estimated that by 1200 A.D., there were 19,000 leper houses and leprosaria in Europe.[8]

The deadliest of the epidemic diseases of the period was the plague. It is hard for us, living at the dawn of the twenty-first century, to imagine the impact of plague on Europe. Three great epidemics of plague occurred: the first began in 543, the second in 1348, and the last in 1664. The worst epidemic occurred in the fourteenth century, when the disease became known as "the black death." An estimated 25 million people died in Europe alone. This is more than twice the number of people who live in the states of New York and California today. Half of the population of London was lost, and in some parts of France only 1 in 10 survived.[10]

The Middle Ages also saw epidemics of other recognizable diseases, including smallpox, diphtheria, measles, influenza, tuberculosis, anthrax, and trachoma. Many other diseases, unidentifiable at the time, took their toll. The last epidemic disease of this period was syphilis, which appeared in 1492. This, like the other epidemics, killed thousands.

Renaissance and Exploration (1500–1700 A.D.)

The Renaissance period was characterized by a rebirth of thinking about the nature of the world and of humankind. There was an expansion of trade between cities and nations and an increase in population concentrations in large cities. This period was also characterized by exploration and discovery. The travels of Columbus, Magellan, and many other explorers eventually ushered in a period of colonialism.

The effects of the Renaissance on community health were substantial. A more careful accounting of disease outbreaks dur-

---

spiritual era of public health A time during the Middle Ages when the causation of communicable disease was linked to spiritual dimensions.

ing this period revealed that diseases such as the plague killed saints and sinners alike. There was a growing belief that diseases were caused by environmental, not spiritual, factors. For example, the term *malaria,* meaning bad air, is a distinct reference to the humid or swampy air which often harbors mosquitoes that transmit malaria.

More critical observations of the sick led to more accurate descriptions of symptoms and outcomes of disease. These observations led to the first recognition of whooping cough, typhus, scarlet fever, and malaria as distinct and separate diseases.[8]

Epidemics of smallpox, malaria, and plague were still rampant in England and throughout Europe. In 1665, the plague took 68,596 lives in London, which at the time had a population of 460,000 (a loss of almost 15% of the population). Explorers, conquerors, and merchants and their crews spread disease to colonists and indigenous people throughout the New World. Smallpox, measles, and other diseases ravaged unprotected natives.

The Eighteenth Century

The eighteenth century was characterized by industrial growth. In spite of the beginnings of recognition of the nature of disease, living conditions were hardly conducive to good health. Cities were overcrowded, and water supplies were inadequate and often unsanitary. Streets were usually unpaved, filthy, and heaped with trash and garbage. Many homes had unsanitary dirt floors.

Workplaces were unsafe and unhealthy. A substantial portion of the work force was made up of the poor, including children, who were forced to work long hours as indentured servants. Many of these jobs were unsafe or involved working in unhealthy environments, such as textile factories and coal mines.

One medical advance, made at the end of the eighteenth century, deserves mention because of its significance for public health. In 1796, Dr. Edward Jenner successfully demonstrated the process of vaccination as a protection against smallpox. He did this by inoculating a boy with material from a cowpox (*Vaccinia*) pustule. When challenged later with material from a smallpox (*Variola*) pustule, the boy remained healthy.

Dr. Jenner's discovery remains as one of the great discoveries of all time for both medicine and for public health. Prior to Dr. Jenner's discovery, millions died or were severely disfigured by smallpox. The only known prevention had been "variolation," inoculation with smallpox material itself. This was a risky procedure because people sometimes became quite ill with smallpox. Nonetheless, during the American Revolution, General George Washington ordered the Army of the American Colonies "variolated." He did this so that he could be sure an epidemic of smallpox would not wipe out his colonial forces.[8] Interestingly enough, the average age at death for one living in United States was then 29 years.

Following the American Revolution, George Washington ordered the first United States census for the purpose of apportionment of representation in the House of Representatives. The census, first taken in 1790, is still conducted every 10 years and serves as an invaluable source of information for health planning.

As the eighteenth century came to a close, a young United States faced numerous disease problems, including continuing outbreaks of smallpox, cholera, typhoid fever, and yellow fever. Yellow fever outbreaks usually occurred in port cities such as Charleston, Baltimore, New York, and New Orleans, where ships arrived to dock from tropical

America. The greatest single epidemic of yellow fever in America occurred in Philadelphia in 1793, where there were an estimated 23,000 cases including 4,044 deaths in a population estimated at only 37,000.[12]

In response to these continuing epidemics and the need to address other mounting health problems, such as sanitation and protection of the water supply, some of America's largest cities founded municipal boards of health. By 1799, Boston, Philadelphia, New York, and Baltimore all had boards of health (see Box 1.1).

The Nineteenth Century

During the first half of the nineteenth century, few remarkable advancements in public health occurred (see Figure 1.6). Living conditions in Europe and England remained unsanitary, and industrialization led to an even greater concentration of the population in cities. However, better agricultural methods led to improved nutrition for many.

During this period, America enjoyed westward expansion, characterized by a spirit of pioneering, self-sufficiency, and rugged individualism. The federal government's approach to health problems was characterized by the French term *laissez faire,* meaning noninterference. There were few health regulations or health departments in rural areas. Health quackery thrived; this was truly a period when "buyer beware" was good advice.

Epidemics continued in major cities in both Europe and America. In 1849, a cholera epidemic struck London. Dr. John Snow studied the epidemic and hypothesized that the disease was being caused by the drinking water from the Broad Street pump. He obtained permission to remove the pump handle, and the epidemic was abated (see Figure 1.7). Snow's action was remarkable because it predated the discovery that microorganisms can cause disease. The predominant theory of contagious disease at the time was the "miasmas theory." According to this theory, vapors, or miasmas, were the source of many diseases. The miasmas theory remained popular throughout much of the nineteenth century.

In the United States, in 1850, Lemuel Shattuck drew up a health report for the Commonwealth of Massachusetts that outlined the public health needs for the state. It included recommendations for the establishment of boards of health, the collection of vital statistics, the implementation of sanitary measures, and research on diseases. Shattuck also recommended health education and controlling exposure to alcohol, smoke, adulterated food, and nostrums (quack medicines).[10] Although some of his recommendations took years to implement (the Massachusetts Board of Health was not founded until 1869), the significance of Shattuck's report is such that 1850 is a key date in American public health; it marks the beginning of the **modern era of public health.**

Real progress in the understanding of the causes of many communicable diseases occurred during the last quarter of the nineteenth century. One of the obstacles to progress was the theory of spontaneous generation, the idea that living organisms could arise from inorganic or nonliving matter. Akin to this idea was the thought that one type of contagious microbe could change into another type of organism.

In 1862, Louis Pasteur of France proposed his germ theory of disease. Throughout the 1860s and 1870s, he and others carried out experiments and made observations

---

modern era of public health   The era of public health that began in 1850 and continues today.

BOX 1.1
History of Health Education

One can assume that health education, at least on an informal basis, is as old as human life on earth and basically followed the history of health and efforts to promote it.* There is evidence, via historical artifacts, that people were concerned about health, illness, and death from the earliest days. It is only logical that information about health was shared by these people. The earliest recorded efforts to influence health behavior through education dates back to Biblical times.

It is difficult to pinpoint the beginning of health education in the United States as we know it today. However, the evolution of health education is tied to the evolution of education in general in this country.* Below is a listing of a number of significant events in the development of health education in America.*†‡

- Benjamin Franklin founded the Academy (the first secondary education in America) and advocated a healthful situation and physical exercise (1751).
- William A. Alcott, who many regard as the father of school health education, wrote a prize-winning book on the healthful construction of schoolhouses (1859).
- Horace Mann (1796–1859), secretary of the first state board of education in the United States (Massachusetts), was an early proponent of health and physical education.
- Harvard and Amherst Colleges offered the first health instruction classes (early 1800s).
- William Homes McGuffey (1800–1873) included good health practices in his readers.
- Lemuel Shattuck (1793–1859) completed a report on public health suggesting needs for sanitary science education (1850).
- The American Public Health Association was founded (1870). The first United States school health instruction centered on alcohol, drugs, and narcotics with impetus from Women's Christian Temperance Union (late 1800s).

- The first school nurse was added to a school staff in New York City (1899).
- The joint committee on Health Problems in Education of the National Education Association and the American Medical Association was established (1911).
- Health was noted as one of the seven Cardinal Principles of Secondary Education by the National Education Association (1918).
- The first true school health instruction as it is known today started at the end of World War I, emphasizing healthful living and not physiology (1918).
- The first professional preparation program for health educators was begun at Columbia University by Thomas D. Wood, M.D., who many regard as the father of health education (1922).
- Schools of public health began to regularly include health education in their curricula (1925–1940).
- Health education was beginning to be a recognized subject in the K–12 curriculum (1940).
- Health education began to be commonly given a distinct identity entirely separate from its parent, physical education, in universities (1950).
- School Health Education Study (SHES), directed by Elena M. Sliepcevich and financed by the Bronfman Foundation, was a scientific study to determine the status of health education in the schools of America. This led to the development of a conceptual-based health education curriculum (1962).

*Butler, J. T. (1994). *Principles of Health Education and Health Promotion.* Englewood, Colo.: Morton.
†Means, R. K. (1975). *A History of Health Education in the United States.* Thorofare, N.J.: Charles B. Slack.
‡Rash, K. J., and M. R. Pigg (1979). *The Health Education Curriculum.* New York: John Wiley & Sons.

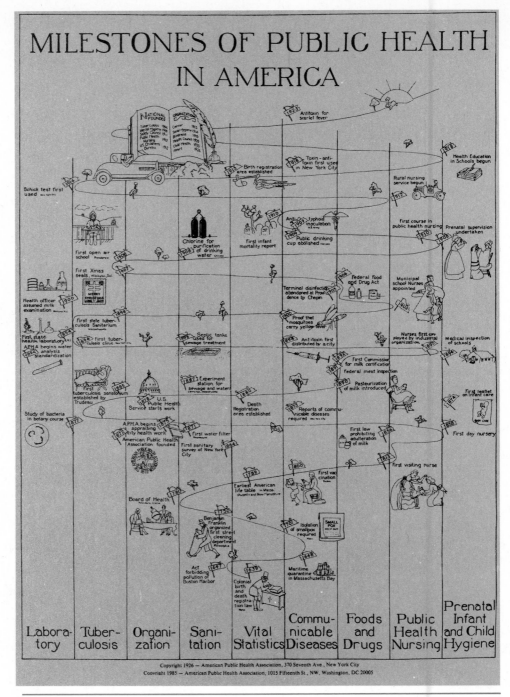

FIGURE 1.6

Milestones of public health in America.

From: American Journal of Public Health *(Dec. 1985). 75(15): 1361–1504.*

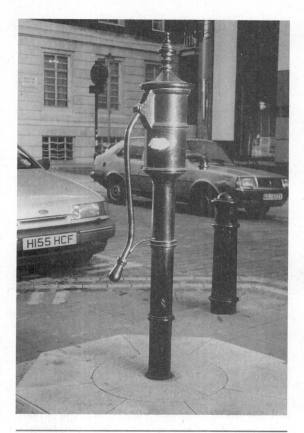

FIGURE 1.7

London, England, 1849. John Snow interrupted a cholera epidemic by removing the handle from this pump, located on Broad Street.

that supported this theory and disproved spontaneous generation. Pasteur is generally given credit for providing the death blow to the theory of spontaneous generation.

It was the German scientist Robert Koch who developed the criteria and procedures necessary to establish that a particular microbe, and no other, causes a particular disease. His first demonstration was in 1876, with the anthrax bacillus. Between 1877 and the end of the century, the identity of numerous bacterial disease agents was established, including those that caused gonorrhea, typhoid fever, leprosy,

tuberculosis, cholera, diphtheria, tetanus, pneumonia, plague, and dysentery. This period (1875–1900) has become to be known as the **bacteriological period of public health.**

Although most scientific discoveries in the late nineteenth century were made in Europe, there were significant public health achievements occurring in America as well. The first law prohibiting the adulteration of milk was passed in 1856, the first sanitary survey was carried out in New York City in 1864, and the American Public Health Association was founded in 1872. The Marine Hospital Service (forerunner of the United States Public Health Service) gained new powers of inspection and investigation under the Port Quarantine Act of 1878.[10] In 1890, the pasteurization of milk was introduced, and in 1891, meat inspection began. In 1895, the first nurses were hired by industry, and septic tanks were introduced for sewage treatment. In 1900, Major Walter Reed of the United States Army announced that yellow fever is transmitted by mosquitoes.

The Twentieth Century

As the twentieth century began, life expectancy was still less than 50 years.[13] The leading causes of death were communicable diseases—influenza, pneumonia, tuberculosis, and infections of the gastrointestinal tract. Other communicable diseases such as typhoid fever, malaria, and diphtheria also killed many people.

There were other health problems. Thousands of children were afflicted with conditions characterized by noninfectious diarrhea or by bone deformity. Although the symptoms of pellagra and rickets were

---

bacteriological period of public health The period 1875–1900, during which the causes of many bacterial diseases were discovered.

known and described, the causes of these ailments remained a mystery at the turn of the century. Discovery that these conditions resulted from vitamin deficiencies was slow because some scientists were searching for bacterial causes.

Vitamin deficiency diseases and one of their contributing conditions, poor dental health, were extremely common in the slum districts of both European and American cities. The unavailability of adequate prenatal and postnatal care meant that deaths associated with pregnancy and childbirth were high.

Health Resources Development Period (1900–1960)

Much growth and development took place during the 60-year period from 1900 to 1960. Because of the growth of health care facilities and providers, this period of time is referred to as the **health resources development period.** The period can be further divided into the reform phase (1900–1920), the 1920s, the Great Depression and World War II, and the postwar years.

The Reform Phase (1900–1920)

By the beginning of the twentieth century, there was a growing concern about the many social problems in America. The remarkable discoveries in microbiology made in the previous years had not dramatically improved the health of the average citizen. By 1910, the urban population had grown to 45% of the total population (up from 19% in 1860). Much of the growth was the result of immigrants who came to America for the jobs created by new industry (see Figure 1.8). Northern cities were also swelling from the northward migration of black Americans

from the southern states. Many of these workers had to accept poorly paying jobs involving hard labor and low wages. There was a deepening chasm between the upper and lower classes, and social critics began to clamor for reform.

The years 1900–1920 have been called the **reform phase of public health.** The plight of the immigrants working in the meat packing industry was graphically depicted by Upton Sinclair in his book *The Jungle.* Sinclair's goal was to draw attention to unsafe working conditions. What he achieved was greater governmental regulation of the food industry through the passage of the Pure Food and Drugs Act of 1906.

The reform movement was broad, involving social and moral as well as health issues. Edward T. Devine noted in 1909 that "Ill health is perhaps the most constant of the attendants of poverty."[13] The reform movement finally took hold when it became evident to the majority that neither the discoveries of the causes of many communicable diseases nor the continuing advancement of industrial production could overcome continuing disease and poverty. Even by 1917, the United States ranked fourteenth out of sixteen "progressive" nations in the maternal death rate.[13]

Although the relationship between occupation and disease had been pointed out 200 years earlier in Europe, occupational health in America in 1900 was an unknown quantity. However, in 1910, the first International Congress on Occupational Diseases was held in Chicago.[14] That same year, New York State passed a tentative Workman's Compensation Act, and over the next ten years most other states passed similar laws.[14] Also

---

health resources development period The years 1900–1960, a time of great growth in health care facilities and providers.

reform phase of public health The years 1900–1920, characterized by social movements to improve health conditions in cities and in the workplace.

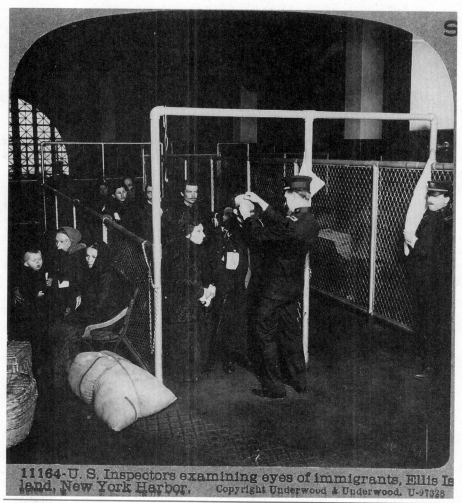

11164-U. S. Inspectors examining eyes of immigrants, Ellis Island, New York Harbor,   Copyright Underwood & Underwood. U-97328

FIGURE 1.8

Ellis Island immigration between 1860 and 1910 resulted in dramatic increases in urban populations in America.

in 1910, the United States Bureau of Mines was created and the first clinic for occupational diseases was established at Cornell Medical College, New York.[13] By 1910, the movement for healthier conditions in the workplace was well established.

This period also saw the birth of the first national-level volunteer health agencies. The first of these was the National Association for the Study and Prevention of Tuberculosis, which was formed in 1902. It arose from the first local voluntary health agency, the Pennsylvania Society for the Prevention of Tuberculosis, organized in 1892.[15] The American Cancer Society, Inc., was founded in 1913. That same year, the Rockefeller Foundation was established in New York. This philanthropic foundation has funded a great many public health projects, including work on hookworm and pellagra, and the development of a vaccine against yellow fever.

Another movement that began about this time was that of public health nursing. The first school nursing program was begun in New York City in 1902. In 1918, the first School of Public Health was established at Johns Hopkins University in Baltimore. This was followed by establishment of another school at Harvard University in 1923.

These advances were matched with similar advances by governmental bodies. The Marine Hospital Service was renamed the Public Health and Marine Hospital Service in 1902 in keeping with its growing responsibilities. In 1912, it became the United States Public Health Service.[10]

By 1900, 38 states had state health departments. The rest followed during the first decades of the twentieth century. The first two local (county) health departments were established in 1911, one in Guilford County, North Carolina, and the other in Yakima County, Washington.

The 1920s

In comparison with the preceding period, the 1920s represented a decade of slow growth in public health, except for a few health projects funded by the Rockefeller and Millbank foundations. Prohibition resulted in a decline in the number of alcoholics and alcohol-related deaths. While the number of county health agencies had risen to 467 by 1929, 77% of the rural population still lived in areas with no health services.[15] The life expectancy in 1930 had risen to 59.7 years.

The Great Depression and World War II

Until the Great Depression (1929–1935), individuals and families in need of social and medical services were dependent on friends and relatives, private charities, voluntary agencies, community chests, and

churches. By 1933, after three years of economic depression, it became evident that private resources could never meet the needs of all the people who needed assistance. The drop in tax revenues during the depression also reduced health department budgets and caused a virtual halt in the formation of new local health departments.[15]

Beginning in 1933, President Franklin D. Roosevelt created numerous agencies and programs for public works as part of his New Deal. Much of the money was used for public health, including the control of malaria, the building of hospitals and laboratories, and the construction of municipal water and sewer systems.

The Social Security Act of 1935 marked the beginning of the government's major involvement in social issues, including health. This act provided substantial support for state health departments and their programs, such as maternal and child health and sanitary facilities. As progress against the communicable diseases became visible, some turned their attention toward other health problems, such as cancer. The National Cancer Institute was formed in 1937.

America's involvement in World War II resulted in severe restrictions on resources available for public health programs. Immediately following the conclusion of the war, however, many of the medical discoveries made during wartime made their way into civilian medical practice. Two examples are the antibiotic penicillin, used for treating pneumonia, rheumatic fever, syphilis, and strep throat, and the insecticide DDT, used for killing insects that transmit diseases.

During World War II, the Communicable Disease Center was established in Atlanta, Georgia. Now called the National Centers for Disease Control and Prevention, it has become the premier epidemiological center of the world.

The Postwar Years

Following the end of World War II, there was concern about medical care and the adequacy of the facilities in which that care could be administered. In 1946, Congress passed the National Hospital Survey and Construction Act (Hill-Burton Act). The goal of the legislation was to improve the distribution and enhance the quality of hospitals. From 1946 through the 1960s, hospital construction occurred at a rapid rate with relatively little thought given to planning. Likewise, attempts to set national health priorities or establish a national health agenda were virtually nonexistent.

The two major health events in the 1950s were the development of a vaccine to prevent polio and President Eisenhower's heart attack. The latter event helped America to focus on its Number 1 killer, heart disease. When the president's physician suggested exercise, some Americans heeded his advice and began to exercise on a regular basis.

Period of Social Engineering (1960–1975)

The 1960s marked the beginning of a period when the federal government once again became active in health matters. The primary reason for this involvement was the growing realization that many Americans were still not reaping any of the benefits of 60 years of medical advances. These Americans, most of whom were either poor or elderly, either lived in underserved areas or simply could not afford to purchase medical services.

In 1965, Congress passed the Medicare and Medicaid bills (Amendments to the Social Security Act of 1935). **Medicare** assists in the payment of medical bills for the elderly, **Medicaid** for the poor. These pieces

---

Medicare Government health insurance for the elderly and disabled.
Medicaid Government health insurance for the poor.

of legislation helped provide medical care for millions who would not otherwise have received it, and they also had the effect of improving standards in health care facilities. Unfortunately, the influx of federal dollars accelerated the rate of increase in the cost of health care for everyone. As a result, the 1970s, 1980s, and now the 1990s have seen repeated attempts and failures to bring the growing costs of health care under control.

Health Promotion Period (1975–1990)

By the mid-1970s, it had become apparent that the greatest potential for saving lives and reducing health care costs in America was to be achieved through health promotion and disease prevention. In the late 1970s, the Centers for Disease Control conducted a study that examined **premature deaths** (deaths prior to age 65) in the United States in 1975. That study revealed that approximately 48% of all premature deaths could be traced to one's life-style or health behavior. Life-styles characterized by a lack of exercise, high-fat diets, smoking, uncontrolled hypertension, and the inability to control stress were found to be contributing factors to premature mortality.

The federal government issued its first set of health objectives in 1980 in a document called *Promoting Health/Preventing Disease: Objectives for the Nation.*[16] This document proposed a total of 226 objectives divided into three main areas—preventive services, health protection, and health promotion. These objectives, many of which were based on the 1979 United States Surgeon General's report, *Healthy People,*[17] provided the bases for the nation's health plan for the 1980s.

In 1985, when progress toward achieving the objectives was checked, it appeared that only about one-half of the objectives

---

premature deaths Deaths prior to age 65.

established in 1979 would be reached by 1990; another one-fourth would not be reached; and progress on the rest could not be judged because of a lack of data. Objectives that were reached or nearly reached were control of high blood pressure; control of infectious diseases; and the reduction of tobacco, alcohol, and drug use. Objectives not reached were those in the areas of prenatal care, infant health, nutrition, physical fitness and exercise, family planning, sexually transmitted diseases, and occupational safety and health.[18]

The 1980 planning process demonstrated the value of setting goals and listing specific objectives as a means of measuring progress in the nation's health and health care services. Thus, the process was repeated in the late 1980s as a guide for the 1990s. The plan was entitled *Healthy People 2000: National Health Promotion and Disease Prevention Objectives.*[19]

Community Health in the 1990s

As we enter the last half of 1990s, it is widely held that while decisions about health are an individual's responsibility to a significant degree, society has an obligation to provide an environment in which achievement of good health is possible and encouraged. Further, many recognize that certain segments of our population whose disease and death rates exceed the general population may require additional resources, including education, to achieve good health.

The American people face a number of serious public health problems. These include health care costs that are out of control, growing environmental concerns, the ever-present life-style diseases, new communicable diseases that are epidemic, and serious substance abuse problems. In the paragraphs that follow, we have elaborated on each of these problems briefly because they seem to represent a significant portion of the community health agenda for the remainder of the 1990s.

Health Care Delivery

Health care delivery is arguably the single greatest community health challenge in the 1990s. While Americans have the highest quality of health care available anywhere in the world, many Americans are beginning to realize that we have health care we cannot afford. At first, it was beyond the reach of only the unemployed; then it became inaccessible to the underemployed, those between jobs, and those without health insurance. By the mid-1990s it is rapidly becoming beyond the reach of fully employed middle-class Americans. After all, who can afford to pay the full medical bill for a family member who loses a two- to three-year battle with cancer? Even the 20% left unpaid by many insurance plans is staggering.

The exorbitant cost of health care is distorting the entire economy in America. In 1993, health care expenditures made up about 14% of America's gross domestic product, up from 12.2% in 1990. In 1991, national health care expenditures totaled $752 billion, an average of $2,868 per person.[20] That figure was expected to grow to $1.6 trillion by the year 2000 if left unchecked.[21]

In September 1993, President Clinton introduced a plan to reform the health care system. He called for a health security system similar to our social security system, in which health care would be made available to every American. The president's plan was expected to undergo long debate in Congress.

Environmental Problems

Millions of Americans live in communities where the air is unsafe to breathe, the water is unsafe to drink, or solid waste is disposed of improperly. With a few minor exceptions, the rate at which we pollute our environment continues to increase. Many

Americans still believe that our natural resources are unlimited and that their individual contributions to the overall pollution are insignificant. In actuality, we must improve upon our efforts in resource preservation and energy conservation if our children are to enjoy an environment as clean as ours.

Life-Style Diseases

The leading causes of death in the United States today are not the communicable diseases that were so feared 100 years ago but chronic illnesses resulting from unwise life-style choices. The four leading causes of death in the 1990s are heart disease, cancer, stroke, and unintentional injuries. Although it is true that everyone has to die from some cause sometime, too many Americans die prematurely (prior to age 65) because of their unhealthy life-styles. It is estimated that better behavioral and life-style choices by Americans could prevent 40% to 70% of all premature deaths, one-third of all acute disabilities, and two-thirds of chronic disabilities.[22]

Communicable Diseases

While communicable diseases no longer constitute the leading causes of death in the United States, they remain the primary reason for days missed at school or at work. The success in reducing the life-threatening nature of these diseases has made many Americans complacent about obtaining vaccinations or taking other precautions against contracting these diseases. With the exception of smallpox, none of these diseases has been eradicated.

Moreover, new communicable diseases continue to appear, demonstrating that communicable diseases still represent a serious community health problem in America. Legionnaire's disease, toxic shock syndrome, Lyme disease, and acquired immunodeficiency syndrome (AIDS) are diseases that were unknown only 20 years ago.

The first cases of AIDS were reported in June 1981.[23] By August 1989, 100,000 cases had been reported[24] and it only took an additional two years to report the second 100,000 cases.[25] By September 1993, there were over 315,000 cases of the disease (see Figure 1.9).

Alcohol and Other Drug Abuse

"Abuse of legal and illegal drugs has become a national problem that costs this country thousands of lives and billions of dollars each year. Alcohol and other drugs are often associated with accidents, domestic violence, and violent crimes."[26] Federal, state, and local governments and private agencies are attempting to address supply and demand problems associated with the abuse of alcohol and other drugs, but a

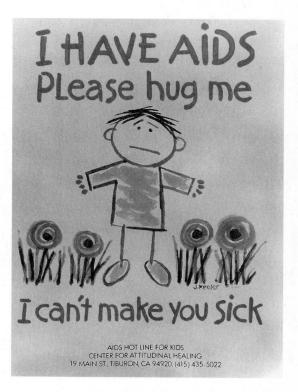

FIGURE 1.9

AIDS is the most feared communicable disease today.

significant challenge remains for America in the 1990s.

OUTLOOK FOR COMMUNITY HEALTH IN THE TWENTY-FIRST CENTURY

So far in this chapter, we have discussed community health, past and present. Now we will describe what community health leaders in the United States and elsewhere in the world hope to achieve in the coming years.

World Planning for the Year 2000

World health leaders recognized the need to plan for the twenty-first century at the thirtieth World Health Assembly of the World Health Organization (WHO), held in 1977. At that assembly, delegations from governments around the world set as a target "that the level of health to be attained by the turn of the century should be that which will permit all people to lead a socially and economically productive life."[27] This target goal became known as "Health for All by the Year 2000." The following year in Alma-Ata, USSR, the joint WHO/UNICEF (United Nation Children's Fund) International Conference adopted a Declaration on Primary Health Care as the key to attaining the goal of "Health for All by the Year 2000." At the thirty-fourth World Health Assembly in 1981, delegates from the member nations unanimously adopted a "Global Strategy for Health for All by the Year 2000." That same year, the United Nations General Assembly endorsed the "Global Strategy" and urged other international organizations concerned with community health to collaborate with WHO.[27]

The underlying concept of "Health for All by the Year 2000" is that health resources should be distributed in such a way that essential health care services are accessible to everyone. The "Global Strategy" to achieve this goal involves the development of a health system infrastructure in every country. This infrastructure would include primary health care services and programs in health promotion, disease prevention, diagnosis, therapy, and rehabilitation. These programs are to be country-specific, have a high degree of community involvement, and be aimed at individuals, families, and communities.[27]

The United States' Plan for Health in the Year 2000

In addition to its participation in WHO's "Health for All by the Year 2000," the United States has its own plan for the year 2000. The plan, called *Healthy People 2000: National Health Promotion and Disease Prevention Objectives,*[19] is based on current health statistics and projections developed by the Bureau of the Census and the National Center for Health Statistics (see Figure 1.10). Some the projections for the United States in the year 2000 are:

1. The population will grow, reaching nearly 270 million, including 6 million new immigrants.[28]
2. The number of husband-wife households will continue to decline from 58% (1985) to only 53%.[29]
3. The median age of Americans will rise to 36 years, up from 29 years in 1975.[30]
4. The number of Americans over the age of 65 will increase to 35 million, 13% of the total population.[30]

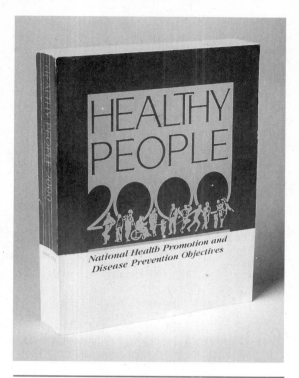

FIGURE 1.10

Healthy People 2000 contains the federal government's public health objectives for the remainder of this century.

5. Racial and ethnic composition of Americans will change. The percentage of whites will drop from 76% (1990) to 72% in the year 2000 while the percentage of blacks will increase from 12.4 to 13.1%, Hispanics from 8 to 11.3%, and other racial groups (including American Indians, Alaskan Natives, Asians, and Pacific Islanders) from 3.5 to 4.3%.[30, 31]

6. The percentage of women in the work force will grow from 45% (1988) to 47%.[32]

Healthy People 2000: National Health Promotion Disease Prevention Objectives begins with three broad goals for community health: (1) to increase the span of healthy life for Americans; (2) to reduce health disparities among Americans; and (3) to achieve access to preventive services for all Americans. A total of 22 priority areas are listed (see Table 1.1). These fall under four categories of activity—three retained from the previous plan: preventive services, health protection, and health promotion—and a new area, surveillance and data systems. This latter category is aimed at improving our national disease-tracking processes and measuring our success in attaining the objectives for the year 2000. Throughout this text, we will refer to examples of *Healthy People 2000* objectives.

As the year 2000 approaches, it appears that the people of the United States and the world are most conscious of the importance of health for all. It is now a matter of doing what is necessary to gain and maintain that health. There is much more work ahead.

CHAPTER SUMMARY

A number of key terms are associated with the study of community health. This chapter began with definitions of health (first from the WHO and then from a more recent holistic approach) and *community* (those with something in common); it then detailed differences between *community* (private and governmental efforts) and *public* (governmental) health. These definitions provide the foundation for a discussion of the four factors that affect the health of a community: physical, social and cultural, community organization, and individual behaviors.

Being able to deal with both the present and the future is partially dependent on having an understanding of the past. Thus, the history of community and public health is traced from the earliest civilizations through the present thrust of health promotion and the goal of health for all by the year 2000.

Though the achievements of community health workers has progressed greatly over the

Table 1.1
Healthy People 2000 Priority Areas

Health promotion

1. Physical activity and fitness
2. Nutrition
3. Tobacco
4. Alcohol and other drugs
5. Family planning
6. Mental health and mental disorders
7. Violent and abusive behavior
8. Educational and community-based programs

Health protection

9. Unintentional injuries
10. Occupational safety and health
11. Environmental health
12. Food and drug safety
13. Oral health

Preventive services

14. Maternal and infant health
15. Heart disease and stroke
16. Cancer
17. Diabetes and chronic disabling conditions
18. HIV infection
19. Sexually transmitted diseases
20. Immunization and infectious diseases
21. Clinical preventive services

Surveillance and data systems

22. Surveillance and data systems

Age-related objectives

Children

Adolescents and young adults

Adults

Older adults

Special populations objectives

1. People with low incomes
2. African Americans
3. Hispanic Americans
4. Asians and Pacific Islanders
5. American Indians and Alaskan natives
6. People with disabilities

years, as evidenced by the control of most communicable diseases and increases in the length and quality of life, this nation and the world are not without serious health problems. Great concern still exists for health care; the environment; diseases caused by an impoverished life-style; the spread of new communicable diseases like AIDS, Legionnaire's disease, toxic shock syndrome, and Lyme disease; and the harm caused by alcohol and other drug abuse. The good news is that steps are being taken to deal with these problems throughout the world, via "Health for All by the Year 2000."

SCENARIO: ANALYSIS AND RESPONSE

1. Do you feel the hepatitis problem in day care centers is a personal health concern or a community health concern? Why?

2. Which of the factors noted in this chapter that affect the health of a community play a part in the hepatitis problem faced by Amy and Todd?

3. Why does the hepatitis problem remind us of the health problems faced by people in the country prior to 1900?

4. Under which of the priority areas in *Healthy People 2000* would hepatitis fall? Why?

REVIEW QUESTIONS

1. How does the 1947 WHO definition of *health* differ from the one offered by Payne and Hahn?

2. What is the difference between community health and public health?

3. What is the difference between the domains of personal health and community health?

4. Define the term *community*.

5. What are four major factors that affect the health of a community? Give an example of each.

6. Identify some of the major events of community health in each of the following periods of time:

Early civilizations (prior to 500 A.D.).

Middle Ages (500–1500 A.D.).

Renaissance and Exploration (1500–1700 A.D.).

The eighteenth century.

The nineteenth century.

7. Provide a brief explanation of the origins from which the following twentieth-century periods get their names:

Health resources development period.

Period of social engineering.

Health promotion period.

8. What significance do each of the following play in community health development in recent years?

Healthy People.

Promoting Health/Preventing Disease: Objectives for the Nation.

Healthy People 2000: National Health Promotion and Disease Prevention Objectives.

9. What are the major community health problems that face the United States as we approach the twenty-first century?

10. How is the world planning for the health of people in the year 2000?

ACTIVITIES

1. Write your own definition for *health*.

2. In a one-page paper, explain why heart disease can be both a personal health problem and a community health problem.

3. Select a community health problem that exists in your hometown, then using the factors that affect the health of a community noted in this chapter, analyze and discuss in a two-page paper at least three factors that contribute to the problem in your hometown.

4. Select one of the individuals below (all have been identified in this chapter), go to the library, and do some additional reading, then write a two-page paper on the person's contribution to community health.

Dr. Edward Jenner.

Dr. John Snow.

Lemuel Shattuck.

Louis Pasteur.

Robert Koch.

Major Walter Reed.

Franklin D. Roosevelt.

5. Locate a copy of *Healthy People 2000,* then set up a time to talk with an administrator in your hometown health department. Find out which of the objectives the health department is working on as priorities. Then summarize in a paper what the objectives are, what they are doing about them, and what they hope to accomplish by the year 2000.

REFERENCES

1. World Health Organization (1947). "Constitution of the World Health Organization." *Chronicle of the World Health Organization* 1.

2. Payne, W. A., and D. B. Hahn (1992). *Understanding Your Health,* 3rd ed. St Louis: Mosby-YearBook.

3. Goldsmith, John R., ed. (1986). *Environmental Epidemiology.* Boca Raton, Fl.: CRC Press, pp. 4–5.

4. Helman, C. (1984). *Culture, Health and Illness: An Introduction for Health Professions.* Bristol, Eng.: John Wright & Sons, Stonebridge Press.

5. Amler, R. W., and H. B. Dull (1987). *Closing the Gap: The Burden of Unnecessary Illness.* New York: Oxford Univ. Press.

6. Brager, G., H. Specht, and J. L. Torczyner (1987). *Community Organizing.* New York: Columbia Univ. Press.

7. Ross, M. G. (1967). *Community Organization: Theory, Principles, and Practice.* New York: Harper & Row.

8. Rosen, George (1958). *A History of Public Health.* New York: MD Publications.

9. Burton, L. E., H. H. Smith, and A. W. Nichols (1980). *Public Health and Community Medicine,* 3rd ed. Baltimore: Williams & Wilkins.

10. Picket, George, and John J. Hanlon (1990). *Public Health: Administration and Practice,* 9th ed. St. Louis: Times Mirror/Mosby.

11. Legon, R. P. (1986). "Ancient Greece." *World Book Encyclopedia.* Chicago: World Book.

12. Woodruff, A. W. (1977). "Benjamin Rush, His Work on Yellow Fever and His British Connections." *Amer. J. Trop. Med. Hyg.* 26(5): 1055–1059.

13. Rosen, George (1975). *Preventive Medicine in the United States, 1900–1975.* New York: Science History Publications.

14. Smillie, W. G. (1955). *Public Health: Its Promise for the Future.* New York: Macmillan.

15. Duffy, John (1990). *The Sanitarians: A History of American Public Health.* Chicago: Univ. of Ill. Press.

16. U.S. Dept. of Health and Human Services (1980). *Promoting Health/Preventing Disease: Objectives for the Nation.* Washington, D.C.: U.S. Government Printing Office.

17. U.S. Dept. of Health, Education, and Welfare (1979). *Healthy People: The Surgeon General's Report on Health Promotion and Disease Prevention* (DHEW pub. no. 79-55071). Washington, D.C.: U.S. Government Printing Office.

18. Mason, J. O., and J. M. McGinnis (1990). "Healthy People 2000": An Overview of the National Health Promotion and Disease Prevention Objectives." *Public Health Reports.* 105(5): 441–446.

19. U.S. Dept. of Health and Human Services (1990). *Healthy People 2000: National Health Promotion Disease Prevention Objectives* (DHHS pub. no. PHS 90-50212). Washington, D.C.: U.S. Government Printing Office.

20. U.S. Dept. of Health and Human Services (1993). *Health, United States 1992* (DHHS pub no. PHS 93-1232). Washington, D.C.: U.S. Government Printing Office.

21. Bush, G. W. (1992, Jan.). *State of the Union Address.* Presented to a joint session of Congress. Washington, D.C.

22. U.S. Dept. of Health and Human Services (1990). *Prevention '89/'90.* Washington, D.C.: U.S. Government Printing Office.

23. Centers for Disease Control (1981). "Pneumocystis Pneumonia—Los Angeles." *Morbidity and Mortality Weekly Reports* 30: 250–252.

24. Centers for Disease Control (1989). "First 100,000 Cases of Acquired Immunodeficiency Syndrome—United States." *Morbidity and Mortality Weekly Reports* 38: 561–563.

25. Centers for Disease Control. (1992). "The Second 100,000 Cases of Acquired Immunodeficiency Syndrome—United States, June 1981–December 1991." *Morbidity and Mortality Weekly Reports* 42(2): 28–29.

26. Payne, W. A., D. B. Hahn, and R. R. Pinger (1991). *Drugs: Issues for Today.* St. Louis: Mosby-YearBook.

27. World Health Organization (1990). *Facts About WHO.* Geneva, Switz.: Author.

28. Passel, J. E., and K. A. Woodrow. (Aug. 1986). "Immigration to the United States." Paper presented to the Census Table.

29. Bur. of the Census (1986). *Projections of the Numbers of Households and Families: 1986 to 2000.* Washington, D.C.: U.S. Dept. of Commerce.

30. Spencer, G. (1989). "Projections of the Population of the United States, by Age, Sex, and Race: 1988 to 2080." *Current Population Reports, Population Estimates and Projections* (series P-25, no. 1018). Washington, D.C.: U.S. Dept. of Commerce, Bur. of the Census.

31. Spencer, G. (1986). "Projections of the Hispanic Population: 1983–2080." *Current Population Reports, Population Estimates and Projections* (series P-25, no. 995. Washington, D.C.: U.S. Dept. of Commerce, Bur. of the Census.

32. Kutscher, R. E. (1987, Sept.). "Projections 2000: Overview and Implications of the Projections to 2000." *Monthly Labor Review* 110(9): 3–9.

Chapter 2

ORGANIZATIONS THAT CONTRIBUTE TO COMMUNITY HEALTH

Chapter Outline

Chapter Objectives

After studying this chapter you will be able to:

1. Explain the need for organizing to improve community health.
2. Explain what a governmental (official) health organization is and give an example of one at each of the following levels: international, national, state, and local.
3. Explain the role the World Health Organization plays in community health.
4. Briefly describe the structure and function of the Public Health Service.
5. Explain the relationship between a state health department and a local one.
6. Explain what is meant by the term *comprehensive school health.*
7. Define the term *quasi-governmental* and explain why some health organizations are classified under this term.
8. List the three primary activities of most voluntary health organizations.
9. Identify five major professional health organizations and three foundations that support community health efforts.
10. Explain how philanthropic foundations contribute to community health.
11. Discuss the role that service and religious organizations play in community health.
12. Identify the major reason why corporations are involved in community health and describe some corporate activities that contribute to community health.

Mary and Bill are average, hard-working Americans who hope to make a better future for their children. Mary is a secretary in a company that is well-known for its high-quality glass products. Bill has just been promoted to foreman after having worked on the "line" for 17 years at his company. Their combined income puts them in the middle income bracket. Through their respective employers, both Mary and Bill have benefit packages that include standard health insurance.

For the past few months, Bill has not felt 100% healthy, so he made an appointment to see his physician. After checking Bill over, his doctor referred him to a specialist, who told Bill that he has cancer. His years on the line at the factory may have contributed to his illness, but no one can be sure. The specialist told Bill that the cancer is still in its early stages and that he has a good chance of beating it.

Battling a serious disease like cancer often requires a great many personal and family resources as well as support from the community. The result can be financial and social devastation. Are there organizations in the community to which Mary and Bill can turn for help?

INTRODUCTION

As noted in Chapter 1, the history of community health dates to antiquity. For much of that history, community health issues were addressed only on an emergency basis. For example, if a community faced a drought or an epidemic, a town meeting would be called to deal with the problem. It has been only in the last 150 years that communities have taken explicit actions to deal aggressively with health issues on a continual basis.

Today's communities differ from those of the past in several important ways. Although individuals are better educated, more mobile, and more independent than in the past, communities are less autonomous and more dependent on state and federal funding for support. Contemporary communities are too large and too complex to respond effectively to sudden emergencies or to make long-term improvements in public health without community organization and

careful planning. Better community organization and careful long-term planning are essential to insure that a community makes the best use of its resources for health, both in times of emergency and over the long run.

The ability of today's communities to respond effectively to their own problems is hindered by the following characteristics: (1) highly developed and centralized resources in our national institutions and organizations; (2) continuing concentration of wealth and population in the largest metropolitan areas; (3) rapid movement of information, resources, and people made possible by advanced communication and transportation technologies; (4) limited horizontal relationships between/among organizations; and (5) a system of **top-down funding** (money that comes from either the federal or state government to the local level) for many community programs.[1]

---

top-down funding Money transmitted from federal or state government to the local level.

In this chapter, we discuss organizations that contribute to a community's ability to respond effectively to health-related issues.

CLASSIFICATION OF HEALTH AGENCIES

There are a great many organizations that in some way work to protect and promote the health of the community and its members. These community organizations can be classified as: official, quasi-official, and unofficial, according to their sources of funding and organizational structure.

GOVERNMENTAL (OFFICIAL) HEALTH AGENCIES

Governmental health agencies, or **official health agencies,** as they are sometimes called, are funded primarily by tax dollars and managed by government officials. Each governmental health agency is designated as having authority for some area of health. Such agencies exist at four governmental levels—international, national, state, and local.

International Health Agencies

The most widely recognized international governmental health organization today is the **World Health Organization (WHO)** (see Figure 2.1). Its headquarters are located in Geneva, Switzerland, and there are six regional offices around the world. The names, acronyms, and cities and countries of locations for WHO regional offices are as follows: Africa (AFRO), Brazzaville, Congo; Americas (PAHO), Washington, D.C., United States; Eastern Mediterranean (EMRO), Alexandria, Egypt; Europe (EURO), Copenhagen, Denmark; Southeast Asia (SEARO), New Delhi, India; and Western Pacific (WPRO) Manila, Philippines.[2]

Although the World Health Organization is now the largest international health organization, it is not the oldest. Among the organizations that predate WHO are the *International D'Hygiene Publique,* which was absorbed by the WHO; the Health Organization of the League of Nations, which was dissolved when WHO was created; the United Nations' Relief and Rehabilitation Administration (UNRRA); the United Nations' Children's Fund (UNICEF), which was formerly known as the United Nations' International Children's Emergency Fund; and the Pan American Health Organization (PAHO), which is still an independent organization but is also integrated with WHO in a regional office.

History of WHO

Planning for WHO began when the charter of the United Nations was adopted at an international meeting in 1945. Contained in the charter was an article calling for the establishment of a health agency with wide powers. In 1946, at the World Health Conference, representatives from all United Nations countries succeeded in creating and ratifying the constitution of the WHO. However, it was not until April 7, 1948, that the constitution went into force and the organization officially began its work. April 7 is commemorated each year as World Health Day.[2]

---

governmental health agency (or official health agencies) Health agencies funded primarily by tax dollars.

World Health Organization (WHO) The most widely recognized international governmental health organization.

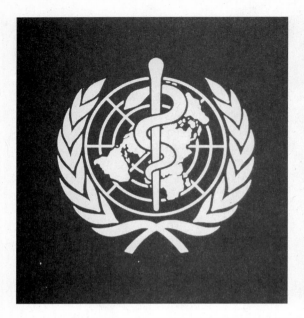 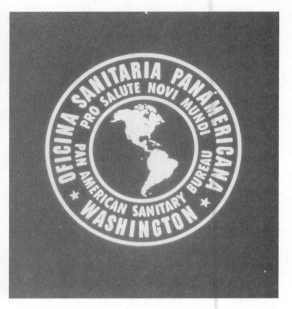

FIGURE 2.1

The emblems of the World Health Organization (left) and the Pan American Sanitary Bureau (right).

Organization of WHO

Membership in WHO is open to any nation that has ratified the WHO constitution and receives a majority vote of the World Health Assembly. The **World Health Assembly** comprises the delegates of the member nations. This assembly, which meets in general sessions annually and in special sessions when necessary, sets policy for the entire organization.

The World Health Organization is administered by a staff that includes a director-general and five assistant directors-general. Great care is taken to insure political balance in staffing WHO positions, particularly at the higher levels of administration.

World Health Assembly A body of delegates of the member nations of the WHO.

Purpose of WHO

The primary objective of WHO as stated in the constitution is the attainment by all peoples of the best possible level of health.[2] The World Health Organization seeks to attain this objective through providing two types of service to member nations: by providing funds to improve the health work force and to control specific diseases and by providing central technical services such as expert advisors and, in some cases, on-the-scene technical service personnel. The work of WHO is financed by its member nations, each of which is assessed according to its ability to pay; the wealthiest countries contribute the greatest portion of the total budget.

Although WHO has sponsored and continues to sponsor many worthwhile programs, we want to mention two that are especially noteworthy. The first was the

BOX 2.1
The Kindest Cut

Once I was in Geneva at the World Health Organization researching a book on communicable diseases. I met Donald Henderson, M.D., director of the smallpox eradication effort.

Not long ago, smallpox was one of the worst diseases anyone could have. About six of every ten who contracted it died. In the United States, even a single known case was regarded as an epidemic.

There is no smallpox known anywhere today. Credit the WHO smallpox vaccination effort. There is still no cure, only prevention; that is, vaccination. At that time, WHO was ready to vaccinate the world, if necessary, to eradicate the disease.

Henderson had been in one high-incidence smallpox region in South America. But few people there were coming to the WHO field station for vaccinations. The warnings about this disease were ho-hum, even though people were seeing smallpox deaths every day.

So, Henderson said, they tried bribery. Not money or goods. They substituted ordinary sewing needles for the standard stainless steel stylets, used to prick under the skin. Then the WHO people spread the word that anyone who came for immunization could keep the needle. Women wanted them for sewing and working of cloth. Men saw them as fine tips for hunting darts.

The sudden fervor and turnout for vaccination rivaled that at any Christmas Eve mass at St. Patrick's Cathedral in New York. Henderson's lesson in resourcefulness for the common good did indeed involve some low-road seduction with rewards, but it was a clear lesson, and one with merit. "Get people to come in for vaccination any way you can. But get them," he said that day in Geneva. "First get them healthy. Then there's time enough to try to educate them about staying healthy."

Henderson is now Deputy Assistant for Health Designate in the U.S. Department of Health and Human Services.

From: Gallagher, Richard (1993). "Resourcerer's Apprentice." *Living: The Magazine of Life* 22(3): 12.

work of WHO in helping to eradicate smallpox. In 1967, smallpox was **endemic** (within people) in 31 countries. During that year, 10–15 million people contracted the disease, and of those, approximately 2 million died and many millions of others were permanently disfigured or blinded. The last known case of smallpox was diagnosed on October 26, 1977, in Somalia.[2] Using the smallpox mortality figures from 1967, it can be estimated that well over 30 million lives have been saved since the eradication (see Box 2.1).

A second noteworthy program of WHO is presently in progress. It is called "Health for All by the Year 2000." This program is a collaborative effort between WHO and the United Nations Children's Fund (UNICEF), agreed upon in 1978 at a conference in Alma-Ata, USSR. It declares that: (1) everyone in the world should have the necessary health services and protection to lead socially and economically productive lives and (2) every community should have the opportunity to determine its health needs and work toward fulfilling those needs.

---

endemic   Within people.

National Health Agencies

Each national government has a department or agency that has primary responsibility for the protection of the health and welfare of its citizens. These national health agencies meet their responsibilities through the promulgation of health policy, enforcement of health regulations, the provision of health services and programs, the funding of research, and the support of their respective state and local health agencies.

In the United States, the primary national health agency is the Department of Health and Human Services. It is important to note, however, that other federal agencies also contribute to the betterment of our nation's health. For example, the Department of Agriculture inspects meat and dairy products and coordinates the Women, Infants, and Children (WIC) food assistance program; the Environmental Protection Agency (EPA) regulates hazardous wastes; the Department of Labor houses the Occupational Safety and Health Administration (OSHA), which is concerned with safety and health in the workplace; and the Department of Commerce, which includes the Bureau of the Census. Each of these departments or agencies is discussed in greater detail in other chapters. A detailed description of the Department of Health and Human Services follows.

Department of Health and Human Services

The **Department of Health and Human Services (DHHS)** is headed by the Secretary of Health and Human Services, who is appointed by the president and is a member of his cabinet. The Department of Health and Human Services was formed in 1980 (during the administration of President Jimmy Carter), when the Department of Health Education and Welfare (USDHEW) was divided into two new departments, DHHS and the Department of Education. With an annual budget in excess of $400 billion, DHHS is by far the largest federal department.

The Department of Health and Human Services comprises four major services: the Public Health Service, the Health Care Financing Administration, the Social Security Administration, and the Administration for Children and Families; and several offices (see Figure 2.2). To support its services, DHHS has ten regional offices located throughout the United States (see Table 2.1).

Public Health Service (PHS)

Although each of the major services in DHHS provides important services, the **Public Health Service (PHS)** contributes most directly to community health. The Public Health Service predates its parent agency by almost 70 years. It emerged in 1912 from the Marine Hospital Service, which was formed in 1798. Over the years, many changes have occurred in the PHS, necessitating dramatic increases in its responsibilities. Today, the Assistant Secretary for Health administers the seven divisions of the PHS while the Surgeon General has responsibility for the Uniformed Public Health Service Officers. The seven divisions are: the National Institutes of Health; Food and Drug Administration; Centers for Disease Control and Prevention; Health Resources and Services Administration; Indian Health Service; Agency for Toxic Substances and Disease Registry; and Substance Abuse and Mental Health Services Administration.

National Institutes of Health (NIH)

The **National Institutes of Health (NIH),** located in Bethesda, Maryland, is the research arm of the PHS. Its mission is the acquisition of new knowledge for the prevention, treatment, and control of dis-

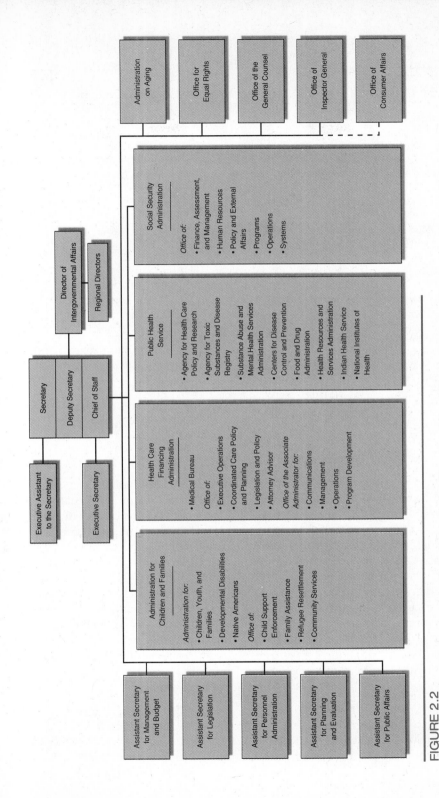

FIGURE 2.2

Organizational chart: Department of Health and Human Services.

Note: In August 1994, President Clinton signed legislation that makes the Social Security Administration an independent agency on March 31, 1995.

Table 2.1

Regional Offices of the U.S. Department of Health & Human Services

Region/Areas Served	Office Address	Telephone Number
Region 1: Connecticut, Maine, Massachusetts, New Hampshire, Rhode Island, Vermont	John F. Kennedy Bldg. Government Center Boston, MA 02203	(617) 565-1500
Region 2: New Jersey, New York, Puerto Rico, Virgin Islands	26 Federal Plaza New York, NY 10278	(212) 264-4600
Region 3: Delaware, Maryland, Pennsylvania, Virginia, West Virginia, District of Columbia	3535 Market St. Philadelphia, PA 19101	(215) 596-6492
Region 4: Alabama, Florida, Georgia, Kentucky, Mississippi, North Carolina, South Carolina, Tennessee	101 Marietta Tower Suite 1403 Atlanta, GA 30323	(404) 331-2442
Region 5: Illinois, Indiana, Michigan, Minnesota, Ohio, Wisconsin	105 W. Adams St. Chicago, IL 60603	(312) 353-5160
Region 6: Arkansas, Louisiana, New Mexico, Oklahoma, Texas	1200 Main Tower Bldg. 11th Flr. Dallas, TX 75202	(214) 767-3301
Region 7: Iowa, Kansas, Missouri, Nebraska	601 East 12th St. Kansas City, MO 64106	(816) 426-2821
Region 8: Colorado, Montana, North Dakota, South Dakota, Utah, Wyoming	1961 Stout St. Denver, CO. 80294	(303) 844-3372
Region 9: Arizona, California, Hawaii, Nevada, American Samoa, Guam, Trust Territory of the Pacific	50 United Nations Plaza San Francisco, CA 94102	(415) 556-6746
Region 10: Alaska, Idaho, Oregon, Washington	Blanchard Plaza Bldg. 2201 6th Ave. Seattle, WA 98121	(206) 442-0420

eases. Although a significant amount of research is carried out by NIH scientists at NIH Laboratories in Bethesda and elsewhere, a much larger portion of this research is conducted by scientists at public and private universities and other research institutions. These scientists receive NIH funding for their research proposals through a competitive grant-application peer-review process. Through this process of proposal-review by qualified scientists, NIH seeks to ensure that federal research monies are spent on the best conceived research projects.

Food and Drug Administration (FDA)

In contrast to the research mission of NIH, the **Food and Drug Administration (FDA)** has a primarily regulatory mission.

The FDA sets health and safety standards for all food, drugs, and cosmetics. The FDA also regulates medical devices, toys, and certain hazardous substances. However, because of the complex nature of its standards and the agency's limited resources, enforcement of many FDA regulations is left to other federal agencies and to state and local agencies. For example, the Department of Agriculture is responsible for the inspection of many foods, such as meat and dairy products. Restaurants, supermarkets, and other food outlets are inspected by state and local health agencies.

Centers for Disease Control and Prevention (CDC)

The **Centers for Disease Control and Prevention (CDC),** located in Atlanta, Georgia, is charged with the surveillance and control of diseases and other health problems in the United States (see Figure 2.3). Once known solely for its work to control communicable diseases, CDC now also maintains, records, and analyzes disease trends and publishes epidemiological reports on all types of diseases, including those that result from life-style, occupational, and environmental causes. Beyond its own specific responsibilities, CDC also supports state and local health departments and cooperates with similar national health agencies of other WHO member nations.

The Centers for Disease Control and Prevention is composed of seven divisions (see Figure 2.4). The major activities of the CDC include: (1) developing disease control programs, (2) maintaining laboratories for diagnostic purposes, (3) keeping supplies of special vaccines and drugs used for rare diseases, (4) developing health education programs, (5) conducting epidemiological investigations, and (6) maintaining disease surveillance data.

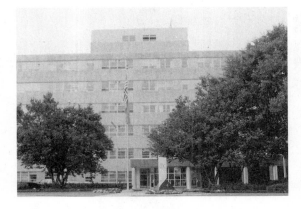

FIGURE 2.3

The Centers for Disease Control and Prevention in Atlanta is one of seven divisions of the Public Health Service.

Health Resources and Services Administration (HRSA)

The **Health Resources and Services Administration (HRSA)** was formed by a union of the Health Resources Administration and Health Services Administration, which occurred in 1982 during Ronald Reagan's presidency. The purpose of HRSA is to improve the nation's health resources and services and their distribution to underserved populations. The Health Resources and Services Administration has three major foci: (1) to provide health care to inner-city and isolated rural residents—a task accomplished through the federal funding of community health centers; (2) to be involved with the Medical Service Corps, which recruits medical professionals to work in underserved areas; and (3) to provide financial assistance for the education and training of health professionals via the Health Professions Education Program.

Indian Health Service (IHS)

The goal of the **Indian Health Service (IHS)** is to raise the health status of the American Indian and Alaskan Native to the highest possible level by providing a comprehensive health services delivery system, which allows these individuals the opportunity for maximum tribal involvement in developing and managing programs to meet their health needs.[3] Though health services have been provided sporadically by the United States government since the early nineteenth century, it was not until 1989 that the IHS was elevated to an agency level within the PHS; prior to that time it was a division in HRSA. (See Chapter 9 for more information on the IHS.)

Substance Abuse and Mental Health Services Administration (SAMHSA)

The **Substance Abuse and Mental Health Services Administration (SAMHSA)** is the primary federal agency charged

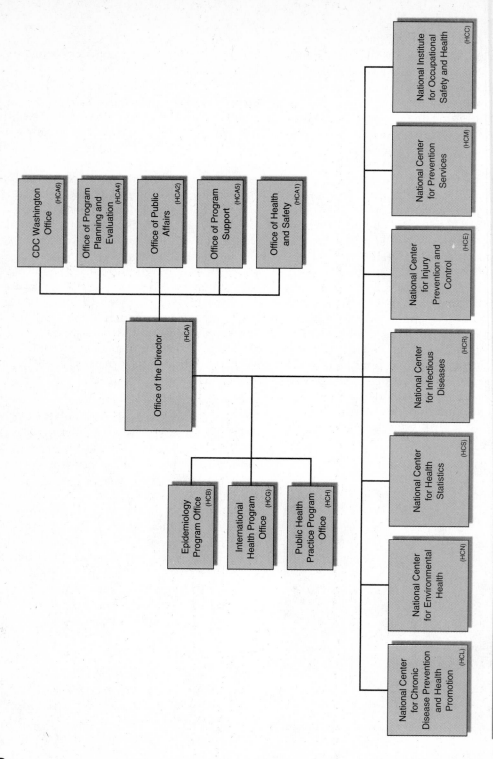

FIGURE 2.4

Organizational Chart: Centers for Disease Control and Prevention (CDC).

with the reduction of the incidence and prevalence of alcohol and other drug abuse and mental disorders. Its missions include the improvement of treatment outcomes for persons suffering from these disorders and the curtailment of the consequences of these problems for families and communities.

Within SAMHSA are three centers: The Center for Substance Abuse Treatment (CSAT), the Center for Substance Abuse Prevention (CSAP), and the Center for Mental Health Services (CMHS). Each of these centers has its own set of missions that contribute to the overall mission of SAMHSA (see Chapter 11).

Agency for Toxic Substances and Disease Registry (ATSDR)

The last and newest division in the PHS is the **Agency for Toxic Substances and Disease Registry (ATSDR).** This agency was created by **Superfund legislation (Comprehensive Environmental Response, Compensation, and Liability Act)** in 1980. It is the legislation enacted to deal with the cleanup of hazardous substances in the environment. ATSDR's mission "is to prevent or mitigate adverse human health effects and diminished quality of life resulting from exposure to hazardous substances in the environment."[4] To carry out its mission and to serve the needs of the American public, ATSDR conducts public health assessments of the effects of hazardous substances released into the environment and keeps exposure and disease registries related to hazardous substances. The agency also provides support to state and local agencies confronted with hazardous-substance emergencies, summarizes and makes available toxicological profiles of hazardous substances, provides health education materials on hazardous-substances and hazardous waste sites, and conducts and sponsors hazardous substances research.[1]

Two specific programs of note from this agency are the National Exposure Registry and ATSDR's 24-hour Emergency Response Line [(404) 639-0615]. The National Exposure Registry was created "to aid in assessing long-term health consequences of exposure to Superfund-related hazardous chemicals. Participation in the program is strictly voluntary and contributes to the body of knowledge about the human health effects of toxic substances."[5] ATSDR's 24-hour Emergency Response Line provides assistance on health issues surrounding the release or threat of release of hazardous materials. Specifically, "the following experts are available for consultation and advice:

- within 10 minutes, an emergency response coordinator;
- within 20 minutes, a preliminary-assessment team, consisting of a toxicologist, chemist, environmental health scientist, physician, and other health personnel as required;
- within 8 hours (if incident necessitates), an on-site response team."[5]

Health Care Financing Administration (HCFA)

The **Health Care Financing Administration (HCFA)** is one of the four major divisions of the DHHS. As its title states, this agency is charged with overseeing the expenditure of all federal monies appropriated for health care services. To accomplish this, HCFA enforces all federal standards pertaining to the quality of health care services. The HFCA also oversees two huge health care service purchasing programs, Medicare and Medicaid. These two programs were created in 1965 to ensure that the el-

---

Superfund legislation   Legislation enacted to deal with the clean up of hazardous substances in the environment.

derly and the disabled (via Medicare) and the poor (via Medicaid) would not be deprived of health care because of cost. Medicare and Medicaid are discussed in detail in Chapter 14.

Social Security Administration (SSA)

The **Social Security Administration (SSA)** is responsible for administering three different programs that provide financial support to special groups of Americans. The largest program, the Social Security system, is a social insurance program that is funded by workers' contributions. Social Security pays benefits to retired and disabled workers and their families and to dependent children or eligible spouses of workers who have died. The other two programs are the **Supplemental Security** income program, which provides cash benefits to elderly, blind, and disabled Americans with minimal resources, and **Aid to Families with Dependent Children (AFDC)** which pays benefits to single mothers and their children who find themselves with minimal resources.

Administration for Children and Families

The **Administration for Children and Families,** the newest division of the DHHS, has the task of coordinating programs that enhance the functioning of the family. These programs include family assistance, refugee resettlement, and child support enforcement.

State Health Agencies

All 50 states have their own state health departments (see Figure 2.5), and although the names of these departments may vary from state to state, their purposes remain the same: to promote, protect, and

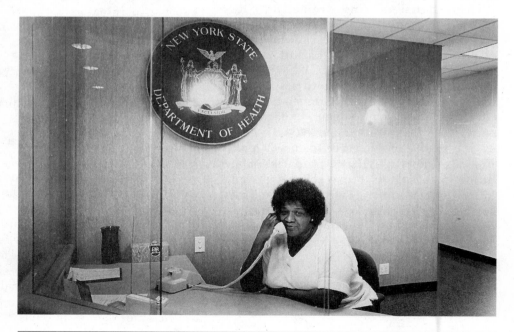

FIGURE 2.5
Each of the 50 states has its own health department.

maintain the health and welfare of their citizens. In this regard, state health departments possess far-reaching powers. For example, state health departments establish and promulgate health regulations that have the force and effect of law throughout the state. State health departments usually must approve appointments of local health officers and can also remove any local health officers who neglect their duties.

The head of the state health department is usually a medical doctor, appointed by the governor, who may carry the title of director, commissioner, or secretary. However, because of the political nature of the appointment, this individual may or may not have extensive experience in community or public health. Unfortunately, political influence sometimes reaches below the level of commissioner to the assistant commissioners and division chiefs. It is the commissioner, assistant commissioners, and division chiefs who set policy and provide direction for the state health department. Middle- and lower-level employees are usually hired through a merit system and may or may not be able to influence health department policy. These employees who carry out the routine work of the state health department are usually professionally trained health specialists such as microbiologists, engineers, statisticians, nurses, and health educators.

Most state health departments are organized into divisions or bureaus that provide certain standard services. A typical organizational chart for a state health department is shown in Figure 2.6. It includes the following divisions: Administration, Communicable Disease Control, Chronic Disease Control, Vital and Health Statistics, Environmental Health, Health Education or Promotion, Health Services, Maternal and Child Health, Mental Health, Occupational and Industrial Health, Dental Health, Laboratory Services, Public Health Nursing, and Veterinary Public Health.

The state health department provides an essential link between federal and local (city and county) health agencies. As such, it serves as a conduit for federal funds aimed at local health problems. Federal funds come to the states as block grants. Funds earmarked for particular health projects are distributed to local health departments by their respective state health departments in accordance with previously agreed upon priorities.

The state health department may also link local needs with federal expertise. For example, epidemiologists from CDC are sometimes made available to investigate local disease outbreaks at the request of the state health department.

Of course, the expertise of the state health department is also at the disposal of local health departments. One particular area where the state health departments can be helpful is laboratory services. Many modern diagnostic tests are simply too expensive for local health departments. Another area is environmental health. Water and air pollution problems usually extend beyond local jurisdictions, and their detection and measurement often require equipment too expensive for local governments to afford. This equipment and expertise are often provided by the state health department. (See Appendix 1 for a listing of all state health departments.)

Local Health Agencies

Local-level governmental health organizations are usually the responsibility of the city or county governments. In large metropolitan areas, community health needs are usually best served by a city health department. In smaller cities with populations of 10,000–50,000, people often come under the

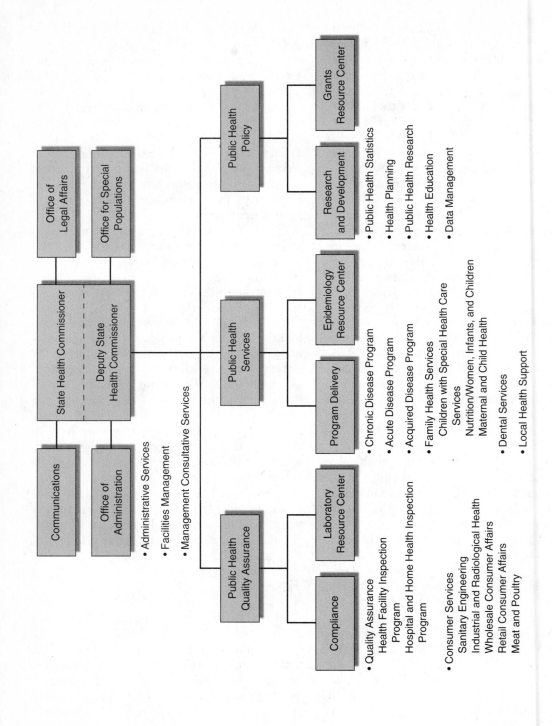

FIGURE 2.6

Organizational Chart: A state health department.

jurisdiction of a county health department. In some rural counties where most of the population is concentrated in a single city, a local health department may have jurisdiction over both city and county residents. In sparsely populated rural areas it is not uncommon to find more than one county served by a single health department.

It is through the local health department (LHD) that health services are provided to the people of the community.[6] A great many of these services are mandated by state laws, which also set standards for health and safety. Examples of mandated local health services include the inspection of restaurants and of public building and public transportation systems, the detection and reporting of certain diseases, and the collection of vital statistics such as births and deaths. Other programs (e.g., safety belt programs, immunization clinics) may be locally planned and implemented. In this regard, local health jurisdictions are permitted to enact ordinances that are stricter than those of the state but cannot enact codes that fall below state standards. It is at this level of governmental health agencies that sanitarians implement the environmental health programs, nurses and physicians offer the clinical services, and health educators present health education and health promotion programs.

Organization of Local Health Departments

Each LHD is headed by a health officer/administrator/commissioner (see Figure 2.7). In most states, there are laws that prescribe who can hold such a position. Those often noted are physicians, dentists, veteri-

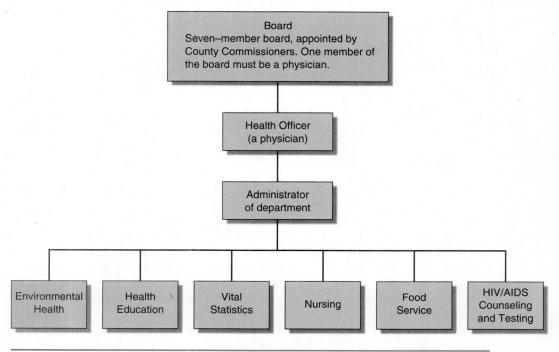

FIGURE 2.7

Organizational Chart: A local health department.

narians, or individuals with masters degrees in public health. If the health officer is not a physician, then a physician is usually hired on a consulting basis to advise as needed. Usually, this health officer is appointed by a board of directors, the members of which are themselves appointed by officials in the city or county government or in some situations elected by the general public. The health officer and administrative assistants may recommend which programs will be offered by the LHDs. However, they may need final approval from a board of directors. Although it is desirable that those serving on the local health board have some knowledge of community health programs, most states have no such requirement. Sometimes politics plays a role in deciding the make-up of the local health board.

The local health officer, like the state health commissioner, has far-reaching powers including the power to arrest someone who refuses to undergo treatment for a communicable disease (TB for example) and who thereby continues to spread disease in the community. The local health officer has the power to close a restaurant on the spot if it has serious health law violations or to impound a shipment of food if it is contaminated. Because most communities cannot afford to employ a full-time physician, the health officer is usually hired on a part-time basis. In such cases, the day-to-day activities of the LHD are carried out by an administrator trained in public health. The administrator is also hired by the board of directors based upon qualifications and the recommendation of the health officer.

In 1974, in its most recent statement, the American Public Health Association (APHA) indicated that it is important for local health departments to coordinate the inputs of the federal and state agencies with the private sector in order to produce comprehensive health services for its citizens. Such services should include community health services, environmental health services, mental health services, and personal health services[6] (see Box 2.2).

A major portion of the funding for the programs and services of the LHDs comes from local property taxes. However, most LHDs also receive some state and federal tax dollars. A limited number of local health department services are provided on a "fee-for-service" basis. For example, there is usually a fee charged for birth and death certificates issued by the LHD. Also, in some communities, minimal fees are charged to offset the cost of providing immunizations, lab work, or inspections. Seldom do these fees cover the actual cost of the services provided. Therefore, income from service fees makes up a very small portion of any local health department budget.

Comprehensive School Health

Few people think of public schools as official health organizations. Consider, however, that schools are funded by tax dollars, are under the supervision of an elected school board, and include as a part of their mission the improvement of the health of those in the school community. Because school attendance is required throughout the United States, the potential for school health programs to make a significant contribution to community health is enormous. However, because of the lack of financial commitment over the years, the full potential of school health programs has never been reached. If communities were willing to finance comprehensive school health programs for grades K–12, the contribution of schools to community health could be almost unlimited.

What exactly is meant by comprehensive school health? The Joint Committee on

---

BOX 2.2
Healthy People 2000—Objectives

8.14 Increase to at least 90% the proportion of people who are served by a local health department that is effectively carrying out the core functions of public health. (Baseline data not yet available.)

Note: The core functions of public health have been defined as assessment, policy development, and assurance. *Local health department* refers to any local component of the public health system, defined as an administrative and service unit of local or state government concerned with health and carrying some responsibility for the health of a jurisdiction smaller than a state.

10.14 Establish in 50 states either public health or labor department programs that provide consultation and assistance to small business to implement safety and health programs for their employees. (Baseline data not yet available.)

20.16 Increase to at least 90% the proportion of public health departments that provide adult immunization for influenza, pneumococcal disease, hepatitis B, tetanus, and diphtheria. (Baseline data not yet available.)

20.17 Increase to at least 90% the proportion of local health departments with ongoing programs for actively identifying cases of tuberculosis and latent infection in populations at high risk for tuberculosis. (Baseline data not yet available.)

21.7 Increase to at least 90% the proportion of people who are served by a local health department that assesses and assures access to essential clinical preventive services. (Baseline data not yet available.)

22.1 Develop a set of health status indicators appropriate for federal, state, and local health agencies and establish use of the set in at least 40 states. (Baseline: No such set exists.)

Baseline data source: National Center for Health Statistics, CDC.

For Further Thought

There are a number of objectives related to the work of local health departments. Of those listed above, which do you think is the most important for a local health department to carry out? Why?

Health Education Terminology has defined a comprehensive school health program as an "organized set of policies, procedures, and activities designed to protect and promote the health and well being of students and staff which has traditionally included health services, healthful school environment, and health education. It should also include, but not be limited to, guidance and counseling, physical education, food service, social work, psychological services, and employee health promotion."[7]

As stated above, there are three essential components in every comprehensive school health program: health education, healthful school environment, and health services. (These topics will be discussed in much greater detail in Chapter 6.) Health instruction should be based on a well-conceived, carefully planned curriculum that has an appropriate scope (coverage of topics) and logical sequencing. Instructional units should include cognitive (knowledge), affective (attitudes), and psychomotor (behavioral) components. The healthful school environment should provide a learning environment that is both physically and mentally safe and healthy. Finally, each school's health program should provide the essential health services, from emergency care through health appraisals, to ensure that students will be healthy learners.

QUASI-GOVERNMENTAL HEALTH ORGANIZATIONS

The **quasi-governmental health organizations**—organizations that have some official health responsibilities but operate, in part, like voluntary health organizations—make important contributions to community health. They derive some of their funding and legitimacy from governments, and carry out tasks that may be normally thought of as government work, yet they operate independently of government supervision. In some cases, they also receive financial support from private sources and become involved in unofficial tasks. Examples of quasi-official agencies are the American Red Cross, the National Science Foundation, and the National Academy of Sciences.

The American Red Cross

The American Red Cross (ARC), founded in 1881 by Clara Barton (see Figure 2.8), is a prime example of an organization that has quasi-governmental status. It has certain official responsibilities

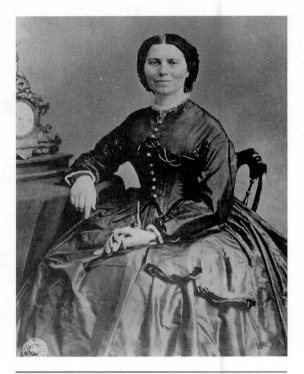

FIGURE 2.8

The American Red Cross was founded by Clara Barton in 1881.

placed on it by the federal government, but it is funded by voluntary contributions. Official duties of the ARC include: (1) acting as the official representative of the United States government during such natural disasters as floods, tornadoes, hurricanes, and fires (Disaster Services); and (2) serving as the liaison between members of the active armed forces and their families during emergencies (Services to the Armed Forces and Veterans). In this latter capacity, the ARC can assist an active-duty member of the armed services in contacting his/her family in case of an emergency, or vice versa.

In addition to these official duties, the ARC also engages in many nongovernmental services. These include blood drives, safety

---

quasi-governmental health organizations Organizations that have some responsibilities assigned by the government but operate more like voluntary agencies.

services (including water safety, first aid, and CPR instruction), nursing and health services, youth services, community volunteer services, and international services.

The ARC was granted a charter by Congress in 1900, and the ARC and the federal government have had a special relationship ever since. The President of the United States is the honorary chairman of the ARC. The United States Attorney General and Secretary of the Treasury are honorary counselor and treasurer, respectively.

The ARC should not be confused with the International Committee of the Red Cross (ICRC), a totally separate organization. The ICRC was founded in 1863 by several Swiss men in Geneva, Switzerland, to provide humane services in times of conflict (war). The leader of this group, Henri Dunant, brought delegates together from 12 nations in 1864 to what is now known as the first Geneva Convention to sign the Geneva Treaty. The ICRC, which has headquarters in Geneva, Switzerland, and is still governed by the Swiss, continues to work today during times of disaster and international conflict. For example, during the Persian Gulf Conflict in 1990–1991, the ICRC was involved in exchanges of prisoners of war.

In addition to the ICRC, there is a league of Red Cross societies, which comprises Red Cross organizations of various countries (in Moslem countries, it is the Red Crescent) that have ratified the Geneva Treaty. The United States first ratified the treaty in 1882.

Other Quasi-Governmental Organizations

Two other examples of quasi-governmental organizations in the United States are the National Science Foundation (NSF) and the National Academy of Sciences (NAS). The purpose of NSF is the funding and promotion of scientific research and the development of individual scientists. It receives and disperses federal funds but operates independently of governmental supervision. Chartered by Congress in 1863, the NAS acts as an advisor to the government on questions of science and technology. Included in its membership are some of America's most renowned scientists. Although neither of these agencies exists specifically to address health problems, both organizations fund projects, publish reports, and take public stands on health related issues.

NONGOVERNMENTAL (UNOFFICIAL) HEALTH AGENCIES

Nongovernmental or unofficial health agencies are funded by private donations or, in some cases, by membership dues. There are thousands of these organizations, all with one thing in common: they arose because there was an unmet health need. The agencies operate, for the most part, free from governmental interference as long as they meet Internal Revenue Service guidelines with regard to their specific tax status. In the sections below we discuss the following types of nongovernmental health agencies: voluntary, professional, philanthropic, service, religious, and corporate.

Voluntary Health Agencies

Voluntary health agencies are an American creation. Each of these agencies

---

voluntary health agencies Organizations created by concerned citizens to deal with a health need not met by governmental health agencies.

was begun by one or more concerned citizens who felt that a specific health need was not being met by existing governmental agencies. In a sense, these new voluntary agencies arose by themselves, in much the same way as a "volunteer" tomato plant arises in a vegetable garden. New voluntary agencies continue to be born each year. Examples of recent additions to the perhaps 100,000 agencies already in existence are A Better Way, Mothers Against Drunk Driving (MADD), and Students Against Driving Drunk (SADD). A discussion of the commonalities of voluntary health agencies follows.

Organization of Voluntary Health Agencies

Most voluntary agencies exist at three levels—national, state, and local. At the national level, policies that guide the agency are formulated. A significant proportion of the money raised locally is forwarded to the national office, where it is allocated according to the agency's budget. Much of the money is designated for research. By funding research, the agencies hope to discover the cause of and cure for a particular disease or health problem. There have been some major successes. The March of Dimes, for example, helped to eliminate polio as a major disease problem in the United States through its funding of immunization research.

There is not always a consensus of opinion about budget decisions made at the national level, some believing that less should be spent for research and more for treating those afflicted with the disease. Another disagreement regards how much of the fund should be sent to the national headquarters in the first place. Others complain that when an agency achieves success, as the March of Dimes did in its fight against polio, it should dissolve. This does not usually occur; instead, successful agencies often find

a new health concern. The March of Dimes now fights birth defects; and when the Tuberculosis Society got that disease under control, it changed its name to the American Lung Association in order to fight all lung diseases.

The state-level offices of voluntary agencies are analogous to the state departments of health in the way that they link the national headquarters with local offices. The primary work at this level is to coordinate local efforts and to insure that policies developed at the national headquarters are carried out. The state-level office may also provide training services for employees and volunteers of local-level offices and are usually available as consultants and problem solvers.

The local-level office of each voluntary agency is usually managed by a paid staff worker who has been hired either by the state-level office or by a local board of directors. Members of the local board of directors usually serve in that capacity on a voluntary basis. Working under the manager of each agency are local volunteers, who are the backbone of voluntary agencies. It has been said that the local level is where the "rubber meets the road." In other words, this is where most of the money is raised, most of the education takes place, and most of the service is rendered. Volunteers are of two types, professional and lay. Professional volunteers have had training in a medical profession, while lay volunteers have no medical training. The paid employees help to facilitate the work of the volunteers with expertise, training, and other resources.

Purpose of Voluntary Health Agencies

Voluntary agencies share three basic objectives: (1) to raise money to fund research, (2) to provide education both to professionals and to the public, and (3) to provide service to those individuals and families that are afflicted with the disease or health problem.

Fund raising is a primary activity of many voluntary agencies. While in the past this was accomplished primarily by door-to-door solicitors, today mass-mailing and telephone solicitation are more common. Some agencies sponsor special events like golf outings, dances, or dinners. One type of special event that is very popular today is the "a-thon." Examples include bike-a-thons, rock-a-thons, telethons, skate-a-thons, and dance-a-thons. These money-making "a-thons" seem to be limited in scope only by the creativity of those planning them. In addition, some of these agencies have become United Way (see Box 2.3) agencies and receive some funds derived from the annual United Way campaign, which conducts fund-raising efforts at worksites.

Over the years, the number of voluntary agencies (see Figure 2.9) formed to help meet special health needs has continually increased. The three largest (in terms of dollars raised) voluntary agencies in the United States today are the American Cancer Society (see Box 2.4), the American Heart Association, and the American Lung Association. Appendix 2 provides a selected list of voluntary health agencies.

Professional Health Organizations/Associations

Professional health organizations and associations are made up of health professionals who have completed specialized

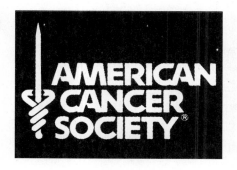
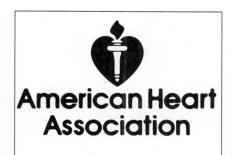
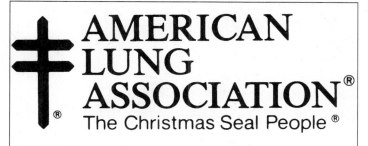

FIGURE 2.9

Voluntary health organizations, such as the ones represented in this picture, make significant contributions to community health.

BOX 2.3
Facts About United Way of America and Local United Ways

United Way of America is the national service and training center supporting local, community-based United Ways which make up the United Way system. United Way of America is governed by a volunteer board. It does not raise or allocate funds but provides to local United Ways assistance that includes the following:

1. A national advertising and promotion program.
2. A partnership with the National Football League.
3. Training for United Way professionals and volunteers.
4. Support to national companies that want to cultivate a year-round relationship with United Ways among employees in corporate locations throughout the country.
5. A national database for several types of information, including fund-raising and fund distribution statistics.
6. A national network allowing United Ways to share best practices and other information.
7. A unified voice in national government relations.

The United Way system comprises more than 2,100 local United Way organizations throughout America. Each local United Way is an independent, separately incorporated community organization governed, like the the United Way of America, by a local board of volunteers. In addition, each United Way has a professional staff to carry out the daily functions of the organization.

The primary focus of each United Way is to work to meet the health and human care needs of people in its community. This is accomplished through the distribution of funds to local agency service providers. The funds are obtained through a single communitywide fund-raising campaign.

Besides raising funds to be distributed to local agency service providers, local United Way volunteers also:

1. Assess community needs and resources available to address them.
2. Bring community organizations and people together for cooperative efforts in community problem solving.
3. Recruit and train other volunteers.
4. Put people in touch with the services they need.
5. Offer management and technical help to a wide range of community agencies.

In 1991, United Ways collectively raised $3.17 billion from individuals, corporations, small businesses, and foundations. In turn, the money raised helped to support approximately 44,000 agencies and chapters throughout the country. Some of the agencies are nationally known charitable organizations with local chapters. Others are smaller, one-of-a-kind local agencies. United Way support has been flexible over the years, supporting not only historical agencies but also those that address newly emerging needs.

Overall, the United Way agencies have played important roles in community health since 1918.

Source: United Way of America (Aug. 1992). *Fact Sheets.* Alexandria, Va.: Author.

education and training programs and have met the standards of certification for their respective fields. Their mission is to promote high standards of professional practice for their specific profession, thereby improving the health of society by improving the people in the profession. Professional organizations are funded primarily by member-

BOX 2.4
A Closer Look at One Voluntary Health Agency: The American Cancer Society

The American Cancer Society (ACS) first opened its doors in 1913. At that time, it was known as the American Society for the Control of Cancer. Today, with offices in every state and Guam, ACS is one of our largest voluntary health organizations. In spite of its success, its mission has remained constant since its founding. It is "dedicated to eliminating cancer as a major health problem by preventing cancer, saving lives from cancer, and diminishing suffering from cancer through research, education, and service."[8]

The mission of ACS includes both short- and long-term goals. Its short-term goals are to save lives and diminish suffering. This is accomplished through education and service. Its long-term goal, the elimination of cancer, is being approached through the society's support of cancer research.

The American Cancer Society's educational programs are targeted at two different groups—the general public and the health professionals who treat cancer patients. The public education program promotes the following skills and concepts to people of all ages: (1) taking the necessary steps to prevent cancer, (2) knowing the seven warning signals, (3) understanding the value for regular checkups, and (4) coping with cancer. The society accomplishes this by offering free public education programs, supported by up-to-date literature and audiovisual materials, whenever and wherever they may be requested. These programs may be presented in homes, worksites, churches, clubs, organizations, and schools. From time to time, the society also prepares public service messages for broadcasting or televising.

The Society's professional education program is aimed at the professionals who work with oncology patients. The objective of this program is to motivate "medical and allied health professionals to use the latest and best possible cancer detection, diagnostic, and patient management techniques."[9] Such education is provided through professional publications, up-to-date audio visual materials, conferences, and grants that fund specialized education experiences.

The ACS offers service and rehabilitation programs that ease the impact of cancer on those affected. The services offered include information and referral to appropriate professionals, home care supplies and equipment for the comfort of patients, transportation of patients to maintain their medical and continuing care programs, and specialized education programs for cancer patients to help them cope and feel better about themselves. There are also rehabilitation programs that provide social support for all cancer patients and specific programs for those who have had a mastectomy, laryngectomy, or ostomy.

"The aim of the Society's research program is to determine what causes cancer and to support efforts to prevent and cure cancer."[8] As such, the society provides research funds to many cancer researchers in a variety of settings. The ACS is the largest source of private cancer research funds in the United States, second only to the National Cancer Institute for all groups, public or private, in funding cancer research.

All ACS programs—education, service, and research—are planned primarily by the volunteers of the society. The society does employ staff members to carry out the day-to-day operations and to help advise and suppport the work of the volunteers, but the ratio of volunteers to paid staff is about 900 to 1.[9] This arrangement of volunteers and staff working together has created a very strong voluntary health agency.

ship dues. Examples of such organizations are the American Medical Association, the American Dental Association, the American Nursing Association, the American Public Health Association, the Association for the Advancement of Health Education, and the Society of Public Health Educators.

Although each professional organization is unique, most provide similar services to their members. These include the certification of continuing-education programs for professional renewal, the hosting of annual conventions where members share research results and interact with colleagues, and the publication of professional journals and other reports. Some examples of journals published by professional health associations are the *Journal of the American Medical Association,* the *American Journal of Public Health,* and *The Journal of Health Education.*

Another important activity of some professional organizations is lobbying. The American Medical Association, for example, has a powerful lobby nationally and in some state legislatures. Their purpose is to affect legislation in such a way as to benefit their membership and their profession. Many professional health organizations provide the opportunity for benefits including group insurance and discount travel rates. There are hundreds of professional health organizations in the United States, and it would be difficult to describe them all here.

Philanthropic Foundations

Philanthropic foundations have made and continue to make significant contributions to community health in the United States and throughout the world. These foundations support community

---

philanthropic foundation An endowed institution that donates money for the good of humankind.

health by funding programs and research on the prevention, control, and treatment of many diseases. Foundation directors, sometimes in consultation with a review committee, determine the types of programs that will be funded. Some foundations fund an array of health projects while others have a narrower scope of interests. Some foundations, such as the Rockefeller Foundation, fund international health projects while others restrict their funding to domestic projects. The geographical scope of domestic foundations can be national, state, or local. Local foundations may restrict their funding to projects that benefit local citizens.

The activities of these foundations differ from those of the voluntary health agencies in two important ways. First, foundations have money to give away, and therefore no effort is spent on fund raising. Second, foundations can afford to fund long-term or innovative research projects that might be too risky or expensive for voluntary or even government-funded agencies. The development of a vaccine for yellow fever by a scientist funded by the Rockefeller Foundation is an example of one such long-range project.

Some of the larger foundations, in addition to the Rockefeller Foundation, that have made significant commitments to community health are: the Commonwealth Fund, which has contributed to community health in rural communities, improved hospital facilities, and tried to strengthen mental health services; the Ford Foundation, which has contributed greatly to family-planning efforts throughout the world; the Robert Wood Johnson Foundation, which has worked to improve access to medical and dental care throughout the United States; the Henry J. Kaiser Family Foundation, which has supported the development of health maintenance organizations (HMOs) and community health promotion; the W. K. Kellogg Foundation, which has funded many diverse health programs that address human issues and provide a practical solution; and the Milbank Memorial Fund, which has primarily funded preventive-medicine projects.

Service and Religious Organizations

Service and religious organizations have also played a part in community health over the years (see Figure 2.10). Examples of service groups involved in community health are the Jaycees, Kiwanis Club, Fraternal Order of Police, Rotary Club, Elks, Lions,

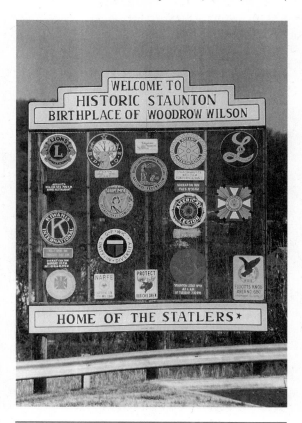

FIGURE 2.10

Community service groups contribute needed resources for the improvement of the health of the community.

Moose, Shriners, and American Legion. Members of these groups enjoy social interactions with people of similar interests while fulfilling the groups' primary reason for existence—service to others in their communities. Although health may not be the specific focus of their mission, many of these groups make important contributions in that direction by raising money and funding health-related programs. Their contributions are sometimes substantial. Examples of such programs include the Shriners' children's hospitals and burn centers, the Lions' contributions to pilot (lead) dog programs and other services for the blind such as the provision of eyeglasses for school-aged children unable to afford them, and the Lions' contributions to the school health curriculum via the educational program "Quest: Skills for Living."

The contributions of religious groups to community health have also been substantial. Such groups have been effective avenues for promoting health programs because they: have had a history of volunteerism and preexisting reinforcement contingencies for volunteerism, can influence entire families, and have accessible meeting-room facilities.[10] One way in which these groups contribute is through donations of money for the less fortunate. Examples of religious organizations that solicit donations from their members include the Protestants' One Great Hour of Sharing, the Catholics' Relief Fund, and the United Jewish Appeal. Other types of contributions by religious groups include: (1) the donation of space for voluntary health programs such as blood donations, Alcoholics Anonymous, and other support groups; (2) sponsorship of food banks and shelters for the hungry, poor, and homeless; (3) sharing the doctrine of good personal health behavior; and (4) allowing community health professionals to deliver their programs through the congregations. This latter contribution has been especially useful in black American communities because of the importance that the churches play in the culture of this group of people.

It should also be noted that some religious groups have hindered the work of community health workers. Almost every community in the country can provide an example where a religious organization has protested the offering of a school district's sex education program, picketed a health clinic, or spoke out about homosexuality.

Corporate Involvement in Community Health

In recent years, Corporate America has become increasingly involved in community health for a number of reasons but primarily because of the rapidly rising cost of health care. Many corporations today find that their single largest annual expenditure is for employee health care. Consider, for example, the cost of manufacturing a new car. The cost of health benefits for those who build the car now exceeds the cost of the raw materials for the car itself.

In an effort to reduce their health care costs, many companies support health-related programs both at and away from the worksite. Worksite programs aimed at trimming employee medical bills have been expanded beyond the traditional safety awareness programs and first aid services to include such programs as substance abuse counseling, nutrition education, smoking cessation, stress management, and physical fitness programs. Many companies are also implementing health promotion policies and enforcing state and local laws that prohibit (or severely restrict) smoking on company grounds or that require the use of safety belts at all times in all company-owned vehicles.

Many corporations are now also sponsoring health enhancing activities away from the worksite. These activities go beyond traditional sponsorship of youth baseball and may include recycling efforts, community health fairs, and screening programs for specific health problems. Although it is true that some of these programs may be among the first to be cut during tough economic times, they represent a positive step in corporate America's committment to community health.

CHAPTER SUMMARY

Contemporary society is too complex to respond effectively to community health problems on either an emergency or a long-term basis. This fact necessitates organizations and planning for health in our communities.

In this chapter, we have described the different types of organizations that contribute to the promotion, protection, and maintenance of health in a community. These organizations can be classified into three groups according to their sources of funding and organizational structure: governmental, quasi-governmental, and nongovernmental. Governmental health agencies exist at the local, state, federal, and international levels and are funded primarily by tax dollars. The quasi-governmental agencies, such as the American Red Cross, share attributes with both the governmental and nongovernmental agencies. Nongovernmental or unofficial organizations include voluntary and professional associations, philanthropic foundations, and service and religious groups. Corporate America has also become more involved in community health, both at the worksite and in the community.

SCENARIO: ANALYSIS AND RESPONSE

After having read this chapter, please respond to the following questions in reference to the scenario at the beginning of the chapter.

1. Select two local health agencies that might be of assistance to Mary and Bill as they fight Bill's cancer, and describe their services.

2. Are there any state or federal agencies that might be able to help them? Explain your answer.

3. Should Mary and Bill expect significant financial support from the local agencies? Why or why not?

REVIEW QUESTIONS

1. What characteristics of modern society necessitate planning and organization for community health?

2. What is the World Health Organization and what does it do?

3. What is the largest federal department in the United States and what major services does it provide?

4. What is the Public Health Service?

5. Explain the major functions of the Centers for Disease Control and Prevention.

6. How do state and local health departments interface?

7. What is meant by the term *comprehensive school health program?* What are the major components of it?

8. What is meant by the term *quasi-governmental agency?* Name one such agency.

9. What are the major differences between a governmental (official) health organization and a voluntary health agency?

10. What does a health professional have to gain from being a member of a professional health organization?

11. How do philanthropic foundations contribute to community health? List five well-known foundations.

12. How do service and religious groups contribute to the health of the community?

13. Why has corporate America become involved in community health?

ACTIVITIES

1. Using a local telephone book, list all the health-related organizations that service your community. Divide your list by the type of health organizations according to their classification in this chapter.

2. Make an appointment to interview someone at one of the organizations identified in Activity 1. During your visit, find answers to the following questions:

   How did the organization begin?

   What is its mission?

   How is it funded?

   How many people (employees and volunteers) work for the organization, and what type of education/training do they have?

   What types of programs and services does the organization provide?

3. Obtain organizational charts from the U.S. Department of Health and Human Services (a copy is in this chapter), your state department of health, and your local health department. Compare and contrast these charts and describe their similarities and differences.

4. Call a local voluntary health organization in your community and ask them if you could volunteer to work 10–15 hours during this academic term. Then volunteer the hours.

5. Carefully review your community newspaper each day for an entire week. Keep track of all articles or advertisements that make reference to local health organizations. Summarize your findings in a one-page paper. (If you don't subscribe, copies of newspapers are available in libraries.)

REFERENCES

1. Green, L. W. (1990). "The Revival of Community and the Public Obligation of Academic Health Centers." In

R. E. Bulger and S. J. Reiser, eds. *Integrity in Institutions: Humane Environments for Teaching, Inquiry and Healing.* Iowa City: Univ. of Iowa Press, pp. 163–180.

2. World Health Organization (1990). *Facts About WHO.* Geneva, Switz.: Author.

3. U.S. Dept. of Health and Human Services (1992). *Comprehensive Health Care Program for American Indians and Alaska Natives.* Washington, D.C.: U.S. Government Printing Office.

4. Agency for Toxic Substances and Disease Registry (1990). *ATSDR Fact Sheet,* Atlanta, Ga.: Author.

5. Ramsey, T. L., ed. (March 1991). *Hazardous Substances and Public Health.* (Available from Agency for Toxic Substances and Disease Registry, PHS, DHHS.)

6. American Public Health Association (1975). "The Role of Official Local Health Agencies." *American Journal of Public Health,* 65(2): 189–193.

7. Joint Committee on Health Education Terminology (1991). "Report of the 1990 Joint Committee on Health Education Terminology." *The Journal of Health Education* 22(2): 105.

8. American Cancer Society (1993). *Cancer Facts and Figures—1993.* Atlanta, Ga.: Author.

9. American Cancer Society (1986). *American Cancer Society: What Is It, What It Does, How It Began, Who Directs It, Where Is It Going.* New York: Author.

10. Lasater, T. M., B. L. Wells, R. A. Carleton, and J. P. Elder (1986). "The Role of Churches in Disease Preventive Research Studies." *Public Health Report* 101(2): 125–131.

Chapter 3

EPIDEMIOLOGY: THE STUDY OF DISEASE, INJURY, AND DEATH IN THE COMMUNITY

Chapter Outline

Chapter Objectives

After studying this chapter you will be able to:

1. Define the terms *epidemic, epidemiology,* and *epidemiologist* and explain their importance in community health.
2. Discuss how the practice of epidemiology has changed since the days of Benjamin Rush and John Snow.
3. Explain why rates are important in epidemiology and list some of the commonly used rates.
4. Define incidence and prevalence rates and provide examples of each.
5. Calculate a variety of rates from the appropriate data.
6. Discuss the importance of disease reporting to a community's health and describe the reporting process.
7. Identify sources of standardized data used by epidemiologists, community health workers, and health officials and list the types of data available from each source.
8. List and describe the three types of epidemiological studies and explain the purpose of each.

Scenario

The picnic seemed to be a success; students from both residence halls appeared to have a good time. For a while it seemed almost too warm, but there were plenty of cold drinks available and by late afternoon it had become quite pleasant. The games were fun too . . . frisbee, softball, and volleyball. Then there was the picnic itself, turkey, potato salad, bread and butter, milk, and dessert. But that was earlier in the afternoon.

At 8 o'clock, that same night, instead of studying as John had planned, he was lying on his bed with a stomach ache. He was experiencing severe diarrhea and had made several hurried trips to the bathroom in the last half-hour.

The telephone rang and it was Michael, John's roommate. He had gone to his girlfriend's house after the picnic to work on a class project with her. He and Caroline were both sick with stomach cramps and diarrhea, and Michael was calling to ask whether John was sick too. As John was answering, he realized that he needed to run to the bathroom again. He quickly hung up, promising to call back soon. On his way to the bathroom, John began to think about what a coincidence it was that all three of them were sick with the same symptoms and at about the same time. Could they have become ill from food they ate at the picnic? There were about 50 people at the picnic; how many others might be sick? Was it the heat? Was it the food? Is this an epidemic? A half-hour later, John called Michael back to tell him that he had decided to go to the campus health center.

Elsewhere . . .

This had turned out to be an interesting volunteer experience. As a requirement for her community health class, Kim had agreed to volunteer at the local health department. The spring semester was almost over now and she was writing a final report of her activities. During the term, she had spent Friday afternoons accompanying a sanitarian on his inspections of restaurants and retail food stores. She had also helped him complete his reports on substandard housing and malfunctioning septic tanks.

Dr. Turner, the health officer, had given Kim permission to use one of the department's personal computers for preparing her final report. Since it was Sunday evening, she was alone in the health department office when the telephone rang. She briefly considered not answering it but finally picked up the receiver. It was Dr. Lee from the University Health Center. He said he was calling in the hope that someone might be there because he needed to reach Dr. Turner immediately. He said that he had admitted six students to the infirmary with severe stomach cramps, vomiting, and diarrhea. The students had been at a picnic earlier, and he thought they could have food poisoning. He called to ask Dr. Turner to investigate this outbreak and asked Kim to try to reach him as soon as possible.

INTRODUCTION

When you become ill and visit a doctor, the first thing the physician does is take measurements and collect information. The measurements include your temperature, heart rate, and blood pressure. The information includes time of onset of your illness, where you have traveled, and what you might have eaten. Next you may be given a physical examination and asked to provide a specimen such as urine or blood for laboratory examination. The information gathered helps the physician understand the nature of your illness and prescribe an appropriate treatment.

While a primary care physician is concerned with the course of disease in an individual patient, an epidemiologist is concerned with the course of disease in a population. When illness, injury, or death occur at unexpected or unacceptable levels in a community or population, epidemiologists seek to collect information about the disease status of the community. First, epidemiologists want to know *how many* people are sick. Second, they want to know *who* is sick—the old? the young? males? females? rich? poor? They also want to know *when* the people became sick, and finally, *where* the sick people live or have traveled. In summary, epidemiologists want to know what it is that the sick people have in common. For this reason, epidemiology has sometimes been referred to as *population medicine.*

Definition of Epidemiology

Before we discuss the types of questions an epidemiologist asks, we need a definition of the term *epidemiology*. **Epidemiology** is "the study of the distribution and determi-

nants of diseases and injuries in human populations."[1] The term *epidemiology* is derived from Greek words that can be translated into the phrase, the study of that which is upon the people. The goal of epidemiology is to limit disease, injury, and death in a community by intervening to prevent or limit outbreaks or epidemics of disease and injury. This is accomplished by describing outbreaks and designing studies to analyze health problems and validate new controls and treatments. Through these practices, epidemiologists contribute to our knowledge of how diseases begin and spread through populations and how they can be prevented or controlled.

The question might be asked, how many cases are required before a disease outbreak is considered an epidemic—10 cases? 100 cases? 1,000 cases? The answer is that it depends upon the disease and the population, but *any unexpectedly large number of cases of a disease* in a particular population at a particular time and place can be considered an **epidemic.** Some recent epidemics in the United States are presented in Table 3.1.

The question might be asked, what are diseases called that occur regularly in a population and are not epidemic? These diseases are referred to as **endemic diseases.** Whether a disease is epidemic or endemic depends on the disease and the population. Heart disease is endemic in America, while in many regions of equatorial Africa, malaria is endemic.

While an **epidemiologist** studies outbreaks of disease, injury, and death in human populations, *epidemics,* an *epizootiologist* studies disease outbreaks in animal

---

epidemiology The distribution and determinants of diseases and injuries in human populations.

epidemic An unexpectedly large number of cases of disease in a particular population.
endemic disease A disease that occurs regularly in a population as a matter of course.
epidemiologist One who practices epidemiology.

Table 3.1

Recent Epidemics in the United States

Disease	Cases in Previous Years	Epidemic Period	Number of Cases
St. Louis encephalitis	5–72	1975	1,815[2]
Legionnaires' disease	Unknown	1976	235[3]
Toxic shock syndrome	11–272	1980	877[4]
Plague	13–19	1983	40
Lyme disease	Unknown	1982–1992	49,872[5]
AIDS	Unknown	1981–1993	315,000[6,7]

populations, *epizootics*. Some diseases, such as bubonic plague and St. Louis encephalitis, may begin as epizootics but later become epidemics. When both animals and humans are involved in a disease outbreak, the term *epizoodemic* is appropriate. Occasionally, an epidemic will spread over a wide area, perhaps even across an entire continent or around the world. Such a widespread epidemic is termed a **pandemic.** The influenza pandemic of 1918 is an example (see Figure 3.1). The disease spread from France to Spain and then to England and the rest of Europe. It spread to China and West Africa and eventually reached the United States, Australia, and New Zealand. An estimated 25 million people died over several years as a result of this pandemic. The current outbreak of acquired immunodeficiency syndrome (AIDS) is another example of a pandemic.

History of Epidemiology

If one searches diligently, it is possible to trace the roots of epidemiological thinking back to the "Father of Medicine," Hippocrates, who as early as 300 B.C. suggested

pandemic An outbreak of disease over a wide geographical area such as a continent.

a relationship between the occurrence of disease and the physical environment.[8] For example, cases of a disease fitting the description of malaria were found to occur in the vicinity of marshes and swamps.

With the fall of the classical civilizations of Greece and Rome and the return in Europe to a belief in spiritual causes of disease, few advances were made in the field of epidemiology. To be sure, epidemics continued to occur. There were two waves of plague—one in 542–543 and another in 1348–1349.[9] There were also epidemics of leprosy, smallpox, malaria, and, later, syphilis and yellow fever.

Epidemics occurred in the New World as well. One such epidemic of yellow fever struck Philadelphia in 1793, causing the death of 4,044 people. Yellow fever was epidemic again in Philadelphia in 1797, 1798, and in 1803.[10] Dr. Benjamin Rush, a prominent Philadelphia physician and signatory of the Declaration of Independence, was able to trace the cases of yellow fever to the docks where ships arrived from tropical ports. However, his conclusion that the disease was caused by vapors arising from decaying coffee beans in port warehouses was incorrect. He could not have known that yellow fever is caused by a virus and is carried by the yellow fever mosquito, *Aedes aegypti*, facts that were discovered by Walter Reed and his associates a century later.

In 1849, some fifty years after the yellow fever outbreaks in Philadelphia, cholera became epidemic in London. A prominent physician, John Snow, investigated the outbreak by interviewing numerous victims and their families. He concluded that the source of the epidemic was probably water drawn from a particular communal well on Broad Street. Snow extinguished the epidemic when he removed the pump handle from the Broad Street pump and forced people to obtain their water elsewhere.[11]

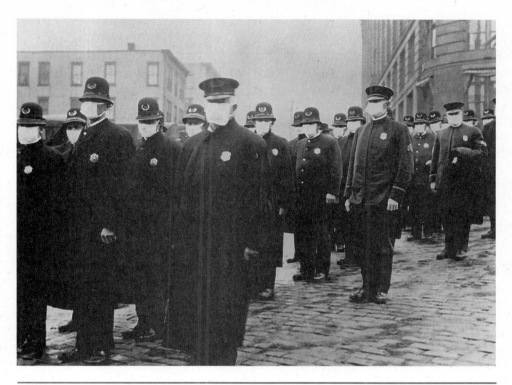

FIGURE 3.1

More than 25 million people died during the influenza pandemic of 1918–1919.

John Snow's interruption of the London cholera epidemic in 1849 is a classic example of how epidemiological methods can be used to limit disease and deaths. His achievement was even more remarkable because it occurred 30 years before Louis Pasteur proposed his "germ theory of disease."

From its early use for the description and investigation of communicable diseases, epidemiology has developed into a sophisticated field of science. Epidemiological methods are used to evaluate everything from the effectiveness of vaccines to the causes of occupational illnesses and traffic deaths.

A knowledge of epidemiology is important for the community health worker who wishes to establish the presence of a set of needs or conditions for a particular health service or program or to justify a request for funding. Likewise, epidemiological methods are used to evaluate the effectiveness of programs already in existence and to plan to meet anticipated needs for facilities and personnel.

THE IMPORTANCE OF RATES

Epidemiologists are concerned with numbers. Of prime importance is the number of **cases** (people who are sick) and, of course,

cases People afflicted with a disease.

the number of deaths. These numbers alone, however, are not enough to provide a description of the extent of the disease in a community. Epidemiologists must also know the total number in the susceptible population so that rates can be calculated. A **rate** is the number of events (births, cases of disease, or deaths) in a given population over a given period or at a given point in time. The three types of rates that are of greatest interest to epidemiologists are **natality (birth) rates, morbidity (sickness) rates,** and **mortality** or **fatality (death) rates.**

Why are rates important? Why not simply enumerate the sick or dead? The answer is that rates allow a comparison of outbreaks that occur at different times or in different places. For example, by using rates it is possible to determine whether there are more cases of gonorrhea per capita this year than there were last year or whether there are more homicides per capita in city A than in city B.

For example, suppose you wish to compare transportation deaths associated with travel by autos and airplanes. To examine this hypothetical situation, consider that for a given time period 1,000 people died in auto crashes while 50 people died in airplane crashes. Without calculating rates, one might assume that auto travel is more dangerous than air travel. However, if you knew the population exposed (100,000 people for auto travel versus 1,000 people for air travel) you could calculate fatality rates, the number of deaths divided by the population, for each mode of travel (see Table 3.2).[12]

Table 3.2
Number of Deaths and Death Rates for Two Modes of Travel

	Source of Fatalities	
	Auto	*Airplane*
Number of fatalities per year	1,000	50
Number exposed to risk	100,000	1,000
Rate of fatality	0.01 (1/100)	0.05 (5/100)

These rates have greater meaning, because they are based upon the **population-at-risk,** those who are susceptible to disease or death from a particular cause. In this case, the fatality rates are 1/100 for autos, and 5/100 for airplanes, indicating that in this hypothetical example air travel is five times more dangerous than auto travel.

Incidence, Prevalence, and Attack Rates

Three important types of morbidity rates are incidence rates, prevalence rates, and attack rates. An **incidence rate** is defined as the number of new cases of a disease in a population-at-risk in a given time period. An example would be the number of *new* cases of influenza in a community in a week. Those who became ill with influenza during the previous week and remain ill during the week in question are not counted in an incidence rate. Incidence rates are important in the study of **acute diseases,** diseases in which the peak severity of symptoms occurs and subsides within days or weeks. These diseases usually move quickly

---

rate The number of events that occur in a given population in a given period of time.
natality (birth) rate The number of live births divided by the total population.
morbidity rate The rate of illness in a population.
mortality (fatality) rate The number of deaths in a population divided by the total population.

---

population-at-risk Those in the population who are susceptible to a particular disease or condition.
incidence rate The number of *new* cases of a disease in a population-at-risk during a particular period of time, divided by the total number in that same population.
acute disease A disease that lasts three months or less.

through a population. Examples of acute diseases are the common cold, influenza, chicken pox, measles, and mumps.

Prevalence rates are calculated by dividing *all* current cases of a disease (*old and new*) by the total population. Prevalence rates are useful for the study of **chronic disease,** diseases that usually last three months or longer. In these cases, it is more important to know how many people are currently suffering from a chronic disease—such as arthritis, heart disease, cancer, or diabetes—than it is to know when they became afflicted. Furthermore, with many chronic diseases, it is difficult or impossible to determine the date of onset of disease. Since a preponderance of health services and facilities are used for the treatment of persons with chronic diseases and conditions, prevalence rates are more useful than incidence rates for the planning of public health programs, personnel needs, and facilities.

An **attack rate** is a special incidence rate calculated for a particular population for a single disease outbreak and expressed as a percent. For example, suppose a number of people who traveled on the same airline flight became ill and epidemiologists suspected that the cause of these illness was associated with the flight itself. An attack rate could be calculated for the passengers on that flight to express the percent who became ill. Furthermore, attack rates could be calculated for various subpopulations such as those seated at various locations in the plane, those who selected specific entrees from the menu, those of particular age

Table 3.3
Crude Rates

$$\text{Crude birth rate} = \frac{\text{Number of live births}}{\text{Estimated midyear population}} \times 1{,}000$$

$$\text{Crude death rate} = \frac{\text{Number of deaths (all causes)}}{\text{Estimated midyear population}} \times 1{,}000$$

groups, or those who boarded the flight at specific stops. Differences in attack rates for different subpopulations might indicate to the epidemiologists the source or cause of the illness.

Crude and Specific Rates

Incidence and prevalence rates can be expressed in two forms—crude and specific. **Crude rates** are those in which the denominator includes the total population. The most important of these are the crude birth rate and the crude death rate. The **crude birth rate** is the number of live births in a given year, divided by the midyear population. The **crude death rate** is the total number of deaths in a given year from all causes, divided by the midyear population (see Table 3.3). Crude rates are relatively easy to obtain and are useful when comparing similar populations. But they can be misleading when populations differ in age structure or some other attribute. For example, the crude birth rate is normally higher in younger populations, which have a higher proportion people of reproductive age, than in populations with more elderly people.

---

prevalence rate   The number of *new and old* cases of a disease in a population in a given period of time, divided by the total number of that population.
chronic disease   A disease or health condition that lasts longer than three months.
attack rate   An incidence rate calculated for a particular population for a single disease outbreak and expressed as a percentage.

crude rate   A rate in which the denominator includes the total population.
crude birth rate   The number of live births per 1,000 in a population in a given period of time.
crude death rate (CDR)   The number of deaths (from all causes) per 1,000 in a population in a given period of time.

Table 3.4
Important Rates in Epidemiology

Rate	Definition	Examples (U.S. 1992)
Crude birth rate	$\dfrac{\text{Number of live births}}{\text{Estimated midyear population}} \times 1{,}000$	16.0/1,000
Crude death rate	$\dfrac{\text{Number of deaths (all causes)}}{\text{Estimated midyear population}} \times 1{,}000$	8.5/1,000
Age-specific death rate	$\dfrac{\text{Number of deaths, 35–44}}{\text{Estimated midyear population, 35–44}} \times 1{,}000$	2.3/1,000
Infant mortality rate	$\dfrac{\text{Number of deaths under 1 year of age}}{\text{Number of live births}} \times 1{,}000$	8.5/1,000
Neonatal mortality rate	$\dfrac{\text{Number of deaths under 28 days of age}}{\text{Number of live births}} \times 1{,}000$	5.4/1,000
Cause-specific death rate	$\dfrac{\text{Number of deaths (diabetes mellitus)}}{\text{Estimated midyear population}} \times 100{,}000$	17.2/100,000

Conversely, the crude death rate would be expected to be higher in an older population. Crude rates are usually reported as events per 1,000 people.

Specific rates measure morbidity and mortality for particular populations or for particular diseases. One could, for example, calculate the age-specific mortality rate for a population of 35- to 44-year-olds by dividing the number of deaths in that age group by the midyear population of 35- to 44-year-olds. Similarly, one could calculate race- and sex-specific mortality rates.

A very important specific rate is the **cause-specific mortality rate (CSMR),** which measures the death rate for a specific disease. This can be calculated by dividing the number of deaths due to a particular

disease by the total population. Because fewer people can be expected to die from each cause than to die from all causes, CSMRs are usually reported per 100,000 population. Table 3.4 depicts some commonly used rates in epidemiology.

Two other important measures of disease are the **case fatality rate (CFR)** and the **proportionate mortality ratio (PMR).**[13] The CFR is simply the percentage of cases that result in death. It is a measure of the severity of a disease and is directly related to the virulence of the disease agent. It is calculated by dividing the number of deaths from a particular disease in a specified period of time by the number of cases of that same disease in the same time period. The resulting fraction is multiplied by 100

---

specific rate   A rate that measures the rate of a specific disease in a population.
cause-specific mortality rate (CSMR)   The death rate due to a particular disease.

case fatality rate (CFR)   The percentage of cases of a particular disease that result in death.
proportionate mortality ratio (PMR)   The percentage of overall mortality in a population that is attributable to a particular cause.

and reported as a percentage. For example, if there were 200 cases of a severe illness and 10 of them resulted in death, the CFR would be: 10 ÷ 200 × 100 = 5%.

The PMR describes the relationship between the number of deaths from a specific cause to the total number of deaths attributable to all causes. It is calculated by dividing the number of deaths assigned to a particular disease by the total number of deaths from all causes in the same population during the same period of time. It is also reported as a percentage. For example, in the United States, there were 725,010 deaths due to cardiovascular diseases in 1990, and 2,162,000 total deaths reported that same year.[14] The PMR for cardiovascular disease can be calculated as follows: 725,010 ÷ 2,162,000 × 100 = 33.5%. In other words, heart disease was responsible for one of every three deaths in the United States in 1990.

REPORTING OF BIRTHS, DEATHS, AND DISEASES

It is important to epidemiologists that births, deaths, and cases of diseases be recorded promptly and accurately. Physicians, clinics, and hospitals are required by law to report all births and deaths as well as all cases of certain **notifiable diseases** to their local health departments. Notifiable diseases are infectious diseases that can become epidemic and for which health officials maintain weekly records. The Centers for Disease Control and Prevention (CDC) issues a list of notifiable diseases for which

they request reports from each state health department (see Table 3.5). Individual states may require the reporting of additional diseases that are of local public health concern. Local health departments are required to summarize all records of births (see Figure 3.2), deaths, and notifiable diseases and report them to their respective state health departments. State health departments summarize these reports and relay them to the CDC through the **National Electronic Telecommunications System (NETS).** The reporting scheme for notifiable disease is shown in Figure 3.3.

The CDC summarizes state and territorial data and uses it to plan epidemiologic research, conduct investigations, and issue reports. One series of reports, published weekly by the CDC, is called the *Morbidity and Mortality Weekly Report (MMWR)*. Copies of the *MMWR* are available to the public at the government documents areas of certain larger libraries.

Unfortunately, the information reported is not always as good as it should be. One study estimated that local health departments may receive notification of only 35% of the cases of some communicable diseases and that many physicians are not familiar with the requirement of reporting. Clinics may not report each and every case of measles or gonorrhea. Doctors' offices and clinics may be understaffed or simply too busy to keep up with reporting. In other cases, patients recover—with or without treatment—before a diagnosis is confirmed. Changes in local and state government administration or other key personnel often interfere with the timely reporting of disease data. The accuracy of disease reporting also depends on the type of disease. In this

---

notifiable diseases Infectious diseases for which health officials request or require reporting for public health reasons.

National Electronic Telecommunications System (NETS) The electronic reporting system used by state health departments and CDC.

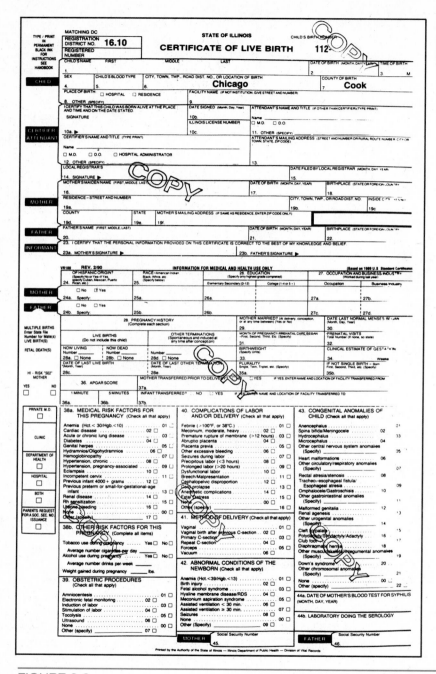

FIGURE 3.2

Birth certificates are issued by local health departments that have jurisdiction where the birth occurred.

Table 3.5

Summary—Cases of Specified Notifiable Diseases, United States, Cumulative, Week Ending December 26, 1992 (52nd week)[6]

	Cum. 1992		Cum. 1992
AIDS	42,978	Measles:	
Anthrax	1	Imported	130
		Indigenous	2,068
Botulism: foodborne	19	Plague	12
Infant	59		
Other	4	Poliomyelitis, paralytic	—
Brucellosis	87	Psittacosis	86
Cholera	102	Rabies, human	—
Congenital rubella syndrome	9	Syphilis, primary and secondary	32,637
Diphtheria	4	Syphilis (congenital) age <1 yr	1,639
Encephalitis, post-infectious	108	Tetanus	39
Gonorrhea	471,488	Toxic shock syndrome	218
Haemophilus influenzae-flu		Trichinosis	39
(invasive disease)	1,222	Tuberculosis	22,592
Hansen disease	148	Tularemia	153
Leptospirosis	46	Typhoid fever	376
Lyme disease	7,777	Typhus fever, tick-borne (RMSF)	489

regard, serious diseases are more likely to be reported than milder ones. Rabies cases, for example, are almost 100% reported while German measles cases may be only 80% to 90% reported. Therefore, morbidity data—while useful for reflecting disease trends—cannot always be considered to be precise counts of the actual number of cases of diseases.

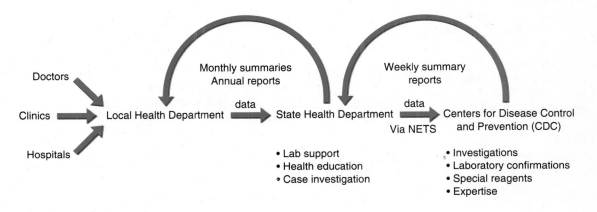

FIGURE 3.3

Scheme for the reporting of notifiable diseases.

SOURCES OF STANDARDIZED DATA

Because demographic and epidemiologic data are used in the planning of public health programs and facilities, students of community health should be aware of the sources of these standardized data. Students can obtain standardized data for use in community health work from the following sources: the *U.S. Census,* the *Statistical Abstract of the United States,* the *Monthly Vital Statistics Report,* and *Morbidity and Mortality Weekly Reports.*

The **U.S. census,** taken every ten years, is an enumeration of the population living in the United States. George Washington ordered the first census in 1790 for the purpose of apportioning representation to the House of Representatives. The most recent census, taken in 1990, was much more complex than the one carried out 200 years earlier. Data were gathered about income, employment, family size, education, type of dwelling, and many other social indicators (see Figure 3.4); copies are available in most libraries.

Census data are important to health workers because they are used for calculating disease and death rates and for program planning. The U.S. census is carried out by the Bureau of the Census, located in the U.S. Department of Commerce.

Another Bureau of the Census publication is the *Statistical Abstract of the United States (SA).* This book, published annually, "is the standard summary of statistics on the social, political and economic organization of the United States."[15] Information is divided into sections under headings such as Population, Vital Statistics, Health and

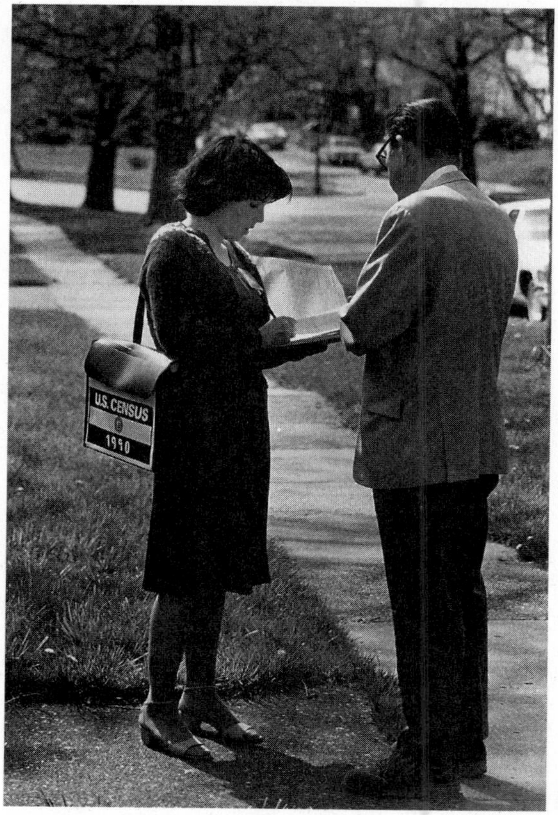

FIGURE 3.4

A census worker collects data used to calculate disease rates.

Nutrition, Education, Law Enforcement, Courts and Prisons, and many more. Data contained in the *SA* are extremely useful and are reasonably up-to-date. (A new edition is published each January and includes data for years up to two years prior to the publication date.) The *SA* can be purchased from the Government Printing Office for about $30 and is available in most libraries.

The National Center for Health Statistics (NCHS), of the Centers for Disease Control and Prevention, provides the most up-to-date national vital statistics available. These appear in the *Monthly Vital Statistics*

U.S. census The enumeration of the population of the United States that is conducted every ten years.

Report, published by the NCHS in Hyattsville, Maryland. **Vital statistics** are statistical summaries of vital records, records of major life events. Listed are live births, deaths, marriages, divorces, and infant deaths. Death rates are also calculated by race and age, and in some issues, by cause. Selected issues also provide mortality data for specific causes: for example, diabetes, drug overdoses, and heart disease. Copies of this publication are available in government document areas of university and large public libraries and can be acquired by writing directly to the NCHS (6525 Belcrest Rd., Hyattsville, MD 20782).

Reported cases of specified notifiable diseases are reported weekly in the *Morbidity and Mortality Weekly Report (MMWR)* published by the Massachusetts Medical Society. Morbidity data are listed by state and by region of the country. The report is prepared by the Centers for Disease Control and Prevention, based upon reports from state health departments. The report is printed and distributed through an agreement with the Massachusetts Medical Society, publishers of the *New England Journal of Medicine.* Each weekly issue also contains several reports of outbreaks of disease, environmental hazards, unusual cases, or other public health problems. The *MMWR* and its annual summary reports are available in most hospitals and university libraries and by subscription from the Massachusetts Medical Society (P.O. Box 9120, Waltham, MA 02254-9120).

Each of these sources of national data have specific value and usefulness to those in the public health field. Students interested in studying local health problems can obtain data from state and local health de-

partments, hospitals, volunteer agencies, and disease registries. The study and analysis of these data provide a basis for planning appropriate health programs and facilities in your communities.

EPIDEMIOLOGICAL STUDIES

When disease and/or death occurs in unexpected or unacceptable numbers, investigations may be carried out by epidemiologists. These investigations may be descriptive, analytical, or experimental in nature, depending upon the objectives of the specific study.

Descriptive Studies

Descriptive studies seek to describe the extent of an outbreak with regard to person, time, and place. They are designed to answer the questions *who, when,* and *where.* To answer the first question, epidemiologists first take a "head count" to determine how many cases of a disease have occurred. At this time, they also try to determine who is ill: children, seniors, men, women, or both. The data they gather should permit them to develop a summary of cases by age, sex, race, marital status, and type of employment.

To answer the second question (*when*), epidemiologists must determine the time of the onset of illness for each case. The resulting data can be used to prepare an **epidemic curve,** a graphic display of the cases

---

vital statistics Statistical summaries of records of major life events, such as births, deaths, marriages, divorces, and infant deaths.

descriptive study An epidemiological study that describes an epidemic with respect to person, place, and time.

epidemic curve A graphic display of the cases of disease according to the time or date of onset of symptoms.

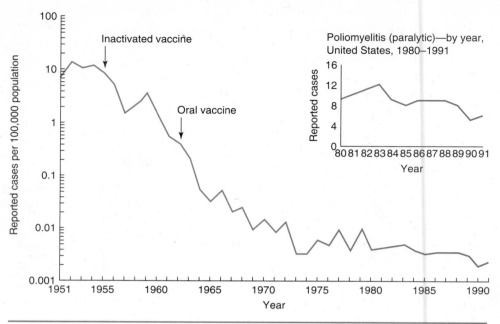

FIGURE 3.5

Secular display: Incidence of poliomyelitis by year, United States, 1951–1991. *Source: CDC.*

of disease by the time or date of the onset of their symptoms. There are three types of epidemic curves commonly used in descriptive studies: secular, seasonal, and single epidemic curves. The secular display of a disease shows the distribution of cases over many years (e.g., cases of paralytic poliomyelitis for the period 1951–1991; see Figure 3.5). Secular graphs illustrate the long-term trend of a disease. A graph of the case data by season or month is usually prepared to show cyclical changes in the numbers of cases of a disease. Cases of arthropod-borne viral infections, for example, peak in the late summer months, following the seasonal rise in populations of the mosquitoes that transmit them (see Figure 3.6).

Epidemic curves for single epidemics vary in appearance with each disease outbreak, but two classical types exist. The

first is the **point source epidemic curve** (see Figure 3.7). In a point source epidemic, each case can be traced to an exposure to the same source—spoiled food, for example. Since the epidemic curve shows cases of a disease by time or date of the onset of their symptoms, the epidemic curve for a single epidemic can be used to calculate the **incubation period,** the period of time between exposure to an infectious agent and the onset of symptoms. The incubation period, together with the symptoms, can often help epidemiologists determine the cause of the disease.

---

point source epidemic curve An epidemic curve depicting a distribution of cases which all can be traced to a single source of exposure.
incubation period The period between exposure to a disease and the onset of symptoms.

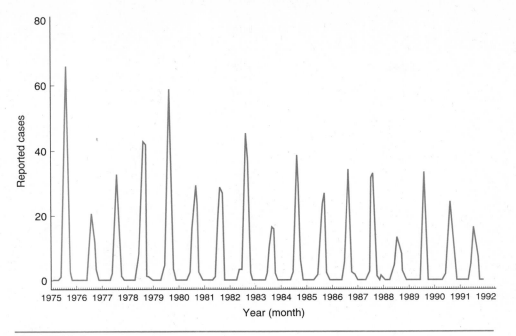

FIGURE 3.6

Seasonal (cyclical) epidemiologic graph: Reported cases of arthropod-borne viral infections (California serogroup), by month, United States, 1975–1991. *Source: CDC.*

The second type of epidemic curve for a solitary outbreak is a **propagated epidemic curve.** In this type of epidemic, primary cases appear first at the end of the incubation period following exposure to an infected source. *Secondary cases* arise after a second incubation period and represent exposure to the primary cases; *tertiary cases* appear even later because of exposure to secondary cases, and so on. Because new cases give rise to more new cases, this type of epidemic is termed a *propagated epidemic.* Epidemics of communicable diseases like chicken pox follow this pattern (see Figure 3.8).

Lastly, epidemiologists must determine *where* the outbreak occurred. To determine

where the illnesses may have originated, the residential address and travel history of each case are recorded. This information provides a geographic distribution of cases and helps to delineate the extent of the outbreak. By plotting cases on a map, along with natural features such as streams and human-made structures such as factories, it is sometimes possible to learn something about the source of the disease.

A descriptive study is usually the first epidemiologic study carried out on a disease. Detectable patterns of cases may provide investigators with ideas that can lead to a hypothesis about the cause or source of a disease.

As important and useful as they are, descriptive studies have limitations as to their usefulness. These limitations are that descriptive studies are usually not applicable

propagated epidemic curve An epidemic curve depicting a distribution of cases traceable to multiple sources of exposure.

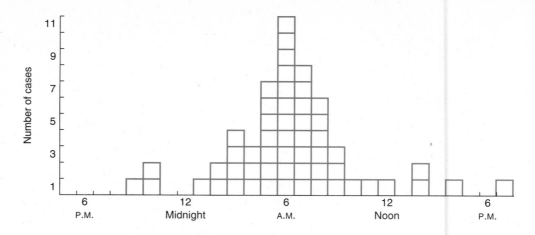

FIGURE 3.7

Point source epidemic curve: Cases of gastroenteritis following ingestion of a common food source.
Source: CDC.

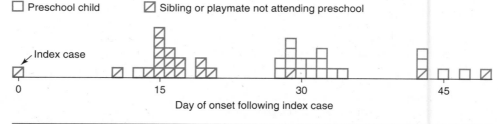

FIGURE 3.8

Propagated epidemic curve: Cases of chicken pox during April–June. *Source: CDC.*

to outbreaks elsewhere. Also, the investigation of a single epidemic cannot provide information about disease trends. Lastly, with few exceptions, descriptive studies by themselves rarely identify with certainty the cause of an outbreak.

Analytical Studies

A second type of epidemiological studies is the **analytical study.** The purpose of

analytical studies is to test hypotheses about relationships between health problems and possible **risk factors,** factors that increase the probability of disease. While analytical studies are usually not conducted by front-line community health workers, it is important that students of community health understand how they are carried out and what kinds of data they generate. Only through such an understanding, can those who work in commu-

---

analytical study An epidemiological study aimed at testing hypotheses.

risk factors Factors that increase the probability of disease, injury, or death.

nity health interpret the findings of these studies to others in the community, who may then apply the knowledge to improve their own health and that of the community.

An example of an analytical study might be one designed to discover whether diabetes (health problem) is associated with obesity (possible risk factor), or whether lung cancer (health problem) is associated with cigarette smoking (possible risk factor). It is important to remember that associations that are discovered through analytical epidemiologic studies are not always cause-and-effect associations.

There are two types of analytical studies, retrospective and prospective. **Retrospective studies** are epidemiological studies that compare people with disease (cases) to healthy people of similar age, sex, and background (controls), with respect to prior exposure to possible risk factors. These **case/control studies** are aimed at identifying familial, environmental, or behavioral factors that are more common or more pronounced in the case group than in the control group. Such factors could be associated with the disease under study. For example, epidemiologists might wish to study the factors associated with cervical cancer in women.

To carry out this study, epidemiologists would identify a number of women with cervical cancer (cases) and an equal or larger number of healthy women (controls). Medical histories for each group would be obtained and compared. In this hypothetical example, an examination of the histories suggests that cigarette smoking is more prevalent in the case group. If exposure to the possible risk factor (smoking) is significantly greater in the cases (of cervical cancer) than in the controls, an association is said to exist. This association may or may not be one of cause and effect. Further studies are usually needed to confirm initial findings. Retrospective studies almost never prove causation by themselves. Instead, they usually indicate the direction for future studies.

Prospective studies or **cohort studies** are epidemiological studies in which the researcher selects a **cohort**, a large number of healthy subjects that share a similar experience such as year of birth or high school graduation. Subjects in this cohort are then classified on the basis of their exposure to one or more possible causative factors such as cigarette smoking, dietary habits, or other factors. The entire cohort is observed for a number of years to determine the rate at which disease develops in each subgroup that was classified by exposure factor.

It is important to note the difference in the type of results obtained from retrospective and prospective studies and the advantages and disadvantages of each type of study. In retrospective studies, results obtained are not true incidence rates because disease was already present at the beginning of the study; that is, there were cases and controls to begin with, rather than a population-at-risk. For this reason, retrospective studies can only provide a probability statement about the association between factor and disease. This probability

---

case/control study (retrospective study) A study that seeks to compare those diagnosed with a disease with those who do not have the disease for prior exposure to specific risk factors.

---

cohort study (prospective study) An epidemiological study in which a cohort is classified by exposure to one or more specific risk factors and observed into the future to determine the rates at which disease develops in each class.
cohort A group of people who share some important demographic characteristic, year of birth for example.

statement can be stated mathematically as an **odds ratio.** The following is a hypothetical example of a such a probability statement: lung cancer patients have a probability of having smoked cigarettes that is 11 times greater than that of the control group. The odds ratio in this case is 11:1. (For a more detailed description of how to calculate an odds ratio and relative risk, see Appendix 3.)

In prospective studies, one begins with a population-at-risk, and therefore, one is able to calculate the risk for developing disease associated with each factor examined. This **relative risk** states the relationship between the risk for acquiring the disease in the presence of the risk factor to the risk of acquiring the disease in the absence of the risk factor. An example of a relative risk statement is: smokers are 11 times more likely to develop lung cancer than are non-smokers.

Although prospective studies yield a relative risk, they have three distinct disadvantages: (1) they are expensive, (2) they usually take many years to complete, and (3) they are not very useful for studying rare diseases because the disease may not develop in the cohort. Retrospective studies, on the other hand, are less expensive to carry out, can be completed more quickly, and are useful for studying rare diseases because one can select cases. Unfortunately, however, they cannot yield a true risk for acquiring a disease.

---

odds ratio A probability statement about the association between a particular disease and a specific risk factor, resulting from a retrospective (case/control) study.

relative risk A statement of the relationship between the risk of acquiring a disease when a specific risk factor is present and the risk of acquiring that same disease when the risk factor is absent.

Experimental Studies

Experimental studies are carried out in order to identify the cause of a disease or to determine the effectiveness of a vaccine, therapeutic drug, or surgical procedure. The central feature of experimental studies is the *control of variables* surrounding the experimental subjects. These subjects may be humans but more often are animals such as laboratory mice, rats, or monkeys. The use of research animals in experimental studies is necessary to determine the safety and effectiveness of new therapeutic agents or medical procedures with minimum risk to human health.

Whether animals or humans are used, every effort is made to reduce unwanted variability associated with the experimental subjects. In the case of animal studies, the variables over which the experimenter may wish to exert control include age, sex, diet, and environmental conditions. In addition to controlling variables, three other principles are essential to properly designed experimental studies: *control groups, randomization,* and *blindness.*

The use of *control groups* means that the experimental treatment (intervention) such as drug, vaccine, smoke-free environment, or special diet is withheld from a portion of the subjects. These subjects belong to the control group, which receives blank doses or treatments, called **placebos.** In order for a treatment regimen to be considered effective or a factor to be considered causally related, it must affect the *treatment group* significantly differently (usually determined using a statistical test) from the control group.

---

experimental study An epidemiological study carried out under controlled conditions.

placebo A blank treatment.

Randomization refers to the practice of assigning subjects to treatment or control groups in a completely random manner. This can be done by assigning numbers to subjects by having numbers selected randomly. Numbers can be selected randomly from a table of random numbers, by drawing lots, or by using a computer-generated list of random numbers. That is, each research subject, human or animal, has an equal chance of being placed in the treatment group.

Blindness refers to the practice in which the researcher remains uninformed and unaware of the identities of treatment and control groups throughout the period of experimentation and data gathering. This prevents the researcher from looking favorably or unfavorably on the responses of any particular subject or group while gathering data during the experiment. Thus, the researcher can remain unbiased.

When studies involve human subjects, it is important that the subjects also remain uninformed as to whether they have been placed in the treatment group or control (placebo) group. Such a procedure is referred to as *double-blind* (neither researcher nor subjects know who is receiving the treatment) and often involves the use of a placebo (see Figure 3.9), such as a saline injection or sugar pill. The use of a placebo prevents subjects from determining by observation whether or not they are receiving treatment. This is important because human thought processes are such that some people begin to feel better if they believe they have received a treatment. In order for a vaccine or therapeutic drug to be labeled as effective, it must consistently perform better than a placebo.

An example of just such an experiment was performed by Tonnesen and his colleagues, who studied the effectiveness of a 16-hour nicotine patch on smoking cessation.[16] They used a double-blind randomized

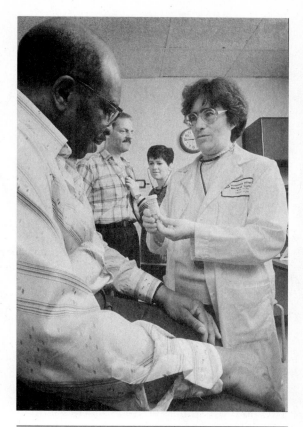

FIGURE 3.9

The use of a placebo (blank treatment) is standard procedure in a controlled, experimental study.

design to compare the effects of a nicotine skin patch with those of a placebo skin patch. Subjects were assigned to the active treatment or the placebo according to computer-generated random numbers. There were 145 subjects who received a nicotine patch and 144 who received the placebo. Subjects were scheduled for visits 1, 3, 6, 12, 26, and 52 weeks after the first visit—the day smoking cessation was to begin. Table 3.6 presents the results of cessation for each group 6, 12, 26, and 52 weeks after the study began.

Table 3.6
Percentage of Subjects Abstaining from Smoking 6, 12, 26, and 52 Weeks After the Start of the Program[16]

	Number of People Remaining in Abstinence	
Week Number	*Nicotine Patch*	*Placebo Patch*
6	53	17
12	41	10
26	24	5
52	17	4

The results of this study indicated that there was a significant difference between the effectiveness of the nicotine patch and the placebo patch with regard to smoking cessation (see Table 3.6).[16]

Controlling variables, the use of treatment and control groups, randomization, and blindness are techniques aimed at insuring objectivity and avoiding bias in experimental studies. Through strict adherence to these principles, researchers hope to achieve experimental results that accurately reflect what occurs in a natural setting.

By carrying out carefully planned descriptive studies, epidemiologists define outbreaks of disease, injury, and death in specific populations and develop hypotheses about the causes of these outbreaks. By designing and carrying out analytical and experimental studies, epidemiologists test these hypotheses. In the next chapter, we will examine how this knowledge is used to prevent and control diseases in the community.

CHAPTER SUMMARY

Epidemiology is the study of the distribution and determinants of disease and injuries in the com-

munity. It is an old science that has become more sophisticated in recent years.

Rates of birth, death, injury, and disease are essential tools for epidemiologists. Incidence rates are a measurement of the number of *new* cases of disease, injury, or death in a population over a given period of time while prevalence rates measure *all* cases. An attack rate is a special kind of incidence rate used for a single outbreak.

Cases of certain diseases—notifiable diseases—are reported by doctors, clinics, and hospitals to local, state, and federal health agencies. These reports assist epidemiologists who study disease trends. Epidemiologists also consult the data available from the *U.S. Census,* the *Statistical Abstract of the United States,* the *Monthly Vital Statistics Report, Morbidity and Mortality Weekly Report,* and other standardized sources of statistical data.

Epidemiologists conduct three general types of studies to learn about disease and injury in populations. Descriptive studies describe the extent of outbreaks with regard to person, place, and time. Analytical studies test hypotheses regarding associations between diseases and risk factors. Experimental studies examine the effects of specific factors under carefully controlled conditions. The purpose of each of these studies is to help determine the cause of disease, injury, and death in the community and to provide information that will assist in controlling current outbreaks and preventing future ones.

SCENARIO: ANALYSIS AND RESPONSE

Assume that you were Kim and you were able to reach Dr. Turner, the local health officer. He then asked whether you would like to help in the investigation of the food-borne outbreak mentioned in the scenario. You agreed to help. So far, you have learned that on Sunday, May 28, 49 people were at a picnic where they had eaten, beginning about noon. People began to report their illnesses later that night. Dr. Turner developed a food-borne outbreak investigation work sheet, which you helped to complete by making numerous phone calls and house visits with the public health nurse. The histories of people attending the picnic appear in Table A. Using Table B, the *Epidemic Curve Tally Sheet,* you tally the cases by hour of onset of illness. Using the results of the tally, you establish the incubation period—the range of hours (after the meal) over which symptoms started. Next, you prepare a graph to illustrate the epidemic curve of the outbreak. Try to answer the following questions:

1. What is the incubation period?

2. Does the curve you prepared suggest a single- or multiple-exposure epidemic?

3. Based solely on the incubation period, can you make a guess as to the cause of the outbreak?

Unfortunately, by the time the investigation began, all the picnic food had been discarded and no samples were available for laboratory testing. In order to determine which food at the picnic

Table A
Histories Obtained from Persons Eating Picnic Lunch

Person No.	Bread	Butter	Turkey	Potato Salad	Milk	Jell-O	Ill*	Not Ill
1			x	x	x		7:30	
2	x	x		x	x			x
3	x	x	x	x	x	x	8:00	
4			x		x	x		x
5			x	x	x		9:15	
6			x	x	x		7:40	
7	x	x		x	x			x
8	x	x	x	x	x	x	8:10	
9			x		x	x		x
10			x	x	x	x	10:15	
11	x			x		x		x
12	x	x	x	x	x	x	8:30	
13			x		x			x
14	x	x	x	x	x	x	9:30	
15	x	x		x	x	x		x
16	x			x		x		x
17	x	x	x	x	x	x	8:35	
18			x		x			x
19	x	x	x	x	x	x	10:05	
20	x	x		x	x	x		x
21			x		x	x	9:15	
22	x	x		x	x	x		x
23	x	x			x	x	8:30	
24	x	x			x	x		x

(continued)

Table A (continued)

Person No.	Bread	Butter	Turkey	Potato Salad	Milk	Jell-O	Ill*	Not Ill
25	x	x	x	x	x	x	12:30 A.M.	
26			x		x	x	9:20	
27	x	x		x	x	x		x
28	x	x	x		x	x	8:40	
29	x	x			x	x		x
30	x	x	x	x	x		12:15 A.M.	
31			x	x	x		7:30	
32	x	x		x	x			x
33	x	x	x	x	x	x	8:00	
34			x		x	x		x
35			x	x	x		10:30	
36			x	x	x		7:30	
37	x	x		x	x			x
38	x	x	x	x	x	x	8:05	
39			x		x	x		x
40			x	x	x	x	9:45	
41	x			x		x		x
42	x	x	x	x	x	x	8:30	
43			x		x			x
44	x	x	x	x	x	x	9:30	
45	x	x		x	x	x		x
46	x			x		x		x
47	x	x	x	x	x	x	8:30	
48			x		x	x		x
49	x	x	x	x	x	x	10:10	

*All time is P.M. unless otherwise indicated.

might have caused the outbreak, you need to calculate attack rates for people eating each food as well as for people not eating each food. Using Table C, the Attack Rate Work Sheet, calculate the attack rates for those who ate and did not eat each food served.

4. Which food would you most suspect of causing the illness?

5. Based on this information, what might the causative agent have been? (Answers to these problems can be found in Appendix 4.)

REVIEW QUESTIONS

1. What is an epidemic? a pandemic? Name some diseases that become epidemic from time to time. Why are epidemiologists sometimes interested in epizootics?

2. What is meant by the term *endemic disease*? Can you give examples of such diseases?

3. What is the difference between natality, morbidity, and mortality? Why are rates important in community health?

Table B
Epidemic Curve Tally Sheet

Time of Onset Period	Tally	Number	Incubation
7:00–7:59			
8:00–8:59			
9:00–9:59			
10:00–10:59			
11:00–11:59			
12:00–12:59			

4. What is the difference between crude and specific rates?

5. Why are prevalence rates more useful than incidence rates for measuring of chronic diseases?

6. What is an infant mortality rate? Why is it such an important rate in community health?

Table C
Attack Rate Work Sheet

Food	Persons Eating Food			
Rate	Total	Ill	Well	Attack
Bread				
Butter				
Turkey				
Potato salad				
Milk				
Jell-O				

Food	Persons Not Eating Food			
Rate	Total	Ill	Well	Attack
Bread				
Butter				
Turkey				
Potato salad				
Milk				
Jell-O				

7. What are notifiable diseases? Give some examples.

8. What is the U.S. Census? How often is it conducted? What types of data does it gather?

9. What types of information are available from the *Statistical Abstract of the United States?*

10. What kinds of data would you expect to find in the Centers for Disease Control's *Morbidity and Mortality Weekly Report?*

11. In a descriptive epidemiological study, what types of information are gathered by the epidemiologist?

12. What is the purpose of an analytical study? Contrast retrospective and prospective studies with regard to methodology and usefulness.

13. How do experimental studies differ from analytical studies? What value do they have in epidemiology? To what four principles must researchers adhere in order to properly carry out an experimental study?

ACTIVITIES

1. When you hear the word *epidemic,* what disease comes to your mind first? Ask this question of ten people you know, allowing them time to think and give you an answer. Try to find people of different ages as you complete your informal poll. List their answers on paper. Are there any answers that surprise you? Does your list include both classic and contemporary epidemic diseases?

2. Look at the data in Table D. What conclusion can you draw about the risk for acquiring tuberculosis for populations in each age group? Write down your answer. Now examine Table E. Which age groups exhibit the highest disease rates? Explain why it is important to calculate rates to report disease outbreaks accurately.

3. There are 346 students at Hillside School. During March and April, 56 pupils were absent with chicken pox. What is the attack

Table D
Reported Tuberculosis Cases, by Age Group Low Socioeconomic Area, City of Dixon, 1960

Age Group in Years	Number of Cases
0–4	7
5–14	7
15–24	6
25–34	10
35–44	6
45–54	9
55–64	8
65 +	7

rate for chicken pox at Hillside School? The 56 pupils who were absent had 88 brothers and sisters at home. Of the 88 siblings, 19 developed chicken pox. What was the secondary attack rate? Of the 75 total cases of chicken pox, 1 child died. Calculate the case fatality rate for chicken pox in this epidemic.

4. In an epidemic in Sample City (population 100,000—60,000 males and 40,000 females), there were 600 cases (350 males, 250 females) of a severe disease. There were 70 deaths (all males) due to this disease and 880 deaths due to causes other than the specific disease. Calculate the following: crude death rate, cause specific mortality rate, case fatality rate, cause-specific morbidity rate for females, and case fatality rate for males.

5. Visit, call, or write your state or local health department. Ask for the total number of birth and death certificates issued for the latest year for which complete data are available. Assuming no migration into or out of your state or county, what is the natural rate of population increase (number of births minus number of deaths)? Try to obtain an estimate of the total population of the state or county for the same year. Calculate a crude birth rate and a crude death rate (number of births and deaths) per 1,000 population.

6. Visit your campus library and locate the *American Journal of Epidemiology*. Examine several recent issues, taking note of the different types of articles as they appear in the Table of Contents. Select six articles and read the abstracts. On a piece of paper, list the titles of these articles. Were these de-

Table E
Reported Tuberculosis Cases and Incidence Rates per 100,000 Population, Low Socioeconomic Area, City of Dixon, 1960

Age Group in Years	Number of Cases	Population of Age Group	Rate*
0–4	7	8,638	81.0
5–14	7	13,098	53.4
15–24	6	10,247	58.5
25–34	10	8,680	115.2
35–44	6	7,528	79.7
45–54	9	6,736	133.6
55–64	8	4,534	176.4
65 +	7	4,075	171.8
Total	60	63,536	94.4

*Example: 7 cases ÷ 8,638 population × 100,000 = 81.0

scriptive, analytical, or experimental studies? After each title you listed, put either the letter D (descriptive), A (analytical), or E (experimental) to denote the type of study you examined.

REFERENCES

1. Mausner, J. S., and S. Kramer (Mausner and Bahn) (1985). *Epidemiology—An Introductory Text.* Philadelphia: W. B. Saunders, p. 1.

2. Monath, T. P. *St. Louis Encephalitis* (1980). Washington D.C.: American Public Health Association, p. 240.

3. Centers for Disease Control (1991). "Summary of Notifiable Disease, United States, 1991." *Morbidity and Mortality Weekly Report* 40(53): 59.

4. Centers for Disease Control (1981). "Toxic Shock Syndrome—United States, 1970–1980." *Morbidity and Mortality Weekly* Report 30(3): 25–33.

5. Centers for Disease Control and Prevention (1993). "Lyme Disease—United States, 1991–1992." *Morbidity and Mortality Weekly Report* 42(18): 345–348.

6. Centers for Disease Control (1992). "The Second 100,000 Cases of Acquired Immunodeficiency Syndrome—United States, June 1991–Dec. 1991." *Morbidity and Mortality Weekly Report* 41(2): 28–29.

7. Centers for Disease Control and Prevention (Feb. 1993). *HIV/AIDS Surveillance Report,* pp. 1–23.

8. Markellis, V. C. (Dec. 1985–Jan. 1986). "Epidemiology: Cornerstone for Health Education." *Health Education,* pp. 15–17.

9. Gale, A. H. *Epidemiologic Disease* (1959). London: Pelican Books, p. 25.

10. Woodruff, A. W. (1977). "Benjamin Rush, His Work on Yellow Fever and His British Connections." *American J. Trop. Med. Hyg.* 26(5): 1055–1059.

11. Snow, John (1963). "The Broad Street Pump." In B. Roueche, *Curiosities of Medicine.* Boston: Little, Brown.

12. Mausner, J. S., and S. Kramer (Mausner and Bahn) (1985). *Epidemiology: An Introductory text.* Philadelphia: W. B. Saunders, p. 5.

13. Morton, R. F., J. R. Hebel, and R. J. McCarter (1990). *A Study Guide to Epidemiology and Biostatistics.* Rockville, Md.: Aspen Publishing, p. 25.

14. National Center for Health Statistics (1991). "Annual Summary of Births, Marriages, Divorces, and Deaths: United States, 1990." *Monthly Vital Statistics Report* 39(13). Hyattsville, Md.: Public Health Services.

15. U.S. Bur. of the Census (1990). *Statistical Abstract of the United States: 1989,* 109th ed. Washington D.C.: U.S. Government Printing Office.

16. Tonnesen, P., J. Norregaard, K. Simonsen, and U. Sawe (1991). "A Double-Blind Trial of a 16-Hour Transdermal Nicotine Patch in Smoking Cessation. *New England Journal of Medicine* 325(5): 311–315.

Chapter 4

EPIDEMIOLOGY: PREVENTION AND CONTROL OF DISEASES AND HEALTH CONDITIONS

Chapter Outline

Chapter Objectives

After studying this chapter you will be able to:

1. Explain the differences between communicable and noncommunicable diseases and between acute and chronic diseases and give examples of each.
2. Describe and explain communicable and multicausation disease models.
3. Explain how communicable diseases are transmitted in a community using the "chain of infection" model and use a specific communicable disease to illustrate your explanation.
4. Explain why noncommunicable diseases are a community health concern and give some examples of important noncommunicable diseases.
5. Explain the difference between primary, secondary, and tertiary prevention of disease and give examples of each.
6. List and explain the various criteria that communities might use to prioritize their health problems in preparation for the allocation of prevention and control resources.
7. List and discuss important measures for preventing and controlling the spread of communicable diseases in a community.
8. List and discuss approaches to noncommunicable disease control in the community.
9. Outline a chronic, noncommunicable disease control program that includes primary, secondary, and tertiary disease prevention components.

Bob had always been an active and athletic person. He lettered in three sports in high school and played varsity tennis in college. Following graduation last May, he was lucky enough to land a job with one of the Fortune 500 companies in nearby Indianapolis. He shares an apartment with Chuck, a business colleague, and both work long hours in the hope that hard work will mean success and advancement. Neither seems to find time to exercise regularly, and both rely increasingly on "fast-food" restaurants. Bob is beginning to wonder whether he is compromising his health for financial success.

When he first came to the company, he took the stairs between floors two at a time and was never winded, even after climbing several flights. Now he becomes tired after two flights.

INTRODUCTION

Chapter 3 discussed the measurement and reporting of disease and the use of rates and ratios to describe disease incidence and prevalence. Then, an explanation was given of how epidemiologists describe disease outbreaks by person, place, and time and how they search for causal associations through analytical and experimental studies.

In this chapter, the discussion of epidemiology continues with a classification of diseases and other health conditions. This is followed by a discussion of communicable and noncommunicable diseases and the ways in which communities prioritize their health problems. Then, the approaches to disease prevention and control—primary, secondary, and tertiary prevention—are introduced.

CLASSIFICATION OF DISEASES AND HEALTH PROBLEMS

Diseases and health problems can be classified in several meaningful ways. The public often classifies diseases by organ or organ system, such as kidney disease, heart disease, respiratory infection, and so on. Another method of classification is by causative agent: viral disease, chemical poisoning, physical injury. In this scheme, causative agents may be biological, chemical, or physical. Biological agents include viruses, rickettsiae, bacteria, protozoa, fungi, and metazoa (multicellular organisms). Chemical agents include drugs, pesticides, industrial chemicals, food additives, air pollutants, and cigarette smoke. Physical agents that can cause injury or disease include various forms of energy such as heat, ultraviolet light, radiation, noise vibrations, and speeding or falling objects (see Table 4.1). In community health, diseases are usually

Table 4.1
Causative Agents for Diseases and Injuries

Biological Agents	Chemical Agents	Physical Agents
Viruses	Pesticides	Heat
Rickettsiae	Food additives	Light
Bacteria	Pharmacologics	Radiation
Fungi	Industrial chemicals	Noise
Protozoa	Air pollutants	Vibration
Metazoa	Cigarette smoke	Speeding objects

classified as acute or chronic, or communicable (infectious) or noncommunicable (noninfectious).

Communicable versus Noncommunicable Diseases

Another important classification system divides diseases into communicable and noncommunicable diseases. **Communicable (infectious) diseases** are those diseases for which biological agents or their products are the cause and which are transmissible from one individual to another. The disease process begins when the agent is able to lodge and grow or reproduce within the body. The process of lodgment and growth of a microorganism or virus in the host is called **infection.**

Noncommunicable (noninfectious) diseases or illnesses are those that cannot be transmitted from an infected person to a susceptible, healthy one. Delineating the causes of noncommunicable diseases is often more difficult because several, or even many, factors may contribute to the development of a given noncommunicable health condition. The contributing factors may be genetic, environmental, or behavioral in nature. For this reason, many noncommunicable health conditions are called multicausation diseases. An example of such is heart disease. Genetics, environmental factors such as stress, and behavioral choices such as diet and exercise all can contribute to heart disease.

communicable disease (infectious disease) An illness caused by some specific biological agent or its toxic products that can be transmitted from an infected person, animal, or inanimate reservoir to a susceptible host.
noncommunicable disease (noninfectious disease) A disease that cannot be transmitted from infected host to susceptible host.

Acute versus Chronic Diseases and Illnesses

In the acute/chronic classification scheme, diseases are classified by duration of symptoms. Acute diseases, as defined in Chapter 3, are those conditions in which the peak severity of symptoms occurs within three months (usually sooner) and recovery in those who survive, is usually complete. Examples of acute communicable diseases include the common cold, influenza (flu), chicken pox, measles, mumps, Rocky Mountain spotted fever, and plague. Examples of acute noncommunicable illnesses are appendicitis, trauma (injury) from auto crashes, acute alcohol intoxication, and sprained ankles (see Table 4.2).

Chronic diseases or conditions are those in which symptoms continue longer than three months and in some cases for the remainder of one's life (see Figure 4.1). Recovery is slow and sometimes incomplete. These diseases can be either communicable or noncommunicable. Examples of chronic

Table 4.2
Classification of Diseases

Types of Diseases	Examples
Acute Diseases	
Communicable	Common cold, pneumonia, mumps, measles, pertussis, typhoid fever, cholera
Noncommunicable	Appendicitis, poisoning, trauma (due to automobile accidents, fire, etc.)
Chronic Diseases	
Communicable	AIDS, Lyme disease, tuberculosis, syphilis, rheumatic fever following streptococcal infections
Noncommunicable	Diabetes, coronary heart disease, osteoarthritis, cirrhosis of the liver due to alcoholism

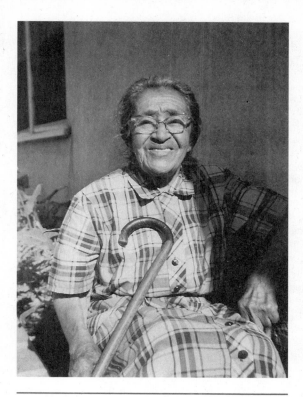

FIGURE 4.1

Arthritis is a noninfectious chronic condition that can persist for one's entire life.

communicable diseases are AIDS, tuberculosis, herpes virus infections, syphilis, and Lyme disease. Chronic noncommunicable illnesses include hypertension, hypercholesterolemia, coronary heart disease, diabetes, and many types of arthritis and cancer.

COMMUNICABLE DISEASES

While **infectivity** refers to the ability of a biological agent to lodge and grow in a host,

---

infectivity   The ability of a pathogen to lodge and grow in the host.

---

the term **pathogenicity** refers to an infectious disease agent's ability to produce disease. Selected pathogenic agents and the diseases they cause are listed in Table 4.3. Under certain conditions, pathogenic, biological agents can be transmitted from an infected individual in the community to an uninfected, susceptible one. Noncommunicable diseases are unable to be so transmitted. Communicable disease agents may be further classified, as will be explained later, according to the manner in which they are transmitted.

The elements of a simplified **communicable disease model**—agent, host, and environment—are presented in Figure 4.2. These three factors seem to sum up the minimal requirements for the occurrence and spread of communicable diseases in a population. In this model, the **agent** is the element that must be present in order for disease to occur. For example, the influenza virus must be present for a person to become ill with influenza (flu). The **host** is any susceptible organism—a single-celled organism, a plant, an animal, or a human—invaded by an infectious agent. The **environment** includes all other factors—physical, biological, or social—that inhibit or promote disease transmission. Communicable disease transmission occurs when a susceptible host and a pathogenic agent exist in an environment conducive to disease transmission.

Chain of Infection

Communicable disease transmission is a complicated but well-studied process that

---

pathogenicity   The capability of a communicable disease agent to cause disease in a susceptible host.

agent (pathogenic agent)   The cause of the disease or health problem.

host   A person or other living organism that affords subsistence or lodgment to a communicable agent under natural conditions.

Table 4.3

Biological Agents of Disease

Type of Agent	Name of Agent	Disease

Viruses	Varicella virus
	Human immunodeficiency
	  virus (HIV)
	Rubella virus
		Chicken pox
		Acquired immunodeficieny
		  syndrome (AIDS)
		German measles

Rickettsiae	Rickettsia rickettsii	Rocky Mountain spotted fever
Bacteria	Vibrio cholera Clostridium tetani Yersinia pestis Borrelia burgdorferi	Cholera Tetanus (pertussis) Plague Lyme disease
Protozoa	Entamoeba histolytica Plasmodium falciparum Trypanosoma gambiense	Amoebic dysentery Malaria African sleeping sickness
Fungi and Yeasts	Tinea cruris Tinea pedis	Jock itch Athletes foot
Nematoda (worms)	Wuchereria bancrofti Onchocerca volvulus	Filariasis (elephantiasis) Filariasis (river blindness)

is best understood through a conceptual model known as the **chain of infection** (see Figure 4.3). Using the chain of infection model, one can visualize the step-by-step process by which communicable diseases spread from an infected person to an uninfected person in the community. The pathogenic (disease-producing) agent leaves its **reservoir** (infected host) via a **portal of exit. Transmission** occurs in either a direct or indirect manner, and the pathogenic agent enters a susceptible host through a **portal of entry** to establish disease. As an example, let us follow the common cold through the chain of infection. The agent, the cold virus, leaves its reservoir, the throat of an infected person, perhaps when the host sneezes. The portal of exits are the nose and mouth. Transmission may be direct if saliva droplets enter the respiratory

tract of a susceptible host at close range or indirect if droplets dry and become airborne. The portal of entry could be the nose or mouth of a susceptible host, and a new infection is established.

There are many variations in the chain of infection, depending upon the disease agent, environmental conditions, infectivity, and host susceptibility. For example, the

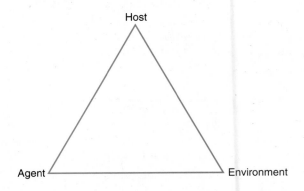

FIGURE 4.2

Communicable disease model.

---

chain of infection A model to conceptualize the transmission of a communicable disease from its source to a susceptible host.

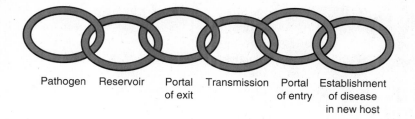

FIGURE 4.3

Chain of infection.

reservoir for a disease may be a case, a person who has the disease, or a **carrier**—one who is well but infected and capable of serving as a source of infection. A (disease) carrier could be one who is incubating the disease, such as a person who is HIV positive but has no signs of AIDS, or one who has recovered from the disease (is asymptomatic), as in typhoid fever. For some diseases, the reservoir is not humans but animals. Diseases for which the reservoir resides in animal populations are called **zoonoses.** Plague, rabies, Rocky Mountain spotted fever, and Lyme disease are examples of zoonoses. Diseases for which humans are the only known reservoir, like measles, are known as **anthroponoses.**

Portals of exit (see Figure 4.4) and entry vary from disease to disease. Natural portals of exit and examples of diseases that use them are the respiratory tract (cold, influenza, measles, tuberculosis, whooping cough), urogenital tract (gonorrhea, syphilis, herpes, AIDS), digestive tract (amoebic dysentery, shigellosis, polio, typhoid fever, and cholera), and skin (ringworm, jock itch).

The skin is actually a good barrier to infection, but it can be bypassed by a hypodermic needle or when there is an open wound. Blood-sucking insects and ticks make their own portals of entry with mouth parts that penetrate the skin. Finally, many diseased organisms can cross the placenta from mother to fetus (rubella virus, syphilis spirochetes, and hepatitis B virus).

Modes of Transmission

Communicable disease transmission may be direct or indirect. **Direct transmission** implies the immediate transfer of the disease agent by direct contact between the infected and the susceptible individuals through such acts as touching, biting, kissing, sexual intercourse, or by direct projection (droplet spread) by coughing or sneezing within a distance of one meter.[1] Examples of diseases for which transmission is usually direct are AIDS, syphilis, gonorrhea, rabies, and the common cold.

Indirect transmission may be one of three types: air-borne, vehicle-borne, or vector-borne. **Air-borne transmission** is the

---

carrier A person or animal that harbors a specific communicable agent in the absence of discernible clinical disease and serves as a potential source of infection to others.

zoonosis A communicable disease transmissible under natural conditions from vertebrate animals to man.

anthroponosis A disease that infects only humans.

---

direct transmission The immediate transfer of an infectious agent by direct contact between infected and susceptible individuals.

indirect transmission Communicable disease transmission involving an intermediate step.

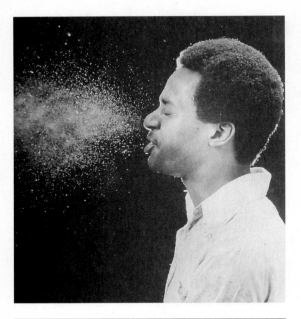

FIGURE 4.4

Portal of exit: The causative agents for many respiratory diseases leave their host via the mouth and nose.

dissemination of microbial aerosols to a suitable portal of entry, usually the respiratory tract. Microbial aerosols are suspensions of dust or droplet nuclei made up wholly or in part of microorganisms. These particles may remain suspended and infective for long periods of time. Tuberculosis, influenza, histoplasmosis, and legionellosis are examples of air-borne diseases.

In **vehicle-borne transmission,** contaminated materials or objects (fomites) serve as **vehicles,** nonliving objects by which communicable agents are transferred to a susceptible host. The agent may or may not have multiplied or developed on the vehicle. Examples of vehicles include toys, handkerchiefs, soiled clothes, bedding, food

service utensils, and surgical instruments. Also considered vehicles are water, milk, food, or biological products such as blood, serum, plasma, organs, and tissues. Almost any disease can be transmitted by vehicles, including those for which the primary mode of transmission is direct, such as dysentery and hepatitis.

Vector-borne transmission is disease transfer by a living organism such as a mosquito, fly, or tick. Transmission may be mechanical, via the contaminated mouth parts or feet of the **vector,** or biological, involving multiplication or developmental changes of the agent in the vector before transmission occurs. In **mechanical transmission,** multiplication and development of the disease organism do not usually occur. For example, organisms that cause dysentery, polio, cholera, and typhoid fever have been isolated from such insects as cockroaches and houseflies and could presumably be deposited on food prepared for human consumption.

In **biological transmission,** multiplication and/or developmental changes of the disease agent occur in the vector before transmission occurs. Biological transmission is much more important than mechanical transmission in terms of its impact on community health. Examples of biological vectors include mosquitoes, fleas, lice, ticks, flies, and other insects. By far, mosquitoes are the most important vectors of human disease. They transmit the viruses that cause yellow fever and dengue fever as well as 200 other viruses. They also transmit malaria, which infects 100 million people in the world each year (mostly in tropical areas), killing at least 1 million of them. Ticks, another important vector, transmit Rocky

---

vehicle Inanimate materials or objects than can serve as a source of infection

vector A living organism, usually an arthropod, that can transmit a communicable agent to susceptible hosts (e.g., mosquitoes, ticks, lice, fleas).

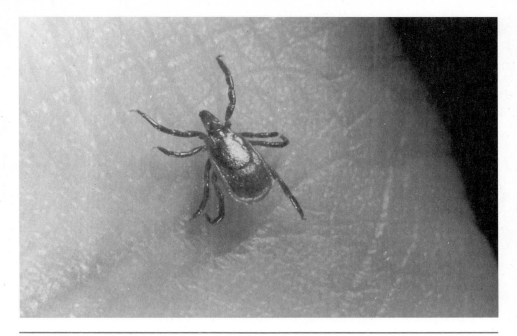

FIGURE 4.5

The Lyme disease tick, *Ixodes scapularis,* is an important disease vector (adult, female).

Mountain spotted fever, relapsing fever, and Lyme disease (see Figure 4.5). Other insect vectors (and the diseases they transmit) are flies (African sleeping sickness, onchocerciasis, loaiasis, and leishmaniasis), fleas (plague, murine typhus), lice (epidemic typhus, trench fever), and kissing bugs (Chagas' disease).

NONCOMMUNICABLE DISEASES

While communicable diseases remain an important concern for communities, certain noncommunicable diseases, such as heart disease, stroke, and cancer, now rank high among the nation's leading causes of death. While these diseases are not infectious, they nonetheless can occur in epidemic propor-

tions. Furthermore, the chronic nature of many of these diseases means that they can deplete a community's resources quite rapidly.

The complex **etiologies**—causes—of many of the noncommunicable diseases, such as coronary heart disease, are best illustrated by the **multicausation disease model** (see Figure 4.6). In this model, the human host is pictured in the center of the environment in which he or she lives. Within the host, there exists a unique genetic endowment which is inalterable. The host exists in an environment comprising a multitude of factors that can contribute to the disease process. These environmental

etiology   The cause of a disease.
multicausation disease model   A visual representation of the host together with various internal and external factors that promote and protect against disease.

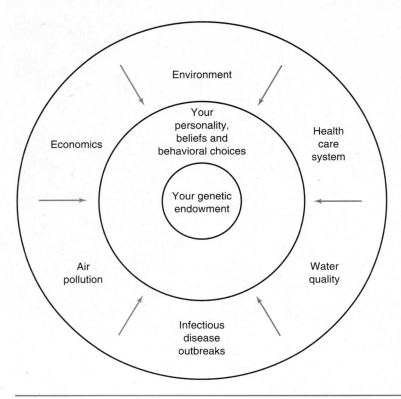

FIGURE 4.6

Multicausation disease model.

factors may be physical, chemical, biological, or social in nature.

Physical factors include the latitude, climate, and physical geography of where one lives. The major health risks in the tropics—communicable and parasitic diseases—are different from those in temperate regions with cold winters—difficulty in finding food and remaining warm. Chemical factors include not only natural chemical hazards of polluted water and air but also the added pollutants of modern society. Biological hazards include communicable disease agents such as pathogenic viruses, bacteria, and fungi. Social factors include one's choice of occupation, recreational ac-

tivities, and living arrangements. Poor choices in life can increase one's risk factors, which is detrimental to one's health.

Diseases of the Heart and Blood Vessels

Diseases of the heart and blood vessels, cardiovascular diseases (CVDs), are a leading cause of death in the United States. Coronary heart disease (CHD), is the Number 1 killer of Americans. In 1992 alone, more than 720,000 people died of heart disease in the United States.[2]

The American Heart Association lists five types of cardiovascular diseases (CVD):

coronary heart disease (CHD), hypertension, stroke, rheumatic heart disease, and congenital heart disease.[3] **Coronary heart disease,** sometimes called *coronary artery disease,* is characterized by damage to the coronary arteries, the blood vessels that carry oxygen-rich blood to the heart muscle. Damage to the coronary arteries usually evolves from the condition known as *atherosclerosis,* a narrowing of the blood vessels. This narrowing usually results from the build up of fatty deposits on the inner walls of arteries. When blood flow to the heart muscle is severely reduced or interrupted, a heart attack can occur. If heart damage is severe, the heart may stop beating—a condition known as cardiac arrest.

Over the past 40 years, the understanding of the process involved in coronary artery disease has become more complete. Numerous risk factors, factors that increase the likelihood of experiencing coronary artery disease, have been identified. While some of these factors cannot be altered by changes in life-style or behavior, others can. Factors that cannot be altered include one's age, sex, race, and the genetic tendency toward developing the disease. Factors that can be modified include cigarette smoking, high blood pressure, high blood cholesterol, physical inactivity, obesity, diabetes, and stress.

Cerebrovascular disease (stroke) is the third leading cause of death in the United States. Strokes killed more than 143,000 people in 1992.[2] During a stroke, or cerebrovascular accident, the blood supply to the brain is interrupted.

The risk factors for developing cerebrovascular disease are similar to those for CHD and include both hereditary and environmental factors. Hypertension and cigarette smoking are especially important risk factors for cerebrovascular disease.

Malignant Neoplasms

More than 500,000 people died from malignant neoplasms (cancer), in 1992, making this the second leading cause of death in the United States.[2] **Malignant neoplasms** occur when cells lose control over their growth and division. Normal cells are inhibited from continual growth and division by virtue of their contact with adjacent cells. Malignant (cancerous) cells are not so inhibited; they continue to grow and divide, eventually piling up in a "new growth," a neoplasm or tumor. As this growth continues, parts of the neoplasm can break off and be carried to distant parts of the body, where they can lodge and continue to grow. When this occurs, the cancer is said to have **metastasized.** When malignant neoplasms have spread to distant parts of the body and established new tumors, the disease is said to be *advanced.* The more the malignancy spreads, the more difficult it is to treat.

Common sites where malignant neoplasms occur include the lungs, colon and rectum, breasts, uterus, ovaries, mouth, prostate gland, bladder, pancreas, and skin. Lung cancer is the leading cause of cancer deaths in both sexes. There were an estimated 140,000 lung cancer deaths in 1990 alone. It has been estimated that 85% of these deaths can be attributed to cigarette smoking.[4] Alcohol and smokeless tobacco contribute to cancers of the mouth, throat, larynx, esophagus, and liver.

Approximately 600,000 new cases of non-melanoma skin cancer are detected

---

malignant neoplasm Uncontrolled new tissue growth resulting from cells that have lost control over their growth and division.

metastasis The spread of cancer cells to distant parts of the body by the circulatory or lymphatic system.

each year in the United States. Almost all of these cases are attributable to exposure to the sun, and yet many people continue to sunbathe, believing that a tanned body is a healthy one. The number of cases of non-melanoma skin cancer are expected to rise if the ozone layer in the atmosphere continues to be eroded (see Chapter 16). This is an example of how environmental policy impacts on public health.

Other Noncommunicable Disease Problems

Other noncommunicable diseases of major concern are: (1) chronic obstructive pulmonary disease and allied conditions (the fourth leading cause of death), (2) diabetes mellitus (the seventh leading cause of death), and (3) chronic liver disease and cirrhosis (the eleventh leading cause of death). Each of these chronic noncommunicable diseases and those listed in Table 4.4, places a burden not only on the afflicted individuals and their families but on the community's health resources as well.

Table 4.4
Some Noncommunicable Health Conditions That Affect Americans

Allergic disorders

Arthritis

Cerebral palsy

Endogenous depression

Epilepsy

Fibrocystic breast condition

Lower back pain

Multiple sclerosis

Osteoporosis

Premenstrual syndrome

Sickle cell trait and sickle cell disease

PRIORITIZING PREVENTION AND CONTROL EFFORTS

Communities are confronted with a multitude of health problems—communicable and noncommunicable diseases, unintentional injuries, violence, substance abuse problems, and so on. How can health officials make logical and responsible choices about the allocation of community resources to prevent or control these problems? Which problems are indeed the most urgent? Which problems will benefit the most from timely intervention? Several criteria are used to judge the importance of a particular disease to a community. Among these are: (1) the number of people who die from a disease, (2) the number of years of potential life lost attributable to a particular cause, and (3) the economic costs associated with a particular disease or health condition.

Leading Causes of Death

The National Center for Health Statistics regularly publishes a list of the leading causes of death. For more than 50 years, the leading cause of death in America has been heart disease. At least one in every three deaths can be attributed to diseases of the heart. Cancers (malignant neoplasms) represent the second leading killer; nearly one in four deaths is the result of cancer. Cerebrovascular disease (stroke) ranks third, chronic obstructive pulmonary diseases rank fourth, and accidents rank fifth (see Table 4.5).[2]

One might prioritize expenditures of health care resources solely on the basis of the number of deaths, but in doing so one would spend 68% of the health budget on these four health problems alone. Very little

Table 4.5
Death Rates and Percentages of Total Deaths for the 15 Leading Causes of Death: United States, 1992

[Rates per 100,000 population, all races, both sexes]

Rank	Cause of death (Ninth Revision, International Classification of Diseases, 1975)	Number	Death rate	Percent of total deaths
—	All causes	2,177,000	853.8	100.0
1	Diseases of heart	720,480	282.5	33.1
2	Malignant neoplasms, including neoplasms of lymphatic and hematopoietic tissues	521,090	204.3	23.9
3	Cerebrovascular diseases	143,640	56.3	6.6
4	Chronic obstructive pulmonary diseases and allied conditions	91,440	35.8	4.2
5	Accidents and adverse effects	86,310	33.8	4.0
—	Motor vehicle accidents	41,710	16.4	1.9
—	All other accidents and adverse effects	44,600	17.5	2.0
6	Pneumonia and influenza	76,120	29.8	3.5
7	Diabetes mellitus	50,180	19.7	2.3
8	Human immunodeficiency virus infection	33,590	13.2	1.5
9	Suicide	29,760	11.7	1.4
10	Homicide and legal intervention	26,570	10.4	1.2
11	Chronic liver disease and cirrhosis	24,830	9.7	1.1
12	Nephritis, nephrotic syndrome, and nephrosis	22,400	8.8	1.0
13	Septicemia	19,910	7.8	0.9
14	Atherosclerosis	16,100	6.3	0.7
15	Certain conditions originating in the perinatal period	15,790	6.2	0.7
—	All other causes	298,430	117.0	13.7

Note: Rates have been recomputed based on revised population estimates.

or perhaps none of the resources would be available for infant and childhood nutrition programs, for example, which have been shown to prevent more serious health care problems in later life. Nor would there be any funds available for the treatment of those with debilitating diseases such as chronic arthritis or mental illness.

Years of Potential Life Lost

Another approach toward prioritizing a community's health care problems is by calculating the number of **years of potential life lost (YPLL)** for each death that occurs from a specific disease. This calculation is made by subtracting the age at death from 65 for all deaths that occur, regardless of cause. For example, in 1990, a total of 12,237,379 years of potential life were lost by people who died before they reached 65 years of age.[5] Using this approach, diseases

---

years of potential life lost   The number of years of life lost when death occurs before the age of 65.

Table 4.6
Years of Potential Life Lost Before Age 65

(by cause of death—United States, 1990)

Cause of Death	YPLL in 1990	Percentage of Total
All causes (total)	12,237,379	100
Unintentional injuries	2,235,335	17.5
Malignant neoplasms	1,846,719	15.1
Suicide/homicide	1,493,672	12.2
Diseases of the heart	1,375,923	11.2
Congenital anomalies	666,684	5.4
HIV (including AIDS)	660,261	5.4

that kill people of all ages become as important as those that kill primarily the elderly. Using this approach, unintentional injuries—which accounted for 17.5% of the all YPLL—was the most serious community health problem in 1990 (see Table 4.6). This cause was followed by malignant neoplasms (15.1%), suicide/homicide (12.2%), diseases of the heart (11.2%), congenital anomalies (5.4%), and HIV infections including AIDS (5.4%).

Economic Cost to Society

Still another way to evaluate the impact of a particular disease or health problem is to estimate the economic cost to the country or community. Economic cost data are hard to come by, and sometimes even experts cannot agree on the estimates obtained. An example of such an estimate is the cost to society resulting from the use and abuse of alcohol and other drugs, a whopping $400 billion annually, more than $1 billion per day.[6] This figure includes not only the cost of treatment and the loss of productivity but also the cost of law enforcement, courts, jails, and social work.

PREVENTION, INTERVENTION, CONTROL, AND ERADICATION OF DISEASES

The goals of epidemiology are to prevent, control, and in rare cases, to eradicate dis-

---

BOX 4.1
Community Health in Your World: Smallpox Eradication

October 1992 marked 15 years since the last naturally acquired case of smallpox in the world. This last case occurred in Somalia in October 1977.[1] Although two cases of smallpox were reported in the United Kingdom in 1978, these were associated with a research laboratory and did not represent a natural recurrence.

Smallpox is caused by the *Variola* virus. In its severe form, it is a disfiguring and deadly disease. Manifestations of the disease include fever, headache, malaise, and prostration. A rash appears and covers the body, and there is bleeding into the skin, mucous linings, and genital tract. The circulatory system is also severely affected. Between 15 and 40 percent of cases die, usually within two weeks. Survivors are terribly scarred for life and sometimes blinded.

Mass vaccinations and case finding measures by the World Health Organization with financial support from the United States led to the eradication of smallpox from the world. Why was it possible to eradicate smallpox? Why have we been unable to eradicate any other diseases since 1977? Do you think we will ever be able to do so? If so, what disease will be eliminated next?

eases and injuries. **Prevention** implies the planning for and taking of action to prevent or forestall the occurrence of an undesirable event and is therefore more desirable than **intervention,** the taking of action during an event. That is, vaccination for a disease is superior to taking an antibiotic after one becomes ill.

Control is a general term for the containment of a disease and can include both prevention and intervention measures. The term *control* is often used to mean the limiting of transmission of a communicable disease in a population. **Eradication** is the uprooting or total elimination of a disease from the human population. It is an elusive goal, only rarely achieved in public health. Smallpox is the only communicable disease that has been eradicated (see Box 4.1).

LEVELS OF PREVENTION

There are three levels of application of preventive measures in disease control: primary, secondary, and tertiary. The purpose of **primary prevention** is to forestall the onset of illness or injury during the prepathogenesis period (before the disease process begins). Examples of primary prevention include health education and health promotion programs, safe-housing projects, and character building and personality de-velopment programs. Other examples are the use of immunizations against specific diseases, the practice of personal hygiene such as hand washing, the use of rubber gloves, and the chlorination of the community's water supply. These are illustrated in Figure 4.7.

Unfortunately, disease or injury cannot always be avoided. Chronic diseases in particular sometimes cause considerable disability before they are detected and treated. In these cases, prompt *intervention* can prevent death or limit disability. The goal of **secondary prevention** is the early diagnosis and prompt treatment of diseases before the disease becomes advanced and disability becomes severe.

Examples of secondary prevention measures include personal and medical screenings. The goal of these screenings is not to prevent the onset of disease but rather to detect its presence during early pathogenesis, thus permitting early intervention (treatment) and limiting disability.

The goal of **tertiary prevention** is to retrain, reeducate, and rehabilitate the patient who has already incurred disability. Tertiary preventive measures include those that are applied after significant pathogenesis has occurred.

Prevention of Communicable Diseases

Prevention and control efforts for communicable diseases include primary, secondary, and tertiary approaches.

---

prevention   The planning for and taking of action to forestall the onset of a disease or other health problem.
intervention   Efforts to control a disease in progress.
eradication   The complete elimination or uprooting of a disease (e.g., smallpox eradication).
primay prevention   Preventive measures that forestall the onset illness or injury during the prepathogenesis period.

---

secondary prevention   Preventive measures that lead to an early diagnosis and prompt treatment of a disease or injury to limit disability and prevent more severe pathogenesis.
tertiary prevention   Measures aimed at rehabilitation following significant pathogenesis.

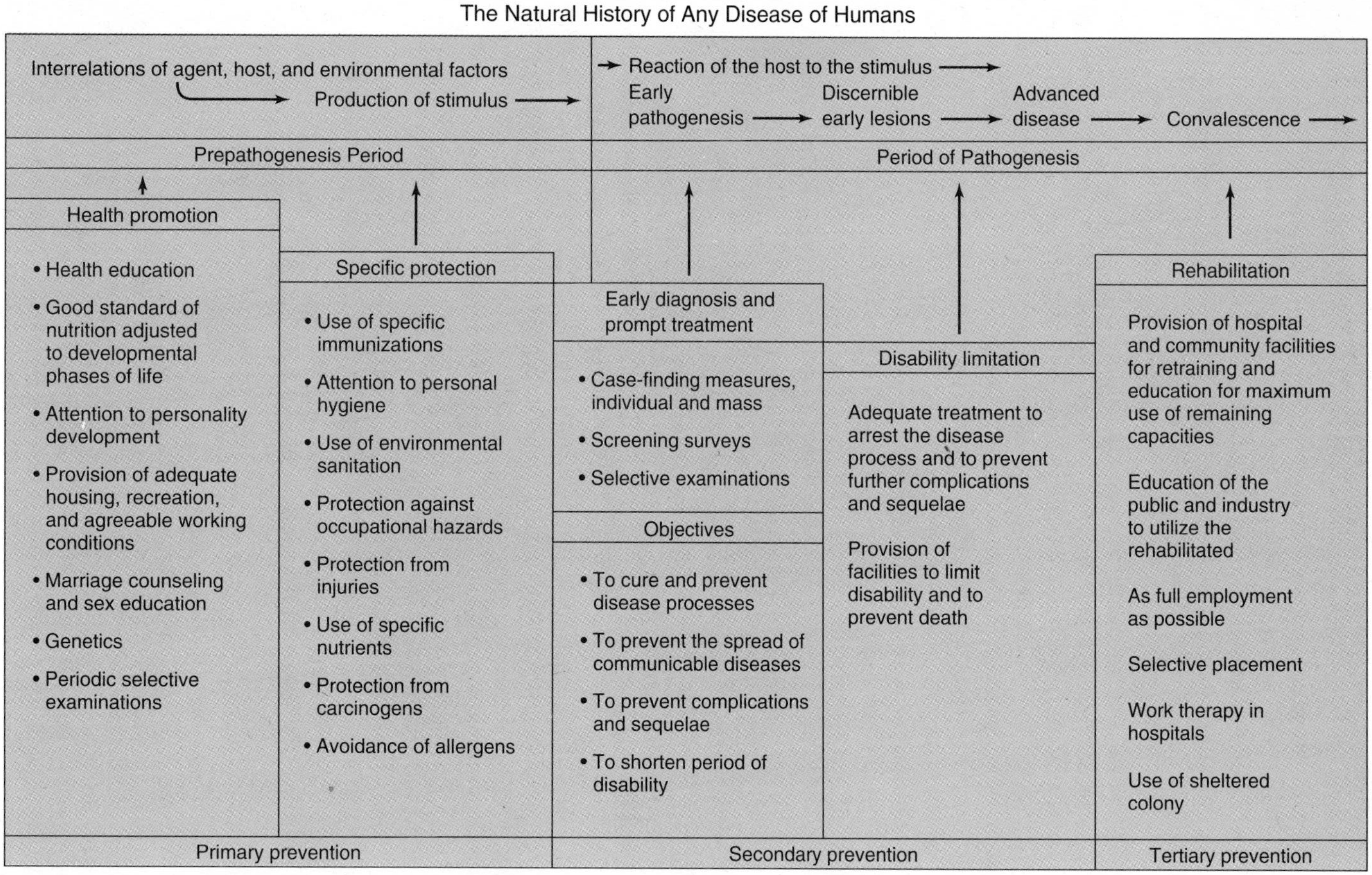

The Natural History of Any Disease of Humans

Interrelations of agent, host, and environmental factors → Production of stimulus → | Reaction of the host to the stimulus → Early pathogenesis → Discernible early lesions → Advanced disease → Convalescence →

Prepathogenesis Period | **Period of Pathogenesis**

Health promotion	Specific protection	Early diagnosis and prompt treatment	Disability limitation	Rehabilitation
• Health education	• Use of specific immunizations	• Case-finding measures, individual and mass	Adequate treatment to arrest the disease process and to prevent further complications and sequelae	Provision of hospital and community facilities for retraining and education for maximum use of remaining capacities
• Good standard of nutrition adjusted to developmental phases of life	• Attention to personal hygiene	• Screening surveys	Provision of facilities to limit disability and to prevent death	Education of the public and industry to utilize the rehabilitated
• Attention to personality development	• Use of environmental sanitation	• Selective examinations		As full employment as possible
• Provision of adequate housing, recreation, and agreeable working conditions	• Protection against occupational hazards	**Objectives**		Selective placement
• Marriage counseling and sex education	• Protection from injuries	• To cure and prevent disease processes		Work therapy in hospitals
• Genetics	• Use of specific nutrients	• To prevent the spread of communicable diseases		Use of sheltered colony
• Periodic selective examinations	• Protection from carcinogens	• To prevent complications and sequelae		
	• Avoidance of allergens	• To shorten period of disability		

Primary prevention	Secondary prevention	Tertiary prevention

FIGURE 4.7

Applications of levels of prevention.

Primary Prevention of Communicable Diseases

The primary prevention measures for communicable diseases can best be visualized using the chain of infection (see Figure 4.8). In this model, prevention strategies are evident at each link in the chain. Successful application of each strategy can be seen as weakening a link, with the ultimate goal of breaking the chain of infection, or interrupting the disease transmission cycle. Examples of community measures include chlorination of the water supply, the inspection of restaurants and retail food markets, immunization programs that reach all citizens, the maintenance of a well-functioning sewer system, the proper disposal of solid waste, and the control of vectors and rodents. To these can be added personal efforts at primary prevention including hand washing, the proper cooking of food, adequate clothing and housing, the use of condoms, and ob-

taining all the available immunizations against specific diseases.

Secondary Prevention of Communicable Diseases

Secondary preventive measures against communicable diseases for the individual involve either: (1) self-diagnosis and self-treatment with nonprescription medications or home remedies or (2) diagnosis and treatment with an antibiotic prescribed by a physician. Secondary preventive measures undertaken by the community against infectious diseases are usually aimed at controlling or limiting the extent of an epidemic. Examples include carefully maintaining records of cases and complying with the regulations requiring the reporting of notifiable diseases (see Chapter 3) and investigating cases and contacts—those who may have become infected through close contact with known cases.

Occasionally, secondary disease control measures may include isolation and quaran-

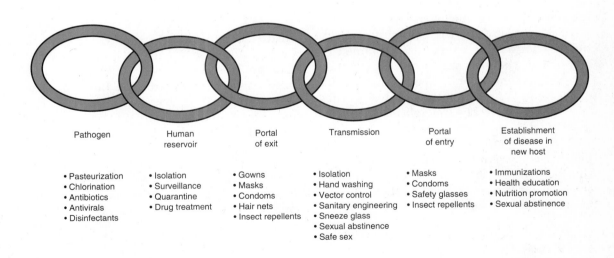

FIGURE 4.8

Chain of infection model showing disease prevention and control strategies.

tine. These are two quite different practices, that are often confused. **Isolation** is the separation, for the period of communicability of infected persons or animals from others so as to prevent the direct or indirect transmission of the communicable agent to a susceptible person. **Quarantine** is the limitation of freedom of movement of well persons or animals that have been exposed to a communicable disease until the incubation period has passed. Further control measures may include **disinfection,** the killing of communicable agents outside of the host, and mass treatment with antibiotics. Lastly, public health education and health promotion should be used as both primary and secondary preventive measures.

Tertiary Prevention of Communicable Diseases

Tertiary preventive measures for the control of communicable diseases for the individual include convalescence from infection, recovery to full health, and return to normal activity. In some cases, such as paralytic poliomyelitis, return to normal activity may not be possible even after extensive physical therapy. At the community level, tertiary preventive measures are aimed at preventing the recurrence of an epidemic. The proper removal, disinfection, and burial of the dead is an example. Tertiary prevention may involve the reapplication of primary and secondary measures in such a way as to prevent further cases. For example, in some countries, such as Japan and the Republic of Korea, people with colds or the flu wear gauze masks in public to reduce the spread of disease.

---

isolation　The separation of infected persons from those who are susceptible.

quarantine　Limitation of freedom of movement of those who have been exposed to a disease.

disinfection　The killing of communicable disease agents outside the body.

Applying Preventive Measures in the Control of a Communicable Disease: AIDS

Acquired immunodeficiency syndrome (AIDS) is a progressive disease that is caused by human immunodeficiency virus (HIV) infection. Individuals are usually infected when they come in contact with the virus through sexual activity or intravenous drug use. It usually takes between three and six months for antibodies to appear in the blood of an infected person. When this happens, these people are referred to *HIV positive* or *seropositive.* From that point, it usually takes eight to ten years, sometimes as long as twenty years, for persons to display symptoms of the illness. Once they do, they are referred to as *HIV positive with symptoms.* They then usually have up to two years before they are diagnosed with AIDS. Their diagnosis is then referred to as *HIV positive with AIDS.* Death usually occurs within five years from this time (see Figure 4.9).

Human immunodeficiency virus (HIV), the causative agent of acquired immunodeficiency syndrome (AIDS), is responsible for a pandemic of unprecedented size. The World Health Organization estimates that 8–10 million adults are currently infected with HIV and that by the year 2000, 40 million people may be infected[7] (see Box 4.2). The reservoir for HIV virus is the infected human population; there are no known animal or insect reservoirs. Referring to the chain of infection, HIV normally leaves its infected host (reservoir) during sexual activity. The portal of exit is the urogenital tract. Transmission is direct and occurs when reproductive fluids or blood are exchanged with the susceptible host. In the case of injection drug users, however, transmission is indirect, by contaminated needles (vehicle). The portal of entry is usually either genital, oral, or anal in direct (sexual) transmission or transdermal in the case of injection drug users or

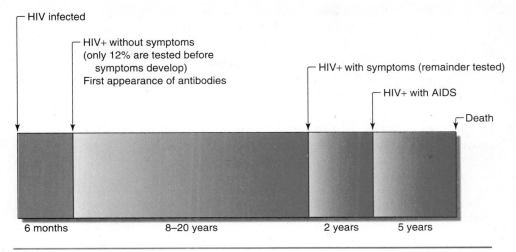

FIGURE 4.9

A time-line for HIV infections. (*Prepared by Wayne A. Payne.*)

blood transfusion recipients. Transmission can also occur during medical procedures if there is an accidental needle stick or some other type of contamination.

A closer examination of the chain of infection reveals that prevention or control measures can be identified for each link. The pathogen in the diseased host can be held in check by the appropriate drug. Outside the host, measures such as sterilizing needles and other possible vehicles and disinfecting surfaces readily kill the virus and reduce the likelihood of transmission by contamination. The infected host (reservoir) can be identified through blood tests and educated to take precautions against the careless shedding of live virus through unsafe sex and needle sharing. Portals of exit can be neutralized by the use of condoms. Transmission can be stopped by the practice of abstinence or reduced by limiting the number of sexual partners. In the case of injection drug users, abstinence from such drug use would preclude transmission by needles. Urogenital portals of entry can be protected through sexual ab-

stinence and the use of female condoms (See Figure 4.10).

For those working in the health professions, the risk of acquiring HIV infection in the workplace is of particular concern. In 1987, the Centers for Disease Control published recommendations for precautions to be taken by health care workers when dealing with blood and other body fluids of *all* patients. Because the precautions were recommended for implementation with *all* patients, regardless of whether they were diagnosed with a communicable disease, they were entitled *Universal Precautions (UP)* or *Universal Blood and Body Fluid Precautions.*[8]

The **Universal Precautions** guideline recommends that all health care workers use appropriate barriers to prevent skin and mucous membrane exposure when contact with blood or other body fluids is anticipated. These barriers include gloves, masks and pro-

Universal Precautions Disease prevention guidelines for those who may come into contact with human body fluids, involving the use of appropriate barriers to reduce or eliminate exposure to these fluids.

BOX 4.2
Healthy People 2000—Objective

18.1 Confine annual incidence of diagnosed AIDS cases to no more than 98,000 cases. (Baseline: an estimated 44,000 to 50,000 diagnosed cases in 1989)

Special Population Targets

Diagnosed AIDS Cases	1989 Baseline	2000 Target
18.1a Gay and bisexual men	26,000–28,000	48,000
18.1b Blacks	14,000–15,000	37,000
18.1c Hispanics	7,000–8,000	18,000

Note: Targets for this objective are equal to upper bound estimates of the incidence of diagnosed AIDS cases projected for 1993.

Baseline data source: Center for Infectious Diseases, CDC.

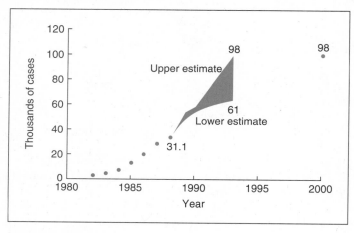

Incidence of AIDS cases.

For Further Thought

If you had the opportunity to pass one law to help stop the spread of AIDS, what would it be? Why?

tective eyewear, and gowns or aprons (see Figure 4.11). Hand washing and changing gloves after each patient are also essential. Another aspect of the UPs deals with needle, scalpels, and other sharp instruments. (Because of the possibility of accidental needle sticks, needles are *not* to be recapped.) All "sharps" are to be placed in puncture resistant containers for disposal or reprocessing.

These guidelines also included precautions for dentistry, dialysis, mortician services, and housekeeping. Guidelines for the management of infected and exposed health care workers were also delineated. The guidelines have been endorsed by the American Hospital Association and mandated by the Occupational Safety and Health Administration.[9]

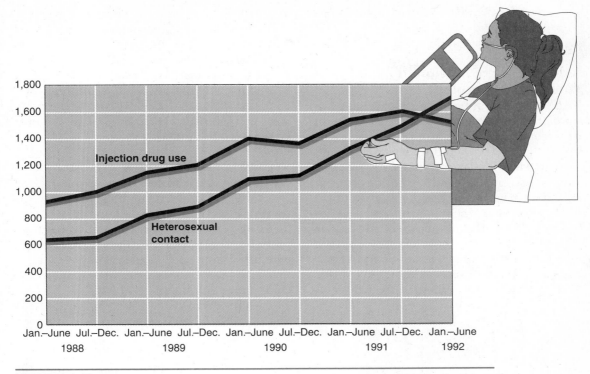

FIGURE 4.10

AIDS among U.S. women attributed to injection drug use (IDU) and heterosexual contact, by half-year diagnosis, 1988–1992.

From: Morbidity and Mortality Weekly Report, *July 23, 1993.*

Prevention of Noncommunicable Diseases

Both the individual and the community can contribute substantially to the prevention and control of multicausation diseases. The community can provide a prohealth environment—physical, economic, and social—in which it becomes easier for individuals to achieve a high level of health.

Primary Prevention of Noncommunicable Diseases

Primary preventive measures for noncommunicable diseases include adequate food and energy supplies, good opportunities for education, employment, and housing, and efficient community services. Beyond this foundation, a community should provide health promotion and health education programs, health and medical services, and protection from environmental and occupational hazards.

Individuals can practice primary prevention by obtaining a high level of education that includes a knowledge about health and disease and the history of disease of others in one's family. In particular, the individual should take responsibility for eating properly, exercising adequately, maintaining appropriate weight, and avoiding the overuse of alcohol and other drugs.

Individuals can also protect themselves from injury by wearing safety belts, safety goggles, and sunscreen lotions.

Secondary Prevention of Noncommunicable Diseases

Secondary preventive measures the community can take include the provision of mass screenings for chronic diseases (see Figure 4.12); case-finding measures; and the provision of adequate health personnel, equipment, and facilities for the community. Secondary prevention responsibilities of individual citizens include personal screenings such as self-examination of breasts or testes (for cancer of these organs) and the hemocult test (for colorectal cancer); and medical screenings such as the Pap test (for cervical cancer), the PSA test for cancer of the prostate, mammography, and screenings for diabetes, glaucoma, or hypertension. Participating in such health screenings and having regular medical and dental checkups represent only the first step in the secondary prevention of noncommunicable diseases. This must be followed by the pursuit of definitive diagnosis and prompt treatment of any diseases detected.

Tertiary Prevention of Noncommunicable Diseases

Tertiary preventive measures for a community include adequate emergency medical personnel, services, and facilities to meet the needs of those citizens for whom primary and secondary preventative measures were unsuccessful. Examples include ambulance services, hospitals, physicians and surgeons, nurses, and other allied health professionals. Interestingly, most communities are doing a more-than-adequate job in tertiary prevention. Many experts feel that most communities in America need to reallocate resources from tertiary prevention to primary and secondary preventive measures.

Tertiary prevention for the individual often requires significant behavioral or lifestyle changes. Examples include strict adherence to prescribed medications, exercise programs, and diet. For example, a heart attack patient could receive nutrition education and counseling and be encouraged to participate in a supervised exercise program, thus maximizing the use of remaining capabilities. This could lead to a resumption of employment and the prevention of a second heart attack. For certain types of noncommunicable health problems, such as those involving substance abuse, regular attendance at support group meetings or counseling sessions may constitute an important part of a tertiary prevention program.

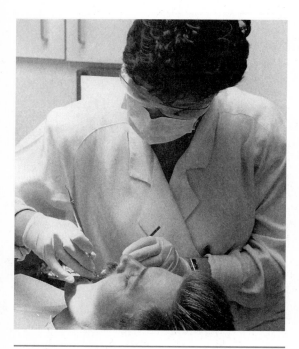

FIGURE 4.11

For health professionals, portals of entry can be protected by gloves, a mask, and safety glasses.

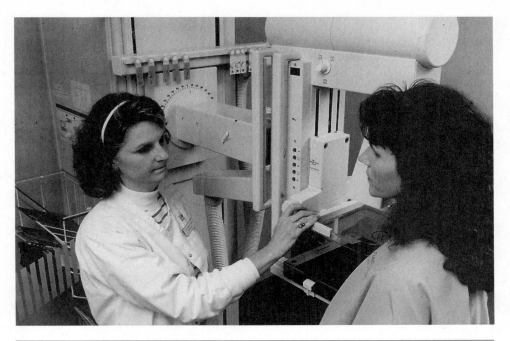

FIGURE 4.12

Mammography, used for screening and early detection of breast cancer, is an example of secondary prevention.

Application of Preventive Measures in the Control of a Noncommunicable Disease: CHD

Coronary heart disease (CHD) is America's Number 1 killer. Many factors contribute to one's risk of developing this disease. Both the community and the individual can contribute to the prevention of CHD (see Box 4.3).

The Community's Role

The community must recognize the importance of preventing chronic disease; intervention following a crisis, such as a heart attack, is the least effective and most expensive way to provide help to a CHD patient. While individual behavioral changes hold the best prospects for reducing the preva-

lence of heart disease in this country, communities can provide a supporting environment for these behavioral changes. For example, the community can support restricting smoking areas and can provide a clear message to youth that smoking is damaging to health. Communities can provide adequate opportunity for health screening for risk factors such as hypertension and serum cholesterol levels. Communities can promote and assist in the development of areas for recreation and exercise, such as safe paths for jogging or cycling and lighted sidewalks for walking. Exercise reduces obesity and increases the high-density lipoproteins (HDLs) in the blood, thereby lowering risk for a heart attack. Last, communities should promote sound nutrition, throughout the lifespan, but particularly in schools.

BOX 4.3
Healthy People 2000—Objective

15.1   Reduce coronary heart disease deaths to no more than 100 per 100,000 people. (Age-adjusted baseline: 135 per 100,000 in 1987)

	Coronary Deaths (per 100,000)	*Special Population Target*		
		1987 Baseline	*2000 Target*	*Percent Decrease*
15.1a	Blacks	163	115	29

Baseline data source: National Vital Statistics System (special analysis), CDC.

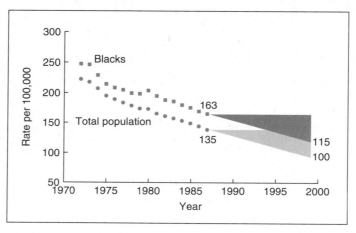

Age-adjusted coronary heart disease death rates.

For Further Thought

What rationale can you provide for the fact that black Americans have a considerably greater number of heart disease deaths than the total population?

The Individual's Role

The risk factors for CHD are multiple. Some of these risk factors are unmodifiable while other risk factors can be modified (reduced) to improve one's health. Each person can increase his or her resistance to CHD by knowing the difference between the types of risk factors and adopting behaviors that prevent or postpone the onset of CHD.

Each person is endowed with a unique genetic code. An individual's innate resistance or susceptibility to heart disease is encoded in the genes. **Unmodifiable risk factors** for CHD include one's race, gender, personality type, age, and basic metabolic rate. Inherited too is one's baseline serum cholesterol level. That is, children whose parents had high serum cholesterol levels

---

unmodifiable risk factors   Factors contributing to the development of a noncommunicable disease that cannot be altered by modifying one's behavior or environment.

are at risk for those same higher levels, independent of their diet.

Modifiable risk factors for CHD include environmental and behavioral factors over which the individual has some control. Modifiable risk factors that would increase the likelihood of CHD include smoking, a diet too rich in fats, lack of exercise, obesity, uncontrolled hypertension, and too much stress. Although none of these factors alone is likely to cause a premature heart attack, each can contribute to the likelihood of CHD.

CHAPTER SUMMARY

Diseases can be classified as communicable or noncommunicable, and acute or chronic. Acute diseases last for less than three months, whereas chronic diseases continue longer than three months. Communicable diseases are caused by biological agents and are transmissible from a source of infection to a susceptible host. Noncommunicable diseases are often caused by a multitude of factors, genetic, behavioral, and environmental. Several of the noncommunicable diseases rank among the leading causes of death in America.

There are three levels of disease prevention: primary, secondary, and tertiary. Both the spread of communicable diseases and the prevalence of noncommunicable diseases can best be reduced by the appropriate application of primary, secondary, and tertiary preventive measures by the community and the individual.

The process of communicable disease transmission is best understood by the chain of infection model. Prevention of communicable disease transmission can then be visualized as breaking one or more links in this chain. The prevention and control of noncommunicable diseases require both individual and community efforts.

---

modifiable risk factor Factors contributing to the development of a noncommunicable disease that can be altered by modifying one's behavior or environment.

SCENARIO: ANALYSIS AND RESPONSE

1. If Bob's roommate, Chuck, were to begin to show signs of the flu, what could Bob do to lessen his chances of becoming infected himself? (Hint: Think about the chain of infection.)

2. As an accountant, Bob spends most of his day behind a desk. Identify primary, secondary, and tertiary preventive measures Bob could take to reduce his risk for heart disease.

REVIEW QUESTIONS

1. What are some of the ways in which diseases and health problems are classified in community health?

2. Contrast the terms *acute disease* and *chronic disease*. Give three examples of each type of disease.

3. Contrast the terms *communicable disease* and *noncommunicable disease*. Give three examples of each type of disease.

4. What is the difference between a communicable agent and a pathogenic agent?

5. What are the components of a simplified communicable disease model?

6. List some examples of environmental factors that can influence the occurrence and spread of disease.

7. Draw and explain the model for multicausation diseases.

8. What is the difference between prevention and intervention?

9. Explain the difference between primary, secondary, and tertiary prevention and give an example of each.

10. What is the "chain of infection" model of disease transmission? Draw the model and label its parts.

11. Again referring to the "chain of infection," indicate how prevention and control strategies

could be implemented to interrupt the transmission of the disease gonorrhea. Are most of these strategies primary, secondary, or tertiary prevention measures?

12. Define the following terms: *case, carrier, vector, vehicle.*

13. List five examples each of vector-borne diseases and non-vector-borne diseases.

14. Explain the difference between the public health practices of isolation and quarantine.

15. Apply the principles of prevention and the examples given in this chapter to outline a prevention strategy for breast cancer that includes primary, secondary, and tertiary prevention components.

ACTIVITIES

1. Call your state health department and find out which are the top communicable disease problems reported in your state. Which are the rarest? Is Lyme disease reportable?

2. List some of the infections you have had. How were these infections transmitted to you—directly, by vehicle, or by vector? Talk to someone who is very old about diseases they can recall from their youth and how these diseases affected them and their families. Take notes on the response and hand in or share orally in class.

3. Look up the word *plague* in an encyclopedia. After reading about the disease, see if you can complete a "chain of infection" model for plague. Identify the causative agent, the vector, the reservoir, and the mode of transmission. What types of prevention and control

strategies were used in the past to stop the spread of this disease? What can be done differently today if there is an epidemic of plague?

4. Think about automobile accidents. List some primary, secondary, and tertiary preventive measures the community and you can take to reduce the number and seriousness of injuries caused by auto accidents.

REFERENCES

1. Benenson, A. S., ed. (1990). *Control of Communicable Diseases in Man,* 15th ed. Washington, D.C.: American Public Health Assn.

2. National Center for Health Statistics (1993). "Annual Summary of Births, Marriages, Divorces, and Deaths: United States, 1992." *Monthly Vital Statistics Report* 41(13), suppl. Hyattsville, Md.: Public Health Service.

3. American Heart Association (1989). *1990 Heart and Stroke Facts.* Dallas: Author.

4. American Cancer Society (1991). *Cancer Facts and Figures—1990.* Atlanta: Author.

5. Centers for Disease Control and Prevention (1991). "Years of Potential Life Lost Before Age 65—United States, 1990 and 1991." *Morbidity and Mortality Weekly Report* 42(13): 251–253.

6. Center for Substance Abuse Prevention (1993). "Prevention Works: A Discussion Paper on Preventing Alcohol, Tobacco, and Other Drug Abuse Problems." Rockville, Maryland: DHHS pub. no. (SMA) 93-2046.

7. Centers for Disease Control (1991). "The HIV/AIDS Epidemic—The First 10 Years." *Morbidity and Mortality Weekly Report* 40(22): 357.

8. Centers for Disease Control (1987). "Recommendations for Prevention of HIV Transmission in Health Care Settings." *Morbidity and Mortality Weekly Report* 36(25): 15–165.

9. American Hospital Association (1991). *Universal Precautions: Policies, Procedures and Resources.* Gina Pugliese, ed. Chicago: American Hospital Publishing, pp. 2–3.

Chapter 5

COMMUNITY ORGANIZATION AND HEALTH PROMOTION PLANNING: TWO IMPORTANT TOOLS OF COMMUNITY HEALTH

Chapter Outline

Chapter Objectives

After studying this chapter you will be able to:

1. Define *community organization* and *community development*.
2. Summarize the steps necessary for organizing a community.
3. Identify the assumptions that underlie the process of community organization.
4. Briefly explain the difference between locality development, social planning, and social action approaches to community organization.
5. List the steps for a hypothetical model for community organization.
6. Explain the difference between health education and health promotion/disease prevention.
7. Define the term *needs assessment*.
8. Briefly explain the five steps used in assessing needs.
9. State and summarize the steps involved in creating a health promotion/disease prevention program.
10. Explain the difference between goals and objectives.
11. List the different types of intervention strategies.
12. Explain the purposes of pilot testing in program development.
13. State the difference between formative and summative evaluation.

It was becoming obvious to many that the suburb of Kenzington now had a drug problem, but few wanted to admit it. The community's residents liked their quiet neighborhoods, and most never thought that drugs would be a problem. In fact, the problem really sneaked up on everyone. The town only had one bar, and while occasionally someone drank too much, the bar's patrons usually controlled their drinking and didn't bother anyone. Occasionally, two or three high school seniors would be caught drinking beer purchased at a store in a nearby town. But these isolated incidents gave no indication of Kenzington's impending drug problem.

Within the past year, the climate of the town had changed considerably. Incidents of teenagers being arrested for possession of alcohol or even other drugs, such as marijuana, were being reported more regularly in the newspaper. There seemed to be more reports of burglaries, too. There had even been a robbery and two assaults reported within the last month. The population of young adults in the community seemed to be increasing, and many of these seemed to be driving impressive cars and wearing fancy clothes. All of these signs suggested the possibility of a drug problem and the need to do something about it.

INTRODUCTION

In order to deal with the health issues that face many communities, community health professionals must possess specific knowledge and skills. They need to be able to identify problems, develop a plan to attack each problem, gather the resources necessary to carry out that plan, implement the plan, and then evaluate the results to determine the degree of progress that has been achieved. In the previous two chapters, we described epidemiological methods as essential tools of the community health professional. In this chapter, we present two other important capabilities each successful community health worker must master: the skills to organize a community and to plan a health promotion program.

---

community organization Planned action to influence social problems.

COMMUNITY ORGANIZATION

Community health problems can be small and simple or large and complex. Small, simple problems that are local and involve few people can be solved with the effort of a small group of people and a minimal amount of organization. Large, complex problems that involve large communities require significant skills and resources for their solution. For these larger problems a considerable effort has to be expended to organize the community to work together to implement a lasting solution to the problem.

Community organization is "intervention whereby individuals, groups, and organizations engage in planned action to influence social problems. It is concerned with the enrichment, development, and/or change of social institutions."[1] It is a process of organizing time, people, and resources. It

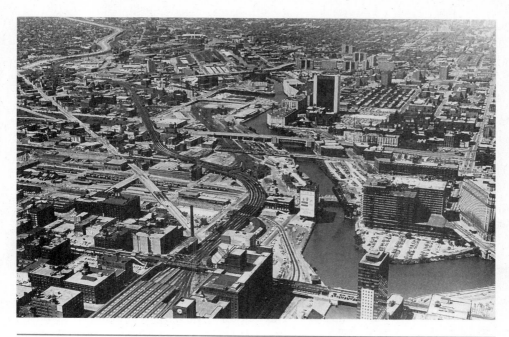

FIGURE 5.1

In today's complex communities, it is not uncommon for people never to meet their neighbors.

is not a science but an art of consensus-building within a democratic process.[2]

Community Organization versus Community Development

Community organization is often confused with another process, community development. Both are social processes, but in community development, economic development is of prime importance. **Community development** has been formally defined as "a mass process designed to create conditions of economic and social progress for a whole community with its active participa-

community development A process to create conditions of economic and social progress for the whole community.

tion and the fullest possible reliance on the community's initiative."[3]

In recent years, the need to organize communities seems to have increased. Advances in electronics (television), communications (telephones and FAX machines), other household appliances (air conditioners), and increased mobility (automobiles) have resulted in a loss of a sense of community. Individuals are much more independent than ever before. The days when people knew everyone on their block are past. Today it is not uncommon for people never to meet their neighbors (see Figure 5.1). In other cases, people see or talk to their neighbors only once or twice each year. Because of these changes in community social structure, it now takes specific skills to organize a community to act together for the collective good. It should be noted that the usefulness of community organization skills extends beyond community health. The process is used by those in the fields of social work, political science, and many different disciplines to unite community members to deal with a problem.

Assumptions for Community Organization

According to Ross,[2] those who organize communities do so while making certain assumptions. The assumptions Ross outlines can be summarized as follows:

1. Communities of people can develop the capacity to deal with their own problems.
2. People want to change and can change.
3. People should participate in making, adjusting, or controlling the major changes taking place in their communities.
4. Changes in community living that are self-imposed or self-developed have a meaning and permanence that imposed changes do not have.
5. A "holistic approach" can successfully address problems with which a "fragmented approach" cannot cope.
6. Democracy requires cooperative participation and action in the affairs of the community, and people must learn the skills that make this possible.
7. Frequently, communities of people need help in organizing to deal with their needs, just as many individuals require help in coping with their individual problems.

Methods of Community Organization

There is no single, preferred method for organizing a community. In fact, a careful review reveals that several different approaches have been successful, leading Rothman and Tropman to state, "We would speak of community organization methods rather than the community organization method."[4]

Some of the early methods of formalizing community organization employed revolutionary techniques.[5] In the 1960s, when there was much unrest in America and the target of organizing efforts was authority at every level, revolutionary techniques were appropriate. Today in America, it is the lack of effective government that is the problem, and revolutionary methods are used very little. They are still seen elsewhere in the world in countries that are struggling with political oppression. Many can still remember the Tienamin Square incident in China and the revolution in Moscow.

In the United States today, the primary methods of community organization are locality development, social planning, and social action.[4] Locality development is based on the concept of broad self-help participation from the local community; one example of this method is the Peace Corps. Peace Corps volunteers help the local citizens to develop new skills and to become more self-sufficient (see Figure 5.2).

Social planning is a method of community organization that involves a technical process of problem solving. It involves various levels of participation from many people. The United Way is a good example. Much of the United Way's work is conducted by volunteers with a variety of skills and abilities, who donate their time to raise money for social programs in the community.

The third method, social action, is a technique that has been useful in helping to organize disadvantaged segments of the population. It often involves trying to redistribute power or resources, which allows for institutional or community change. This method is not used as much as it once was, but it was useful during the civil rights movements and in other settings where peo-

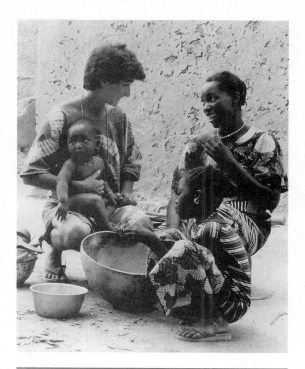

FIGURE 5.2

Peace Corps volunteers working in developing areas to help others.

ple have been oppressed. A more recent example of the method was the 1993 march for gay rights, which occurred in Washington, D.C., shortly after President Clinton was inaugurated.

Each of the above-noted approaches to community organization varies slightly from the others. However, they all revolve around a common theme: the work and resources of many have a much better chance of solving a problem than the work and resources of a few. It is beyond the scope of this textbook to explain each of these approaches to community organization in detail. Instead, we present below a generalized but hypothetical model of community organization that draws upon elements from each of the three approaches.

A PROCESS FOR ORGANIZING A COMMUNITY

McKenzie and Jurs synthesized the work of several others to create a ten-step generalized or hypothetical approach to community organization (see Figure 5.3).[6] The steps are briefly reviewed in the sections that follow.

Recognition of a Problem

The process of community organization begins when someone recognizes that a problem exists in a community and decides to do something about it. For the purposes of this discussion, let us assume the problem is violence. People in most communities would like to have a violence-free community, but it would be most unusual to live in a community that was without at least some level of violence. But how much violence is too much? At what point is a community willing to organize to deal with the problem? In a small-town community, an acceptable level of violence would be very low, while in a large city, an acceptable level would be much higher. However, most people would agree that the Los Angeles riots following the verdict in the Rodney King case in summer of 1992 exceeded an acceptable level.

The people who first recognize a problem in the community and decide to act can be members of the community or individuals from outside the community. If those who initiate community organization are members of the community, then the movement is referred to as being **grass-roots, citizen initiated,** or organized from the **bottom up.** Community members who might recognize that violence is a problem could include teachers, police officers, or other concerned citizens. When community

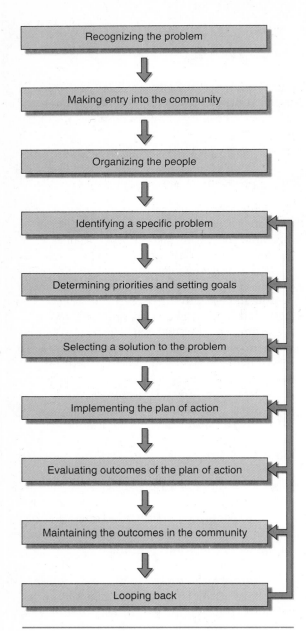

FIGURE 5.3

Summary of steps in community organization.

From: McKenzie, J. F., and J. L. Jurs (1993). Planning, Implementing, and Evaluating Health Promotion Programs: A Primer. *New York: Macmillan, p. 126.*

organization is initiated by individuals from outside of the community, the problem is said to be organized from the **top down** or **outside in.** Individuals from outside the community who might initiate organization could include a judge who presides over cases involving violence, a state social worker who handles cases of family violence, or a politically active group that is against violent behavior wherever it happens. In cases where the person who recognizes the community problem is not a community member, efforts must be made to make those within the community aware of the problem.[7]

Gaining Entry into the Community

After a problem is recognized, the community must be properly informed. This may seem like a relatively easy matter, but an error by organizers at this step could ruin the chances of successfully organizing the community. This may be the most crucial step in the whole process.

Gaining entry into the community is best accomplished through the community's most influential members, the **gatekeepers.** Gatekeepers are those who control, both formally and informally, the political climate of the community.[8] These "power brokers" know their community, how it functions, and how to accomplish tasks within it. Long-time residents are usually able to identify the gatekeepers of their community. These people usually include politicians, leaders of activist groups, business and education leaders, and clergy, to name but a few.

Community organizers must approach such figures on the gatekeepers' own terms

---

gatekeepers Those who control, both formally and informally, the political climate of the community.

and "play" the gatekeepers' "ball game." However, before approaching these important individuals, organizers must study the community well. They need to know where the power lies, what type of politics must be used to solve a problem, and whether the particular problem they wish to solve has ever been dealt with before in the community.[8] In the violence example, community organizers need to know: (1) who is causing the violence and why, (2) how the problem has been addressed in the past, (3) who supports and who opposes the idea of addressing the problem, and (4) who could provide more insight into the problem. This is a critical step in the community organization process because failure to study the community carefully in the beginning may lead to a delay in organizing it later and a subsequent waste of time and resources.

Once the organizers have a good understanding of the community, they are then ready to approach the gatekeepers. In keeping with the violence example, the gatekeepers would probably include the police department, elected officials, school board members, social service personnel, members of the judicial system, and possibly some of those who are creating the violence.

When the top-down approach is being used, organizers might find it advantageous to enter the community through a well-respected organization or institution that is already established in the community, such as a church, a service group, or another successful local group. If such an organization/institution can be convinced that the problem exists and needs to be solved, it can help smooth the way for gaining entry and achieving the remaining steps in the process.

Organizing the People

Obtaining the support of community members to deal with the problem is the next step in the process. It is best to begin by organizing those who are already interested in seeing that the problem is solved. This core group of community members, sometimes referred to as "executive participants,"[1] will become the "backbone" of the work force and will end up doing the majority of the work. For our example of community violence, the core group could include law enforcement personnel, former victims of violence and their families (or victims' support groups), parent-teacher organizations, and public health officials. It is also important to recruit people from the subpopulation that are most directly affected by the problem. For example, if most of the violence in a community is directed toward teenagers, teenagers need to be included in the core group. If elderly persons are impacted, they need to be included.

Although the formation of the core group is essential, this group is usually not large enough to do all the work itself. Therefore, one of the core group's tasks is to recruit more members of the community to the cause. By broadening the constituency, the core group can spread out the workload and generate additional resources to deal with the problem.

However, recruiting additional workers can often be difficult. Over the last 30 years, the number of people in many communities interested in volunteering their time has decreased. Today, if you ask someone to volunteer, you may hear the reply, "I'm already too busy." There are two primary reasons for this response. First, there are many families in which both husband and wife work outside the home. Between 1970 and 1990, the proportion of married women with preschool-aged children in the labor force doubled from 30% to 59%. Also during this same period of time, the proportion of married women with children of school age in the labor force jumped from 49% to 75%. In 1990, 70% of married couples with children reported that both the husband and wife were employed.[9] Second, there are more single-parent households. Between 1970 and 1988, the number of single parents who maintained their own households and had their own children living with them rose from 3.8 million to 9.4 million. Today they constitute about one-fourth of all family households with children, and most are headed by women.[10]

Therefore, when organizers are expanding their constituencies, they should be sure to: (1) identify people who are impacted by the problem that they are trying to solve, (2) provide "perks" for or otherwise reward volunteers, (3) keep volunteer time short, (4) match volunteer assignments with the ability and expertise of the volunteers, and (5) consider providing appropriate training to make sure volunteers are comfortable with their tasks. For example, if the organizers need someone to talk with law enforcement groups, it would probably be a good idea to solicit the help of someone who feels comfortable around such groups and who is respected by them, such as another law enforcement person.

When the core group has been expanded to include these other volunteers, the larger group is sometimes referred to as an *association, task force,* or *coalition.* Of these three groups, the coalition is the most formal. A **coalition** can be defined as a temporary union of two or more individuals and/or organizations to achieve a common purpose (often, to compensate for deficits in power, resources, and expertise). A larger group with more resources, people, and energy has a greater chance of solving a community problem than a smaller less-powerful group (see Figure 5.4).

coalition A temporary union of two or more individuals and/or organizations who work together—often to compensate for separate shortcomings in power, resources, or expertise—to achieve a common goal.

Identifying the Specific Problem

After the organizers have expanded the working group, the next task is to isolate and define more carefully the specific problem (or problems) that need to be resolved. In our violence example, the coalition should ask the question, "Is violence really the problem, or is it merely a symptom of a more serious underlying problem?" Sometimes a noisy minority or a powerful majority can overshadow the real needs. There are some who will work very hard not to let the truth be known. Archer and Fleshman have indicated that most community problems are complex and the reality is that someone usually benefits if a problem remains unsolved.[11]

To delineate the "real" problem, the right questions need to be asked and the corresponding data collected and analyzed. These actions are collectively referred to as a **needs assessment, community analy-**

Table 5.1
Sources of Needs Assessment Data

1. Service needs or real needs (seen through the eyes of the planners)
   a. Epidemiological data from government agencies.
   b. Records of health and health care.
   c. Results of health risk appraisals or health hazard appraisals.
   d. Information from significant others.
   e. Examining current literature.
2. Service demands or wants, or perceived or felt needs (seen through the eyes of those in the target population):
   a. Community forum with target population.
   b. Focus groups within target population.
   c. Opinion leaders' survey.
   d. Survey of target population.
   e. Observation of target population.

From: McKenzie, J. F., and J. L. Jurs (1993). *Planning, Implementing, and Evaluating Health Promotion Programs: A Primer.* New York: Macmillan.

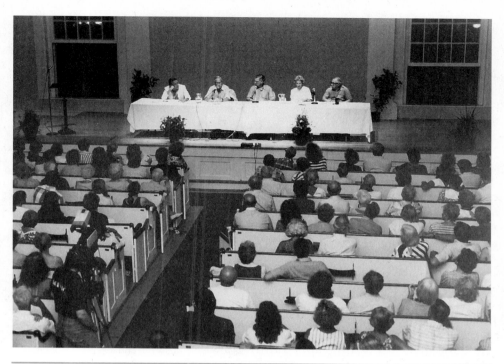

FIGURE 5.4

Coalition building is an important step in successful community organization.

sis,[12] or **community diagnosis.**[13] (See Table 5.1 for sources of needs assessment data.) Great care must be taken to assure that the needs assessment data are collected in a representative and unbiased manner. This activity, if conducted properly, will not only help to identify the specific problem, but will also describe the community's cultural values—those things that are most important to the community. [Note: Needs assessment is discussed in greater length in the second half of this chapter, with regard to program planning.]

Determining Priorities and Setting Goals

An analysis of the needs data should result in the identification of the real problems to be addressed. However, more often than not, the resources needed to solve all identified problems are not available. Therefore, the problems that have been identified must be prioritized. This prioritization is best achieved through general agreement or consensus so that "**ownership**" can take hold. It is critical that those in the coalition feel that they "own" the problem and want to see it solved. Without this sense of ownership, they will be unwilling to give of their time and energy to solve it. For example, if a few highly vocal members in the coalition intimidate people before a consensus is actually reached into voting for certain activities to be the top priorities for solving the violence problem, it is unlikely that those who disagreed on this assignment of priorities will work enthusiastically to help solve the problem. They may even leave the coalition because they feel no ownership in the decision-making process.

Once the problems have been prioritized, goals need to be identified that will serve as guides for problem solving. The practice of consensus building should again be employed during the setting of goals. The goals, which will become the foundation for all the work that follows, can be thought of as the "hoped-for end result." In other words, once community action has occurred, what will have changed? In the community where violence is a problem, the goal may be to reduce the number of violent crimes or eliminate them altogether. Sometimes at this point in the process, some members of the larger group drop out because they do not see their priorities or goals included on consensus lists. Unable to feel ownership, they are unwilling to expend their resources on this process. Because there is strength in numbers, efforts should be made to keep them in. One strategy for doing so is to keep the goal list as long as possible.

Arriving at a Solution and Selecting Intervention Activities

There are alternative solutions to every community problem. A solution involves selecting one or more intervention activities (see Table 5.2). Each type of intervention activity has advantages and disadvantages. The coalition must try to agree upon the best solution and then select the most advantageous intervention activity or activities. Again, the group must work toward consensus through compromise. If the educators in the group were asked to provide a recommended solution, they might suggest offering more preventive-education programs; law enforcement personnel might recommend more enforceable laws; judges might want more space in the jails and pris-

ons. The protectionism of the subgroups within the larger group is often referred to as **turfism.** It is not uncommon to have turf struggles when trying to build consensus.

The Final Steps in the Process—Implementing, Evaluating, Maintaining, Looping Back

The last four steps in this generalized or hypothetical approach to community organization include implementation of the intervention activity that was selected in the previous step, evaluating the outcomes of the

---

Table 5.2
Methods of Intervening to Solve Problems

Intervention activities

1. Traditional educational activities—examples include using audiovisual materials and equipment, printed educational materials, classroom teaching strategies and techniques, and strategies and techniques for outside the classroom.

2. Behavior modification activities—include modifying behavior to stop smoking, starting to exercise, managing stress, and regulating diet.

3. Environmental change activities—include no-smoking signs or putting only "healthy" foods in vending machines.

4. Regulatory activities—include laws, policies, position statements, regulations, and rules to change health behavior.

5. Community participation activities to influence public policy—include mass mobilization; social action; community planning; community service development; community education; and community advocacy, such as a letter-writing campaign.

6. Activities affecting organization culture—include activities that work to change norms and traditions.

7. Communication activities—include mass media, billboards, booklets, bulletin boards, fliers, direct mail, newsletter, pamphlets, posters, video and audio materials.

8. Economic and other incentives—include money and other material items.

9. Social activities—include support groups, social activities, and social networks.

plans of action, maintaining the outcomes over time, and if necessary, going back to a previous step in the process—"looping back"—to modify or restructure the work plan to organize the community. (See Box 5.1 for an example of this process.)

BOX 5.1
Organizing to Eliminate Drugs

Accessibility, poverty, and high incidence of youth unemployment made the residents of Omaha, Nebraska's public housing developments easy targets for outside drug dealers. The area was caught by surprise. Between 1987 and 1989, drug arrests in the area increased by 75%, guns became evident, and children were becoming "runners" for the drug dealers. By the late 1980s, it was obvious that there was a serious problem.

The problem was evident to the residents of the development, but it was a top-down community organization effort that began to turn things around. The leadership came from Omaha Housing Authority (OHA) Executive Director Robert Armstrong. It was his belief that the drug problem was really a symptom of the residents' feelings of fear and hopelessness and their lack of opportunity. Therefore, the OHA staff began efforts to organize residents, police, and service providers to attack the problem. A multifaceted, community-based approach revolving around collaboration and communication was begun in order to empower the residents. Great care was given to actively involve the residents in seeking solutions. Residents had major roles in planning and implementing various programs and policies.

The resulting activities of the community organization effort included:

1. Tough management policies against crime and drug dealing that allowed OHA to evict residents who broke the policies.
2. A curfew for youth, ages 17 and under, and issuance of photo ID cards to adult residents.
3. Increased police foot patrol in the area and a base station where an OHA security co-

ordination acted as a liaison between the residents and police.
4. Social activities between police and youth in the community to allow the youth to see off-duty police officers as "real people."
5. Efforts to encourage youth to study and to urge parents to stay active in their children's education, thus creating a positive home environment for learning, and keeping youngsters in school.
6. The development of study centers to provide tutoring for children.
7. The development of the OHA Foundation to provide funds not only for emergency assistance but also for college scholarships and rewards for school attendance and good grades.
8. The creation of an OHA sports recreation program for youths.
9. The development of Operation Shadow Program, where children aged 6–12 can "shadow" OHA staff after school for four hours a day, two or three times per week.
10. The establishment of First Step, a "one-stop shopping" system for human services, which eliminated barriers of red tape and fragmentation. Some services included were visiting nurses; health and nutrition screening; health, drug prevention, and treatment services; and WIC.
11. The development of a wide range of summer programs that included jobs, internships, and employment training.

From: U.S. Dept. of Housing and Urban Development (1992). *Together We Can . . . Create Drug-Free Neighborhoods* (pub. no. HUD-1364-PIH). Washington, D.C.: U.S. Government Printing Office.

Special Note About Community Organization

Before we leave the process of community organization, it should be noted that no matter what approach is used in organizing a community—locality development, social planning, social action, or the generalized approach outlined here—not all problems can be solved. In other cases, repeated attempts may be necessary before a solution is reached. And it is important to remember that if a problem exists in a community, there are probably some people who benefit from its existence and who may work toward preventing a successful solution to the problem. Whether or not the problem is solved, the final decision facing the coalition and its organizers is whether to disband the group or reorganize to take on a new problem or attack the first problem from a different direction.

HEALTH PROMOTION AND DISEASE PREVENTION PROGRAMMING

In Chapters 2 to 4, we discussed how communities describe, analyze, and intervene to solve existing health problems such as disease outbreaks or other community problems. However, the 1979 Surgeon General's Report on Health Promotion and Disease Prevention, *Healthy People* (see Figure 5.5), charted a new course for community health—away from curing diseases and toward preventing diseases and promoting health. Health promotion and disease prevention programming have now become important tools of community health professionals. The second half of this chapter presents the process of health promotion/ disease prevention programming.

Basic Understanding of Program Planning

Prior to discussing the process of program planning, two relationships must be presented. They are the relationships between health education and health promotion/disease prevention, and program planning and community organization.

Health education and *health promotion/disease prevention* are terms that are sometimes used interchangeably. This is incorrect because health education is only a part of health promotion/disease prevention.

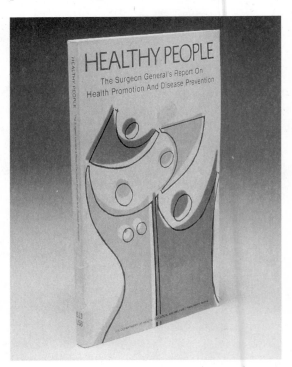

FIGURE 5.5

Healthy People, the 1979 Surgeon General's report on health promotion and disease prevention, chartered a new course for community health.

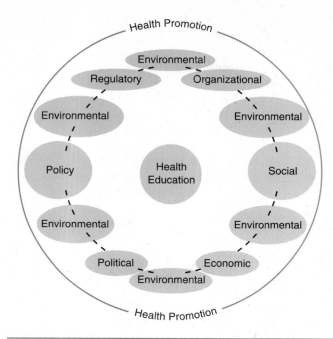

FIGURE 5.6

Relationship of health education and health promotion.

From: McKenzie, J. F., and J. L. Jurs (1993). Planning, Implementing, and Evaluating Health Promotion Programs: A Primer. *New York: Macmillan, p. 4.*

The Joint Committee on Health Education Terminology defines the process of **health education** as the "continuum of learning which enables people, as individuals and as members of social structures, to voluntarily make decisions, modify behaviors, and change social conditions in ways which are health enhancing."[14] The Committee defined **health promotion and disease prevention** as "the aggregate of all purposeful activities designed to improve personal and public health through a combination of strategies, including the competent implementation of behavioral change strategies, health education, health protection mea-

sures, risk factor detection, health enhancement and health maintenance."[14] From these definitions, it is obvious that the terms are not the same and that *HP/DP* is a much more encompassing term than *health education.* Figure 5.6 provides a graphic representation of the relationship between the terms.

The first half of this chapter described the process of community organization—the process by which individuals, groups and organizations engage in planned action to influence social problems. Program planning may or may not be associated with community organization. **Program planning** is a process in which an intervention is planned

health promotion and disease prevention The aggregate of all purposeful activities designed to improve personal and public health.

program planning A process by which an intervention is planned to help meet the needs of a target population.

to help meet the needs of a specific group of people. It may take a community organization effort to be able to plan such an intervention. The antiviolence campaign used earlier in the chapter is such an example, where many resources of the community were brought together in order to create interventions (programs) to deal with the violence problem. However, program planning need not be connected to community organization. For example, a community organization effort is not needed before a company offers a smoking cessation program for its employees or a church offers a stress management class for its members. In such cases, only the steps of the program planning process need to be carried out. They are described below.

CREATING A HEALTH PROMOTION/DISEASE PREVENTION (HP/DP) PROGRAM

The process of developing a HP/DP program, like the process of community organization, involves a series of steps. Success depends upon many factors, including the assistance of a professional experienced in program planning (see Box 5.2).

Several successful models have been developed to assist those who wish to create or develop a HP/DP program. These include the PRECEDE/PROCEED Model,[15] probably the best known and most often used (see Figure 5.7);[16] the Model for Health Education Planning;[17] the Model for the Analysis of Health Education Planning and Resource Development;[18] the Comprehensive Health Education Model;[15] and the Generic Health/Fitness Delivery System.[19]

Each of these planning models has its strengths and weaknesses, and each has distinctive components that makes it unique. In addition, each of the models has been used to plan HP/DP programs in a variety of settings with many successes and a few failures.

It is not absolutely necessary that the beginning community health student have a thorough understanding of the five models mentioned here, but it is important to know the basic steps in the planning process. Therefore, we have drawn on each of these models to create a generalized HP/DP program planning model. The steps of this generalized model are presented in Figure 5.8 and explained below.

Assessing the Needs of the Target Population

In order to create a useful and effective program for the **target population,** those whom the HP/DP program is intended to serve, planners must determine the needs and wants of these people. This procedural step is referred to as a needs assessment, a community diagnosis,[12] or a community analysis.[13] **Needs assessment** is "the process by which the program planner identifies and measures gaps between what is and what ought to be."[20] The purpose is to determine whether the needs of the people are being met (see Figure 5.9).

As they begin the needs assessment process, planners must remember that the needs of the target population can depend on the one who is identifying those needs. There are two basic ways of examining the needs. The first is through the eyes of the

---

target population Those whom the program is intended to serve.
needs assessment Gaps between what is and what ought to be.

BOX 5.2
Program Planning in Union County, Indiana

Union County is a small (approximate population, 7,000), rural county in eastern Indiana with few health resources. The health department has three employees, two full-time and one half-time; a full-time clerk; a half time sanitarian; and a full-time nurse, who is also the administrator. There are two doctors in the county, no hospitals, and few health service agencies.

At a professional meeting in fall 1992, the nurse of the health department, who was looking for program planning assistance, was introduced to a faculty member from Ball State University who was looking for a community in need of some assistance in program planning. It was a win-win meeting for both the nurse and the professor. The county would get much needed help and the professor found a perfect classroom for his students.

The planning process began with several meetings between the nurse, faculty member, and university students. Much effort was put into making the students as knowledgeable as possible about the community with which they were to work. Students listened to presentations about the county, read literature from the Chamber of Commerce, studied Indiana Department of Health health statistics for the county, and reviewed data for the county from the 1990 census.

Once the students had a good understanding of the county, the needs assessment process began. Based upon the resources available, students decided to collect data with original instruments from county opinion leaders, identified by the nurse, and randomly, via telephone interview, from county residents.

Analysis of the needs assessment data, along with other information provided, allowed the students to identify a list of needs of the county's residents. For each need, students then developed goals and objectives. With solid goals and objectives, students either individually or in groups of up to three people planned appropriate interventions for the county and presented their plans to the County Health Department. At this point, the academic term ended and with it the students' program planning efforts. Thus the final steps in the program planning process—implementation of the intervention and the evaluation—became the responsibility of the County Health Department personnel.

Though the link between the County Health Department and the university was a bit unusual, the steps followed in this planning process provide a fairly typical picture of the steps professionals would follow in planning a program.

---

planners. Windsor and colleagues have referred to these needs as **service needs or real needs.**[20] These are the needs that health professionals believe the target population must have met in order to resolve a health problem. The second way of examining the needs is through the eyes of those in

the target population. Windsor and colleagues have referred to these as **service demands or wants** or as **perceived or felt needs.**[20] These are the needs that those in the target population feel must be met in order to resolve a health problem. Both types of needs are important, and both must

---

service needs or real needs Needs that health professionals believe the target population must have met in order to resolve a problem.

perceived or felt needs Needs that those in the target population believe must be met in order to resolve a problem.

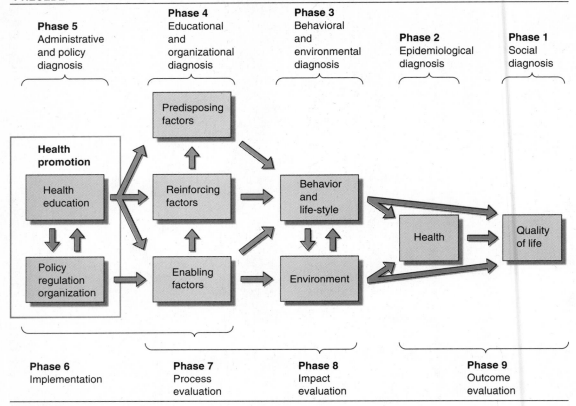

FIGURE 5.7

The PRECEDE/PROCEED Model for health promotion planning and evaluation.

From: Health Promotion Planning: An Educational and Environmental Approach *(p. 23) by L. W. Green and M. W. Kreuter, 2nd ed., 1991, Mountain View, Calif.: Mayfield Publishing. Copyright 1991 by Mayfield Publishing Reprinted by permission.*

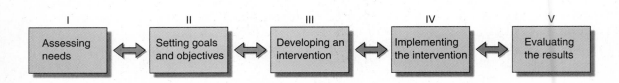

FIGURE 5.8

A generalized model for program planning.

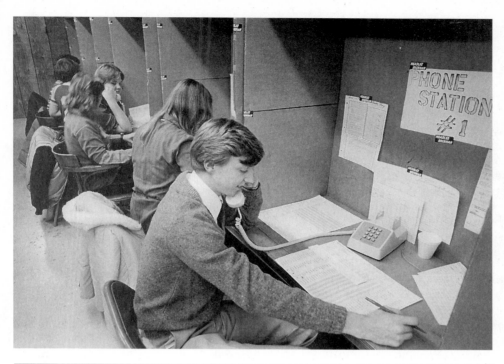

FIGURE 5.9

A telephone survey is a common form of data collection for a health needs assessment.

be identified in order for true needs of the target population to be identified.

For those interested in a detailed explanation of the process of conducting a needs assessment, an extensive account is available.[21] Presented below is a simplified five-step approach.[6]

Step 1: Determining the Present State of Health of the Target Population

Determining the health status of the target population involves either collecting health data first hand (primary data) or identifying existing health data (secondary data). Sources of existing health data include local, state, and federal agencies, hospitals, disease registries, volunteer health agencies and health risk appraisals (see Table 5.1). This first step should uncover the health deficits of the target population.

Step 2: Identifying Existing Programs

Following the determination of the current health status of a target population and the establishment of particular health deficits, it is important to identify existing HP/DP programs that deal with these deficits. If it can be determined that existing programs are dealing effectively with them, similar services should not be recommended. The community's resources are too valuable to waste through the duplication of services. The identification of existing health programs or services is best accomplished through networking with health agencies in the community, talking with related coalitions, or personal investigative work.

Step 3: Comparing Health Deficits with Existing Programs

The actual need for a new health promotion/disease prevention program is determined by comparing deficits in the health status of the target population as determined in Step 1 with the available services provided by existing HP/DP programs as determined by Step 2. These unmet needs provide the basis for the creation of a new HP/DP program.

Step 4: Dealing with the Problems

Invariably, more than one unmet need exists and planners need to prioritize unmet needs. In conducting this step, planners may want to consider: (1) the importance of the need, (2) how changeable the need is, and (3) whether adequate resources are available to deal with the problem. Figure 5.10 presents a 2×2 matrix that can be used in making priority decisions.

Step 5: Validating the Need

The final step in this process is to double-check to confirm that the identified need is indeed a need of the target population. For example, a limited amount of data may indicate that the primary need of the target group is weight management. However, more extensive data or more comprehensive networking may indentify another problem such as stress, diabetes, or malnutrition. Before this step is completed, planners must make sure they have indeed identified a true need. In short, all work should be double-checked.

Setting Goals and Objectives

Once the needs have been well defined and prioritized, the planners can set goals and develop objectives for the program. The goals and objectives should be thought of as the foundation of the program. The remaining portions of the programming process—intervention development, implementation, and evaluation—will be designed to achieve the goals by meeting the objectives.

	Important	Less important
Changeable		
Not changeable		

FIGURE 5.10

Priority decision making.

From: McKenzie, J. F., and J. L. Jurs (1993). Planning, Implementing, and Evaluating Health Promotion Programs: A Primer. *New York: Macmillan, p. 13.*

The words *goals* and *objectives* are often used interchangeably, but there is really a significant difference between the two. "A goal is a future event toward which a committed endeavor is directed; objectives are the steps taken in pursuit of a goal."[17] To further distinguish between goals and objectives, McKenzie and Jurs[6] have stated that goals: (1) are much more encompassing and global than objectives, (2) are written to cover all aspects of a program, (3) provide overall program direction, (4) are more general in nature, (5) usually take longer to complete, (6) are usually not observed but inferred,[22] and (7) often are not easily measured. Goals are easy to write and include two basic components—who will be affected and what will change because of the program. Here are some examples of program goals:

1. To help employees learn how to manage their stress.

2. To reduce the number of teenage pregnancies in the community.

3. To help cardiac patients and their families deal with the life-style changes that occur after a heart attack.

Objectives are more precise and can be considered the steps to achieve the program goals. Since some program goals are more complex than others, the number and type of objectives will vary from program to program. For example, the process of getting a group of people to exercise is a more complex activity than trying to get a group to learn the four food groups. The more complex a program, the greater the number of objectives needed. To deal with these different types of programs, McKenzie and Jurs[6] adapted a hierarchy of program objectives first developed by Parkinson & Associates.[23] Table 5.3 presents a list of the hierarchy and an example of an objective at each of the levels within the hierarchy.

Table 5.3
Hierarchy of Program Objectives

Level	Example Objective
1. Increase awareness	After reading the American Cancer Society's brochure on skin cancer, all the employees will be able to identify their own risks for the disease.
2. Increase knowledge	On a written test, students will be asked to list with 100% accuracy the four major food groups.
3. Change attitudes	During a neighborhood meeting, residents will be able to talk about their views on the issue of the development of a new landfill.
4. Develop health skills	After the class on recycling, participants will be able to accurately sort a bag of trash into the appropriate recyclable containers.
5. Access to health care	Upon completing of orientation on "How to Create Your Own Screening Program," the employees of Delaware County Schools will be able to plan and implement their own screening program.
6. Change behavior	Six months after the community recycling meetings, 35% of the neighborhoods will have an active recycling program.
7. Risk-reduction	The collective safe behavior of those in the "Safe Driving Classes" will reduce the health risk of the group by 50% over the preprogram evaluation figures.
8. Change in health status	The teachers participating in the school site wellness program will use 15% fewer sick days after the program than before it.

From the examples presented in Table 5.3 it should be obvious that the hierarchy goes from less-complex to more complex levels. Thus it takes less energy and fewer resources to increase awareness than to improve health status. Close examination of the example objectives reveals that the objectives are written in behavioral form, stating specific changes the program is expected to bring about in the target population. The objectives are written so that the level of their attainment is observable and measurable.

A final note about objectives. In Chapter 1, the three national health goals from *Healthy People 2000* are listed.[24] Selected objectives from this publication are presented in boxes in the other chapters (see Box 5.3). These goals and objectives provide a good model for developing goals and objectives for a new program. In fact, these goals and objectives can be adapted to most community health programs by referring to *Healthy Communities 2000: Model Standards.*[25]

Developing an Intervention

The next step in the programming process is to design activities that will help the target population meet their objectives and, in the process, achieve their goals. These activities are collectively referred to as the intervention or **treatment.** This intervention or treatment constitutes the program that the target population will experience.

The number of activities in an intervention may be many or only a few. Although no minimum number has been established, it has been shown that multiple activities are often more effective than a single activ-

ity. For example, if planners wanted to change the attitudes of community members toward a new landfill, they would have a greater chance of doing so by distributing pamphlets door to door, writing articles for the local newspaper, *and* speaking to local service groups, than by performing any one these activities by itself. "In other words, 'dosage' is important in health promotion/disease prevention. Few people change their behavior based on a single exposure (or dose); instead, multiple exposures (doses) are generally needed to change most behaviors. It stands to reason that 'hitting' the target population from several angles or through multiple channels should increase the chances of making an impact."[6]

The choice of activities for an intervention depends on a number of variables. Some types of activities work better with groups than with individuals. Activities aimed at groups are referred to as **macro intervention activities** while those aimed at individuals are called **micro intervention activities.** The intervention activities designed to solve problems associated with community organization, as presented in Table 5.2, are the same activities being discussed here.

Implementing the Intervention

The moment of truth is when the intervention is implemented. **Implementation** is the actual carrying out or putting into practice the activity or activities that make up the intervention. It is at this point that the planners will learn whether the product (intervention) they developed will be useful

---

treatment An activity or activities designed to create change in people

macro intervention activities Activities aimed at groups of people.
micro intervention activities Intervention activities aimed at individuals.
implementation Putting a planned program into action.

BOX 5.3
Healthy People 2000—Objectives

8.6 Increase to at least 85% the proportion of workplaces with 50 or more employees that offer health promotion activities for their employees, preferably as part of a comprehensive employee health promotion program. (Baseline: 65% of worksites with 50 or more employees offered at least one health promotion activity in 1985; 63% of medium and large companies had a wellness program in 1987.)

Baseline data sources: For worksites with 50 or more employees, the National Survey of Worksite Health Promotion Activities, ODPHP; for medium and large companies, the Health Research Institute biennial survey.

8.7 Increase to at least 20% the proportion of hourly workers who participate regularly in employer-sponsored health promotion activities. (Baseline data not yet available.)

8.8 Increase to at least 90% the proportion of people aged 65 and older who had the opportunity to participate during the preceding year in at least one organized health promotion program through a senior center, lifecare facility, or other community-based setting that serves older adults. (Baseline data not yet available).

8.12 Increase to at least 90% the proportion of hospitals, health maintenance organizations, and large groups practices that provide patient education programs, and to at least 90% the proportion of community hospitals that offer community health promotion programs addressing the priority health needs of their communities (Baseline: 66% of 6,821 registered hospitals provided patient education services in 1987; 60% of 5,677 community hospitals offered community health promotion programs in 1987.)

Baseline data source: American Hospital Association Annual Survey.

For Further Thought

If you had the opportunity to write one more objective dealing with the implementation of health promotion programs for use in *Healthy People 2000,* what would it be? What is your rationale for selecting such an objective?

---

in producing the measurable changes as outlined in the objectives.

To ensure a smooth-flowing implementation of the intervention, it is wise to **pilot test** it at least once and sometimes more than once. A pilot test is a trial run. It is when the intervention is presented to just a few individuals who are either from the intended target population or from a very similar population. For example, if the intervention is being developed for fifth-graders

in a particular school, it might be pilot tested on fifth-graders with similar educational backgrounds and demographic variables but from a different school.

The purpose of pilot testing an intervention is to determine whether there are any problems with it. Some of the more common problems that pop up are those dealing with the design or delivery of the intervention, but any part of it could be flawed. For example, it could be determined during pilot testing that there is a lack of resources to carry out the intervention as planned or that

pilot test A trial run of an intervention.

those implementing the intervention need more training. When minor flaws are detected and they can be corrected easily, the intervention is then ready for full implementation. However, if a major problem surfaces—one that requires time and resources to correct—it is recommended that the intervention be pilot tested again with the improvements in place before implementation.

An integral part of the piloting process is collecting feedback from those in the pilot group. By surveying the pilot group, planners can identify popular and unpopular aspects of the intervention, how the intervention might be changed or improved, and whether the facilitators were effective. This information can be useful in fine-tuning this intervention or in developing future programs.

Once the intervention has been pilot tested and corrected as necessary, it is ready to be disseminated and implemented. Rather than implementing the intervention over an entire target population at once, it is advisable for planners to phase it in gradually. **Phasing in** refers to a step-by-step implementation in which the intervention is introduced first to smaller groups instead of the entire target population. Common criteria used for selecting participating groups for phasing in include participant ability, number of participants, program offerings, and program location.[6]

The following is an example of phasing in by location. Assume that a local health department wants to provide smoking cessation programs for all the smokers in the community (target population). Instead of initiating one big intervention for all, planners could divide the target population by residence location. Facilitators would begin implementation by offering the smoking

cessation classes on the south side of town during the first month. During the second month, they would continue the classes on the south side and begin implementation on the west side of town. They would continue to implement this intervention until all sections of the town were included.

Evaluating the Results

The final step in the basic HP/DP program planning model is the evaluation. Although evaluation is the last step in this model, it really takes place in all steps of program planning. Indeed, it is very important that planning for evaluation occurs during the first stages of program development, not just at the end.

Evaluation is the process by which community health planners determine the value or worth of the objective of interest by comparing it against a **standard of acceptability.** Common standards of acceptability include, but are not limited to, mandates (policies, statues, laws), values, norms, and comparison groups.

Evaluation can be categorized further into summative and formative evaluation. **Formative evaluation** is done during the planning and implementing processes to improve or refine the program. For example, validating the needs assessment and pilot testing are both forms of formative evaluation. **Summative evaluation** begins with the development of goals and objectives and is conducted after implementation to deter-

---

phasing in Implementation of an intervention with a series of small groups instead of the entire population.

evaluation Determining the value or worth of an objective of interest.

standard of acceptability A comparative mandate, value, norm, or group.

formative evaluation The evaluation that is conducted during the planning and implementing processes to improve or refine the program.

summative evaluation The evaluation that determines the impact of a program on the target population.

mine the impact of the program on the target population.

Like other steps in our program planning model, this step can be broken down into smaller steps. The mini-steps of evaluation include planning the evaluation, collecting the necessary valuative data, analyzing the data, and reporting and applying the results.

Planning the Evaluation

As noted earlier, planning for summative evaluation begins with the development of the goals and objectives of the program. These statements put into writing what should happen as a result of the program. Also in this planning mini-step, it should be determined who will evaluate the program: an internal evaluator (one who already is in-

volved in the program) or an external evaluator (one from outside the program). In addition, this portion of the evaluation process should identify an evaluation design and a timeline for carrying out the evaluation.

Collecting the Data

Data collection includes deciding how to collect the data (e.g., with a survey, from existing records, by observation, etc.), determining who will collect them, pilot testing the procedures, and performing the actual data collection (see Figure 5.11).

Analyzing the Data

Once the data are in hand, they must be analyzed and interpreted. Also, it must be decided who will analyze the data and when the analysis is to be completed.

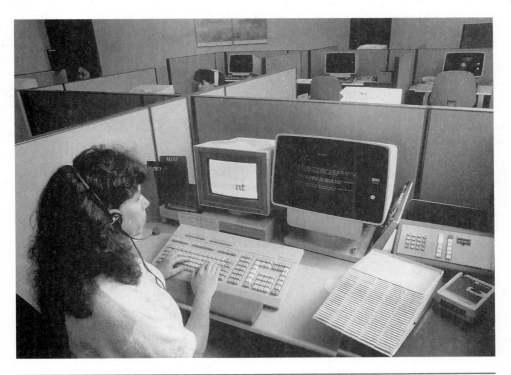

FIGURE 5.11

Data entry and analysis are important components of evaluation.

Reporting Results

The interpretation report should be written. Decisions must be made (if they have not been made already) regarding who should write the report, who should receive the report, in what form, and when.

Applying the Results

With the findings in hand, it then must be decided how they will be used. When time, resources, and effort are spent on an evaluation, it is important that its results be useful for reaching a constructive end, and for deciding whether to continue or discontinue the program or to alter it in some way.

CHAPTER SUMMARY

This chapter presented two important tools of community health practice—community organization and program planning. Community organization, the process by which individuals, groups, and organizations engage in planned action to influence social problems, can be accomplished through one of three models: locality development, social planning, or social action. Each of these models differs a bit from the others, but all contain the basic steps of recognizing the problem, gaining entry into the community, organizing the people, identifying a specific problem, determining priorities and setting goals, arriving at a solution, implementing an intervention, evaluating the efforts, and maintaining the change.

Program planning, a process in which an intervention is planned to help meet the needs of a target population, may or may not be associated with program planning. In either case, it too has several steps. These include assessing the needs, setting goals and objectives, developing an intervention, implementing the intervention, and evaluating the results.

A knowledge of community organization and program planning is essential for community health workers whose job it is to promote and protect the health of the community.

REVIEW QUESTIONS

1. What is the difference between community organization and community development?

2. What are the assumptions (identified by Ross) under which organizers work when bringing a community together to solve a problem?

3. What is the difference between top-down and bottom-up community organization?

4. What is meant by the term *gatekeepers?* Who would they be in your community?

5. Identify the ten steps in the generalized approach to community organization presented in this chapter.

6. What is a needs assessment? Why is it important in the health promotion/disease prevention programming process?

7. What are the five major steps in program development?

8. What are the differences between goals and objectives?

9. What are intervention activities? Give five examples.

10. What is meant by the term *pilot testing?* How is it useful when developing an intervention?

11. Name and briefly describe the five major components of evaluation.

ACTIVITIES

1. From your knowledge of the community in which you live (or from the telephone book yellow pages), generate a list of seven to ten agencies that might be interested in creating a coalition to deal with community drug problems. Provide a one-sentence rationale for why each might want to be involved.

2. Ask your instructor or church leader if he or she is aware of any community organization efforts in a local community. If you are able to identify such an effort, make an appointment—either by yourself or with some of your classmates—to meet with the person

who is leading the effort and ask the following questions:

What is the problem that faces the community?

What is the goal of the group?

What steps have been taken so far to organize the community, and what steps are yet to be taken?

Who is active in the core group?

Did the group conduct a needs assessment?

What intervention will be/has been used?

Is it anticipated that the problem will be solved?

3. Using a smoking cessation program, write one program goal and an objective for each of the levels mentioned in this chapter.

4. Visit a voluntary health agency in your community, either by yourself or with your classmates. Ask employees if you may review any of the standard health promotion/disease prevention programs the agency offers to the community. Examine the program materials, locating the five major components of a program discussed in this chapter. Then in a two-page paper, summarize your findings.

SCENARIO: ANALYSIS AND RESPONSE

The town of Kenzington sounds like a good candidate for a community organization effort. Assume that Kenzington is the town in which you now live. Based upon what you know about the problem in the scenario and what you know about your town, answer these questions.

1. What is the real problem?

2. What strategy might you use to gain entry into the community? Why did you select this strategy?

3. Who do you think the gatekeepers are in the community?

4. What groups of people in the community might be most interested in solving this problem?

5. What groups might have a vested interest in seeing the problem remain unsolved?

6. What will be the name of your task force?

7. What do you think the priorities and goals of this task force should be?

8. What interventions would be useful in dealing with the problem?

9. How would you evaluate your efforts to solve the problem?

10. What strategies might you recommend to make the solution lasting?

REFERENCES

1. Brager, G., H. Specht, and J. L. Torczyner (1987). *Community Organizing*. New York: Columbia Univ. Press, p. 55.

2. Ross, M. G. (1967). *Community Organization: Theory, Principles, and Practice*. New York: Harper and Row, pp. 86–92.

3. United Nations (1955). *Social Progress Through Community Development*. New York: Author, p. 6.

4. Rothman, J., and J. E. Tropman (1987). "Models of Community Organization and Macro Practice Perspectives: Their Mixing and Phasing." In F. M. Cox, J. L. Erlich, J. Rothman, and J. E. Tropman, eds. *Strategies of Community Organization: Macro Practice* (pp. 3–26). Itasca, Ill: F. E. Peacock, pp. 4–5.

5. Alinsky, S. D. (1971). *Rules for Radicals: A Pragmatic Primer for Realistic Radicals*. New York: Random House.

6. McKenzie, J. F., and J. L. Jurs (1993). *Planning, Implementing, and Evaluating Health Promotion Programs: A Primer*. New York: Macmillan.

7. Perlman, J. (1978). "Grassroots Participation from Neighborhood to Nation." In S. Langton, ed. *Citizen Participation in America* (pp. 65–79). Lexington, Mass.: Lexington Books.

8. Braithwaite, R. L., F. Murphy, N. Lythcott, and D. S. Blumenthal (1989). "Community Organization and Development for Health Promotion Within an Urban Black Community: A Conceptual Model." *Health Education,* 20(5): 56–60.

9. U.S. Dept. of Commerce, Bur. of the Census (1992). *Statistical Brief: Family Life Today. . . and How It Has Changed* (SB/92-13). Washington, D.C.: U.S. Government Printing Office.

10. U.S. Dept. of Commerce, Bur. of the Census (1989) *Statistical Brief: Single Parents and Their Children* (SB-3-89). Washington, D.C.: U.S. Government Printing Office.

11. Archer, S. E., and R. P. Fleshman (1985). *Community Health Nursing.* Monterey, Calif.: Wadsworth Health Sciences.

12. Green, L. W., M. W. Kreuter, S. G. Deeds, and K. B. Partridge (1980). *Health Education Planning: A Diagnostic Approach.* Palo Alto, Calif.: Mayfield.

13. Dignan, M. B., and P. A. Carr (1987). *Program Planning for Health Education and Health Promotion.* Philadelphia: Lea and Febiger.

14. Joint Committee on Health Education Terminology (1991). "Report of the 1990 Joint Committee on Health Education Terminology." *Journal of Health Education* 22(2): 103.

15. Sullivan, D. (1973). "Model for Comprehensive, Systematic Program Development in Health Education. *Health Education Report* 1(1) (Nov.–Dec.): 4–5.

16. Green, L. W., and M. W. Kreuter (1991). *Health Promotion Planning: An Educational and Environmental Approach,* 2nd ed. Mountain View, Calif.: Mayfield.

17. Ross, H. S., and P. R. Mico (1980). *Theory and Practice in Health Education.* Palo Alto, Calif.: Mayfield, p. 219.

18. Bates, I. J., and A. E. Winder (1984). *Introduction to Health Education.* Palo Alto, Calif.: Mayfield.

19. Patton, R. W., J. M. Corry, L. R. Gettman, and J. S. Graf (1986). *Implementing Health/Fitness Programs.* Champaign, Ill.: Human Kinetics.

20. Windsor, R. A., T. Baranowski, N. Clark, and G. Cutter (1984). *Evaluation of Health Promotion and Education Programs.* Palo Alto, Calif.: Mayfield.

21. Gilmore, G., M. D. Campbell, and B. L. Becker (1989). *Needs Assessment Strategies for Health Education and Health Promotion.* Indianapolis: Benchmark Press.

22. Jacobsen, D., P. Eggen, and D. Kauchak (1989). *Methods for Teaching: A Skills Approach,* 3rd ed. Columbus, Oh.: Merrill, an imprint of Macmillan.

23. Parkinson, R. S., & Associates (1982). *Managing Health Promotion in the Workplace: Guidelines for Implementation and Evaluation.* Palo Alto, Calif.: Mayfield.

24. U.S. Dept. of Health and Human Services (1990). *Healthy People 2000: National Health Promotion Disease Prevention Objectives* (DHHS pub. no. PHS-90-50212). Washington, D.C.: U.S. Government Printing Office.

25. American Public Health Assn. (1991). *Healthy Communities 2000: Model Standards,* 3rd ed. Washington, D.C.: Author.

Chapter 6

THE SCHOOL HEALTH PROGRAM: A COMPONENT OF COMMUNITY HEALTH

Chapter Outline

Chapter Objectives

After studying this chapter you will be able to:

1. Define *comprehensive school health program.*
2. List the ideal members of a school health team.
3. Explain why a school health program is important.
4. Identify the two major foundations of a comprehensive school health program.
5. Define *written school health policies* and explain their importance to the school health program.
6. Explain processes for developing and implementing school health policies.
7. List the four major components of a comprehensive school health program.
8. Describe the role of the school health coordinator.
9. Identify those services offered as part of school health services and explain why the school is a logical place to offer such services.
10. Describe three models for offering school health services.
11. Explain what is meant by *healthful school environment* and discuss the two major environments.
12. Differentiate between health instruction and school health education.
13. List the three major instructional patterns for teaching health.
14. Identify major school health curricula.
15. Identify and briefly explain three issues that are faced by school health advocates.

Seldom does an elementary school teacher have a typical day. Each day seems to bring a variety of new experiences. Take for example the day Mrs. Graff experienced last Wednesday. Even before the first bell at 8:30 A.M. she was summoned to the hallway, where one of her second-graders became ill and threw up. Remembering her teachers' in-service workshop on HIV and AIDS, Mrs. Graff put into action her new knowledge of universal precautions[1] for handling spilled blood and body fluids. She remembered she was to:

1. Put on disposable gloves (latex or vinyl).
2. Use paper towels to absorb the spill.
3. Place the used towels in a leak-proof plastic bag (extreme spills require a *RED* plastic bag).
4. Flood the area with a bleach solution (one part bleach to ten parts water), alcohol, or a dry sanitary absorbent agent.
5. Clean the area with paper towels, vacuum, or a broom and dust pan.
6. Place used towels, vacuum cleaner bag, or waste in a leak-proof plastic bag.
7. Remove gloves—pull inside out.
8. Place used gloves in a bag and tie.
9. Wash hands with soap and water for at least ten seconds.

After that incident, her day seemed to be going along well until two of Mrs. Graff's students began fighting in the lunch room. They were arguing over who had the healthier lunch. It seemed that Billy thought that his candy bar and cupcake were healthier than Tommy's bag of potato chip doodles. Mrs. Graff was skillful in helping to settle the dispute.

After lunch, Mrs. Graff began her lesson on drug education. She wasn't ten minutes into her lesson when the school nurse stuck her head in the door and asked if Mrs. Graff could send five students for their annual vision screening. Reluctantly, Mrs. Graff excused five of her students.

During the last half-hour of the school day, Mrs. Graff provided the children with quiet time so that they could read or work on some of their homework. Just before the last bell was to ring, Annie brought a sandwich bag with about 20 or so very small bugs up to Mrs. Graff's desk. When Mrs. Graff inquired where the bugs came from, Annie responded, "I picked them out of the hair of the girl sitting in front of me."

Just another "typical day" for Mrs. Graff.

---

[1]From the poster "Universal Precautions: Procedures for Handling Spilled Blood and Body Fluids." Indianapolis: Indiana State Dept. of Health.

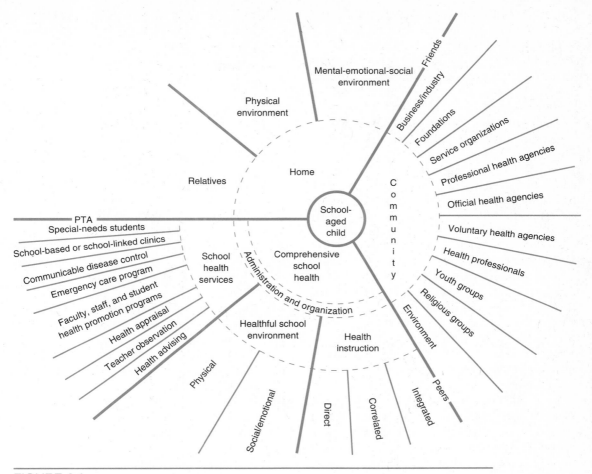

FIGURE 6.1

Influences on the health of a child.

INTRODUCTION

The school health program is an important component of community health. Though the primary responsibility for the health of school-aged children lies with their parents/guardians, the schools have immeasurable potential for affecting the health of children, their families, and eventually the health of the community (see Figure 6.1). In this chapter, we explore the reasons why school health is important, discuss the com-

ponents of school health, and present some of the issues facing school health today.

Definitions

A **comprehensive school health program** has been defined as "an organized set of

---

comprehensive school health program A program to protect and promote the health and well-being of students and staff, which has traditionally included health services, healthful school environment, and health education.

policies, procedures, and activities designed to protect and promote the health and well-being of students and staff which has traditionally included health services, healthful school environment, and health education. It should also include, but not be limited to, guidance and counseling, physical education, food service, social work, psychological services, and employee health promotion."[1]

The school health program has great potential for impacting the health of many. There are over 46 million school-aged children and 5 million instructional and noninstructional employees in the United States.[2] "The knowledge, attitudes, behavior, and skills developed as a result of effective school health programs enable individuals to make informed choices about behavior that will affect their own health throughout their lives, as well as the health of the families for which they are responsible, and the health of the communities in which they live."[3] However, in practice the quality and quantity of comprehensive school health programs in school districts throughout the United States varies greatly. In the majority of school districts, school health programs are not well defined or coordinated. Less than 5% of the school districts in the United States have comprehensive school health programs. Most school districts have some of the basic components of a comprehensive school health program, but those who work with the components usually work independently of each other and thus miss the chance for an even greater effect. For example, it is not unusual for a health teacher to be talking about the importance of aerobic exercise but never tell the physical education teacher. Similarly, a home economics teacher may be teaching a unit on nutrition while the food service workers prepare meals that do not reflect what is being taught in the classroom. Additionally, there is little coordination between school districts and community

health agencies to improve the health of the school-aged child. Table 6.1 provides some possibilities for such interaction.

The School Health Team

In order for comprehensive school health programs to fulfill their potential, a great deal of time and effort must be expended by those involved in the various components of the program. When these individuals work together to plan and implement a school health program they are referred to as the **school health team.** The ideal team would include representation from: administrators, food service workers, counseling personnel, maintenance workers, medical personnel (especially a school nurse and school physician), social workers, parents, students, teachers (especially those who teach health, physical education, and home economics classes), and personnel from appropriate community health agencies. From this group must come a leader or coordinator. Most often the coordinator of the school health team is a health educator or school nurse. The primary role of this team is to provide coordination of the various components of the comprehensive school health program to help students reach and maintain high-quality health.

The School Nurse

As noted above, the school nurse is one of a couple of people who is positioned to provide leadership for a comprehensive school health program (Figure 6.2). The nurse not only has the medical knowledge but should also have formal training in health education and an understanding of the health needs of all children in kinder-

---

school health team Those individuals who work together to plan and implement the school health program.

Table 6.1

Selected Examples of Exchanges by Functions to Integrate School and Community Programs

Functions	Exchanges		
	One-Way	Two-Way	Multiple
Information	Distribution of materials produced by voluntary health agencies	Delivery of workshops/seminars on parenting health issues by school and agency experts	Distribution to multiple agencies, newsletters, calendars of events and/or directory of services
Service	Screening for health problems by volunteer community lay and/or health professional	Cooperative venture utilizing school setting for training of medical students, nursing students, etc.	Collaborative venture by school and community agencies to provide school clinics
Advising and decision making	Formation of school health advisory council	Collaboration by physician/teacher to improve health status and educational attainment	Formation of an interagency management system
Planning and development	Utilization of school recreational facilities for fitness programming by community residents	Utilization of parents as partners in specific instructional strategies	Development of a consortium to implement validated curriculum
Research and evaluation	Providing access for researchers from higher educational institutions	Cooperative submission of a grant proposal by schools and community agency	Utilization of multiagency task force to gather specific health, epidemiological, and social and economic data on adolescent health problems
Monitoring and reporting	Citizen monitoring of school desegregation	Monitoring referrals of students between health and social service agencies to assure continued treatment	Development of Adolescent Services Network to monitor health/educational needs and referral from one agency to another
Training	Utilization of community professionals as consultants for in-service or instructional programs	Utilization of community agencies as learning laboratories for students who serve as volunteers in service/instructional capacity	Utilization of personnel in adolescent health service network to provide in-service programs for respective members
Advocacy	Utilization of parents as fund raisers	Initiation and development of regional school health education coalition by a state school health education advocacy network	Formation of a coalition to publicize the benefits of comprehensive school health
Electoral/ legislative	Citizen campaigning for individuals running for school board	Campaigning for individual whose platform is supportive of school health	Formation of a coalition to promote legislative mandate

Adapted from: Killip, D. C., Lovick, S. R., Goldman, L., Allensworth, D. D. "Integrated School and Community Programs" from *Journal of School Health*, 1987: 57(10), 437–444.

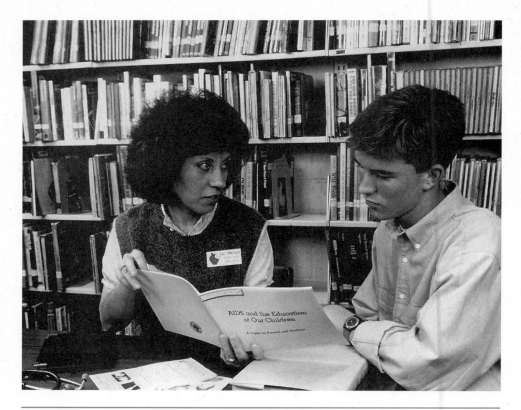

FIGURE 6.2
The school nurse is in a good position to guide the school health program.

garten through the twelfth grade. Some of the key responsibilities of the school nurse as a member of the school health team have been identified.[4] They include:

1. Constructing and/or maintaining health records of all students.
2. Periodically reviewing records to make sure they are accurate and up to date.
3. Dispensing medication to students in accordance with health policies.
4. Providing in-service training on health observation of students to all school personnel.
5. Conducting ongoing follow-up on students referred to health professionals for a potential medical problem.
6. Participating actively in the development of school health policies.
7. Providing or arranging for health counseling for students.
8. Reporting suspected cases of child abuse and/or neglect.
9. Acting as the medical resource person for health education teachers.
10. Identifying students with special medical problems and educating school personnel in how to deal with them.
11. Identifying and using community resources for school health services.

It should be noted that even though school nurses are in a good position to provide leadership to the school team, there are many school districts that do not have the resources to hire a full-time school nurse. It is not uncommon for a school district to contract with an outside health agency like a local health department for nursing services. When this scenario occurs, it is not uncommon for the contracted nurse only to complete the nursing tasks required by state law and not to take on the leadership responsibilities for the school health team. This task may then be fulfilled by a school

health educator. In fact, the health educator may even be responsible when a full-time nurse is present.

The Teacher's Role

Though the school nurse might provide the leadership for a comprehensive school health program, the classroom teachers carry a heavy responsibility in seeing that the program works (see Figure 6.3). On the

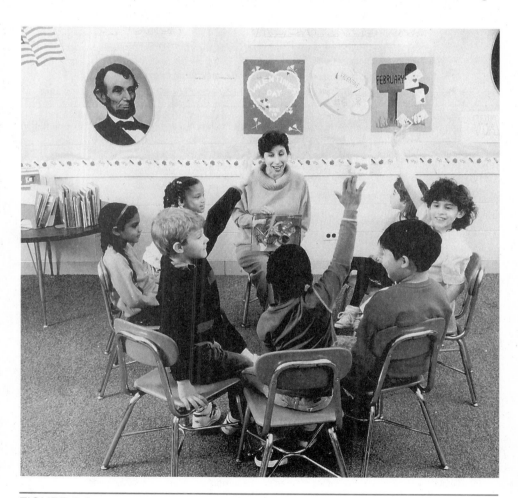

FIGURE 6.3

The classroom teacher's participation is essential for a successful school health program.

Table 6.2

Competencies for Teachers Who Expect to Be
Active Participants in a Comprehensive School Health Program

General

The teacher understands and appreciates:

1. The meaning of health as a multidimensional state of well-being that includes physical, psychological, social, and spiritual aspects.

2. That health of individuals is influenced by the reciprocal interaction of the growing and developing organism and environmental factors and is necessary for optimal functioning as productive members of society.

3. The significance of children's and youths' health problems on learning.

4. The importance and the need for the school health program in today's society.

5. The nature of the total school health program.

6. The role of the teacher in each of the school health program components—services, environment, and instruction.

7. The influence on students of teacher health and teacher health habits.

8. The need for basic scientific information about a variety of health content areas, including dental health; drugs (alcohol, tobacco, and other drugs); care of eyes, ears, and feet; exercise, fitness, rest, and fatigue; prevention and control of diseases and disorders (communicable and chronic); safety and first aid; family health; consumer health; community health; environmental health; nutrition; mental health; anatomy; and physiology.

Health instruction

The teacher:

1. Can identify and use a variety of techniques and procedures to determine the health needs and interests of pupils.

2. Is able to organize the health instruction program around the needs and interests of students and can develop effective teaching units for the grade being taught.

3. Is able to stress the development of attitudes and behaviors for healthful living based on scientific health information.

4. Can distinguish between the various patterns of health instruction and attempts to use the direct approach in teaching whenever possible.

5. Realizes that health education must receive time in the school program along with other subject areas.

6. Possesses current scientific information about a variety of health content areas.

7. Can use a variety of stimulating and motivating teaching techniques derived from fundamental principles of learning.

8. Is able to identify and use "teachable moments" or incidents that occur in the classroom, in the school, or in the community.

9. Uses a variety of teaching aids in the instructional program and is familiar with their sources.

10. Is familiar with the sources of scientific information and the procedures necessary to keep up to date with current health information.

11. Is able to provide a variety of alternative solutions to health problems to enable students to make wiser decisions.

12. Can integrate health into other phases of the curriculum, such as social science, science, and language arts.

13. Uses a variety of evaluative procedures periodically to (a) assess the effectiveness of the program on students and (b) determine the quality and usefulness of teaching aids and materials.

Health services

The teacher:

1. Is familiar with the characteristics of the healthy child and can recognize signs and symptoms of unhealthy conditions; refers problems to the school nurse or other appropriate school personnel.

2. Is familiar with the variety of health appraisal procedures used in schools and uses them to enrich the health instruction program.

3. Acquires limited skill in counseling and guiding students and parents regarding student health problems.

4. Understands the value and purposes of teacher-nurse conferences.

5. Is familiar with the variety of health personnel found in schools, their functions, responsibilities, and usefulness to the teacher.

6. Is able to use information contained on health records.

7. Can identify and follow the policies and procedures in schools with regard to such matters as emergency care, accidents, disease control, and referrals, exclusions, and readmittance of pupils.

8. Can administer immediate care when accidents or illnesses to pupils occur or can act promptly to obtain sources of help within the school.

9. Is able to adjust the school program to the individual health needs of students.

10. Is able to relate the health services program to the health instruction program.

Healthful school living

The teacher:

1. Is familiar with the standards for hygiene, sanitation, and safety needed in schools to provide a safe and healthful environment.

2. Is familiar with the physical and emotional needs of students and adjusts classroom activities to help students satisfy these needs whenever possible.

3. Understands the nature and importance of the food services program and is able to relate it to the instructional program.

4. Is able to recognize hazardous conditions on the playground, in the classroom, and elsewhere in the school and takes appropriate action to eliminate or correct such conditions.

5. Is cognizant of the effect of teacher health, personality, biases, and prejudices on student health and learning and is concerned with the humane treatment of pupils.

6. Integrates healthful environmental aspects into the health instruction program.

Coordination

The teacher:

1. Understands the need for school and community health councils or committees and is willing to participate as a member if requested to do so.

2. Realizes the importance of and need for a coordinator, consultant, or a person with administrative responsibility being in charge of the school health program.

From: Redican, K. J., L. K. Olsen, and C. R. Baffi (1986). *Organization of School Health Programs.* New York: Macmillan, pp. 27–28.

average school day, teachers spend more waking hours with school-aged children than their parents do. A teacher may spend six to eight hours a day with children while parents spend an hour with the child before school and maybe four to five hours with the child after school and before bedtime. Teachers are also in a position to make judgments on the "normal and abnormal" behavior and condition of children since they are able to compare the students in their classroom each day. Table 6.2 presents a suggested list of competencies for teachers who expect to be active and full participants in a comprehensive school health program.[5]

WHY SCHOOL HEALTH?

The primary role of schools is to educate. However, an unhealthy child has a difficult time learning. Consider for example, a child who arrives at school with a slight temperature, runny nose, and without adequate sleep. This child will be unable to concentrate on school work and may infect other children. You, yourself, know how difficult it is to study for a test or even to read this textbook when you do not feel well or are sleepy or hungry (see Box 6.1).

"Health of children and their learning are reciprocally related."[5] Children must be

---

BOX 6.1
It Is Harder to Learn if You Are Not Healthy!

It stands to reason that if children are not healthy it is harder for them to concentrate and in turn to have a meaningful learning experience. One such example of this has been documented by researchers who have studied the impact of breakfast on learning. Now there is scientific evidence to back the claim that "breakfast may be the most important meal of the day."

It was obvious back in the mid-1960s that millions of children were coming to school hungry and ill prepared to learn. As such, in 1966, Congress authorized a two-year pilot School Breakfast Program (SBP) aimed at children from lower-socioeconomic-level families and children who had to travel long distances to school. Congressional amendments extended the SBP through 1975 when it became permanently authorized in PL 94-105. Today, as both a nutrition and education program, the SBP is available to all students nationwide in schools offering the program. In order for schools to receive financial support for the SBP, they must meet minimal nutritional standards as set forth in the SBP meal pattern established by the U.S. Department of Agriculture's Food and Nutrition Service. The

SBP is then offered at no cost, a reduced price, or at full price depending on the students' family size and income.

Because the SBP has been in place for a number of years, several studies have been conducted with those who have participated in SBP. Results of these studies show that students who participate in SBP enhanced their abilities to learn, compared to those who do not. SBP participants showed significantly greater improvements in standardized test scores and decreases in tardiness rates and absenteeism. Beyond the educational benefits, SBP participation has also improved total daily nutrient intake and nutritional status, shown to help control body weight by minimizing impulsive eating, and possibly reducing risk of coronary heart disease by lowering blood cholesterol levels.

The SBP provides a vivid example of: (1) how the school acts as a community health service provider, and (2) how school health education can reach beyond the traditional health education classroom.

Source: National Dairy Council (1993) "Breakfast, Its Effects on Health and Behavior." *Dairy Council Digest* 64(2): 7–12.

BOX 6.2

Healthy People 2000— Objectives

8.4   Increase to at least 75% the proportion of the Nation's elementary and secondary schools that provide planned and sequential kindergarten through 12th grade quality school health education.

(Baseline data not available.)

8.5   Increase to at least 50% the proportion of postsecondary institutions with institutionwide health promotion programs for students, faculty, and staff. (Baseline: At least 20% of higher-education institutions offered health promotion activities for students in 1989–90.)

Baseline data source: American College Health Association

For Further Thought

Assuming money is available, why doesn't every school district in the nation have a K–12 school health education program?

Nevertheless, a comprehensive school health program is not a panacea. There are no quick and easy solutions to improving the overall health of a community. However, a comprehensive school health program provides a strong base upon which to build.

FOUNDATIONS OF THE SCHOOL HEALTH PROGRAM

The true foundations of any school health program are: 1) a well-organized school health team that is genuinely interested in providing a comprehensive program for the students, (2) a school administration that supports such an effort, and (3) school health policies. Every effort should be made to employ personnel who are appropriately trained to carry out their responsibilities as members of the school health team. For example, the Association for the Advancement of Health Education (AAHE) has recommended that the "minimal requirements for school nurses should be state licensure as a registered professional nurse, a baccalaureate degree, including study in health education,"[6] yet many school nurses without college degrees and training in health education are asked to teach. Conversely, certified teachers who lack preparation in health screening procedures are sometimes asked to administer screening tests to students.[7] Qualified personnel are a must!

A highly supportive administration is also a necessity for a quality comprehensive school health program. In almost all organizations—and schools are no different—the administration controls resources. Without leadership and support from top school administrators, it will be an ongoing struggle to provide a quality program.

healthy to obtain the maximum benefit from their educational experiences, but these experiences must also provide them with the knowledge and skills to enable them to live in a healthful manner. A comprehensive school health program provides the integration of education and health.

The importance of the school health program is also evident by its mention in the national health objectives for the year 2000. Of all the objectives listed in the publication *Healthy People 2000: National Health Promotion and Disease Prevention Objectives,* more than one-third can either be directly attained by schools or their attainment can be influenced in important ways by schools[3] (see Box 6.2).

SCHOOL HEALTH POLICIES

School health policies are written statements used to guide all those who work within the program.[7] The written policy also describes the nature of the program and the procedure for its implementation to those outside the program.[8] A well-written school health policy provides a sense of direction, credibility, and a means of accountability for the school health program.

Policy Development

The development of a set of written policies is not an easy task. This challenging and time-consuming task should be executed by the school health team, since the team includes those most knowledgeable about the school health program and also represents many different constituencies in the school community.

The policies should cover all facets of the school health program. See Table 6.3 for a checklist that can be used for developing policies.

Once the policies have been written, it is important that they receive approval at three levels. Approval should come from (1) the school district's medical advisor, (2) the school administration, and (3) the board of education. The approval process provides credibility to the policies as well as legal protection for those who must implement the policies.[8]

Policy Implementation

The development of written policies is an important step to building a solid base for a comprehensive school health program. But if the policies are never implemented, the school district will be no better off than before their development.

Implementation begins with the distribution of the policy to those who will be affected by it—faculty, staff, students, and parents. Some ideas for carrying out this process include: (1) distribution of the policy with a memorandum of explanation, (2) placing the policy in both faculty/staff and student handbooks, (3) presenting it at a gathering of the different groups (e.g., staff or PTO meetings, or an open house), or (4) holding a special meeting for the specific purpose of explaining the policy. News releases might even be considered if the policy includes major changes. Each school district must decide the best way to disseminate its school health policies.

MAJOR COMPONENTS OF A COMPREHENSIVE SCHOOL HEALTH PROGRAM

If implemented appropriately, a comprehensive school health program should impact every employee and student within the school district. In order to do so, the program needs to include four major components: (1) administration and organization, (2) school health services, (3) a healthful school environment, and (4) health instruction. Each of these components is addressed below.

Administration and Organization

Effective administration and organization of the school health program insures that the people and activities that constitute

---

school health policies Written statements that describe the nature and procedures of a school health program.

the program work in a coordinated manner to meet the goals of the program. The responsibility for coordinating the program in each school district should be delegated to a properly trained and thoroughly knowledgeable individual. Logical choices for this position of **school health coordinator,** would be a properly trained school nurse, a health educator, or even a school physician. At the present time, approximately one-half of the states and territories in the United States have school districts who employ school health coordinators. There are only a few states that require such a person.[9]

Schaller[10] presented a list of the functions of a school health coordinator. Below is a revision of this original list of seven functions with several others added to it.

1. Organize and supervise all aspects of the school health program.
2. Organize and supervise those on the school health team as they contribute to the goals of the school health program.
3. Insure that written school health policies are in place and understood by those who they affect.
4. Insure that the school district has an appropriate and functional school health record-keeping system.
5. Coordinate the activities of the program with those in the community—working with health departments, civic and service organizations, professional associations, parents, police, safety specialists, health care providers, private and voluntary agencies, and community health councils.
6. Serve as a consultant to professional and nonteaching personnel on health activities.

7. Help to develop and continually update a progressive, well-coordinated health curriculum in grades K–12.
8. Plan for an in-service education program that keeps those involved with the school health program up to date.
9. Plan for and implement a continuous evaluation of the program.

School Health Services

"**School health services** are that part of the school health program provided by physicians, nurses, dentists, health educators, other allied health personnel, social workers, teachers, and others to appraise, protect and promote the health of students and school personnel."[1] Specifically, those services offered by schools include health appraisals (screenings and examinations), emergency care for injury and sudden illness, prevention and control of communicable disease, provisions for special/handicapped students, health advising, and remediation of detected health problems within the limits of state laws through referral and follow-up by the school nurse and teachers (see Figure 6.4). Over the years, the intent of school health services has been to supplement rather than to supplant the family's responsibility for meeting the health care needs of its children. However, because of the poorer health status of youth, the involvement of youth in high risk behaviors such as smoking, drinking, substance abuse, and unprotected sexual intercourse, such barriers to health care as inadequate health insurance and lack of providers, and inappropriate use of the present health system, local, state and national policy makers are considering a

---

school health coordinator A person who coordinates the school health program for a school district.

school health services Health services provided by school health workers to appraise, protect, and promote the health of students and school personnel.

Table 6.3
A Checklist for Developing Written Policies

	PIP	PN	NA
I. Administration and Organization			
A. Duties and responsibilities of the coordinator of the school health program			
B. Duties and responsibilities of the school health team			
C. Responsibilities of school health personnel			
1. Medical advisor			
2. School nurse			
3. Health instructors			
4. Other teachers			
5. First-aiders			
6. Other related personnel			
7. Volunteers			
D. School health records			
1. Recording of health history			
2. Maintenance of school health records			
a. What will be entered (results of screenings and examination, emergency illness/injury)			
b. Who will enter the information			
3. Information for emergency situations			
4. Recording of student immunizations			
E. General School Health Policies			
1. Use of prescribed medication in the school			
2. Report of child abuse and neglect			
3. Substance use/abuse			
4. Student health insurance			
5. Home health visits			
6. Health policies for after-school activities (including emergency care)			
7. Sending ill/injured students home			
8. Relationships with community health agencies/organizations			
9. In-service health programs for teachers			
II. School Health Services			
A. Emergency care for illness/injury			
1. Duties of school employees in the emergency care program			
2. Responsibility for financial charges incurred in the emergency care process (e.g., transportation fees, hospital charges, etc.)			
3. Use of emergency care room/health clinic			
4. Purchase and availability of emergency care supplies and equipment			
5. Standing orders for common emergency problems			
6. Notification of personnel needed in an emergency situation			
7. Responsibility for transportation of ill/injured student			
8. Completion and filing of accident reports			
9. Procedure for follow-up inquiry into the post-emergency condition of a student			
10. Procedure for readmission of an injured/ill student to school attendance			
11. Universal precautions outlined			
B. Handicapped students			
1. Procedures to adhere to Public Law 94:142			
2. Procedures to adhere to all state laws			
C. Health Appraisal			
1. Medical examinations			
a. Financial responsibilities			
b. Who will perform them			
c. When will they be required (including athletic examinations)			

	PIP	PN	NA
2. Screening programs			
a. Who will perform them			
b. What tests will be given			
c. When will they be given			
d. Follow-up procedures			
3. Dental examinations			
a. Who will perform them			
b. Financial responsibilities			
c. When will they be required			
d. Follow-up procedures			
4. Social and psychological evaluations			
a. Who will perform them			
b. Financial responsibilities			
c. When will they be required			
d. Follow-up procedures			
5. Policy for health referrals to parents			
D. Communicable Disease Control	▓	▓	▓
1. Required immunizations			
2. Student exclusion from when he/she has measles, German measles, chicken pox, scarlet fever, infectious hepatitis, nuisance disease, athlete's foot, impetigo, ringworm, pinkeye, and other communicable disease			
3. Readmittance policy after a communicable disease			
E. Health Advising	▓	▓	▓
1. Who will perform it			
2. When will it be performed			
3. Steps in referral			
4. Procedures for follow-up			
III. School Health Environment	▓	▓	▓
A. Safety Program			
1. Responsibilities of school personnel			
2. Expected student classroom conduct			
3. Maintenance of equipment/instructional materials			
4. Reporting of unsafe conditions in school environment			
B. Safety Patrol and Bus Safety	▓	▓	▓
1. Responsibilities of school personnel			
2. Responsibilities and procedures of students			
C. Emergency Drills (fire, tornado, etc.)	▓	▓	▓
1. Drill procedures			
2. Emergency exit procedures			
3. Procedure to help individuals with special needs in an emergency situation			
D. Food Service	▓	▓	▓
1. Responsibilities of school personnel			
IV. Health Instruction	▓	▓	▓
A. Curriculum guides	▓	▓	▓
1. Procedures for curriculum development and revision			
2. Individual Education Programs for students with special needs			

Code:

PIP = Policy in place
PN = Policy Needed
NA = Not applicable to our district

From: McKenzie, J. F. (1983). "Written Policies: Developing a Solid Foundation for a Comprehensive School Health Program." *Future Focus: Ohio Journal of Health, Physical Education, Recreation and Dance* 4(3):9–11.

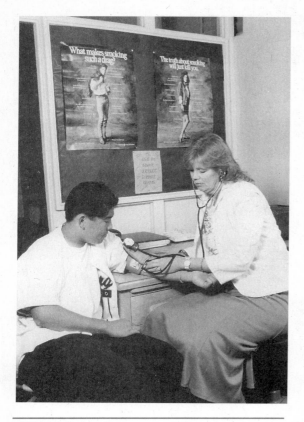

FIGURE 6.4

Health screenings are important components of school health services.

broadening of the role of schools in providing health care.[11]

Because school attendance is required throughout the United States, schools represent our best opportunity to reach many of those children in need of proper health care. "The school's ability to reach children and youth disenfranchised from the health care system and at highest risk for poor health and potentially health-threatening behaviors is unmatched."[11] The advantages[12] of having school health services include:

1. Equitability: School health services provide a point of entry into the health care system for *all* children in school.

2. Breadth of coverage: Many preventive services are provided that are not covered in a majority of health insurance policies.
3. Confidentiality.
4. User friendliness: The school is an environment with which students are familiar and in which they feel comfortable.
5. Convenience: Services are accessible to all students.

Each school district is unique, from the demographics of their students to the availability of its health resources. As such, three models have been developed which describe the delivery of school health services: (1) basic health services, (2) expanded health services, and (3) comprehensive health services (see Figure 6.5). The basic health services model views the school district in the role of health screener. In this model, emphasis is placed on the detection of health problems and the referral to providers in the community for treatment. This is the model most commonly found in the schools today.

The expanded health model builds upon the basic health model and extends it by providing comprehensive care for medically underserved students. This model not only requires more health care provider services in the school but also permits a better opportunity for preventative education.

The comprehensive health model includes the services offered in both the basic and expanded health models but in addition provides comprehensive and self-contained services via a school-based clinic. Such a clinic would employ a number of health care professionals on a full-time basis. The idea of school-based clinics is gaining momentum throughout the country and will be discussed in greater detail later in this chapter.

Healthful School Environment

The term *healthful school environment*, sometimes referred to as *healthful school*

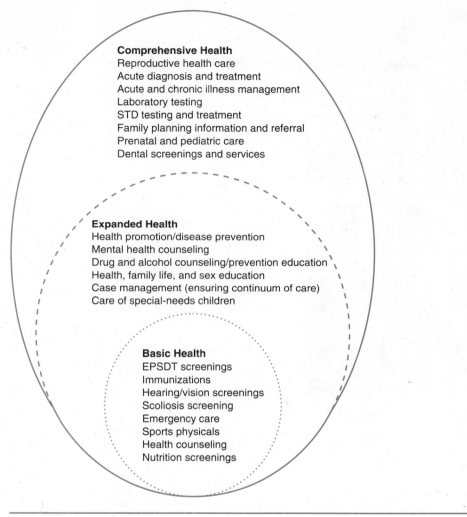

Comprehensive Health
Reproductive health care
Acute diagnosis and treatment
Acute and chronic illness management
Laboratory testing
STD testing and treatment
Family planning information and referral
Prenatal and pediatric care
Dental screenings and services

Expanded Health
Health promotion/disease prevention
Mental health counseling
Drug and alcohol counseling/prevention education
Health, family life, and sex education
Case management (ensuring continuum of care)
Care of special-needs children

Basic Health
EPSDT screenings
Immunizations
Hearing/vision screenings
Scoliosis screening
Emergency care
Sports physicals
Health counseling
Nutrition screenings

FIGURE 6.5

School health services.

From: Schlitt, J. J. (June 1991). "Issue Brief—Bringing Health to School: Policy Implications for Southern States." Washington, D.C.: Southern Center on Adolescent Pregnancy Prevention and Southern Regional Project on Infant Mortality. Printed in Journal of School Health *62(2): 60a–60h.*

living, designates that part of a comprehensive school health program which provides for a safe—both physically and emotionally—learning environment (Figure 6.6). If children are not placed in a safe environment, learning becomes difficult at best. The most recent definition of *healthful envi-* *ronment* was provided by the 1972–1973 Joint Committee on Health Education Terminology. They stated that providing a **healthful school environment** includes "the promotion, maintenance, and utilization of safe and wholesome surroundings, organization of day-by-day experiences and

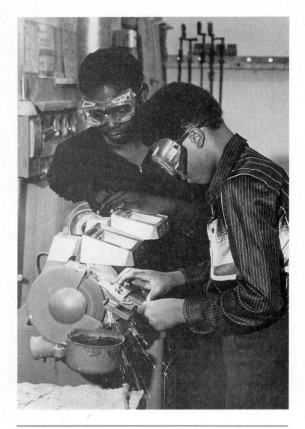

FIGURE 6.6

The school should be a safe and healthful place to learn.

planned learning procedures to influence favorable emotional, physical and social health."[13]

By law, school districts are required to provide a safe school environment. However, the responsibility for maintaining this safe environment should rest with all who use it. Everyone, including those on the board of education, administrators, teachers, custodial staff, and students, must con-

---

healthful school environment The promotion, maintenance, and utilization of safe and wholesome surroundings in a school environment.

tribute to make a school a safer place via their daily actions. An unsafe school environment can exist only if those responsible for it and those who use it let it exist.

The Physical Environment

The physical environment of a school can be divided into two major categories. The first is the actual physical plant, the buildings and surrounding areas and all that come with them. The second is the behaviors of those using the buildings. The factors that must be considered when looking at the physical plant are things like: (1) where the school is located, (2) the age of the buildings, (3) the traffic patterns in and around the school, (4) temperature control, (5) lighting, (6) acoustics, (7) water supply, (8) sanitation, (9) food service, (10) playgrounds, (11) school bus safety, and other items. Each school district should have an appropriate protocol for dealing with and maintaining these aspects of the physical environment.

The behavior of both the school personnel and students in the school environment also has an impact on the safety of the environment. Each year a significant number of students throughout the country are injured on their way to, at, or on their way home from school. Some of these injuries occur from an unsafe physical plant that is in need of repair, but many occur from inappropriate behavior. Unsafe behavior that is observed too frequently in schools includes acts of violence between students and smoking by school employees. Even with such problems, few school employees or students wake up each day with a healthful school environment on their minds. Most do not worry about a safe environment until they are faced with a problem. Every school building in the United States could become a safer environment if greater attention were given to prevention than to cure. Table 6.4 presents a checklist that can be used to provide feedback on a safe learning environment.

The Social/Emotional Environment

Although a safe physical environment is important, a safe social/emotional environment is equally important. Students who are fearful of responding to a teacher's question because the teacher might make fun of them if they answer incorrectly or students who are afraid to say hello to the school principal because he is never nice to anyone are not learning in a healthful social/emotional environment. For many, learning does not come easily and anxiety-producing factors like these can only make it more difficult.

The ways in which school personnel and students treat each other can add much to the teaching/learning process (see Figure 6.7). All individuals within the school should be treated with respect. People should be polite and courteous to each other. This does not mean that high academic standards should not be upheld and that everyone should agree with all that others do, but students and teachers should not be afraid to express themselves in a cooperative, respectful way. For example, think back to your middle school and high school days. Think about the teachers you liked best. Did you like them because they were great teachers and knew their subject well? Or did you like them because of the way they treated and respected you? The social/emotional environment can have a significant impact on the school environment!

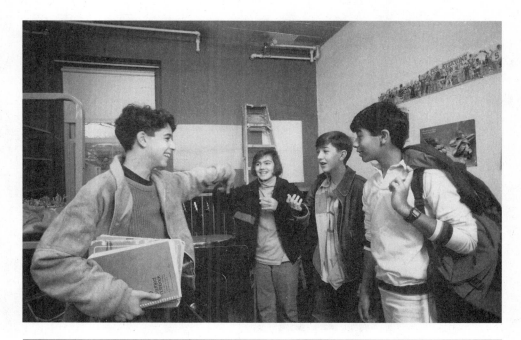

FIGURE 6.7

A healthy social environment, conducive to learning, is an important component of good school health.

Table 6.4

A Self-Awareness Checklist for a Safe Learning Environment

	Yes	No	Comment
1. There are clearly defined written policies regarding the safe conduct of children in the learning environment:			
a. Students have helped develop the policies.			
b. The policies are short and concise.			
c. The policies are discussed with the children.			
d. Parents are apprised of the policies.			
e. The policies are posted in the classroom for all to read.			
f. New policies are developed annually.			
2. The teacher uses constant foresight and prudent behavior inherent in the role of the professional educator by:			
a. Providing appropriate supervision.			
b. Using rational behavior.			
c. Eliminating the presence of any attractive nuisance.			
d. Not allowing student horseplay.			
e. Providing an attractive, pleasant, and safe surrounding.			
f. Providing a good mental/emotional learning environment.			
g. Being (and promote being) polite, patient, and courteous.			
3. The physical learning environment is well maintained:			
a. The area is clean.			
b. Wastes are disposed of properly.			
c. The furniture is maintained and is appropriate for the students.			
d. Classroom services are well maintained (water, electric, heating, lighting, gases, etc.).			
e. Maintenance problems are reported so they can be corrected.			
4. There is an appropriate traffic pattern for the classroom:			
a. The exit(s) is (are) appropriately marked.			
b. More than one exit is available.			
c. Aisle ways are wide enough and clear of obstacles.			
d. There is appropriate space for the learning activities.			
5. Classroom activities are well planned:			
a. Activities are appropriate for the abilities, capacities, skill, and age of the students.			
b. Activities are appropriate for the facility.			
c. The teacher includes the appropriate safety information with classroom activities.			
d. The teacher makes the students aware of the possible dangers in an activity.			
6. The equipment/instructional materials are well maintained:			
a. The equipment/materials are inspected on a regular basis.			
b. The equipment/materials are kept in good condition with the faulty or broken equipment/materials being repaired or discarded.			
c. Policies exist regarding the safe use of all equipment/materials.			
d. The equipment/materials are stored properly when not in use.			
e. Appropriate equipment/materials are always used (e.g., glass vs. plastic).			
f. Students are required to wear appropriate clothing for the activity.			

	Yes	No	Comment
7. Procedures for emergency drills (fire, tornado, etc.) are well defined and practiced on a routine basis:			
a. Teacher and students know emergency drill procedures.			
b. Teachers and students know how to use the fire alarms and fire fighting equipment (extinguishers).			
c. Teacher and students know more than one way to exit building.			
d. Emergency exit plans are posted.			
e. Procedures have been planned for helping students with special needs in emergency drill situations.			
8. Procedures for emergency are well defined.			
a. The teacher's first aid and CPR skills are up to date.			
b. Students, as well as teachers, know what to do in case of sudden illness or injury.			
c. There is a first aid kit available in the room.			
d. The teacher never conducts an activity without a plan for medical assistance if needed.			
e. Accident report forms are completed according to school policy.			
9. The above safety concerns are followed in all areas of the school building, but special concern is given when children are under the supervision of the teacher in special areas (pool, labs, playground, etc.)			

From: McKenzie, J. F., and I. C. Williams (1982). "Are Your Students Learning in a Safe Environment.?" *Journal of School Health* 52(5):284–285.

Health Instruction

Health instruction has been defined as

the development, delivery, and evaluation of a planned curriculum, preschool through 12, with goals, objectives, content sequence, and specific classroom lessons which include, but are not limited to, the following major content areas:

- Community health
- Consumer health
- Environmental health
- Family life
- Mental and emotional health
- Injury prevention and safety
- Nutrition
- Personal health
- Prevention and control of disease
- Substance use and abuse.[1]

Health instruction is only a part of school health education. *School health education* includes all health education in the school (Figure 6.8). For example, health education can take place when the school nurse gives a vision screening test to a student or when coaches talk with their teams about the abuse of drugs. Health education includes health instruction as well as any other activities designed to positively influence the health knowledge and skills of students, parents, and school staff (see Box 6.3).

For health instruction to be effective, it should be well conceived and carefully

---

health instruction The development, delivery, and evaluation of a planned curriculum, preschool through grade 12.

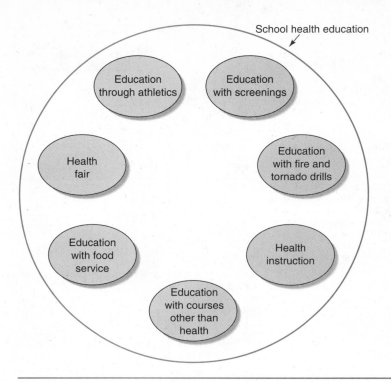

School health education

Education through athletics

Education with screenings

Health fair

Education with fire and tornado drills

Education with food service

Health instruction

Education with courses other than health

FIGURE 6.8

The relationship of school health education and health instruction.

planned. The written plan for school health instruction is referred to as the health **curriculum.** The curriculum not only outlines the **scope** (what will be taught), and the **sequence** (when it will be taught), but also provides (1) objectives, (2) learning activities, (3) possible instructional resources, and (4) methods for determining the extent to which learning objectives were met. If health instruction is to be effective, the health curriculum should include lessons of appropriate scope and sequence for all

grades from kindergarten through the twelfth grade.

Approaches to Designing an Instructional Curriculum

A number of different approaches have been used by schools to develop their health curricula. However, the three primary approaches are direct instruction, correlated instruction, and integrative instruction.

Direct Instruction

The **direct instruction** pattern is one in which health is identified as a separate

---

curriculum   A written plan for instruction.
scope   Part of the curriculum that outlines what will be taught.
sequence   Part of the curriculum that states in what order the content will be taught.

---

direct instruction   A pattern of instruction in which subject matter is identified as a separate subject.

BOX 6.3
Controversy and School Health

Certain topics taught as part of the school health curriculum 30 years ago were labeled "controversial." In some parts of the country, they are still considered controversial today. Many of the topics that are considered a part of a comprehensive sex education unit like abortion, birth control, homosexuality, masturbation, and premarital intercourse still bring citizens to board of education meetings to express their opinions.

A recent incident of such concern occurred in May 1993 in a community of about 75,000 in Indiana, at the Community School Board of Education meeting. At that meeting, the school district's curriculum director made a recommendation, based upon the work of a committee, to adopt a specific middle school health education text. The textbook was one that had been adopted by many school districts throughout the country and published by one of the leading high school textbook companies. However, when some parents in the community discovered the textbook included several "controversial" sex education topics, they appeared at the board of education meeting to express their opinion. Selected parental quotes included: "it's the parents', not the teachers', place to teach about those

subjects"; "This curriculum challenges a lot of those values we have tried to instill. This is not diagramming a sentence or multiplication. It deals with issues such as abortion, homosexuality, and birth control"; "the book is amoral"; and "It [the book] is undermining family values."

This issue was controversial because it had two sides to it. Other parents in the community stated: "It's fine and dandy to say we parents should teach [about sex education], but we're not doing it as a community, and sometimes children don't listen to their parents"; and "I wanted to see a textbook that addressed date rape as well as abstinence."

After considerable discussion and debate, the school district's curriculum director suggested the book adoption be tabled until further study of the matter could be concluded. The board unanimously approved that motion. Though a final decision was not made at the time this book was written, those close to the issue predicted that at a later meeting, the board of education would adopt a different textbook in which the sex education unit was contained in a supplemental book. And as one might guess, the supplemental book would not be adopted.

subject and is allocated a specified amount of teaching time in the school day along with other subjects such as mathematics, English, and science. This pattern provides for the greatest opportunity for a sequential program arranged to consider the needs, interests, and developmental levels of the students.[5] Direct instruction, which is the method of health instruction preferred by school health advocates, is usually provided by a teacher or school nurse trained in health education (i.e., as a college major or minor) or by an elementary

school teacher who has had college course work in health education.

Correlated Instruction

In the **correlated instruction** pattern, health content is integrated into many other subjects and not taught as its own subject. For example, the home economics teachers would be responsible for teaching nutrition and family life education, science teachers

correlated instruction A pattern of instruction in which the subject matter is taught in many other subjects.

would present the disease process, physical education teachers would include information on exercise, and sociology teachers would include information on community health agencies and resources. It should be obvious that this pattern of instruction would require a great deal of coordination and planning to insure that all necessary topics were covered and that the curriculum was properly sequenced. This pattern of health instruction usually uses teachers not formally trained in health education to present the health curriculum.

Integrated Instruction

The **integrated instruction** pattern involves the teaching of health as a vehicle to teach other subjects (see Figure 6.9). For example, a teacher who has the primary task of reading uses a health-related story to teach reading skills. Or a mathematics teacher may use weight maintenance via calorie consumption and expenditure to teach computation. Integrated instruction, like correlated instruction, requires a great deal of planning to insure that an appropriate health curriculum is presented. Two major drawbacks of this approach have been identified "(1) the major emphasis in the learning may be on a special subject area rather than health, and (2) the learning objectives stressed may be on the acquisition of information, factual data, or the skills of writing, reading, or computation rather than healthful living."[5]

Curriculum Development

Each year, many school districts throughout the United States are faced with the task of developing a curriculum to guide health instruction. Such a task can be completed in one of several ways. One, a school district could purchase a prepackaged cur-

riculum that has been developed by nationally recognized specialists. A second means could be to use the state Department of Education's approved curriculum. Another method would be to adopt a new health textbook series and consider the series as a district's curricular guide. Some districts may even develop their own in-house curriculum. Each of these approaches has its strengths and weakness, and school districts have to decide which approach best suits their particular situation. It is not within the scope of this chapter to provide a full discussion of curricular development, and such discussions are available elsewhere. Nonetheless, we do think it is important to present information on some of the major curriculum efforts in health.

Determining what is and what is not a good curriculum can be a difficult process. Some very poor curricula, packaged in a "slick" way, can convince administrators that they have purchased a very fine product. Conversely, some educationally sound programs may not be well packaged. Fortunately, there is a federally funded project that can reduce the guesswork for those who must choose curricula. The **National Diffusion Network (NDN)** provides exemplary and proven curricula for all subjects areas available for schools to review and adopt.

The NDN was created in 1973 under the Secondary Education Act of 1965. The network works in the following way. When a new curriculum has been developed, the funding agency which backed the curriculum development or the curriculum developers themselves may nominate the curriculum for review by NDN if the curriculum is considered exemplary. The NDN defines "exemplary" to be a curriculum that both is educationally effective with the tar-

---

integrated instruction A pattern of instruction in which a certain subject matter is the vehicle used to teach other subjects.

National Diffusion Network (NDN) An organization that reviews and rates curricula.

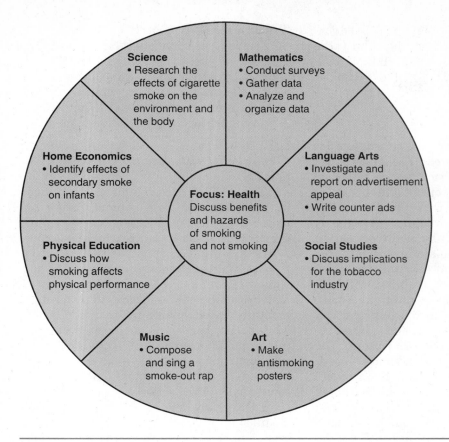

FIGURE 6.9

Sample planning wheel: Smoke Free 2000.

From: Allensworth, D. D. (1993). "Health Education: State of the Art." Journal of School Health *63(1): 16. After Palmer, J. M. (1991). "Planning Wheels Turn Curriculum Around."* Educational Leadership *49(2): 58. Reprinted with permission of the Association for Supervision and Curriculum Development and Joan Palmer. Copyright © 1991 by ASCD. All rights reserved.*

get population and that can be delivered in a cost-effective manner. The NDN considers the nominations, and if then it feels the exemplary criteria are met, the curriculum will be submitted to a panel for review. If approved, it will then be included on the NDN diffusion list. An approved curriculum has the potential to receive several benefits including: (1) eligibility for diffusion funds from NDN or other funding agencies, (2) program recognition both by professionals and by the public through awareness work-shops, (3) inclusion in the federal diffusion system, and (4) enhanced chances for obtaining competitive federal funding.[5] At the present time, only one comprehensive health curriculum is included in the NDN diffusion list, and that is "Growing Healthy."

Another means of judging the worth of a curriculum is to compare it to the *Criteria for Comprehensive Health Education Curricula.* This publication was designed to help school personnel select or develop kindergarten to 12th-grade health education curricula. It is available from the American School Health Association (P.O. Box 708, Kent, OH 44240, (216) 678-1601).

Curriculum Models

"Growing Healthy"

"**Growing Healthy**" is a curriculum for grades K–6 that was created when two previously created curricula—the "School Health Curriculum Project" and the "Primary Grades Health Curriculum Project"—were merged. This curriculum is taught by classroom teachers, not by health education specialists. Teachers planning to use this curriculum must attend an intensive training session. During the training, teachers are presented with the content and with methods for presenting the information. They are also oriented to the organized sequence of presenting the curriculum. The sequence includes: (1) introduction—motivational activities, (2) awareness—body interactions, (3) appreciation—contribution of body parts to well-being, (4) structure and function of the parts of the body being studied, (5) diseases and disorders associated with the parts of the body being studied, (6) prevention of ill health, and (7) a culminating activity that includes the parents of the students.

For more information about this curriculum, contact the National Center for Health Education, 72 Spring St., Suite 208, New York, NY 10012 [Telephone: (212) 334-9470, Fax: (212) 334-9845].

Two noncomprehensive curricula that are also on the NDN diffusion list deserve mention. These are "Have a Healthy Heart" and "Teenage Health Teaching Modules."

"Have a Healthy Heart"

"Have a Healthy Heart" deals with cardiovascular health in grades four through eight. This curriculum was developed by Model Classrooms and was created to supplement a more comprehensive curriculum. A special feature of this curriculum is its aerobic activity component.

"Teenage Health Teaching Modules" (THTM)

The **THTM** curriculum was developed by the Education Development Center between 1979 and 1983, with support from the Centers for Disease Control, because school districts using "Growing Healthy" asked for a compatible curriculum for use at the secondary level. The THTM, which includes 21 instructional modules organized by developmentally based health tasks of concern to adolescents, can stand alone as a curriculum or supplement other curricular materials. Some of the modules were developed to be used in the junior high/middle schools, some for the high schools, and some for either. Obviously, the content of each of the modules is different, but all models are intended to address the following five skill areas: (1) self-assessment, (2) communication, (3) decision making, (4) health advocacy, and (5) healthy self-management. The titles of some of the modules are: "Having Friends," "Living with Feelings and Handling Stress," "Protecting Oneself and Others: Tobacco, Alcohol, and Other Drugs," and "Preventing AIDS."

Like "Growing Healthy," this curriculum has been well received and a comprehensive evaluation[14] has confirmed its effectiveness. It is likely that the distribution of this curriculum will continue to grow over the years.

School Health Education Study

Another well-recognized curriculum that is not included in the NDN diffusion

---

"Growing Healthy" A curriculum for grades K–6, distributed by the National Center for Health Education.

list is the one that resulted from the **School Health Education Study (SHES).** This nationwide study, which began in 1960, was designed to determine the status of health education. The results of the study showed the status to be very poor. As a result, a writing team of health education experts was formed to create an experimental curriculum. This writing team worked closely with public schools in California, Illinois, New York, and Washington to develop a K–12 curriculum that was based on concepts. Health was the unifying concept, and under that came the three key concepts of growing and developing, interacting, and decision making. These key concepts were then followed by ten major health instruction concepts (see Table 6.5) and a number of subconcepts, long-range goals, and behavioral objectives. Though this curriculum was never really widely adopted because of the cost of the final product, it is considered the classic school health curriculum. Today, it is often cited by authors of newer curriculum projects.

Other Curricula

There are a number of other sources for health curricula. As a matter of fact, if we tried to create a list, it would consume many pages of this book and probably still not be entirely inclusive. Here is a list of places where you may be able to find other health curricula. Some of them may be comprehensive (include a variety of topics and for every grade level, K–12) and others may be topic and/or grade-level specific. These other sources include:

1. State departments of education or health: A number of states have either recommended or required a particular

---

Table 6.5

Key Concepts from School Health Education Curriculum Design

Growth and development influences, and is influence by, the structure and functioning of the individual.

Growing and developing follows a predictable sequence yet is unique for each individual.

Protection and promotion of health are individual, community, and international responsibilities.

The potential for hazards and accidents exists, whatever the environment.

There are reciprocal relationships involving man, disease, and environment.

The family serves to perpetuate humankind and to fulfill certain health needs.

Personal health practices are affected by a complexity of forces, often conflicting.

Utilization of health information, products, and services is guided by values and perceptions.

Use of substances that modify mood and behavior arises from a variety of motivations.

Food selection and eating patterns are determined by physical, social, mental, economic, and cultural factors.

From: School Health Education Study (1967). *Health Education: A Conceptual Approach to Curriculum Design.* St. Paul, Minn.: 3 M Educational Press.

---

curriculum. Some states do not have comprehensive curricula but require instruction in some of the more controversial health topics like substance use and abuse and sexuality education.

2. Health agencies and associations: Many of the voluntary health agencies (e.g., American Cancer Society, American Health Association, and American Lung Association) and other health-related associations (e.g., National Dairy Council, American Health Foundation, and United Way) have developed curricula for grades K–12. Most of these are not comprehensive, but they are usually well done, supported by audiovisuals and handouts, and available either at very low or no cost.

School Health Education Study (SHES)   A study that began in 1960 to determine the status of health education in U.S. schools.

3. Commercially produced curricula: These curricula have been developed by private corporations for schools. Two good examples of such curricula are the "Health Activities Project" (HAP) distributed by Hubbard Scientific Company, and a variety of curriculum materials distributed by the Wisconsin Clearinghouse.

ISSUES AND CONCERNS FACING THE SCHOOL HEALTH PROGRAM

Like most other community health programs, the school health program is not without its issues and concerns. "In the 1940's, the three leading school discipline problems were talking, chewing gum, and making noise."[15] Today, many of the problems are health related. In the remainder of this chapter, we will summarize a few of the challenges that still lie ahead of those who work in school health.

Comprehensive School Health Program

A battle that school health advocates continue to fight is the recognition that every school district in the country should have a comprehensive school health program. We have already pointed out that healthy children are better learners and that a comprehensive school health program can contribute to the health of children. More globally, comprehensive school health "facilitates the attainment of the goal of schooling; an educated populace whose health permits continued productivity through the lifespan."[16]

While many Americans support the idea that everyone is entitled to good health, we have not supported through legislation the notion that everyone is entitled to a comprehensive school health program. Obviously, getting legislation passed is a complicated process and is dependent on a number of different circumstances, including but not limited to economics, social action, and politics. This difficult task should not deter those who feel comprehensive school health is vital. It is becoming clearer that many of the answers to current and future health problems lie with the resources found in the school—the one institution of society through which all of us must pass. Here are a few examples of the impact school health can have:

1. At the present time, the key to dealing with the AIDS problem is education.
2. The biggest stride in improving the health of the country will not come from new technology but from the health behavior in which we engage.
3. Many of the primary health care services needed by the children of this country are not available because of the barriers of the health care system.

The need for comprehensive school health should be obvious to all. We have taken the liberty to rephrase a quote from a group of school health experts[14] who say it best—society should not be as concerned with what happens when we implement comprehensive school health as about what is likely to happen if we do not.

Dealing with Controversy in the Curriculum

The words *sexual intercourse, suicide, AIDS, substance use and abuse, sexually transmitted diseases, abortion, contraception,* and *death and dying* get attention. The very nature of the topics covered in health instruction today create controversy. Yet controversy is not new to health instruction; it has followed health instruction ever since it first attempted to deal with the many issues that face youth (see Figure 6.10).

Controversy is a part of health instruction for a number of reasons. Part of it deals with the pressure applied to schools by present-day conservative groups. These groups are interested in discouraging health instruction that includes values-clarification activities and open-ended decision-making processes.[17] Others believe that controversy exists because of the differences in family value systems and religious beliefs. Bensley and Harmon[18] have suggested that controversies fall into two major categories: issues that center around the values and beliefs of the content taught and issues that arise from improper implementation of the curriculum. The former category questions things like: (1) Do students really need to learn in school how to use a condom? (2) Doesn't talk of suicide lead some students to think that it might be the best alterna-

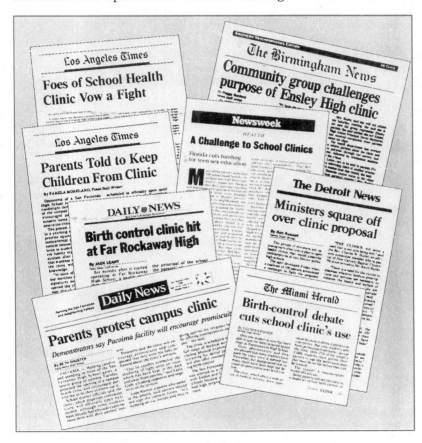

FIGURE 6.10

There are still many controversial issues that surround health education in the schools.

tive for them? (3) Aren't chiropractors just health quacks? (4) Isn't Nancy Reagan's "Just Say No" slogan all that students need to know about drugs? and (5) Why do students need to know about funeral preplanning in high school? These are legitimate concerns, but they are also issues that today's adolescents face. Lack of awareness, knowledge, and skills are not excuses for undesirable health behavior. If the students do not get this information at school, where will they get it? Studies have shown that the institutions of church and family have taught little about the controversial topics included in the health curriculum.

Improper implementation of the curriculum is indeed a concern. Because health is not considered a CORE subject in most school districts, it has received little attention and support. In many school districts throughout the United States, the low priority given to health has meant that much of the health education is provided by individuals other than health education specialists. These people are not incapable of teaching health, but they have not been educated to do so. Therefore, the health curriculum is sometimes improperly implemented and controversy arises.

School districts can help reduce controversy by (1) implementing age-appropriate curricula, (2) using acceptable teaching methods, (3) gaining parent/guardian approval of curricula and teaching methods, (4) developing school policy that allows for parents/guardians to review the curricula and to withdraw their children from lessons that go against family or religious beliefs, (5) implementing a school policy that provides for the handling of concern by parents/guardians,[18] and (6) making sure qualified and interested teachers teach health (see Box 6.3).

School-Based Clinics (SBCs) or School-Linked Clinics (SLCs)

The concept of offering comprehensive health care services through the schools via school-based or school-linked clinics is a relatively new one. In 1970, there was only one U.S. school that had an SBC/SLC.[19] By 1984 that number had jumped to 31, then to 150 in 1989. By early 1991, 306 SBCs and 21 SLCs were operating in 33 states and Puerto Rico. The majority of SBCs/SLCs have functioned as primary health care providers for medically underserved adolescents[20] (51% operate in high schools). However, there are some SBCs/SLCs that operate in middle/junior high (13%) and elementary (14%) schools. Another 22% operate in schools with combined grade levels.[21]

Although there is no single model for SBCs/SLCs, the SBCs/SLCs today share a number of similarities[19] These similarities are that SBCs/SLCs:

1. Are developed to meet the needs of the students within a specific community.
2. Attempt to provide comprehensive health care (including education and counseling) and make necessary referrals to other providers in the community.
3. Are generally located on or adjacent to school property.
4. Maintain confidential students health records.
5. Have representative advising groups.
6. Are mostly staffed by nurse practitioners and either social workers or counselors, although larger SBCs employ full- or part-time physicians.
7. Encourage students to discuss their health concerns with their parents/guardians
8. Require written consent from parents/guardians before care is provided.

As mentioned earlier in the chapter, there are a number of sound reasons why expanded (or comprehensive) school health sources should be offered through the schools. Yet SBCs/SLCs have been the frequent targets of intense criticism at the local and national levels by political and religious groups.[22-24] Much of the controversy surrounding SBCs/SLCs has centered on the issue of reproductive health care, including counseling and the distribution of contraceptive devices and/or prescriptions.[19] However, it has been reported that only approximately 20% of SBCs/SLCs provide reproductive health care.[25] It appears that the same issues that surround the controversy in health instruction are present with SBCs/SLCs.

It is a shame that SBCs/SLCs have met with this resistance. It seems most ironic that at a time when such a large portion of our society is either entirely without or receiving limited health care a means to reach many unserved is meeting with such resistance.

CHAPTER SUMMARY

Those people involved with school health represent a specific population within the community. The potential impact of a comprehensive school health program on the health of children, their families, and the community is great, since the school is the one institution through which we all must pass. To date, the full potential of school health has not been reached, due to lack of support and interest. However, that may change as society continues to struggle with many health issues. If implemented properly, comprehensive school health can improve access to health services, educate students about pressing health issues, and provide a safe and healthy environment in which students can learn and grow.

As we look toward the future a number of issues face school health advocates. These include: support for comprehensive school health, dealing with controversy in the health curriculum, and the implementation of school-based and school-linked clinics.

SCENARIO: ANALYSIS AND RESPONSE

It was obvious that Mrs. Graff had a very full day, which included several issues related to a comprehensive school health program. Based upon what you read in this chapter and other knowledge you have about school health, respond to the following questions:

1. Identify five school health concerns with which Mrs. Graff had to deal.

2. For each of the concerns you identified in question 1, state how written policies may have helped or hindered Mrs. Graff with her responsibilities.

3. How important do you feel is the role of the classroom teacher in making a comprehensive school health program work? Why do you feel this way?

REVIEW QUESTIONS

1. What is meant by the term *comprehensive school health program?*

2. What individuals (name by position) should be considered for inclusion on the school health team?

3. What two foundations are needed to insure a comprehensive school health program? Why?

4. Why are written school health policies needed?

5. Who should approve written school health policies?

6. What are the four major components of a school health program?

7. What is the difference between basic, expanded, and comprehensive health services?

8. Explain the difference between direct, correlated, and integrated instruction models.

9. How does a curriculum get included in the National Diffusion Network?

10. Describe why each of the following are considered important curriculum models: "Growing Healthy," the "SHES Curriculum," "Teenage Health Teaching Models."

11. State three issues facing school health advocates and indicate why they are issues.

ACTIVITIES

1. Make arrangements to observe an elementary classroom in your town for a half-day. While observing, keep a chart of all the activities that take place in the classroom that relate to a comprehensive school health program. Select one activity from your list and write a one-page paper describing the activity, why it was health related, how the teacher handled it, and what could have been done differently to improve the situation.

2. Visit a voluntary health agency in your community and ask the employees to describe the organization's philosophy on health education and inquire into the availability of their health education materials for use in a school health program. Summarize your visit with a one-page reaction paper.

3. Make an appointment to interview either a school nurse or a school health coordinator. During your interview, ask the person to provide an overview of what his/her school offers in the way of a comprehensive school health program. Ask specifically about the four major components of the school health program and the three issues of controversy presented in this chapter. Summarize your visit with a two-page written paper.

4. Make arrangements to interview a school administrator or school board member in a district where a school-based or school-linked clinic exists. Ask the person to describe the process he or she went through to start the clinic, what resistance the district met in do-

ing so, and what the district would do differently if it had to implement it again or start another clinic.

REFERENCES

1. Joint Committee on Health Education Terminology (1991). "Report of the 1990 Joint Committee on Health Education Terminology.'" *Journal of Health Education,* 22(2): 105–106.

2. No author (1991). "Healthy People 2000: National Health Promotion and Disease Prevention Objectives and Healthy Schools." *Journal of School Health* 61(7): 298–299.

3. McGinnis, J. M., and C. DeGraw, (1991). "Healthy Schools 2000: Creating Partnerships for the Decade." *Journal of School Health,* 61(7): 292–296.

4. Redican, K. J., L. K. Olsen, and C. R. Baffi (1986). *Organization of School Health Programs.* New York: Macmillan, p. 5.

5. Cornacchia, H. J., L. K. Olsen, and C. J. Nickerson (1991). *Health in Elementary Schools,* 7th ed. St. Louis: Times Mirror/Mosby, pp. 27–28, 195–196.

6. Association for the Advancement of Health Education (May/June 1992). "School Nurse in Education: AAHE Position Statement. *HE-XTRA* 17(3): 6.

7. Bruess, C. E., and J. E. Gay (1978), *Implementing Comprehensive School Health.* New York: Macmillan.

8. McKenzie, J. F. (1983). "Written Policies: Developing a Solid Foundation for a Comprehensive School Health Program." *Future Focus: Ohio Journal of Health, Physical Education, Recreation, and Dance,* 4(3): 9–11.

9. Maylath, N. S. (1991). "Employment of School Health Coordinators." *Journal of School Health* 61(2): 98–100.

10. Schaller, W. E. (1981). *The School Health Program,* 5th ed. New York: CBS College Publishing.

11. Schlitt, J. J. (June 1991). "Issue Brief—Bringing Health to School: Policy Implications for Southern States." Washington, D.C.: Southern Center on Adolescent Pregnancy Prevention and Southern Regional Project on Infant Mortality. Printed in *Journal of School Health* 62(2): 60a–60h.

12. Klein, J. D., and L. S. Sadowski (1990). "Personal Health Services as a Component of Comprehensive Health Programs." *Journal of School Health* 60(4): 164–169.

13. Joint Committee on Health Education Terminology (1974). "New Definitions: Report of the 1972–73 Joint Committee on Health Education Terminology." *Journal of School Health* 44(1): 33–37.

14. Gold, R. S., G. S. Parcel, H. J. Walberg, R. V. Luepker, B. Portnoy, and E. J. Stone (1991). "Summary and Conclusions of the THTM Evaluation: The Expert

Work Group Perspective." *Journal of School Health* 61(1): 39–42.

15. U.S. Dept. of Health and Human Services, Office for Substance Abuse Prevention (1989). *Drug-Free Committees: Turning Awareness into Action* (DHHS Pub. no. ADM 89-1562). Washington, D.C.: U.S. Government Printing Office.

16. Assn. for the Advancement of Health Education (Oct. 1991). *Position Statement: Comprehensive School Health*. Reston, Va.: Author.

17. Cleary, M. J. (1991). "School Health Education and a National Curriculum: One Disconcerting Scenario." *Journal of School Health* 61(8): 355–358.

18. Bensley, L. B., Jr., and E. O. Harmon (1992). "Addressing Controversy in Health Education." *Update* May/June: 9–10.

19. Council on Scientific Affairs, American Medical Association (1990). "Providing Medical Services Through School-based Health Programs. *Journal of School Health* 60(3): 87–91.

20. Pacheco, M., S. Adelsheim, L. Davis, V. Mancha, L. Aime, P. Nelson, D. Derksen, and A. Kaufmann (1991). "Innovation, Peer Teaching and Multidisciplinary Collaboration: Outreach from a School-based Clinic. *Journal of School Health* 61(8): 367–369.

21. The Center for Population Options (1991). *The Facts: School-based and School-linked Clinics*. Washington, D.C.: Author.

22. Pacheco, M., W. Powell, C. Cole, N. Kalishman, R. Benon, and A. Kaufmann (1991). "School-based Clinics: The Politics of Change." *Journal of School Health* 61(2): 92–94.

23. Rienzo, B. A., and J. W. Bulton (1993). "The Politics of School-based Clinics: A Community-level Analysis." *Journal of School Health* 63(6): 266–272.

24. The School-based Adolescent Health Care Program (1993). *The Answer Is at School: Bringing Health Care to Our Students*. Washington, D.C.: Author.

25. Keenan, T. (1986). "School-based Adolescent Health Care Programs. *Pediatric Nursing* 12(5): 365–369.

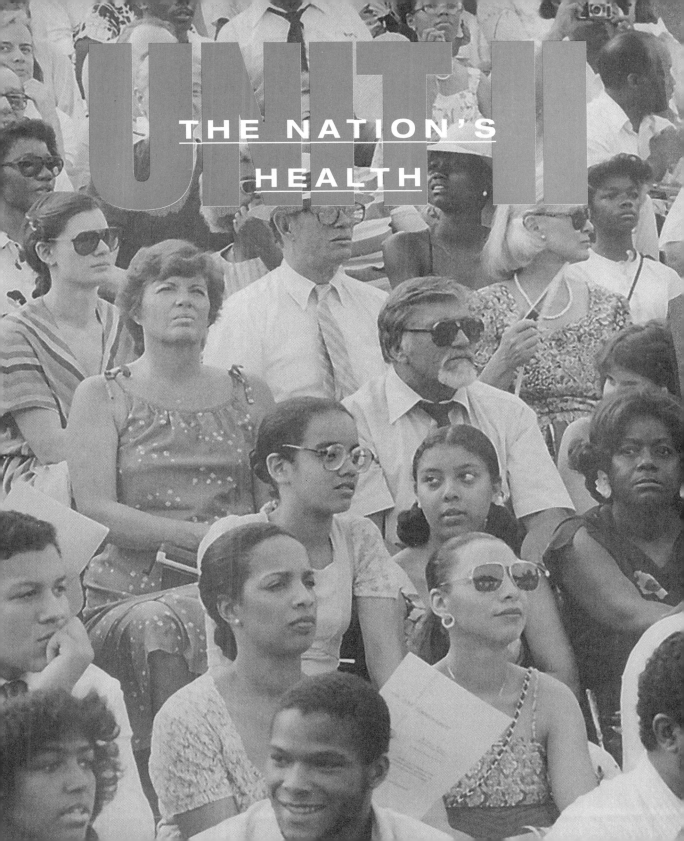

UNIT II

THE NATION'S HEALTH

Chapter 7

A HEALTH PROFILE
OF THE
AMERICAN PEOPLE

Chapter Outline

Chapter Objectives

After studying this chapter, you will be able to:

1. Describe the role health behavior plays in determining health status in the United States today.
2. Explain why morbidity and mortality data are used to measure health status.
3. List the four leading causes of death in the United States today and compare them to the leading causes of death in 1900.
4. Define *life expectancy* and give an example.
5. Identify the American subpopulations with the longest life expectancies and those with the shortest.
6. Explain why years of potential life lost are calculated using age 65 rather than life expectancy figures.
7. Summarize self-assessment of health status data.
8. Explain what data are used to calculate a DALY.
9. List the five age groups for which health data are usually summarized in the United States.
10. Outline the health profiles for the various age groups—infants and children, adolescents and young adults, adults, and seniors—listing the major causes of morbidity and mortality for each group.

Every morning, Fred and Martha begin their day by reading the newspaper over breakfast. They usually finish this task over a second cup of coffee. Whenever either of them comes across an interesting article, he or she will usually share its contents with the other. On this day, Fred began the conversation by asking Martha what she thought of the headlines on the features page that read, "By most measures, the U.S. is the Healthiest Nation in the World."

"What's so newsworthy about that?" Martha replied. "Everyone knows we are. We have by far the best health care system in the world." Fred nodded his head in agreement, and they just went on reading.

INTRODUCTION

How often have you heard someone say, "If you have your health, you have everything." That statement is another way of acknowledging that until people lose their health, it is taken for granted. As Americans, we often forget that when we lose our health, the quality of our lives and sometimes the lives of those around us deteriorates very quickly. Acute or chronic health problems can deplete personal resources (and those of the family), alter personal relationships, lower productivity, cause the loss of a job, affect school work, and seriously alter life-styles. Even minor colds can inhibit one's ability to enjoy life for a week to ten days.

Good health and the quality of life it brings have been much sought after goals ever since people gained freedom from hunger and environmental dangers. Today, more than ever before, these goals are within grasp. Americans are no longer subject to violent epidemics of communicable diseases that were beyond our control in the early 1900s. Sanitation has improved. There is an abundance of healthful food in this country. Americans have available to them the best immunizations and pharmaceuticals in the world. Thus, the United States has arrived at a situation in the 1990s in which the greatest potential for improvement in health status can only be realized through individual behavioral change. Specifically, Americans must be willing to take more responsibility for their own health by eliminating or greatly reducing certain behavioral risk factors such as a lack of exercise; unhealthy diets; the use of alcohol, tobacco, and other drugs; the practice of unprotected sexual activity; and so on. It has been estimated that such behavioral changes on the part of individuals could eliminate 40%–70% of all premature deaths, one-third of all acute disabilities, and two-thirds of chronic disabilities. To be sure, there are other contributors to ill health, such as heredity and environmental and social problems. But, there is little doubt that health promoting behaviors are the key to improving the health status of Americans, both individually and collectively, as we approach the twenty-first century.[1]

In this chapter, we survey the health status of the American people, first by describing the kinds of data used to measure health, and then by presenting a profile of the health of Americans by age group. In many cases, because of the way statistics were kept in the past, data are available only for black Americans and white Americans, and not for other racial groups and Americans of Hispanic origin. We hope that you, the student, will become knowledgeable about specific health problems of each age group, and also become mindful of those populations at special risk, including mothers and infants, children, minorities, and seniors. In the chapters that follow, we will examine the health issues that are particular to these high-risk special populations.

HEALTH STATUS AND ITS MEASUREMENT

In Chapter 1, we offered several different definitions for *health*. Though each of the definitions is easy to understand, none is easily quantifiable. For example, it is very difficult to measure how much health exists in a population, since healthy people do not normally come to the attention of public health officials. Instead, most health statistics, based on the traditional medical model, describe ill health—disease, injury, and death. Thus, as a society, we have chosen to define our health status with its opposite—ill health.[2]

In this chapter, we develop a health profile of Americans using measurements of ill health and death: mortality statistics, life expectancy data, years of potential life lost data, data from the National Health Interview Survey, data from the National Health and Nutrition Examination Survey, and disability-adjusted life years. The most accurate and easily acquired data are those

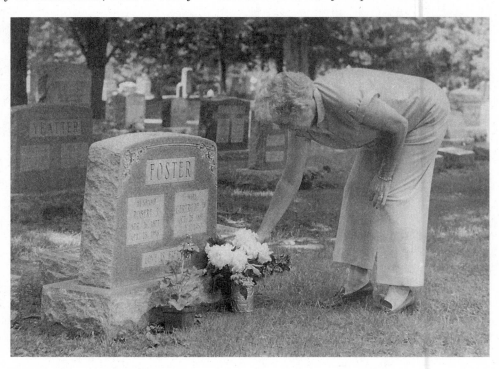

FIGURE 7.1
Mortality is the most reliable single indicator of a population's health status.

for mortality. For this reason, three of the six measurements discussed below are based upon mortality data.

Mortality Statistics

"The transition from wellness to ill health is often gradual and poorly defined. Because death, in contrast, is a clearly defined event, it has continued to be the most reliable single indicator of the health status of a population (see Figure 7.1). Mortality statistics, however, describe only a part of the health status of a population, and often only the end point of an illness process."[3]

In 1990, 2,148,463 deaths were registered in the United States (see Table 7.1). This was 19,536 fewer deaths than were reported in 1988, when the highest annual mortality rate on record was reported. These annual mortality figures have been attributed to normal population growth, the increasing proportion of older persons in the population, and, in 1988, an outbreak of influenza.[4] Even though the total number of deaths had been on the rise until 1988, **death rates** have consistently decreased over time (see Table 7.1).

A study of the mortality statistics for the twentieth century reveals a shift in the leading causes of death. When the century began, communicable diseases such as pneumonia, tuberculosis, and gastrointestinal infections were the leading causes of death (see Table 7.2). However, a century of progress in public health practice and in biomedical research has resulted in a significant reduction in the proportion of deaths from communicable diseases, so that the four leading causes of death today are noncommunicable diseases (see Tables 4.5, 7.3). During this century, life expectancy at birth

increased from 47.3 years in 1900 to 75.7 years in 1991 (see Table 7.4). As we approach the end of the century, the five leading causes of death in America—heart disease, cancer, stroke, chronic obstructive pulmonary disease and unintentional injuries—account for 66–75% of all deaths in the United States.[4]

This domination of annual mortality statistics by noncommunicable-disease causes masks the importance of communicable diseases as causes of deaths in certain age groups. For example, pneumonia and influenza still kill many seniors in this country each year. Also, HIV infection, a communicable disease, was listed as the eighth overall leading cause of death for Americans in 1992. As with pneumonia and influenza, HIV deaths are higher in specific subpopulations—specifically, among white and black males. Still another communicable disease, tuberculosis, is also on the rise; cases per 100,000 population have increased each year since 1988. The causes for the increase in tuberculosis are the AIDS epidemic and the proliferation of drug-resistant strains of the tubercle bacterium.[5] Thus, it is important to remember that viewing the leading causes of death for the entire population does not provide a clear picture of the health of any one segment of the population.

Life Expectancy

Life expectancy is another standard measurement used to compare health status of various populations. Also based on mortality, **life expectancy** is defined as the average number of years a person, from a specific cohort, is projected to live from a given point in time. While life insurance companies are interested in life expectancy at

---

death rate The number of deaths per 100,000 resident population.

life expectancy The average number of years a person is projected to live from a given point in time.

Table 7.1

Deaths, Death Rates, and Age-Adjusted Death Rates, by Race and Sex: United States, Selected Years, 1940–1990

[Rates per 100,000 population in specified group. Rates are based on populations enumerated as of April 1 for census years and estimated as of July 1 for all other years. Beginning 1970, excludes deaths of nonresidents of the United States.]

| Year | All Races | | | White | | | All Other | | | | | |
| | | | | | | | Total | | | Black | | |
	Both Sexes	Male	Female	Both Sexes	Male	Female	Both Sexes	Male	Female	Both Sexes	Male	Female
						Number						
1990	2,148,463	1,113,417	1,035,046	1,853,254	950,812	902,442	295,209	162,605	132,604	265,498	145,359	120,139
1985	2,086,440	1,097,758	988,682	1,819,054	950,455	868,599	267,386	147,303	120,083	244,207	133,610	110,597
1980	1,989,841	1,075,078	914,763	1,738,607	933,878	804,729	251,234	141,200	110,034	233,135	130,138	102,997
1975	1,892,879	1,050,819	842,060	1,660,366	917,804	742,562	232,513	133,015	99,498	217,932	123,770	94,162
1970	1,921,031	1,078,478	842,553	1,682,096	942,437	739,659	238,935	136,041	102,894	225,647	127,540	98,107
1960	1,711,982	975,648	736,334	1,505,335	860,857	644,478	206,647	114,791	91,856	196,010	107,701	88,309
1950	1,452,454	827,749	624,705	1,276,085	731,366	544,719	176,369	96,383	79,986	169,606	92,004	77,602
1940	1,417,269	791,003	626,266	1,231,223	690,901	540,322	186,046	100,102	85,944	178,743	95,517	83,226
						Death Rate						
1990	863.8	918.4	812.0	888.0	930.9	846.9	737.9	851.5	634.2	871.0	1,008.0	747.9
1985	876.9	948.6	809.1	900.4	963.6	840.1	745.0	861.7	638.8	854.8	989.3	734.2
1980	878.3	976.9	785.3	892.5	983.3	806.1	791.7	936.5	660.6	875.4	1,034.1	733.3
1975	878.5	1,002.0	761.4	886.9	1,004.1	775.1	823.1	987.6	673.1	882.5	1,055.4	726.1
1970	945.3	1,090.3	807.8	946.3	1,086.7	812.6	938.4	1,115.9	775.3	999.3	1,186.6	829.2
1960	954.7	1,104.5	809.2	947.8	1,098.5	800.9	1,008.5	1,152.0	872.6	1,038.6	1,181.7	905.0
1950	963.8	1,106.1	823.5	945.7	1,089.5	803.3	1,119.4	1,251.1	993.5	—	—	—
1940	1,076.4	1,197.4	954.6	1,041.5	1,162.2	919.4	1,382.8	1,513.7	1,256.2	—	—	—

| Year | All Races | | | White | | | All Other | | | | | |
| | | | | | | | Total | | | Black | | |
	Both Sexes	Male	Female	Both Sexes	Male	Female	Both Sexes	Male	Female	Both Sexes	Male	Female
						Age-adjusted Death Rate						
1990	520.2	680.2	390.6	492.8	644.3	369.9	686.7	910.2	512.5	789.2	1,061.3	581.6
1985	548.9	723.0	410.3	524.9	693.3	391.0	709.1	931.8	535.7	793.6	1,053.4	594.8
1980	585.8	777.2	432.6	559.4	745.3	411.1	774.2	1,015.1	582.6	842.5	1,112.8	631.1
1975	630.4	837.2	462.5	602.2	804.3	439.0	840.6	1,090.1	634.5	890.8	1,163.0	670.6
1970	714.3	931.6	532.5	679.6	893.4	501.7	983.4	1,231.4	770.8	1,044.0	1,318.6	814.4
1960	760.9	949.3	590.6	727.0	917.7	555.0	1,046.1	1,211.0	893.3	1,073.3	1,246.1	916.9
1950	841.5	1,001.6	688.4	800.4	963.1	645.0	1,225.7	1,358.5	1,095.7	—	—	—
1940	1,076.1	1,213.0	938.9	1,017.2	1,155.1	879.0	1,634.7	1,764.4	1,504.7	—	—	—

From: U.S. Dept. of Health and Human Services, NCHS (Jan 1993). "Advance Report on Final Mortality Statistics 1990." *Monthly Vital Statistics Report* 41(7):14.

every age, health statisticians are usually concerned with life expectancy at birth and at the age of 65 years. It must be remembered that life expectancy is an average for an entire cohort (usually of a single birth year) and is not necessarily a useful prediction for any one individual. Moreover, it certainly cannot describe the quality of one's life. However, the ever-increasing life expectancy for Americans suggests that, as a country, we have managed to control some of those factors that contribute to early deaths.

Table 7.4 provides a summary of life expectancy figures for the United States from 1900 to 1990. The data presented indicate that the overall life expectancy both at birth and at age 65 has consistently increased since 1900, that women are projected to live longer than men, and that whites live longer than blacks.

When compared with the life expectancy figures of other countries (see Table 7.5), the United States figures roughly correspond with those of other countries with well-developed economies. The highest life expectancy figures are reported from Japan while the lowest are reported from the countries with weakly developed economies.

Years of Potential Life Lost

While standard mortality statistics, such as leading causes of death, provide one measure of the importance of various diseases, years of potential life lost (YPLL) provides another, different measure. The YPLL is calculated by subtracting a person's age at death from 65 years. Thus, for a person who dies at age 59, the YPLL are six. In the United States, a death prior to 65 years is considered a premature death. Some ask why the age 65 is used instead of one's actual life expectancy when calculating YPLL. The rationale for using 65 is that for many

Table 7.2
Leading Causes of Death in the United States in 1900

1. Pneumonias
2. Tuberculosis (all forms)
3. Gastrointestinal infections
4. Cardiovascular disease
5. Cerebrovascular disease
6. Kidney diseases
7. Trauma
8. Cancer

years, 65 was the standard age of retirement. While this is no longer true today, full Social Security payments can begin at age 65, and a majority of the work force is retired by this age. Many of us know people who continue to work beyond that age; two examples are former American presidents Reagan and Bush.

YPLL weights deaths such that the death of a very young person counts more than the death of a very old person. Table 7.6 provides a summary of the YPLL for selected causes of death in the United States for selected years between 1970 and 1990. In examining this table, note that the number of YPLL per 100,000 population under 65 years fell by 23% between 1970 and 1980 and by another 12% between 1980 and 1990. Also, note that the greatest number of YPLL for the population as a whole are the result of unintentional injuries and malignant neoplasms (cancer), because these problems often strike people when they are young.

Years of potential life lost from specific causes vary depending upon the gender and race of the subpopulation. For example, the leading cause of YPLL for women is cancer while the leading cause of YPLL for men is unintentional injuries. The YPLL from all causes for blacks are twice those for whites in both genders. Perhaps the most alarming YPLL data are those for the black male population. In this group, more than one-seventh of the YPLL come from homicide and **legal intervention** and nearly another one-seventh come from unintentional injuries.

National Health Interview Survey Data

A fourth means of measuring health is through health interviews. As a part of both the 1986 and the 1991 National Health Interview Survey, conducted by the National Center for Health Statistics, respondents were asked to describe their health status using one of five categories: excellent, very good, good, fair, or poor. As can be seen in Table 7.7, there is little difference between the responses for the two years. Less than 10% of the respondents each year described their health status as either fair or poor, suggesting that most Americans believe they are in good, very good, or excellent health.

It is important to remember that these data were generated by self-reported responses to the National Health Interview Survey and not by actual examinations objectively generated in a clinic. As such, respondents may overreport information such as good health habits or underreport information such as illicit drug use.[3] Such reporting is often dependent on the respondent's perceived social stigma or support for a response and the degree to which people's responses are confidential or anonymous. Furthermore, people have widely divergent views on what constitutes poor or good health. For example, many sedentary, cigarette smoking, high-stress people see themselves as being in good health, while "health nuts" feel their health is deteriorating when they miss a day of exercise. In general, the young assess their health better than the old do, males better than females, whites better than blacks, and those with large family incomes better than those with smaller ones.

National Health and Nutrition Examination Survey

The National Health and Nutrition Examination Survey (NHANES), is conducted by the National Center for Health Statistics to assess the health and nutritional status of the general U.S. population. The data are collected, using a mobile examination center, through direct physical examinations, clinical and laboratory testing, and related procedures, on a representative group of Americans. The examinations result in the most authoritative source of standardized clinical, physical, and physiological data on the American people. Included in the data are the prevalence of specific conditions and diseases and data on blood pressure, serum cholesterol, body measurements, nutritional status and deficiencies, and exposure to environmental toxicants.

Three cycles of the NHANES have been conducted. The first was conducted in 1959 as the Health Examination Survey. The second cycle, conducted in 1970, was expanded to include a nutritional component. The third cycle (NHANES III) began in 1988 and ended in 1994. During that six-year period, approximately 40,000 persons were examined. A special version of this survey, the Hispanic Health and Nutrition Examination Survey, was conducted in 1982–1984. This survey provides data on a 12,000-person sample of three subgroups of the Hispanic population—Mexican Ameri-

---

legal intervention deaths Deaths attributable to police action or legal execution.

Table 7.3

Deaths and Death Rates for the Ten Leading Causes of Death in Specified Race-Sex Groups: United States, 1990

[Rates per 100,000 population in specified group.]

Rank Order*	Cause of Death, Race, and Sex (International Classification of Diseases 9th rev., 1975)		Number	Rate
	All Races, Both Sexes			
...	All causes		2,148,463	863.8
1	Diseases of heart	390–398, 402, 404–429	720,058	289.5
2	Malignant neoplasms, including neoplasms of lymphatic and hematopoietic tissues	140–208	505,322	203.2
3	Cerebrovascular diseases	430–438	144,088	57.9
4	Accidents and adverse effects	E800–E949	91,983	37.0
...	Motor vehicle accidents	E810–E825	46,814	18.8
...	All other accidents and adverse effects	E800–E807, E826–E949	45,169	18.2
5	Chronic obstructive pulmonary diseases and allied conditions	490–496	86,679	34.9
6	Pneumonia and influenza	480–487	79,513	32.0
7	Diabetes mellitus	250	47,664	19.2
8	Suicide	E950–E959	30,906	12.4
9	Chronic liver disease and cirrhosis	571	25,815	10.4
10	Human immunodeficiency virus infection	042–044	25,188	10.1
...	All other causes	Residual	391,247	157.3
	White, Male			
...	All causes		950,812	930.9
1	Diseases of heart	390–398, 402, 404–429	319,362	312.7
2	Malignant neoplasms, including neoplasms of lymphatic and hematopoietic tissues	140–208	232,608	227.7
3	Accidents and adverse effects	E800–E949	51,348	50.3
...	Motor vehicle accidents	E810–E825	27,288	26.7
...	All other accidents and adverse effects	E800–E807, E826–E949	24,060	23.6
4	Cerebrovascular diseases	430–438	48,024	47.0
5	Chronic obstructive pulmonary diseases and allied conditions	490–496	45,234	44.3

Rank Order*	Cause of Death, Race, and Sex (International Classification of Diseases 9th rev., 1975)		Number	Rate
7	Pneumonia and influenza	480–487	4,797	25.1
8	Chronic obstructive pulmonary diseases and allied conditions	490–496	4,182	21.9
9	Certain conditions originating in the perinatal period	760–779	4,001	21.0
10	Diabetes mellitus	250	3,449	18.1
...	All other causes	Residual	33,075	173.2
	All Other, Female			
...	All causes		132,604	634.2
1	Diseases of heart	390–398, 402, 404–429	41,268	197.4
2	Malignant neoplasms, including neoplasms of lymphatic and hematopoietic tissues	140–208	28,062	134.2
3	Cerebrovascular diseases	430–438	10,889	52.1
4	Diabetes mellitus	250	5,519	26.4
5	Accidents and adverse effects	E800–E949	4,459	21.3
...	Motor vehicle accidents	E810–E825	2,045	9.8
...	All other accidents and adverse effects	E800–E807, E826–E949	2,414	11.5
6	Pneumonia and influenza	480–487	3,910	18.7
7	Certain conditions originating in the perinatal period	760–779	3,167	15.1
8	Homicide and legal intervention	E960–E978	2,322	11.1
9	Chronic obstructive pulmonary diseases and allied conditions	490–496	2,318	11.1
10	Nephritis, nephrotic syndrome, and nephrosis	580–589	2,209	10.6
...	All other causes	Residual	28,481	136.2
	Black, Male			
...	All causes		145,359	1,008.0
1	Diseases of heart	390–398, 402, 404–429	37,038	256.8

Cause of Death, Race, and Sex
(International Classification of Diseases 9th rev., 1975)

Rank Order*	Cause of Death	ICD	Number	Rate
6	Pneumonia and influenza	480–487	32,101	31.4
7	Suicide	E950–E959	22,448	22.0
8	Diabetes mellitus	250	16,817	16.5
9	Human immunodeficiency virus infection	042–044	16,106	15.8
10	Chronic liver disease and cirrhosis	571	13,889	13.6
…	All other causes	Residual	152,875	149.7
	White, Female			
…	All causes		902,442	846.9
1	Diseases of heart	390–398, 402, 404–429	318,002	298.4
2	Malignant neoplasms, including neoplasms of lymphatic and hematopoietic tissues	140–208	208,977	196.1
3	Cerebrovascular diseases	430–438	76,502	71.8
4	Pneumonia and influenza	480–487	38,705	36.3
5	Chronic obstructive pulmonary diseases and allied conditions	490–496	34,945	32.8
6	Accidents and adverse effects	E800–E807, E826–E949	25,586	24.0
…	Motor vehicle accidents	E810–E825	12,363	11.6
…	All other accidents and adverse effects	E800–E807, E826–E949	13,223	12.4
7	Diabetes mellitus	250	21,879	20.5
8	Atherosclerosis	440	10,315	9.7
9	Septicemia	038	8,670	8.1
10	Nephritis, nephrotic syndrome, and nephrosis	580–589	8,550	8.0
…	All other causes	Residual	150,311	141.1
	All Other, Male			
…	All causes		162,605	851.5
1	Diseases of heart	390–398, 402, 404–429	41,426	216.9
2	Malignant neoplasms, including neoplasms of lymphatic and hematopoietic tissues	140–208	35,675	186.8
3	Accidents and adverse effects	E800–E949	10,590	55.5
…	Motor vehicle accidents	E810–E825	5,118	26.8
…	All other accidents and adverse effects	E800–E807, E826–E949	5,472	28.7
4	Homicide and legal intervention	E960–E978	10,457	54.8
5	Cerebrovascular diseases	430–438	8,673	45.4
6	Human immunodeficiency virus infection	042–044	6,280	32.9

Cause of Death, Race, and Sex
(International Classification of Diseases 9th rev., 1975)

Rank Order*	Cause of Death	ICD	Number	Rate
2	Malignant neoplasms, including neoplasms of lymphatic and hematopoietic tissues	140–208	31,995	221.9
3	Homicide and legal intervention	E960–E978	9,981	69.2
4	Accidents and adverse effects	E800–E949	8,756	60.7
…	Motor vehicle accidents	E810–E825	4,046	28.1
…	All other accidents and adverse effects	E800–E807, E826–E949	4,710	32.7
5	Cerebrovascular diseases	430–438	7,653	53.1
6	Human immunodeficiency virus infection	042–044	6,097	42.3
7	Pneumonia and influenza	480–487	4,161	28.9
8	Certain conditions originating in the perinatal period	760–779	3,762	26.1
9	Chronic obstructive pulmonary diseases and allied conditions	490–496	3,628	25.2
10	Diabetes mellitus	250	3,049	21.1
…	All other causes	Residual	29,239	202.8
	Black, Female†			
…	All causes		120,139	747.9
1	Diseases of heart	390–398, 402, 404–429	38,073	237.0
2	Malignant neoplasms, including neoplasms of lymphatic and hematopoietic tissues	140–208	25,082	156.1
3	Cerebrovascular diseases	430–438	9,754	60.7
4	Diabetes mellitus	250	5,065	31.5
5	Accidents and adverse effects	E800–E949	3,663	22.8
…	Motor vehicle accidents	E810–E825	1,514	9.4
…	All other accidents and adverse effects	E800–E807, E826–E949	2,149	13.4
6	Pneumonia and influenza	480–487	3,402	21.2
7	Certain conditions originating in the perinatal period	760–779	2,982	18.6
8	Homicide and legal intervention	E960–E978	2,163	13.5
9	Nephritis, nephrotic syndrome, and nephrosis	580–589	2,049	12.8
10	Chronic obstructive pulmonary diseases and allied conditions	490–496	2,027	12.6
…	All other causes	Residual	25,879	161.1

*Rank based on number of deaths. †Black included in All Other.

From: U.S. Dept. of Health and Human Services, NCHS (Jan. 1993). "Advance Report on Final Mortality Statistics 1990." *Monthly Vital Statistics Report* 41(7): 20.

Table 7.4

Life Expectancy at Birth and at 65 Years of Age, According to Race and Sex: United States, Selected years 1900–1991

[Data are based on the National Vital Statistics System.]

Specified Age and Year	All Races Both Sexes	Male	Female	White Both Sexes	Male	Female	Black Both Sexes	Male	Female
At Birth				*Remaining Life Expectancy in Years*					
1900*†	47.3	46.3	48.3	47.6	46.6	48.7	‡33.0	‡32.5	‡33.5
1950†	68.2	65.6	71.1	69.1	66.5	72.2	60.7	58.9	62.7
1960†	69.7	66.6	73.1	70.6	67.4	74.1	63.2	60.7	65.9
1970	70.9	67.1	74.8	71.7	68.0	75.6	64.1	60.0	68.3
1975	72.6	68.8	76.6	73.4	69.5	77.3	66.8	62.4	71.3
1980	73.7	70.0	77.4	74.4	70.7	78.1	68.1	63.8	72.5
1985	74.7	71.1	78.2	75.3	71.8	78.7	69.3	65.0	73.4
1990	75.4	71.8	78.8	76.1	72.7	79.4	69.1	64.5	73.6
Provisional data:									
1990†	75.4	72.0	78.8	76.0	72.6	79.3	70.3	66.0	74.5
1991†	75.7	72.2	79.1	76.4	73.0	79.7	70.0	65.6	74.3
At 65 Years									
1900–1902*†	11.9	11.5	12.2	—	11.5	12.2	—	10.4	11.4
1950†	13.9	12.8	15.0	—	12.8	15.1	13.9	12.9	14.9
1960†	14.3	12.8	15.8	14.4	12.9	15.9	13.9	12.7	15.1
1970	15.2	13.1	17.0	15.2	13.1	17.1	14.2	12.5	15.7
1975	16.1	13.8	18.1	16.1	13.8	18.2	15.0	13.1	16.7
1980	16.4	14.1	18.3	16.5	14.2	18.4	15.1	13.0	16.8
1985	16.7	14.5	18.5	16.8	14.5	18.7	15.2	13.0	16.9
1990	17.2	15.1	18.9	17.3	15.2	19.1	15.4	13.2	17.2
Provisional data:									
1990†	17.3	15.3	19.0	17.3	15.3	19.0	16.1	14.2	17.6
1991†	17.5	15.5	19.2	17.6	15.5	19.3	16.1	14.2	17.5

*Death registration area only. The death registration area increased from ten states and the District of Columbia in 1900 to the coterminous United States in 1933.

†Includes deaths of nonresidents of the United States.

‡Figure is for the all other population.

NOTES: Final data for the 1980s have been revised based on intercensal population estimates and differ from previous editions of Health, United States. Provisional data for 1989–91 were calculated using 1980s-based postcensal population estimates.

From: U.S. Dept. of Health and Human Services (1993). *Health, United States, 1992* [DHHS pub. no. PHS-93-1232]. Washington, D.C.: U.S. Government Printing Office.

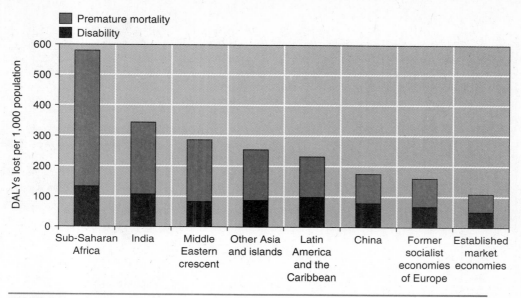

FIGURE 7.2

Burden of disease attributable to premature mortality and disability, by demographic region, 1990.

From: World Development Report 1993: Investing in Health *(1993). New York: Oxford Univ. Press (for the World Bank).*

cans in the Southwest; Cubans in Miami (Dade County), Florida; and Puerto Ricans in the New York City area.

Disability-Adjusted Life Years

The five measurements of health status discussed above are the most commonly used measurements in the United States and other developed countries. However, because mortality does not entirely express the burden of disease (for example, chronic depression and paralysis caused by polio are responsible for great loss of healthy life but are not reflected in mortality tables), the World Health Organization and the World Bank developed a measure called the **disability-adjusted life years (DALYs).**[5] The DALYs combine losses from premature mortality and loss of healthy life resulting from

disability. The calculation of DALYs is an involved process which takes into effect the severity of the health condition, age, and impact on the future (see reference 6 for a more thorough explanation of disability-adjusted life years). Figure 7.2 illustrates the number of DALYs lost per 1,000 population in 1990 from eight demographic regions of the world. Table 7.8 shows the distribution of DALY loss by cause and demographic region for 1990. Please note that included in the "established market economies" region are countries in North America, Western Europe, Australia, New Zealand, and Japan. (Text continues on p. 188.)

---

disability-adjusted life years (DALYS) A measure for the burden of disease that takes into account premature death and disability.

Table 7.5
Life Expectancy Figures in 127 Countries, Selected Years, by Income and Gender

	Under-5 Mortality Rate (per 1,000 live births)		Health and Welfare					Education							
			Life Expectancy at Birth (years)				Maternal Mortality (per 100,000 live births) 1988	Percentage of Cohort Persisting to Grade 4				Females per 100 males			
			Female		Male			Female		Male		Primary		Secondary	
	Female 1991	Male 1991	1970	1991	1970	1991		1970	1986	1970	1986	1970	1990	1970	1990
Low-income economies	96 w	104 w	54 w	58 w	53 w	61 w	308 w	..	..	..	..	..	78 w	..	65 w
China and India	75 w	80 w	57 w	60 w	57 w	64 w	115 w	..	..	..	..	..	79 w	..	65 w
Other low-income	135 w	148 w	47 w	57 w	46 w	54 w	587 w	65 w	66 w	74 w	70 w	61 w	76 w	44 w	66 w
1 Mozambique	265	294	42	48	39	45	..	..	..	..	..	..	76	..	61
2 Tanzania	153	171	47	49	44	46	342	82	90	88	89	65	98	38	74
3 Ethiopia	185	204	44	50	43	47	..	57	56	56	56	46	64	32	67
4 Uganda	175	195	51	47	49	46	550	..	..	..	..	65	..	31	..
5 Bhutan	200	188	41	49	39	47	1,305	..	..	..	..	5	59	3	41
6 Guinea-Bissau	236	262	36	39	35	38	..	..	..	..	..	43	56	62	53
7 Nepal	139	125	42	53	43	54	833	..	..	..	..	18	47	16	..
8 Burundi	169	189	45	50	42	46	..	47	84	45	84	49	84	17	57
9 Chad	197	219	40	49	37	46	..	..	77	..	81	34	44	9	22
10 Madagascar	156	174	47	52	44	50	333	65	..	63	..	86	97	70	99
11 Sierra Leone	341	377	36	45	33	40	600	..	..	..	..	67	70	40	56
12 Bangladesh	136	130	44	52	46	53	..	..	43	..	43	47	81	..	49
13 Lao PDR	153	172	42	52	39	49	561	..	..	..	..	59	77	36	66
14 Malawi	185	205	41	45	40	44	350	55	67	60	72	59	81	36	54
15 Rwanda	209	234	46	48	43	45	300	63	76	65	75	79	99	44	56
16 Mali	180	205	41	50	40	47	2,325	52	68	89	75	55	58	29	48
17 Burkina Faso	189	209	42	50	39	46	810	71	86	68	84	57	62	33	50
18 Niger	303	337	40	48	37	44	..	75	93	74	78	53	57	35	42
19 India	125	123	49	60	50	60	..	42	..	45	..	60	71	39	55
20 Kenya	97	113	52	61	48	57	..	84	78	84	76	71	95	42	78
21 Nigeria	177	195	43	53	40	50	800	64	..	66	..	59	76	49	74
22 China	37	48	63	71	61	67	115	..	76	..	81	..	86	..	72
23 Haiti	145	164	49	56	46	53	600	..	..	..	..	..	93	..	96
24 Benin	157	175	45	52	43	49	161	71	..	75	..	45	..	44	37
25 Central African Rep.	122	136	45	52	40	45	..	67	81	67	85	49	63	20	38
26 Ghana	122	140	51	57	48	53	1,000	77	..	82	..	75	82	35	63
27 Pakistan	139	137	47	59	49	59	270	56	..	60	..	36	52	25	41
28 Togo	131	149	46	56	43	52	..	85	78	88	86	45	65	26	34
29 Guinea	215	239	37	44	35	44	1,247	..	77	..	87	46	46	26	31
30 Nicaragua	59	72	55	68	52	64	300	48	62	45	59	101	104	89	138
31 Sri Lanka	19	25	66	74	64	69	80	94	97	73	99	89	93	101	105
32 Mauritania	188	209	41	49	38	45	800	..	83	..	83	39	69	13	45
33 Yemen, Rep.	148	166	42	52	41	52	330	..	..	..	..	..	..	..	..
34 Honduras	54	66	55	68	51	63	221	..	..	..	..	99	98	79	..
35 Lesotho	146	167	50	58	48	55	220	87	87	70	76	150	121	111	149

		Under-5 Mortality Rate (per 1,000 live births)		Life Expectancy at Birth (years)				Maternal Mortality (per 100,000 live births) 1988	Percentage of Cohort Persisting to Grade 4				Females per 100 males			
				Female		Male			Female		Male		Primary		Secondary	
		Female 1991	Male 1991	1970	1991	1970	1991		1970	1986	1970	1986	1970	1990	1970	1990
36	Indonesia	102	120	49	61	46	58	450	67	82	89	99	84	93	59	82
37	Egypt, Arab Rep.	82	96	52	62	50	60	..	85	..	93	..	61	80	48	76
38	Zimbabwe	50	63	52	62	49	59	77	74	81	80	81	79	99	63	88
39	Sudan	156	176	43	53	41	50	..	..	..	..	..	61	75	40	80
40	Zambia	166	186	48	50	45	47	..	93	..	99	..	80	91	49	59
	Middle-income economies	**44 w**	**54 w**	**62 w**	**71 w**	**58 w**	**65 w**	**107 w**	**78 w**	**87 w**	**76 w**	**90 w**	**86 w**	**91 w**	**94 w**	**104 w**
	Lower-middle-income	**50 w**	**60 w**	**61 w**	**69 w**	**57 w**	**64 w**	**111 w**	**79 w**	**87 w**	**80 w**	**88 w**	**80 w**	**90 w**	**89 w**	**104 w**
41	Bolivia	117	127	48	61	44	57	371	77	..	..	..	69	90	64	..
42	Côte d'Ivoire	144	163	46	53	43	50	..	..	83	83	88	57	71	27	45
43	Senegal	140	160	44	49	42	46	..	..	90	80	94	63	72	39	51
44	Philippines	53	68	59	67	56	63	74	..	85	..	84	..	94	..	..
45	Papua New Guinea	67	81	47	56	47	55	700	76	..	84	..	57	80	37	62
46	Cameroon	112	130	46	57	43	54	..	59	85	58	86	74	85	36	68
47	Guatemala	76	84	54	67	51	62	..	33	..	73	..	79	..	65	..
48	Dominican Rep.	66	72	61	69	57	65	300	55	..	13	..	99	98	..	..
49	Ecuador	56	62	60	69	57	64	156	69	..	70	..	93	..	76	..
50	Morocco	66	79	53	65	50	61	..	78	80	83	81	51	66	40	69
51	Jordan	30	33	..	70	..	66	..	90	97	92	99	78	94	53	96
52	Tajikistan	60	66	..	72	..	67	39	..	..	..	..	85	..	..	..
53	Peru	62	76	56	66	52	62	165	..	..	..	..	85	..	74	..
54	El Salvador	46	50	60	68	56	63	148	61	..	62	..	92	98	77	95
55	Congo	159	177	49	54	43	49	..	86	90	89	98	78	87	43	72
56	Syrian Arab Rep.	37	47	57	69	54	65	143	92	93	95	95	57	87	36	71
57	Colombia	23	29	63	72	59	66	200	57	74	51	72	101	98	73	100
58	Paraguay	38	46	67	69	63	65	300	70	77	71	77	89	93	91	102
59	Uzbekistan	47	59	..	73	..	66	43	..	..	..	..	..	..	..	..
60	Jamaica	16	20	70	76	66	71	115	..	100	..	98	100	99	103	..
61	Romania	28	38	71	73	67	67	..	90	..	89	..	97	106	151	174
62	Namibia	85	97	49	60	47	56	..	..	..	..	..	..	108	..	127
63	Tunisia	40	51	55	68	54	67	127	..	91	..	94	64	85	38	77
64	Kyrgyzstan	45	58	..	70	..	62	43	..	..	..	..	..	..	..	..
65	Thailand	30	40	61	72	56	66	37	71	..	69	..	88	95	69	97
66	Georgia	18	23	..	77	..	69	55	..	..	..	..	..	..	..	..
67	Azerbaijan	34	45	..	75	..	67	29	..	..	..	..	..	..	..	..
68	Turkmenistan	68	83	..	70	..	62	55	..	98	81	98	..	89	..	..
69	Turkey	70	77	59	70	55	64	146	76	..	81	..	73	89	37	63
70	Poland	15	21	74	75	67	67	..	99	..	97	..	93	95	251	266
71	Bulgaria	18	23	74	75	69	68	..	91	91	100	93	94	93	111	198
72	Costa Rica	13	16	69	78	65	74	18	93	91	91	90	96	94	..	103
73	Algeria	77	85	54	67	52	65	..	90	95	95	97	60	81	40	79
74	Panama	24	28	67	75	64	71	60	97	88	97	85	92	93	99	103

(continued)

Table 7.5(continued)

	Health and Welfare							Education							
	Under-5 Mortality Rate (per 1,000 live births)		Life Expectancy at Birth (years)				Maternal Mortality (per 100,000 live births) 1988	Percentage of Cohort Persisting to Grade 4				Females per 100 males			
			Female		Male			Female		Male		Primary		Secondary	
	Female 1991	Male 1991	1970	1991	1970	1991		1970	1986	1970	1986	1970	1990	1970	1990
75 Armenia	24	30	..	75	..	68	35	..	..	..	..	..	..	..	..
76 Chile	18	22	66	76	59	68	40	86	..	83	..	98	95	130	115
77 Iran, Islamic Rep.	83	91	54	65	55	65	120	75	92	74	93	55	86	49	74
78 Moldova	24	32	..	72	..	65	34	..	..	..	..	..	..	..	..
79 Ukraine	18	26	74	75	67	66	33	..	..	..	..	96	..	127	..
80 Mauritius	22	28	65	73	60	67	99	97	99	97	99	94	98	66	100
81 Czechoslovakia	12	17	73	76	67	68	..	96	97	98	97	96	97	183	132
82 Kazakhstan	33	44	..	73	..	64	53	..	..	..	..	..	..	..	..
83 Malaysia	15	21	63	73	60	68	26	..	..	..	..	88	95	69	104
Upper-middle-income	**36 w**	**46 w**	**64 w**	**72 w**	**59 w**	**65 w**	**104 w**	**75 w**	**..**	**70 w**	**94 w**	**94 w**	**95 w**	**101 w**	**102 w**
84 Botswana	36	44	51	70	48	66	..	97	96	90	97	113	107	88	114
85 South Africa	65	79	56	66	50	59	..	..	..	..	..	98	..	95	..
86 Lithuania	15	21	75	76	67	65	29	..	..	..	..	..	..	..	..
87 Hungary	17	23	73	74	67	66	..	90	97	99	97	93	95	202	198
88 Venezuela	35	44	68	73	63	67	55	84	91	61	81	99	99	102	137
89 Argentina	28	32	70	75	64	68	140	92	..	69	..	98	103	156	..
90 Uruguay	21	25	72	77	66	70	36	..	98	..	96	91	95	129	..
91 Brazil	60	73	61	69	57	63	140	56	..	54	..	99	..	99	..
92 Mexico	38	50	64	73	60	67	200	..	73	..	94	92	94	..	92
93 Belarus	15	21	76	76	68	66	25	..	..	..	..	..	..	..	..
94 Russian Federation	21	29	..	74	..	64	49	..	..	..	..	..	..	..	..
95 Latvia	17	23	..	75	..	64	57	..	..	..	..	..	..	..	..
96 Trinidad and Tobago	21	25	68	74	63	69	89	78	..	74	..	97	97	113	102
97 Gabon	144	163	46	55	43	52	..	73	80	78	78	91	..	43	..
98 Estonia	13	19	74	75	66	65	41	..	..	..	..	..	..	..	..
99 Portugal	11	15	71	77	64	70	..	92	..	92	..	95	91	98	116
100 Oman	33	43	49	71	46	67	..	..	97	..	100	16	89	..	82
101 Puerto Rico	16	20	75	80	69	72	21	..	..	..	..	..	..	..	..
102 Korea, Rep.	16	22	62	73	58	67	26	96	100	96	100	92	94	65	87
103 Greece	12	14	74	80	70	75	..	97	99	96	99	92	94	98	103
104 Saudi Arabia	33	44	54	71	51	68	..	93	..	91	..	46	84	16	79
105 Yugoslavia	19	25	70	76	65	70	..	91	..	99	..	91	94	86	98
Low-and middle-income	**80 w**	**89 w**	**56 w**	**63 w**	**54 w**	**62 w**	**238 w**	**61 w**	**76 w**	**64 w**	**80 w**	**70 w**	**81 w**	**60 w**	**73 w**
Sub-Saharan Africa	**167 w**	**186 w**	**45 w**	**52 w**	**42 w**	**49 w**	**686 w**	**66 w**	**71 w**	**69 w**	**72 w**	**60 w**	**76 w**	**40 w**	**67 w**

Health and Welfare   Education

	Under-5 Mortality Rate (per 1,000 live births)		Life Expectancy at Birth (years)				Maternal Mortality (per 100,000 live births) 1988	Percentage of Cohort Persisting to Grade 4				Females per 100 males			
			Female		Male			Female		Male		Primary		Secondary	
	Female 1991	Male 1991	1970	1991	1970	1991		1970	1986	1970	1986	1970	1990	1970	1990
East Asia and Pacific	46 w	58 w	60 w	66 w	58 w	66 w	195 w	..	78 w	..	82 w	..	88 w	..	75 w
South Asia	129 w	127 w	48 w	59 w	50 w	59 w	444 w	45 w	..	48 w	..	55 w	69 w	38 w	54 w
Europe and Central Asia	28 w	35 w	69 w	74 w	64 w	66 w	60 w	90 w	97 w	92 w	98 w	89 w	94 w	137 w	143 w
Middle East and N. Africa	73 w	84 w	54 w	65 w	52 w	63 w	151 w	83 w	90 w	87 w	92 w	54 w	79 w	41 w	72 w
Latin America and Caribbean	48 w	58 w	63 w	71 w	58 w	65 w	162 w	66 w	76 w	60 w	85 w	96 w	97 w	101 w	103 w
Severely indebted	55 w	66 w	62 w	69 w	58 w	64 w	171 w	75 w	80 w	73 w	89 w	87 w	88 w	109 w	115 w
High-income economies	8 w	11 w	75 w	80 w	68 w	73 w	..	95 w	98 w	93 w	97 w	96 w	95 w	95 w	100 w
OECD members	8 w	11 w	75 w	80 w	68 w	73 w	..	95 w	98 w	93 w	97 w	96 w	95 w	95 w	100 w
106 Ireland	9	11	73	78	69	72		..	98	..	97	96	96	124	101
107 Israel	10	14	73	78	70	74		96	97	96	97	92	98	131	116
108 New Zealand	9	13	75	79	69	73		..	98	..	98	94	94	94	98
109 Spain	9	11	75	80	70	74		76	98	76	97	99	93	84	102
110 Hong Kong	5	7	73	80	67	75	4	94	..	92	..	90	..	74	..
111 Singapore	7	9	70	77	65	72	10	99	100	99	100	88	90	103	100
112 United Kingdom	8	10	75	79	69	72		..	97	..	94	95	96	94	96
113 Australia	8	10	75	80	68	73		76	..	74	..	94	95	91	99
114 Italy	10	12	75	81	69	74		..	..	..	..	94	95	86	97
115 Netherlands	8	10	77	80	71	74		99	..	96	..	96	99	91	109
116 Belgium	10	12	75	80	68	73		..	87	..	85	94	97	87	94
117 Austria	9	11	74	80	67	73		95	99	92	98	95	95	95	94
118 France	8	10	76	81	68	73		97	..	90	..	95	94	107	106
119 Canada	8	10	76	81	69	74		95	97	92	93	95	93	95	96
120 United States	9	13	75	79	67	72		..	..	..	..	95	95	93	95
121 Germany*	8	10	74	79	67	73		97	99	96	97	96	96	102	98
122 Denmark	9	11	76	78	71	72		98	100	96	100	97	96	112	106
123 Finland	7	9	74	79	66	73		..	98	..	99	90	95	97	111
124 Norway	9	11	77	80	71	74		99	..	98	..	105	95	97	105
125 Sweden	7	9	77	81	72	75		98	..	96	..	96	95	92	109
126 Japan	5	7	75	82	69	76		100	100	100	100	96	95	101	99
127 Switzerland	8	10	76	81	70	74		94	..	93	..	98	96	93	99
World	69 w	77 w	60 w	65 w	57 w	64 w	237 w	67 w	78 w	70 w	82 w	77 w	84 w	68 w	76 w
Fuel exporters	114 w	127 w	50 w	61 w	48 w	58 w	492 w	75 w	88 w	75 w	88 w	60 w	81 w	51 w	80 w

*Data refer to the Federal Republic of Germany before unification. The letter W means weighted average.

Note: Figures in italics are for years other than those specified. The bold areas are summary measures for groups of economies.

.. means data not available.

From: No author (1993). *World Development Report 1993: Investing in Health.* New York: Oxford Univ. Press (for the World Bank).

Table 7.6

Years of Potential Life Lost Before Age 65 for Selected Causes of Death, According to Sex and Race: United States, Selected Years 1970–1990

[Data are based on the National Vital Statistics System.]

Sex, Race, and Cause of Death	1970	1980	1985	1990
All Races	*Years lost per 100,000 Population Under 65 Years of Age*			
All causes	8,595.9	6,416.0	5,660.2	5,623.0
Diseases of heart	1,108.9	841.3	752.6	632.2
Ischemic heart disease	—	544.3	448.4	350.0
Cerebrovascular diseases	241.1	140.8	119.6	110.7
Malignant neoplasms	1,013.0	907.5	875.3	848.6
Respiratory system	190.7	211.9	207.6	203.0
Colorectal	78.9	68.7	65.1	60.6
Prostate*	8.2	8.5	8.4	8.7
Breast†	115.6	105.5	107.1	109.4
Chronic obstructive pulmonary diseases	73.2	57.2	61.1	61.0
Pneumonia and influenza	392.1	97.5	81.1	81.2
Chronic liver disease and cirrhosis	187.8	145.3	113.7	103.1
Diabetes mellitus	80.6	56.2	54.8	67.0
Human immunodeficiency virus infection	—	—	—	303.4
Unintentional injuries	1,599.1	1,373.1	1,087.9	984.7
Motor vehicle crashes	889.4	840.8	660.8	615.5
Suicide	250.2	309.0	313.5	312.0
Homicide and legal intervention	271.8	373.6	291.7	374.3
White Male				
All causes	9,757.4	7,611.5	6,697.6	6,503.1
Diseases of heart	1,607.4	1,179.1	1,034.8	847.7
Ischemic heart disease	—	869.7	707.8	545.5
Cerebrovascular diseases	215.0	122.6	104.5	93.9
Malignant neoplasms	1,036.9	935.1	887.5	843.1
Respiratory system	287.8	286.0	266.8	251.6
Colorectal	81.2	73.5	71.2	66.1
Prostate	14.4	15.2	15.0	16.2
Chronic obstructive pulmonary diseases	88.8	64.2	63.2	60.3
Pneumonia and influenza	353.2	88.7	77.6	76.3
Chronic liver disease and cirrhosis	209.8	166.9	136.8	132.5
Diabetes mellitus	75.3	52.5	53.9	65.7
Human immunodeficiency virus infection	—	—	—	451.2
Unintentional injuries	2,261.3	2,071.0	1,606.9	1,420.1
Motor vehicle crashes	1,296.5	1,301.7	985.2	886.8
Suicide	369.6	509.0	529.4	532.3
Homicide and legal intervention	201.9	365.4	275.0	313.3
Black Male				
All causes	20,283.5	14,381.9	12,675.5	14,365.8
Diseases of heart	2,022.2	1,661.4	1,561.7	1,387.8
Ischemic heart disease	—	800.9	684.9	552.5
Cerebrovascular diseases	595.6	349.3	295.8	279.9
Malignant neoplasms	1,216.0	1,175.8	1,141.3	1,131.9
Respiratory system	376.7	400.4	386.0	378.2
Colorectal	80.8	76.7	79.4	83.8
Prostate	35.2	34.1	33.1	30.5
Chronic obstructive pulmonary diseases	146.8	110.8	114.6	121.9

Sex, Race, and Cause of Death	1970	1980	1985	1990
	Years Lost per 100,000 Population Under 65 Years of			
Pneumonia and influenza	1,308.9	315.2	254.9	261.4
Chronic liver disease and cirrhosis	463.5	391.9	305.8	242.4
Diabetes mellitus	144.0	102.2	106.1	133.7
Human immunodeficiency virus infection	—	—	—	1,224.5
Unintentional injuries	3,500.6	2,308.9	1,891.1	1,807.4
Motor vehicle crashes	1,466.1	1,022.4	893.7	919.9
Suicide	237.5	323.8	336.9	376.3
Homicide and legal intervention	2,234.6	2,274.9	1,689.1	2,580.7
White Female				
All causes	5,527.4	3,983.2	3,542.3	3,330.7
Diseases of heart	497.4	401.2	369.4	309.6
Ischemic heart disease	—	227.9	195.4	155.9
Cerebrovascular diseases	180.1	111.6	93.0	84.5
Malignant neoplasms	974.6	858.3	846.4	829.1
Respiratory system	89.8	132.6	144.9	150.2
Colorectal	77.0	64.0	57.9	52.2
Breast	233.4	211.7	215.1	217.5
Chronic obstructive pulmonary diseases	46.5	43.0	51.8	52.7
Pneumonia and influenza	247.2	64.0	52.1	50.5
Chronic liver disease and cirrhosis	114.7	79.1	58.9	51.3
Diabetes mellitus	65.1	45.4	43.2	52.0
Human immunodeficiency virus infection	—	—	—	35.0
Unintentional injuries	755.6	647.8	532.4	494.2
Motor vehicle crashes	466.5	437.3	364.2	351.6
Suicide	157.2	145.4	137.7	126.3
Homicide and legal intervention	69.7	109.3	98.1	97.5
Black Female				
All causes	12,188.8	7,927.2	6,961.4	7,382.2
Diseases of heart	1,292.7	937.2	856.7	782.4
Ischemic heart disease	—	382.7	325.1	272.3
Cerebrovascular diseases	564.7	289.0	248.8	235.8
Malignant neoplasms	1,044.8	968.4	936.8	972.7
Respiratory system	89.3	132.8	137.6	149.0
Colorectal	81.4	70.3	74.7	72.9
Breast	209.3	210.9	236.4	264.1
Chronic obstructive pulmonary diseases	93.3	62.5	74.5	80.6
Pneumonia and influenza	888.7	187.4	141.1	145.6
Chronic liver disease and cirrhosis	295.6	210.9	146.7	122.7
Diabetes mellitus	179.7	109.3	100.8	125.8
Human immunodeficiency virus infection	—	—	—	336.7
Unintentional injuries	1,169.9	718.5	616.8	614.4
Motor vehicle crashes	478.4	296.8	283.1	305.6
Suicide	81.9	70.3	59.1	69.8
Homicide and legal intervention	460.3	492.0	399.8	509.8

*Male only.

†Female only.

NOTES: For data years shown, the code numbers for cause of death are based on the International Classification of Diseases, Ninth Revision, International Classification of Diseases codes for human immunodeficiency virus infection not available for use with the National Vital Statistics System until 1987. Years of potential life lost before age 65 provides a measure of the impact of mortality on the population under 65 years of age.

From: U.S. Dept. of Health and Human Services (1993). *Health, United States, 1992* (DHHS pub. no. PHS-93-1232). Washington, D.C.: U.S. Government Printing Office, pp. 216–217.

Table 7.7

Self-Assessment of Health, According to Selected Characteristics: United States, 1986 and 1991

[Data are based on household interviews of a sample of the civilian noninstitutionalized population.]

Characteristic	Total	Excellent		Very Good		Good		Fair or Poor	
		1986	1991	1986	1991	1986	1991	1986	1991
			*Percent Distribution**						
Total†‡	100.0	40.2	39.7	27.3	28.5	22.9	22.6	9.6	9.3
Age									
Under 15 years	100.0	52.7	52.3	27.3	28.0	17.5	17.3	2.6	2.5
Under 5 years	100.0	53.8	52.8	26.5	27.7	16.9	16.8	2.8	2.6
5–14 years	100.0	52.0	52.0	27.7	28.1	17.9	17.5	2.4	2.4
15–44 years	100.0	43.9	42.0	29.4	31.0	21.2	21.2	5.5	5.8
45–64 years	100.0	26.6	28.5	26.1	26.7	29.2	28.1	18.2	16.7
65 years and over	100.0	16.4	15.7	20.8	22.8	32.9	32.4	29.9	29.0
65–74 years	100.0	17.2	17.1	21.5	24.5	33.8	32.3	27.5	26.0
75 years and over	100.0	15.1	13.7	19.7	20.2	31.5	32.6	33.7	33.6
Sex†									
Male	100.0	42.8	41.7	26.6	28.1	21.5	21.3	9.1	8.9
Female	100.0	37.7	37.7	28.0	28.7	24.3	23.8	10.1	9.7
Race†									
White	100.0	41.8	41.2	28.0	28.9	21.6	21.3	8.7	8.6
Black	100.0	29.6	30.4	22.7	25.3	30.5	29.2	17.2	15.1
*Family income†****									
Less than $14,000	100.0	28.4	25.9	22.7	25.3	29.0	28.9	19.9	19.9
$14,000–24,999	100.0	33.6	34.0	27.6	28.5	26.5	26.7	12.3	10.8
$25,000–34,999	100.0	42.1	40.8	27.9	29.2	22.7	22.8	7.4	7.1
$35,000–49,999	100.0	44.2	43.7	29.9	31.4	19.8	19.5	6.1	5.5
$50,000 or more	100.0	52.2	52.1	27.6	28.2	16.3	15.8	3.9	3.9
Geographic Region†									
Northeast	100.0	39.1	42.2	29.9	28.5	22.3	21.8	8.8	7.4
Midwest	100.0	41.2	40.9	27.6	29.9	22.8	21.1	8.4	8.1
South	100.0	37.0	36.2	26.5	27.5	24.5	24.5	12.0	11.7
West	100.0	45.7	41.3	25.7	28.1	20.8	22.0	7.8	8.8
Location of Residence†									
Within MSA	100.0	41.2	40.6	27.6	28.4	22.1	22.1	9.0	8.9
Outside MSA	100.0	36.9	36.3	26.0	28.7	25.6	24.2	11.4	10.7

*Denominator excludes unknown health status.

†Age adjusted.

‡Includes all other races not shown separately and unknown family income.

**Family income categories for 1991. Income categories for 1986 are: less than $11,000; $11,000–19,999; $20,000–29,999; $30,000–39,999; and $40,000 or more.

From: U.S. Dept. of Health and Human Services (1993). *Health, United States, 1992* (DHHS pub. no. PHS-93-1232). Washington, D.C.: U.S. Government Printing Office, p. 101.

Table 7.8
Distribution of DALY Loss
by Cause and Demographic Region, 1990
(percent)

Established Cause	World	Sub- Saharan Africa	India	China	Other Asia and Islands	Latin America and the Caribbean	Middle Eastern Crescent	Formerly Socialist Economies of Europe	Market Economies
Population (millions)	5,267	510	850	1,134	683	444	503	346	798
Communicable diseases	45.8	71.3	50.5	25.3	48.5	42.2	51.0	8.6	9.7
Tuberculosis	3.4	4.7	3.7	2.9	5.1	2.5	2.8	0.6	0.2
STDs and HIV	3.8	8.8	2.7	1.7	1.5	6.6	0.7	1.2	3.4
Diarrhea	7.3	10.4	9.6	2.1	8.3	5.7	10.7	0.4	0.3
Vaccine-preventable childhood infections	5.0	9.6	6.7	0.9	4.5	1.6	6.0	0.1	0.1
Malaria	2.6	10.8	0.3	*	1.4	0.4	0.2	*	*
Worm infections	1.8	1.8	0.9	3.4	3.4	2.5	0.4	*	*
Respiratory infections	9.0	10.8	10.9	6.4	11.1	6.2	11.5	2.6	2.6
Maternal causes	2.2	2.7	2.7	1.2	2.5	1.7	2.9	0.8	0.6
Perinatal causes	7.3	7.1	9.1	5.2	7.4	9.1	10.9	2.4	2.2
Other	3.5	4.6	4.0	1.4	3.3	5.8	4.9	0.6	0.5
Noncommunicable diseases	42.2	19.4	40.4	58.0	40.1	42.8	36.0	74.8	78.4
Cancer	5.8	1.5	4.1	9.2	4.4	5.2	3.4	14.8	19.1
Nutritional deficiencies	3.9	2.8	6.2	3.3	4.6	4.6	3.7	1.4	1.7
Neuropsychiatric disease	6.8	3.3	6.1	8.0	7.0	8.0	5.6	11.1	15.0
Cerebrovascular disease	3.2	1.5	2.1	6.3	2.1	2.6	2.4	8.9	5.3
Ischemic heart disease	3.1	0.4	2.8	2.1	3.5	2.7	1.8	13.7	10.0
Pulmonary obstruction	1.3	0.2	0.6	5.5	0.5	0.7	0.5	1.6	1.7
Other	18.0	9.7	18.5	23.6	17.9	19.1	18.7	23.4	25.6
Injuries	11.9	9.3	9.1	16.7	11.3	15.0	13.0	16.6	11.9
Motor vehicle	2.3	1.3	1.1	2.3	2.3	5.7	3.3	3.7	3.5
Intentional	3.7	4.2	1.2	5.1	3.2	4.3	5.2	4.8	4.0
Other	5.9	3.9	6.8	9.3	5.8	5.0	4.6	8.1	4.3
Total	100.0	100.0	100.0	100.0	100.0	100.0	100.0	100.0	100.0
Millions of DALYs	1,362	293	292	201	177	103	144	58	94
Equivalent infant deaths (millions)	42.0	9.0	9.0	6.2	5.5	3.2	4.4	1.8	2.9
DALYs per 1,000 population	259	575	344	178	260	233	286	168	117

*Less than 0.05%.

Note: DALY, disability-adjusted life year; STD, sexually transmitted disease; HIV, human immunodeficiency virus.

From: No Author (1993). *World Development Report 1993: Investing in Health.* New York: Oxford Univ. Press (for the World Bank).

CREATING A
HEALTH PROFILE
OF AMERICANS

Creating a health profile for Americans requires a clear understanding of the health-related problems and opportunities of all Americans. However, infants do not face the same health concerns as adolescents, and children do not face the same health issues as seniors. Instead, each of these age groups has its own set of health problems and health risks. Therefore, we present in this chapter a health profile for each age group: infants (those less than 1 year old), children (ages 1–14 years), adolescents and young adults (ages 15–24), adults (ages 25–64 years), and older adults (65 and older). These subgroupings have been used by the U.S. government to describe the health status of Americans, for both the *1990 Health Objectives for the Nation* and the *Healthy People 2000* reports. Viewing these age group profiles enables public health workers to detect the sources of diseases, injury, and death for specific target populations and to propose programs to reduce these sources. Effective programs aimed at specific population age groups can reduce the rates of diseases, injury, and death for the entire population.

A HEALTH PROFILE
OF INFANTS
AND CHILDREN

It has been said that the health of a nation can best be judged by the health of its youngest members—the **infants**—those who have not yet reached one year of age

(see Figure 7.3). While the vast majority of infants born in America are healthy at birth, a significant minority are not. As a result, there are many industrialized nations that have better records than the United States when it comes to infant mortality. Infant mortality data for the United States is characterized by a long-standing and serious disparity between the health statistics for white infants and those of color. This disparity is not directly attributable to races, although certain diseases occur more often in certain races. Rather, the disparity can be traced to disparities in the socioeconomic status between segments of the American population. Low income and limited education correlate very highly with poor health status. If the young are indeed the hope for the future, the United States must work hard to insure the health of each infant, regardless of color or socioeconomic status.[7]

If the health of infants is a good measure of the health of a nation, the health of **children** (ages 1–14) could be considered one of several measures used to judge the parenting skills of a nation. Throughout the twentieth century, the health profile of America's children has improved greatly. Childhood mortality dropped 28% from 1977 to 1990, surpassing the national goal for 1990 (see Figure 7.4). The threat of infectious diseases (**childhood diseases**) such as polio, diphtheria, scarlet fever, pneumonia, measles, and whooping cough have nearly disappeared because of widespread immunization[1, 8, 9] (see Figure 7.5 and Box 7.1). However, there is still much to be done to improve the health of American children.

Because maternal and child health is a critical issue in community health, it warrants an entire chapter. Therefore, the reader is directed to Chapter 8 for a full discussion of a health profile of infants and children.

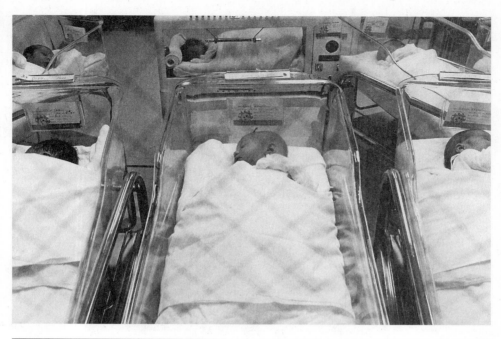

FIGURE 7.3

The health of a nation is often judged by the health of its youngest members.

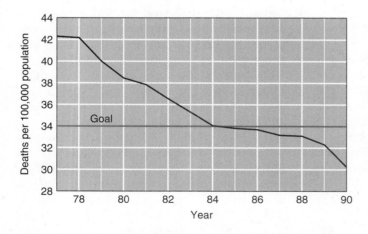

FIGURE 7.4

Death rates for children 1–14 years of age, 1977–1990 and 1990 goal.

From: CDC, NCHS, National Vital Statistics System.

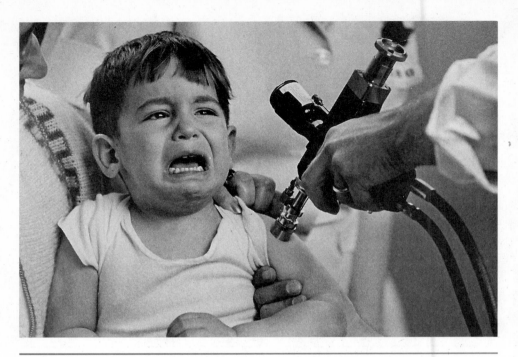

FIGURE 7.5
Immunizations have all but eliminated childhood diseases in the United States.

A HEALTH PROFILE
OF ADOLESCENTS
AND YOUNG ADULTS

Adolescents and young adults are considered to be those people who fall into the 15- to 24-year-old range. With regard to the health profile of this cohort, three major areas stand out: mortality, morbidity from specific infectious diseases, and health behavior and life-style choices.

Mortality

Between 1950 and 1990, the death rate of adolescents and young adults dropped by 19%, from 128.1 to 99.2/100,000.[4] This decline in death rates in adolescents and

young adults, like that for children, can be attributed to the advances in medicine and public health.[10] When subgroups from this age group are examined, it is revealed that white men and blacks of both sexes have higher mortality rates than women and whites respectively.[4]

Mortality from unintentional injuries in this age group has declined during the past 40 years but much more slowly than that for most diseases. Even so, unintentional-injury deaths remain the leading cause of death in adolescents and young adults, accounting for approximately half of all deaths in this age group (see Table 7.9). About three-fourths of these deaths result from motor vehicle crashes and, in more than half of all the fatal crashes, alcohol was a contributing factor. Unlike other mor-

BOX 7.1
Healthy People 2000—Objective

20.1 Reduce indigenous cases of vaccine-preventable diseases as follows:

Disease	1988 Baseline	2000 Target
Diphtheria among people aged 25 and younger	1	0
Tetanus among people aged 25 and younger	3	0
Polio (wild-type virus)	0	0
Measles	3,058	0
Rubella	225	0
Congenital Rubella Syndrome	6	0
Mumps	4,866	500
Pertussis	3,450	1,000

Baseline data source: Center for Prevention Services, CDC.

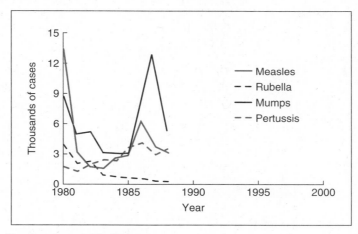

Vaccine-preventable diseases.

For Further Thought

If you were given the opportunity to pass one law that would increase the number of vaccine-preventable diseases, what would it be? Defend your response.

tality data in this age group, white males have a higher rate of death in motor vehicles than black males. The rates for women of both races are lower than those for males of either race.[11]

The most alarming mortality trend in this age group has been the growing number of homicides and suicides. During the period from 1960 to 1988 (see Figure 7.6), homicide and suicides rates increased between 200%

and 300% respectively.[10] Homicide is the second leading cause of death in the 15- to 24-year age group and the leading cause of death among blacks.[11] Between 1985 and 1989, homicides increased 74% among black men in this age group, reaching the highest recorded level in 1989.[12] It is not race, per se, that is a risk factor for violent death but rather socioeconomic status and environment. Differences in homicide rates between races are significantly reduced when socioeconomic factors are taken into account. However, alcohol and drugs are involved in about 60% of all homicides.[11]

Suicide is the third leading cause of death in adolescents and young adults and the second leading cause of death of white males in this age group. The rate among

Table 7.9
Number of Deaths per 100,000 Persons 15–24 Years Old, by Age and Cause of Death: 1960–1988

Cause of Death	1960	1965	1970	1975	1980	1985	1988
15–19 Years Old							
All causes	92.2	95.1	110.3	101.5	97.9	81.2	88.0
Motor vehicle accidents	35.9	40.2	43.6	38.4	43.0	33.9	37.3
All other accidents	16.8	16.5	20.3	19.0	14.9	10.3	9.4
Suicide	3.6	4.0	5.9	7.6	8.5	10.0	11.3
Males, white	5.9	6.3	9.4	13.0	15.0	17.3	19.6
Females, white	1.6	1.8	2.9	3.1	3.3	4.1	4.8
Males, all other races	3.4	5.2	5.4	7.0	7.5	10.0	11.0
Females, all other races	1.5	2.4	2.9	2.1	1.8	2.2	2.6
Homicide	4.0	4.3	8.1	9.6	10.6	8.6	11.7
Males, white	3.2	3.0	5.2	8.2	10.9	7.3	8.1
Females, white	1.2	1.3	2.1	3.2	3.9	2.7	3.0
Males, all other races	27.6	30.6	59.8	47.8	43.3	39.9	64.4
Females, all other races	7.0	7.1	10.1	14.6	10.1	9.4	10.2
Cancer	7.7	7.6	7.3	6.0	5.4	4.6	4.4
Heart disease	6.2	5.3	3.9	3.4	2.3	2.2	2.2
Pneumonia/influenza	2.8	2.1	2.1	1.5	0.6	0.5	0.5
20–24 Years Old							
All causes	125.6	127.3	148.0	138.2	132.7	108.9	115.4
Motor vehicle accidents	42.9	49.3	51.3	40.1	46.8	38.1	39.7
All other accidents	19.6	18.7	22.9	23.5	18.8	14.1	12.4
Suicide	7.1	8.9	12.2	16.5	16.1	15.6	15.0
Males, white	11.9	13.9	19.3	26.8	27.8	27.4	27.0
Females, white	3.1	4.3	5.7	6.9	5.9	5.2	4.4
Males, all other races	7.8	13.1	19.4	23.6	20.9	20.2	20.0
Females, all other races	1.6	4.0	5.5	6.0	3.6	3.5	3.0
Homicide	8.2	10.0	16.0	18.3	20.6	15.1	19.0
Males, white	6.0	7.4	11.1	14.5	19.9	14.6	14.8
Females, white	1.9	2.3	3.5	4.8	5.4	4.3	4.7
Males, all other races	64.2	80.5	136.3	124.9	109.4	72.8	105.6
Females, all other races	16.3	17.3	23.9	23.6	23.3	15.2	19.7
Cancer	9.2	9.0	9.4	7.6	7.2	6.1	5.7
Heart disease	11.3	9.3	6.2	5.4	3.5	3.3	3.6
Pneumonia/influenza	3.2	2.3	2.8	1.9	1.0	0.8	0.9

From: U.S. Dept. of Education (1991). *Youth Indicators: Trends in the Well-Being of American Youth* (pub. no. PIP-91-863). Washington, D.C.: U.S. Government Printing Office, p. 116.

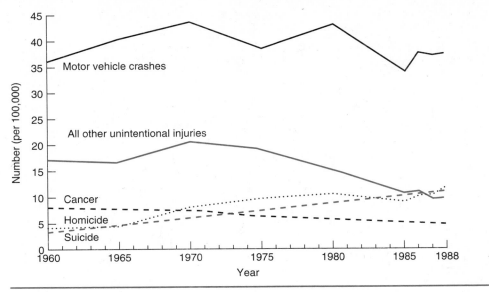

FIGURE 7.6

Number of deaths per 100,000 persons 15–19 years old, by cause of death: 1960–1988.

From: U.S. Dept. of Education (1991). Youth Indications: Trends in the Well-Being of American Youth. *(pub. no. PIP-91-863). Washington, D.C.: U.S. Government Printing Office, p. 116.*

black males is about half that of whites. Suicide rates are increasing faster among 15- to 19-year-olds than among 20- to 24-year-olds. The suicide rate in females, both black and white, is significantly lower than that for males, although young women attempt suicide approximately three times more often than young men.[11]

While the number of completed suicides by adolescents and young adults is alarming, it represents only a fraction of all the suicides contemplated. Data from the Centers for Disease Control and Prevention's Youth Risk Behavior Surveillance System indicate that 29% (females 37%, males 21%) of 15- to 19-year olds in the United States had thought seriously about attempting suicide, 19% (females 25%, males 13%) had made a specific plan to attempt suicide, 7% (females 11%, males 4%) have actually attempted suicide, and 2% (females 2%, males 1%) have made an attempt that resulted in an injury

or poisoning that had to be treated by a doctor or nurse.[13]

"For young people overall, 70% of mortality can be attributed to four causes: motor vehicle crashes (35%), other unintentional injuries (15%), homicide (10%), and suicide (10%)."[14]

Morbidity

While a higher proportion of adolescents and young adults survive to age 24 than ever before, this groups still suffers significantly from a number of different communicable diseases. One of these diseases, measles (rubeola), once thought to be only a childhood disease and close to eradication, made a resurgence in the late 1980s (see Tables 7.10 and 7.11). Measles is a much more severe disease for adolescents and young adults than it is for children. It was first thought that a single vaccination for

Table 7.10
Total Number of Reported Cases
of Selected Youth-Related Diseases, for All Age Groups: 1950–1989

Year	Polio	Measles	Tuberculosis	Gonorrhea	Syphilis	AIDS
1950	33,300	319,124	121,742	286,746	217,558	—
1955	28,985	555,156	77,368	236,197	122,392	—
1960	3,190	441,703	55,494	258,933	122,538	—
1965	61	261,904	49,016	324,925	112,842	—
1970	31	47,351	37,137	600,072	91,382	—
1975	8	24,374	33,989	999,937	80,356	—
1980	9	13,506	27,749	1,004,029	68,832	—
1985	7	2,822	22,201	911,419	27,131	8,249
1987	—	3,655	22,517	*780,905	*35,147	21,070
1988	9	3,396	22,436	719,536	40,117	31,001
1989	5	18,193	23,495	*733,151	*44,540	33,722

—Data not available.

*Civilian cases only.

From: U.S. Dept. of Education (1991). *Youth Indicators: Trends in the Well-Being of American Youth* (pub. no. PIP-91-863). Washington, D.C.: U.S. Government Printing Office, p. 108.

Table 7.11
Number of Reported Cases of Selected Diseases
Among 15- to 24-Year-Olds: 1981–1989

Year	Polio 15–19	Polio 20–24	Measles 15–19	Measles 20–24	Tuberculosis 15–19	Tuberculosis 20–24	Gonorrhea 15–19	Gonorrhea 20–24	Syphilis 15–19	Syphilis 20–24	AIDS 15–19	AIDS 20–24
1981	2	—	466	128	656	1,542	243,432	374,562	4,173	8,792	—	—
1982	—	2	279	92	560	1,407	235,086	363,135	4,517	9,461	—	—
1983	—	2	382	163	530	1,375	220,385	340,378	4,395	9,204	—	—
1984	—	2	676	204	414	1,268	210,530	329,476	3,218	8,069	—	—
1985	—	—	—	251	464	1,208	218,821	341,645	3,132	7,717	30	349
1986	—	—	1,159	304	513	1,206	215,918	337,711	3,133	7,885	47	616
1987	—	—	1,071	187	535	1,241	188,233	292,938	4,331	10,209	70	937
1988	—	—	1,045	239	432	1,184	195,312	230,797	3,969	9,903	100	1,343
1989	—	1	4,403	1,578	514	1,228	*204,023	*225,200	4,408	10,495	108	1,378

—Data not available

*Civilian cases only.

From: U.S. Dept. of Education (1991). *Youth Indicators: Trends in the Well-Being of American Youth* (pub. no. PIP 91-863). Washington, D.C.: U.S. Government Printing Office, p. 108.

Table 7.12
1989 Recommendations for Measles Vaccination
(routine childhood schedule, United States)

Most areas	Two doses*† first dose at 15 months second dose at 4–6 years (entry to kindergarten or first grade)§
High-risk areas¶	Two doses*† first dose at 12 months second dose at 4–6 years (entry to kindergarten or first grade)§
Colleges and other educational institutions post-high school	Documentation of receipt of two doses of measles vaccine after the first birthday† or other evidence of measles immunity**
Medical personnel beginning employment	Documentation of receipt of two doses of measles vaccine after the first birthday† or other evidence of measles immunity**

*Both doses should preferably be given as combined measles, mumps, rubella vaccine (MMR).
†No less than one month apart. If no documentation of any dose of vaccine, vaccine should be given at the time of school entry or employment and no less than one month later.
§Some areas may elect to administer the second dose at an older age or to multiple age groups.
¶A county with more than five cases among preschool-aged children during each of the last five years, a county with a recent outbreak among unvaccinated preschool-aged children, or a country with a large inner-city urban population. These recommendations may be applied to an entire county or to identified risk areas within a county.
**Prior physician-diagnosed measles disease, laboratory evidence of measles immunity, or birth before 1957.

From: No author (1989)."Measles Prevention: Recommendations of the Immunization Practice Committee (ACIP)."
Morbidity and Mortality Weekly Reports 38(5–9): 4.

---

measles (taken concurrently with mumps and rubella, as the MMR vaccination, at 15 months of age) would confer life-long immunity against the disease. However, measles is much more communicable than once believed, so that a second immunization at the time of first entering school is now recommended. "This schedule is expected to provide protection to most persons who do not respond to their initial vaccination."[15] The recommendations for measles vaccination that were adopted in 1989 are given in Table 7.12.

The other diesease that are causing considerable morbidity in adolescents and youth are sexually transmitted diseases (STDs)–diseases that are spread primarily through unprotected sexual activity. Reported cases of gonorrhea, which in-

creased steadily between 1960 and 1975 and remained at near-record levels through 1982, have declined during the past ten years.[5] Syphilis, on the other hand, reached an all-time low in 1985 but then increased each year through 1990. And as might be expected, the number of cases of AIDS has steadily increased in recent years (see Tables 7.10 and 7.11).[10] Overall, it is estimated that each year there are approximately 2.5 million cases of sexually transmitted diseases among teens in the United States.[14]

Health Behaviors and Life-Style Choices

While many behavioral patterns begin during the childhood years (ages 1–14),

Table 7.13

Use of Selected Substances in the Past Month by High School Seniors, According to Sex, Race, and Average Parental Education: United States, 1980–1991

[Data are based on a survey of high school seniors in the coterminous United States]

Substance, Sex, Race, and Average Parental Education	Class of											
	1980	*1981*	*1982*	*1983*	*1984*	*1985*	*1986*	*1987*	*1988*	*1989*	*1990*	*1991*
Cigarettes	*Percent Using Substance in the Past Month*											
All seniors	30.5	29.4	30.0	30.3	29.3	30.1	29.6	29.4	28.7	28.6	29.4	28.3
Male	26.8	26.5	26.8	28.0	25.9	28.2	27.9	27.0	28.0	27.7	29.1	29.0
Female	33.4	31.6	32.6	31.6	31.9	31.4	30.6	31.4	28.9	29.0	29.2	27.5
White	31.0	30.1	31.3	31.3	31.0	31.7	32.0	32.2	32.3	32.1	32.5	31.8
Black	25.2	22.3	21.2	21.2	17.6	18.7	14.6	13.9	12.8	12.4	12.0	9.4
Average parental education*:												
Less than high school	32.7	32.5	32.6	32.7	33.6	32.3	28.6	28.8	28.1	25.4	26.3	31.3
High school graduate	34.2	31.7	32.0	32.2	31.8	32.3	32.3	31.4	29.9	30.8	30.8	28.7
Some college	28.0	28.2	29.0	28.0	28.1	29.7	29.7	28.8	27.8	29.4	29.3	28.4
College graduate	25.7	26.0	25.5	27.8	25.2	27.7	26.4	27.6	28.6	27.0	29.1	26.9
Some postgraduate	24.0	22.5	25.1	25.5	23.7	22.6	26.7	29.3	27.8	26.3	28.6	27.1
Alcohol												
All seniors	72.0	70.7	69.7	69.4	67.2	65.9	65.3	66.4	63.9	60.0	57.1	54.0
Male	77.4	75.7	74.1	74.4	71.4	69.8	69.0	69.9	68.0	65.1	61.3	58.4
Female	66.8	65.7	65.4	64.3	62.8	62.1	61.9	63.1	59.9	54.9	52.3	49.0
White	75.8	75.0	74.2	73.5	72.1	70.2	70.2	71.8	69.5	65.3	62.2	57.7
Black	47.7	45.8	46.2	49.3	42.1	43.6	40.4	38.5	40.9	38.1	32.9	34.4
Average parental education*:												
Less than high school	65.9	62.1	61.3	61.2	58.1	58.7	56.1	56.3	54.5	47.8	47.2	49.9
High school graduate	72.0	70.7	69.4	69.2	67.4	65.9	65.3	67.0	64.6	59.7	57.2	53.3
Some college	73.3	71.5	72.7	70.4	69.6	66.9	66.7	67.2	64.3	62.9	57.7	54.3
College graduate	74.4	73.1	74.5	73.1	69.3	68.9	68.0	68.8	66.0	62.1	60.8	54.8
Some postgraduate	77.2	77.4	74.1	75.0	70.3	67.9	69.9	70.5	67.3	62.2	60.8	58.0
Marijuana												
All seniors	33.7	31.6	28.5	27.0	25.2	25.7	23.4	21.0	18.0	16.7	14.0	13.8
Male	37.8	35.3	31.4	31.0	28.2	28.7	26.8	23.1	20.7	19.5	16.1	16.1
Female	29.1	27.3	24.9	22.2	21.1	22.4	20.0	18.6	15.2	13.8	11.5	11.2
White	34.2	32.4	29.1	26.6	25.3	26.4	24.6	22.3	19.9	18.6	15.6	15.0
Black	26.5	24.9	24.8	26.9	22.8	21.7	16.6	12.4	9.8	9.4	5.2	6.5
Average parental education*:												
Less than high school	29.9	29.7	24.9	26.2	23.8	23.4	21.0	19.9	15.6	13.9	11.4	11.7
High school graduate	34.6	31.5	28.4	27.3	25.4	25.9	24.1	20.9	16.8	16.3	14.3	12.9
Some college	33.6	31.4	29.3	26.1	25.8	26.5	24.1	21.1	17.7	17.9	13.5	13.8
College graduate	33.7	31.9	30.1	26.9	23.3	27.1	23.1	21.1	19.3	17.1	15.0	13.7
Some postgraduate	36.2	31.9	27.7	25.5	23.4	20.6	21.7	21.2	20.6	16.2	15.0	17.6

Table 7.13 (continued)

Substance, Sex, Race, and Average Parental Education	Class of											
	1980	1981	1982	1983	1984	1985	1986	1987	1988	1989	1990	1991
Cocaine	Percent Using Substance in the Past Month											
All seniors	5.2	5.8	5.0	4.9	5.8	6.7	6.2	4.3	3.4	2.8	1.9	1.4
Male	6.0	6.3	5.9	5.7	7.0	7.7	7.2	4.9	4.2	3.6	2.3	1.7
Female	4.3	5.0	3.8	4.1	4.4	5.6	5.1	3.7	2.6	2.0	1.3	0.9
White	5.4	6.1	4.9	4.9	6.0	7.0	6.4	4.4	3.7	2.9	1.8	1.3
Black	2.0	2.1	3.2	3.0	2.4	2.7	2.7	1.8	1.4	1.2	0.5	0.8
Average parental education*:												
Less than high school	3.8	3.9	3.6	4.6	4.5	6.5	5.8	3.4	3.2	3.5	2.0	1.8
High school graduate	4.5	4.9	4.6	4.2	5.9	6.7	6.1	4.1	3.3	2.7	1.8	1.3
Some college	5.8	6.0	5.2	4.7	5.6	6.7	6.7	4.9	3.0	2.6	2.0	1.4
College graduate	5.9	7.6	5.9	6.0	6.2	6.8	6.1	4.2	4.0	3.1	1.2	1.2
Some postgraduate	7.0	7.4	5.4	6.0	6.6	6.4	5.3	4.0	3.6	2.4	2.0	0.9

*Average parental education is calculated by averaging the following respondent-reported parental educational categories: (1) completed grade school or less, (2) some high school, (3) completed high school, (4) some college, (5) completed college, and (6) graduate or professional school after college.

Notes: The Nation's High School Seniors survey excludes high school dropouts (about 15% of the age group during the 1980s) and absentees (about 16–19% of high school students). High school dropouts and absentees have higher drug usage than those included in the survey.

Data from: National Institute on Drug Abuse: Monitoring the Future Study: Annual surveys.

Source: U.S. Dept. of Health and Human Services (Aug. 1993). *Health, United States, 1992* (DHHS pub. no. PHS-93-1232). Washington, D.C.: U.S. Government Printing Office, p. 106.

others begin in adolescence and young adulthood. In these years of experimentation, young people are susceptible to developing deleterious behaviors such as the abuse of alcohol and illicit drugs, including tobacco products, fighting; and carrying of a weapon.

To better track the specific health behaviors among young people, the CDC developed the Youth Risk Behavior Surveillance System (YRBSS). The system currently has three complementary components: national school-based surveys, state and local-based surveys, and a national household-based survey. In the spring of 1991, CDC conducted for the first time the national school-based Youth Risk Behavior Survey. This survey continues to be conducted biannually during odd-numbered years among national probability samples of ninth- through twelfth-grade students from private and public schools. Results of the 1991 survey are included in the sections below. In 1990, CDC began offering to each state and to selected local departments of education the YRBSS questionnaire and fiscal and technical assistance to conduct the Youth Risk Behavior Survey. During 1990, 24 states and eight cities conducted surveys. The third component of YRBSS, national household-based surveys, was initiated when the Bureau of Census incorporated a Youth Risk Behavior Supplement in the 1992 National Health Interview Survey (NHIS).[16] Results of this third component were not available at the time of this writing.

Alcohol and Other Drugs

While for some, the first use of alcohol or other drugs begins during the childhood years, for most, experimentation with these substances reaches its peak during the ages of 15–24 years. National surveys indicate that 28% of eighth graders and 27% of tenth graders have experienced occasions of heavy drinking and 6% and 13% of these same groups, respectively, have used marijuana at least once in the preceding month.[8, 17] While these figures may seem high, they actually represent slight drops from the levels of alcohol and marijuana use by this age group in previous years.

Nonetheless, alcohol use and abuse continue to be major problems for both adolescents and young adults, particularly among high school dropouts. As was reported earlier in this chapter, alcohol contributes significantly to motor vehicle crashes and violence in this cohort. In 1991, about 54% of high school seniors reported drinking during the previous month, while in 1988, 65% of 18- to 24-year-olds reported such behavior. The percentage of 18- to 24-year-olds is higher than all other age groups.[8,9]

The prevalence of illicit drug use by this cohort has declined in recent years. In 1989, 51% of high school seniors reported having used an illicit drug at least once in their lifetime, as compared to 65% in 1980. The percentage of high school seniors who reported having used an illicit drug in the previous 30 days also dropped from 39% in 1980 to 15% in 1991[9] (see Table 7.13). The most popular illicit drug in both years was marijuana. While these trends are positive signs that prevention and control strategies are working, most will agree that alcohol and other drug problems remain a major health concern for this age group. In Chapter 12, a more detailed examination of the problems of alcohol and other drug misuse and abuse are presented.

Tobacco Products

The use of tobacco products represents one of the most serious health problems for this group. In 1991, 17.3% of ninth-graders and 24% of twelfth-graders in the United States reported regular cigarette use. The vast majority of people who become dependent upon nicotine develop that dependency between the ages of 15 and 24 years, most before they reach the age of 20.

Recent data on the use of tobacco products by adolescents and young adults reveal two primary trends: (1) the use of smokable tobacco (cigarettes) per capita has leveled off, and (2) use of **smokeless tobacco** (snuff and chewing tobacco) is on the rise (see Figure 7.7). The percentage of high school seniors reporting daily smoking in the mid- to late- 1970s was just under 30%. Between the late 1970s and the early 1980s, that figure dropped to about 19% and has remained at that level despite numerous education efforts to reduce tobacco use even further. It is important to note, however, that this survey of high school seniors does not include high school dropouts, who have the highest prevalence rates for the cohort.[8] More than 1 million teens begin smoking each year; three-fourths of these have parents who smoke. The most alarming trend is that smokers, especially females, are beginning at younger ages than in the past.[1]

The use of smokeless tobacco among teenage boys has increased dramatically in recent years. Between 1970 and 1986, snuff use increased fifteen-fold and chewing tobacco use four-fold among 17- to 19-year-old men.[8] In 1991, the prevalence rates for ninth-grade boys who use smokeless tobacco was 9%, while that for twelfth grade boys was 10.7%.[17]

Physical Fighting and Weapon Carrying

As is noted in Chapter 17, the concern about violence in the United States, particularly among adolescents and young adults,

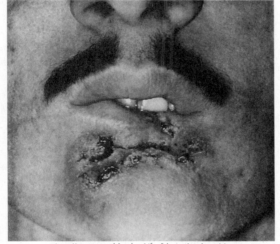

With Smokeless Tobacco, You Could Be His Spittin' Image.

Why would anyone use smokeless tobacco? After all, there's evidence that smokeless can cause cancer. And cancer could claim your cheek. Your jaw. Maybe even your life. So before you have a dip or a chaw, be sure to use your head. While it's still all there.

Don't Use Smokeless. Give Yourself The Chance Of A Lifetime.

AMERICAN CANCER SOCIETY®
For more information call 1 800 ACS-2345.

FIGURE 7.7

Use of smokeless tobacco among adolescents and young adults continues to rise despite educational campaigns to discourage it.

is growing. Data collected for the Centers for Disease Control and Prevention's Youth Risk Behavior Surveillance Systems reveal that 42% (females 34%, males 50%) of the 15- to 19-year-olds had been in at least one physical fight during the previous 12 months. In addition, 26% (females 11%, males 40%) had carried a weapon such as a gun, knife, or club at least 1 day during the previous 30 days. And of those students who carried a weapon, 11% (females 7%, males 12%) most often carried a handgun.[13]

Sexual Activity

Studies have shown that 78% of teenage girls and 86% of teenage boys have engaged in sexual intercourse prior to age 20. The primary health risks associated with such behavior are infection with STDs and unwanted pregnancies, both of which show increasing trends. Each year, more than a million girls in the United States between the ages of 15 and 19 become pregnant; 84% of these pregnancies are unintended. In addition to the health risks associated with teenage pregnancies for both mother and child, there are a number of psychosocial risks for the teenaged mother. She is less likely to complete high school, more likely to be unemployed, and more likely to lack parenting skills.[8]

A HEALTH PROFILE
OF ADULTS

The adult cohort, aged 25–64, represents slightly more than half of the United States population. The health profile of this age group is characterized by mortality from chronic diseases stemming from poor health behavior and poor choices of life-style.

Mortality

As was noted earlier in this chapter, any death that occurs prior to the age of 65 is considered a premature death. Thus any death of an adult (aged 24–64) in the United

States is a premature death. During the 1950s and 1960s, it was revealed that many of the leading causes of death in this age group were the results of preventable conditions associated with unhealthy behaviors and life-styles.

The death rate among adults has improved considerably in the last 45 years, and it is projected to improve further as we move closer to the year 2000. In 1950, the adult mortality rate stood at 687.1/100,000. By 1987, that number had dropped to 423.4/100,000, and by 2000, it is projected to be about 340/100,000 (see Box 7.2). Much of this improvement can be traced to changes in health behavior and life-style. Many adults have quit smoking, and more Americans are exercising regularly and paying attention to proper nutrition than ever before.

Figure 7.8 presents the ten leading causes of death for adults. Noncommunicable health problems dominate the list, headed by cancer and heart disease,

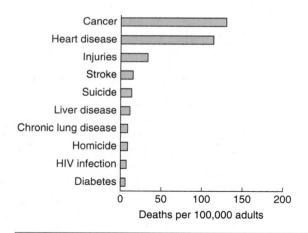

FIGURE 7.8

Leading causes of death of adults aged 25–64 (1987).

From: U.S. Dept. of Health and Human Services (1991). Healthy People 2000: National Health Promotion and Disease Prevention Objectives *[full report with commentary] (DHHS pub. no. PHS-92-1232). Washington, D.C.: U.S. Government Printing Office.*

BOX 7.2
Healthy People 2000—Objective

Reduce the death rate for adults by 20% to no more than 340 per 100,000 people aged 25 through 64.

(Baseline: 423 per 100,000 in 1987.)

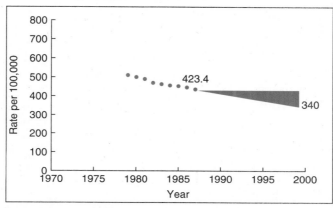

Death rate among adults aged 25–64.

For Further Thought

The health profile of American adults is substantially determined by behavioral risk factors. If you could get adults to change three health behaviors, which ones would you select? Why?

municable health problems dominate the list, headed by cancer and heart disease, which account for between 55% and 60% of all deaths in this age group.

Cancer

Since 1983, the Number 1 cause of death in the adult cohort has been cancers (malignant neoplasms) of various types. (For a review of malignant neoplasms, see Chapter 4.) Actually, cancer death rates have remained relatively steady since 1950 (132.8/100,000 in 1950 compared to 130.0/100,000 in 1986), but declines in cardiovascular deaths have resulted in cancer deaths achieving a Number 1 ranking.[1] The leading cause of cancer deaths and the most preventable type of cancer for both men and women is lung cancer. This trend will continue as large numbers of smokers continue to age. Of all lung cancer deaths, 85% can be attributed to smoking. The second leading cause of death due to cancer is colorectal cancer. Some research has suggested that diets high in fat or low in fiber (such those available from most fast-food restaurants) increase one's risk for this type of cancer.

The other type of cancer that receives much attention is breast cancer. Until it was surpassed by lung cancer in the mid-1980s, it was the leading cause of cancer deaths in women. Although it is less deadly than lung cancer, the number of cases of breast cancer is twice that of lung cancer in women. Because of increased community awareness and the availability of diagnostic screening for breast cancer, survival rates are much higher than for lung cancer. It has been estimated that breast cancer rates could be reduced an additional 30% with fuller participation in regular screening.[8]

Cardiovascular Diseases

Some of the greatest changes in cause-specific mortality rates in adults are those for the cardiovascular diseases. Mortality from diseases of the heart dropped from 243.8/100,000 in 1950 to 118.6/100,000 in 1986, while deaths from strokes dropped from 56.9/100,000 to 16.3/100,000 during the same period of time. These figures represent drops of about 51% and 71% respectively. These changes are due primarily to the numbers of people who have stopped smoking and from those who are exercising and eating better. As mentioned above, the reduction, or postponement, of deaths from heart disease has resulted in cancer becoming the leading cause of deaths in this cohort.

Other Leading Causes of Death

Other leading causes of adult deaths are intentional and unintentional injuries, diseases of the liver and the respiratory system, HIV infections, and diabetes. Deaths from HIV infection are expected to continue to ascend on the list of leading causes of death for adults in the near future. In 1990, HIV infection was the third leading cause of death in 25- to 44-year-olds and tenth for 45- to 64-year-olds.[4]

Health Behaviors and Life-Style Choices

Many of the risk factors associated with the leading causes of mortality and morbidity in American adults are associated with health behavior and life-style choices.

Adults have a unique opportunity to take personal action to substantially decrease their risk of ill health, and in recent years, many have taken such action. Today, more than ever before, adults are watching what they eat, buckling their safety belts, controlling their blood pressure, and exercising with regularity. The prevalence of smoking among adults has declined, as has the incidence of drinking and driving. While these are encouraging signs, there is still much more than can be done.

The best single behavioral change Americans can make to reduce morbidity and mortality is to stop smoking. Smoking is responsible for one in every six deaths in the United States. It is an important risk factor for cancer, heart disease, and stroke. In 1990, 25.4% of those aged 18 years and older smoked. This amounts to about 45.8 million Americans.[18] The proportion of Americans who smoke has dropped considerably since 1965, when 40% of all Americans smoked. While more men (32%) than women (27%) smoke, the gap between the genders is decreasing. In general, smoking rates are higher among blacks, Hispanics, blue-collar workers, and people with fewer years of education.[8]

Four other interrelated risk factors that contribute to disease and death in this cohort are poor eating patterns, lack of exercise, failure to control hypertension, and failure to maintain an appropriate body weight. Dietary factors are associated with five of the ten leading causes of death in this cohort. Many dietary components are involved in the diet-health relationship, but chief among them is the disproportionate consumption of foods high in fat, often at the expense of foods high in complex carbohydrates and dietary fiber. Total dietary fat (saturated and unsaturated) accounts for more than 36% of total calories consumed in the United States. A diet that contains no more than 30% fat is recommended.[8] Currently the largest source of fat in diets comes from cheeses and oils.[1]

In 1990, less than half of those Americans over 18 years of age reported that they exercised regularly at least three times per week, for at least 20 minutes each time, regardless of intensity.[19] It was once thought that **intensity** had to be high in order for cardiovascular benefits from exercise to accrue. But now it is believed than even light to moderate physical activity can have significant health benefits. Reducing inactivity and sedentary life-styles, even through walking for 20 minutes each day, is important to one's health.

Being overweight increases one's chances of a number of health problems including heart disease, some cancers, hypertension, elevated blood cholesterol, diabetes, stroke, gall bladder disease, and osteoarthritis. Approximately one-fourth of American adults are overweight, with a higher percentage of women (27%) being overweight than men (24%). The trend of weight gain increases with age. The key to maintaining an appropriate weight throughout life is a combination of diet and exercise; total reliance on either factor alone makes it a difficult process.[8]

Hypertension, defined by a resting blood pressure reading of 140/90mm of mercury or higher for those under 65 years of age and 160/90 for those 65 and older, afflicts about 58 million Americans, and is considered the most prevalent cardiovascular disease in the United States. Fortunately, once detected, hypertension is a risk factor that is highly modifiable (Figure 7.9).[1] The most desirable means of controlling hypertension is through a combination of diet modification, appropriate physical exercise,

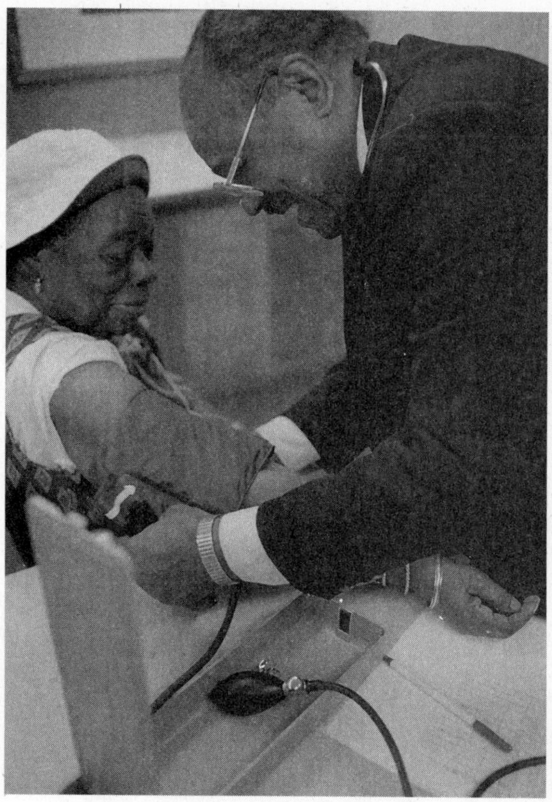

FIGURE 7.9

Hypertension is a highly modifiable risk factor.

and weight management. In cases in which these measures prove ineffective, hypertension can usually still be controlled with medication. Unfortunately, a great many Americans with hypertension are unaware of their problem. The keys to reducing morbidity and mortality resulting from hypertension are mass screenings that result in early detection of previously unidentified cases and their appropriate treatment.

The final health behavior presented for the adult cohort is alcohol consumption. Approximately 70% of adult Americans consume alcohol. While most do so in moderation, about 10% develop serious problems

---

intensity Cardiovascular workload measured by heart rate.

with their alcohol use. It is estimated that the 10% who consume the greatest amount of alcohol consume about 50% of all the alcohol consumed in America. These people are at greatest risk for developing a dependence upon alcohol and for developing such alcohol-related health problems as cirrhosis, alcoholism, and alcohol psychosis.

One does not have to become dependent on alcohol to have a drinking problem. Alcohol contributes to society's problems in a great many other ways. As noted elsewhere, alcohol increases the rates of homicide, suicide, family violence, and unintentional injuries such as those from motor vehicle crashes, boating incidents, and falls. The use of alcohol by pregnant women can cause fetal alcohol syndrome, the leading cause of birth defects in children. Clearly, alcohol consumption adversely affects the health and well-being of Americans.[1,8]

A HEALTH PROFILE OF SENIORS

Seniors are those who have reached their sixty-fifth birthday. The number of seniors in America and their proportion of the total population have increased dramatically during this century. In 1900 there were about 3.25 million seniors, who constituted 1.3% of the total population.[3] In 1991, there were an estimated 31.5 million seniors, who made up 12.6% of the population (see Figure 7.10).

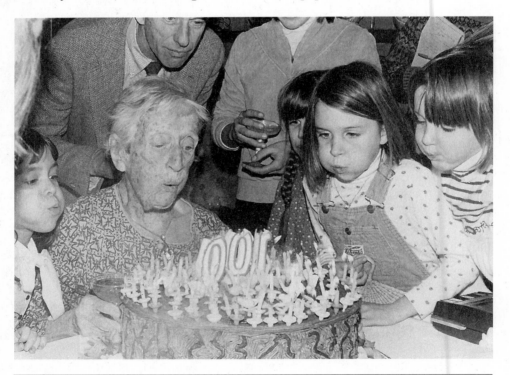

FIGURE 7.10

The proportion of seniors in the United States increased dramatically during the twentieth century.

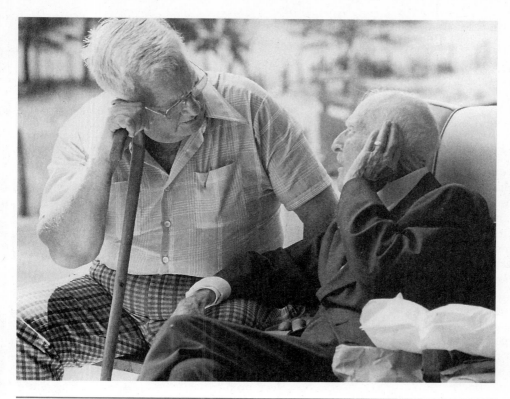

FIGURE 7.11

Physical impairments increase with age.

The fastest growing segment of the senior population comprises those who are more than 85 years old. These people are referred to as **oldest old.** As one might expect, their health status is not as good as their younger counterparts.

In presenting a health profile of the seniors, we will examine life expectancy, mortality, morbidity, and health behavior and life-style choices. This group is discussed in greater detail in Chapter 10.

Life Expectancy

As noted earlier in this chapter, life expectancy is the average number of years of life remaining for a cohort reaching a partic-ular age. The life expectancy of those reaching the age of 65 years has consistently increased since 1900 and, in 1990, had reached 17.3 years (see Table 7.4). Life expectancy is different for each subset of the senior population. Senior women have a greater life expectancy than senior men. White seniors can expect to live longer than black seniors, and black senior men, reaching the age of 65, have the shortest life expectancy of any subset of seniors, 14.2 years.

Though life expectancy measures (on average) how long a person can expect to live, it does not predict or describe the quality of life during those years. Frequently, the quality of life in one's last year is not very high (Figure 7.11). Thus, while it has been indicated that an individual who became 65 years old in 1990 could expect to live another 17.3 years, on average he or she will only have about 12 years of healthy life remaining.

Mortality

The top five causes of death for seniors are heart disease, cancer, stroke, chronic obstructive pulmonary disease, and pneumonia and influenza. Over the past 45 years, the overall age-adjusted mortality rate for seniors has fallen by nearly 20%. The major reason for this has been the declining death rates for heart disease and stroke that were discussed above. Despite such drops, heart disease remains the leading cause of death in this age group.[1, 8] Unlike the death rates for heart disease and stroke, the cancer death rate, especially for lung cancer, has continued to rise in seniors. Heart disease, cancer, and stroke account for 75% of the deaths in this cohort.[1]

Morbidity

The amount and severity of morbidity that seniors face have an impact on the quality of life. In 1988, 37.0% of seniors reported that they were limited to some degree in their activities, compared to only 13.7% of the general population.[3] In 1985, 111 of every 1,000 seniors reported difficulty performing two or more personal-care activities.[8] The causes of this reduced activity can be classified into two types: chronic conditions and impairments.

Chronic Conditions

Chronic conditions are systemic health problems that persist longer than three months such as hypertension, arthritis, heart disease, diabetes, and emphysema (see Table 7.14). The actual number of chronic conditions increases with age, and as such, these problems become increasingly prevalent with age. Chronic conditions of seniors vary by gender and race. More men experience life-threatening acute

Table 7.14
Number of Selected Reported Chronic Conditions per 1,000 Persons Aged 65 and Over, by Race and Age: United States, 1988

Type of Chronic Condition	White			Black		
	Total	65–74 Years	75 Years and Over	Total	65–74 Years	75 Years and Over
Arthritis	489.0	452.0	547.0	487.7	429.0	586.2
High blood pressure (Hypertension)	358.8	357.6	360.5	530.6	524.8	538.9
Heart disease	302.9	278.6	341.0	224.1	202.0	261.6
Ischemic heart disease	146.1	136.1	161.7	*44.1	*26.4	*74.4
Diabetes	83.9	86.3	80.1	187.4	185.5	190.5
Chronic bronchitis	66.6	68.1	64.3	*48.7	*46.9	*51.9
Hardening of the arteries	61.9	50.5	79.6	60.0	*51.5	*74.4
Cerebrovascular disease	48.2	36.7	66.3	67.5	*64.0	*73.3
Emphysema	39.2	37.7	41.7	*22.5	*19.8	*25.9
Kidney trouble	25.6	21.7	32.0	*23.3	*15.2	*37.2

*Numerator has a relative standard error of more than 30%.

From: U.S. Dept. of Health and Human Services (1991). *Health Status of Minorities and Low-Income Groups, 3rd ed.* Washington, D.C.: U.S. Government Printing Office, p. 304.

illnesses (i.e., heart disease and hypertension-induced stroke), while more women experience physically limiting chronic illness (i.e., osteoporosis and arthritis). Blacks are more likely to experience arthritis and hypertension than whites.[1]

Impairments

Impairments are deficits in the functioning of one's sense organs or limitations in one's mobility or range of motion. Like chronic conditions, impairments are far more prevalent in older seniors. As is noted in Table 7.15, the three primary impairments are hearing impairments, cataracts, and orthopedic impairments. Again, rates differ by race, but unlike chronic conditions, impairments are affected by two other variables, previous income level (see Table 7.16) and previous occupational exposure. This latter variable also correlates highly with income in old age.[3]

Health Behaviors and Life-Style Choices

There is no question that health behavior and social factors play a significant role in helping seniors maintain health in later life.[3] Some seniors believe that they are too old to gain any benefit from changing their health behaviors. This, of course, is not true; it is never too late to make a change for the better.

In interviews, seniors generally report more favorable health behaviors than their

---

Table 7.15

Number of Selected Reported Impairments per 1,000 Persons, by Race and Age: United States, 1988

| | White | | | Black | | |
| | 65 Years and Over | | | 65 Years and Over | | |
Type of Impairment	Total	65–74 Years	75 Years and Over	Total	65–74 Years	75 Years and Over
	Number of Impairments per 1,000 Persons					
Visual impairment	90.4	67.1	126.9	101.6	*83.8	*131.9
Color blindness	13.9	17.3	*8.5	*5.4	*3.3	*9.0
Cataracts	170.0	120.0	248.1	147.4	100.3	228.9
Glaucoma	37.1	27.8	51.7	90.0	*77.2	*112.7
Hearing impairment	327.9	286.5	392.6	201.2	152.5	284.1
Tinnitus	88.2	93.4	79.9	*54.6	*66.0	*33.8
Speech impairment	13.2	13.9	*12.2	*16.2	*16.5	*14.7
Absence of extremities (excludes tips of fingers or toes only)	19.1	21.6	15.3	*33.3	*36.3	*28.2
Paralysis of extremities, complete or partial	17.4	21.0	*11.8	*19.6	*23.1	*12.4
Deformity or orthopedic impairment	166.1	155.9	182.1	121.2	107.6	*145.4
Back	83.7	77.9	92.9	*56.2	*58.1	*53.0
Upper extremities	26.1	26.4	25.7	*20.4	*5.3	*46.2
Lower extremities	73.7	70.8	78.2	62.5	*66.7	*55.2

*Numerator has a relative standard error of more than 30%.

From: U.S. Dept. of Health and Human Services (1991). *Health Status of Minorities and Low-Income Groups,* 3rd ed. Washington, D.C.: U.S. Government Printing Office, p. 305.

Table 7.16
Number of Selected Reported Impairments per 1,000 Persons, by Family Income and Age: United States, 1988

	Family income											
	Less than $10,000			$10,000–19,999			$20,000–34,999			$35,000 or More		
	65 Years and Over			65 Years and Over			65 Years and Over			65 Years and Over		
Type of Impairment	Total	65–74 Years	75 Years and Over	Total	65–74 Years	75 Years and Over	Total	65–74 Years	75 Years and Over	Total	65–74 Years	75 Years and Over
Visual impairment	111.1	82.2	138.7	102.7	87.7	129.0	68.4	45.5	119.3	70.2	75.8	*54.6
Color blindness	*8.0	*8.0	*7.9	18.0	*21.3	*12.2	*7.1	*7.0	*6.8	*21.9	*30.3	*—
Cataracts	182.6	137.1	226.0	174.0	139.4	234.4	130.8	78.4	247.4	149.6	122.9	218.6
Glaucoma	40.1	*28.3	51.4	37.8	29.6	51.6	42.7	*27.9	*75.8	57.2	*53.1	*68.0
Hearing impairment	307.8	243.5	369.5	364.0	335.7	413.6	259.0	239.4	302.7	314.4	331.6	270.1
Tinnitus	89.5	101.5	78.1	100.8	95.1	110.8	84.3	100.7	*47.9	74.2	87.8	39.2
Speech impairment	*17.2	*23.0	*12.1	*8.9	*7.2	*11.8	*6.4	*6.1	*7.5	*15.8	*21.9	*—
Absence of extremities (excludes tips of fingers or toes only)	*20.5	*24.6	*16.5	31.4	43.1	*10.8	*20.4	*15.3	*31.7	*2.9	*4.0	—
Paralysis of extremities, complete or partial	*14.1	*20.0	*8.3	*14.2	*20.0	*3.9	*25.2	*30.4	*13.7	*—	*—	*—
Deformity or orthopedic impairment	182.2	178.6	185.7	178.6	163.7	204.7	136.1	127.2	156.0	140.1	163.6	*79.4
Back	93.6	92.1	94.9	97.6	90.6	110.4	56.2	58.9	*50.3	52.4	55.9	42.3
Upper extremities	23.7	*17.6	*29.5	32.2	33.5	*29.7	28.1	*25.1	*35.4	*18.1	*20.8	*11.3
Lower extremities	84.1	85.5	82.9	79.0	75.6	84.9	60.5	56.1	*70.2	79.4	93.0	43.3

*Numerator has a relative standard error of more than 30%.

From: U.S. Dept. of Health and Human Services (1991). Health Status of Minorities and Low-Income Groups, 3rd ed. Washington, D.C.: U.S. Government Printing Office, p. 306.

younger counterparts. They are less likely to: (1) consume large amounts of alcohol, (2) smoke cigarettes, and (3) be overweight or obese. However, it should be noted that many of those who drank to excess, smoked, and were overweight or obese died before 65 and thus were unavailable for interview.[3]

Health behavior, like chronic conditions and impairments, differs by gender and race. Senior men consume alcohol more regularly than senior women, and senior whites and Hispanics consume alcohol more regularly than blacks. But higher percentages of Hispanics and blacks reported consuming five or more drinks in one day at least five times more in the past year than did whites.[3]

With regard to smoking, a greater percentage of senior black men (27.8%) and Hispanics (20.0%) report being current smokers than whites (18.9%). In women, the order changes; 14.5% of blacks, 13.3% of whites and 6.9% of Hispanics reported being current smokers. A close look at obesity in seniors reveals that women and blacks are more likely to be obese; 10.9% of senior white males versus 18.6% of senior black males are obese, while 18.8% of senior white females versus 38.5% of senior black females are obese.[3]

CHAPTER SUMMARY

The health profile of Americans has improved in recent years, but there is still room for further improvement. Health status can be measured in a number of different ways including mortality statistics, life expectancy, years of potential life lost, and health surveys. Using these and other data, health profiles can be created for Americans in each of five age groups. Each of these age groups has a unique and characteristic set of health concerns. For example, the health of infants is influenced to a significant degree by the behavior and environmental exposure of the mother during pregnancy. The greatest threats

to children are no longer communicable diseases but social morbidities. Seventy percent of adolescent and young adult mortality can be attributed to motor vehicles, other unintentional injuries, homicide, and suicide. This age group remains at considerable risk from STD morbidity.

Reductions in deaths from cardiovascular diseases in the adult cohort have been substantial, but health problems resulting from unhealthy behaviors, like smoking and drinking, can be reduced further. Seniors are living longer than ever before, but inevitably must face death. Chronic conditions and impairments often lower the quality of life in the last few years. In the end, the leading causes of death for this group are heart disease and cancer.

No matter how the health profile of Americans is broken down and described, we can summarize it by saying that the health of Americans has come a long way in the past 50 years, but there is still room for improvement!

SCENARIO: ANALYSIS AND RESPONSE

1. Do you agree with Martha and Fred that the United States is the healthiest nation in the world? Why or why not?

2. What makes a nation healthy?

3. Is a high-technology health care system the best measure of the health status of a country? Why or why not?

4. If you were asked to create a single index to measure the health status of a country, what variables would you include in it?

REVIEW QUESTIONS

1. What role does health behavior play in determining health status?

2. Why do you suppose Americans seem to be more interested in curing disease than in preventing it?

3. In general, contrast the leading causes of death in the United States in 1900 with those

in 1992. Are there any trends apparent from available data?

4. Why is life expectancy often calculated both at birth and at age 65?

5. In the United States, which segment of the population has the longest life expectancy? The shortest?

6. What are years of potential life lost? How does calculating YPLL assist in developing a health profile?

7. What can be said about the reliability of self-reported health data?

8. What is DALY?

9. The health of what age group is often used to judge the health of a nation?

10. The health of what age group is used to assess, in part, the parenting skills of a nation?

11. How would you summarize the health profile of each of these age groups of Americans?

Adolescents and young adults

Adults

Seniors

ACTIVITIES

1. Obtain a copy of the results of the Behavioral Risk Factor Surveillance Survey for your state. Review the data presented and then prepare a two-page summary on the "Health Behavior Profile" of your state.

2. Using the data presented in Table 7.4, determine (as best you can) the life expectancy of your siblings, parents, and grandparents *at birth*. If your grandparents are older than 65, determine what their life expectancy was when they *turned* 65.

3. Interview a group of seniors (approximately 15) about their present health status. Ask them questions about their health behavior and health problems. Then summarize the data you collect in writing and compare it to the information in this chapter about seniors. How are the data similar? How do they differ?

4. Write a two-page paper that presents ideas on how the health profile of Americans can be improved. Make sure your paper includes at least one idea for each of the five cohorts presented in this chapter.

REFERENCES

1. U.S. Dept. of Health and Human Services (1990). *Prevention '89/90': Federal Programs and Progress.* Washington, D.C.: U.S. Government Printing Office.

2. Cohen, H. J. (1991). "My Grandmother Said, 'If You Have Your Health, You Have Everything.' What Did She Mean?" In M. Feinleib, ed. *Vital and Health Statistics: Proceedings of 1988 International Symposium on Data on Aging* (DHHS pub. no. PHS-91-1482.) Washington, D.C.: U.S. Government Printing Office, pp. 5–9.

3. U.S. Dept. of Health and Human Services (1991). *Health Status of Minorities and Low-Income Groups,* 3rd ed. Washington, D.C.: U.S. Government Printing Office.

4. U.S. Dept. of Health and Human Services (1993). "Advance Report of Final Mortality Statistics, 1990." *Monthly Vital Statistics Report* 41(7): 4–12.

5. Centers for Disease Control (1992). "Summary of Notifiable Diseases, United States—1991." MMWR 40(53): 1–63.

6. No author (1993). *World Development Report 1993: Investing in Health.* New York: Oxford Univ. Press (for the World Bank).

7. U.S. Dept. of Health and Human Services (1990). *Child Health USA '90* (pub. no. HRS-M-CH 90-1). Washington, D.C.: U.S. Government Printing Office.

8. U.S. Dept. of Health and Human Services (1991). *Healthy People 2000: National Health Promotion and Disease Prevention Objectives* [full report, with commentary (DHHS pub. no. PHS-91-50212). Washington, DC: U.S. Government Printing Office.

9. U.S. Dept. of Health and Human Services, Center for Health Statistics (1993). *Health, United States, 1992* (DHHS pub. no. PHS-92-1232). Washington, D.C.: U.S. Government Printing Office.

10. U.S. Dept. of Education (1991). *Youth Indicators: Trends in the Well-Being of American Youth* (pub. no. PIP 91-863). Washington, D.C.: U.S. Government Printing Office.

11. U.S. Dept. of Health and Human Services (1991). *Healthy Children 2000: National Health Promotion and Disease Prevention Objectives Related to Mothers, Infants, Children, Adolescents, and Youth* (DHHS pub. no. HRSA-M-CH-91-2). Washington, D.C.: U.S. Government Printing Office.

12. Smith, S. (1992). "National Center for Health Statistics Data Line." *Public Health Reports* 107(5): 599–601.

13. No author (1992). "Behaviors Related to Unintentional and Intentional Injuries Among High School Students—United States, 1991." *Journal of School Health* 62(9): 439–443.

14. Lavin, A. T., G. R. Shapiro, and K. S. Weill (1992). "Creating an Agenda for School-based Health Promotion: A Review of 25 Selected Reports." *The Journal of School Health* 62(6): 212–228.

15. Centers for Disease Control (1989). "Measles Prevention: Recommendations of the Immunization Practices Advisory Committee (ACP)." *MMWR* 38(S-9): 1–18.

16. Kolbe, L. J., L. Kann, and J. L. Collins (1993). "Overview of the Youth Risk Behavior Surveillance System." *Public Health Reports* 108 (Suppl. 1): 2–10.

17. Kann, L., W. Warren, J. L. Collins, J. Ross, B. Collins, and L. J. Kolbe (1993). "Results from the National School-based 1991 Youth Risk Survey and Progress Toward Achieving Related Health Objectives for the Nation." *Public Health Reports* 108 (Suppl. 1): 47–55.

18. The American Cancer Society (1993). *Cancer Facts and Figures—1993*. Atlanta: Author.

19. Centers for Disease Control (1991). "Behavioral Risk Factor Surveillance, 1986–1990." *MMWR* 40(SS-4): 1–47.

Chapter 8

MATERNAL, INFANT, AND CHILD HEALTH

Chapter Outline

Chapter Objectives

After studying this chapter you will be able to:

1. Define *maternal and child health.*
2. Explain the importance of maternal and child health as indicators of a society's health.
3. Define *maternal mortality rate.*
4. Define *prenatal care.*
5. Discuss reasons for the lack of prenatal care and the influence this has on pregnancy outcome.
6. Explain the reasons for differences between infant mortality rates in the United States and those for other countries.
7. Explain the differences among infant mortality, neonatal mortality, and postneonatal mortality.
8. List the major factors that contribute to infant mortality.
9. List the major reasons for birth defects.
10. List and describe possible causes and risk factors of SIDS.
11. Identify the major causes of childhood morbidity and mortality.
12. Identify reasons for the current increase in preventable childhood diseases.
13. List the immunizations required in order for a two-year-old child to be considered fully immunized.
14. Explain how health insurance and health care services impact childhood health.
15. Identify programs developed to improve maternal and child health.
16. Define *family planning.*
17. Define *legalized abortion* and discuss Roe vs. Wade, Pro-Life and Pro-Choice movements.
18. Briefly explain what WIC programs are and who they serve.
19. Outline the suggested schedule for immunizations.
20. Identify three groups who are recognized as child advocates.
21. Briefly describe the problems associated with child care.
22. Explain the Family and Medical Leave Act.

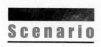
Susan is 18 years old and graduated from high school last June. She lives in a small town with a population of about 2,700 people. The town is so small that the people rely very heavily on the city 25 miles away for shopping, recreation, and health care. Susan had dated the same boy in high school for the past two years but had no plans to marry him. Just before graduation, she learned that she was pregnant. Last week, she completed her seventh month of pregnancy and went into premature labor. She was rushed to the emergency room of a hospital for what became the premature birth of her baby. While Susan was in recovery, doctors determined that her baby was not normally developed. When asked whether she had received any prenatal care, Susan replied, "No, I couldn't afford it; besides, I didn't know where to go to get help."

INTRODUCTION

Maternal, infant, and child health encompasses the health of women of childbearing age from prepregnancy, through pregnancy, labor and delivery, and the postpartal period. It also includes the health of the child prior to birth through adolescence.[1] In this chapter, we examine the risk factors associated with maternal, infant, and child morbidity and mortality, define and discuss commonly used rates for the measurement of maternal, infant, and child health, and review selected programs aimed at improving the health of women of childbearing age, infants, and children.

Maternal, infant, and child health are important to a community for several reasons. First, maternal and infant mortality are regarded as accurate indicators of a community's overall health. Inadequate sanitation, poor nutrition, and high rates of communicable diseases, coupled with a lack of health care services in a community, are precursors to high rates of maternal, infant,

and early childhood mortality. Second, we now know that prompt intervention with services for the health of women, infants, and children reduces the necessity to provide more costly medical or social assistance to these same members of society later.

MATERNAL HEALTH

Maternal health encompasses the health of women in the childbearing years, including those in the prepregnancy period, those who are pregnant, and those who are caring for young children (see Figure 8.1). In the United States, maternal health has improved steadily over the past 20 years, but significant differences remain among the various subpopulations.

Maternal Mortality Rates

The **maternal mortality rate** is defined as the number of mothers dying per 100,000 live births in a given year. The number does not include all deaths occurring to pregnant women but only those deaths assigned to complication of pregnancy, childbirth, and puerperium. The

---

maternal, infant, and child health The health of women of childbearing age and that of the child through adolescence.

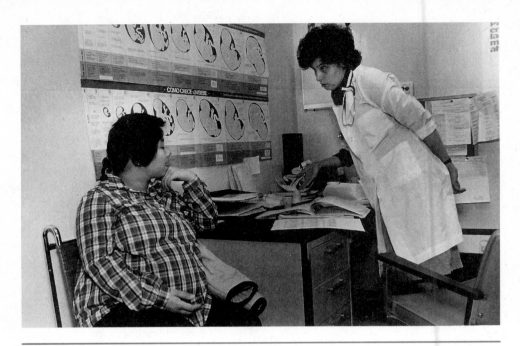

FIGURE 8.1
Maternal health encompasses the health of women in the childbearing years.

maternal mortality rate for the United States declined from 21.5 in 1970 to 7.6 in 1990.[2, 3] (See Figure 8.2.) This decline is the result of a drop in the number of pregnancy complications, such as hemorrhage, toxemia, and infections, and the improved availability of effective contraception and legalized abortion. Complications associated with pregnancy have been reduced by new screening procedures and high-technology equipment, such as amniocentesis, sonograms, and fetal monitors.

While there has been significant improvement in the maternal mortality rate for the population as a whole, mortality rates for certain subpopulations of American women remain much too high. For example, in 1990, the maternal mortality rate for black Americans, 21.7/100,000, was more than four times that for white Americans, 5.1/100,000 (Figure 8.2).[2]

Factors Associated with Maternal Morbidity and Mortality

The two factors most often associated with maternal morbidity and mortality are the lack of prenatal care and the teenage status of the mother. Upon closer examination, one finds numerous underlying causes including low education and achievement, sociocultural and language factors, poverty, and shortcomings of the health care delivery system.

Prenatal Health Care

Prenatal health care is the medical care received by the pregnant woman from

---

prenatal health care Medical care provided to a pregnant woman from the time of conception until the birth process occurs.

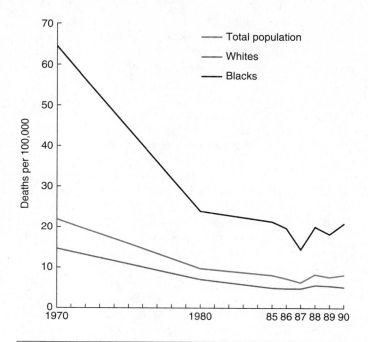

FIGURE 8.2

Maternal mortality rates by race, United States, 1970–1990.

Source: U.S. Dept. of Health and Human Services (1993). Health, United States, 1992 and Healthy People 2000 Review (DHHS pub. no. PHS-93-1232). Washington, D.C.: U.S. Government Printing Office.

the time of conception until the birth process occurs. In addition to clinical and laboratory services, prenatal health care includes education about nutrition, avoidance of drug use, risky sexual behavior involving STD transmission, and avoidance of exposure to toxic substances. Such care in 1993 could be provided for approximately $700 per expectant mother.

Early and regular prenatal care, beginning during the first trimester of pregnancy, can help insure good health for both mother and child and minimize the factors that lead to low birth weight. A pregnant woman who receives no prenatal care is three times as likely to give birth to a **low-birth-weight**

low-birth-weight infant One that weighs less than 2,500 grams, or 5.5 pounds, at birth.

infant as one who receives the appropriate care and four times as likely to have her baby die in infancy.

Low birth weight is costly, both emotionally and economically. In 1990, the hospital-related costs of caring for all low-birth-weight infants during the neonatal period totaled more than $2 billion—or $21,000 for each baby—instead of $2,900 for the average delivery.[4] Overall, the costs of managing a low-birth-weight infant immediately after delivery ranges between $30,000 and $70,000. Long-term costs may be five to ten times that amount.[5]

Unfortunately, approximately 24% of pregnant women in 1990 in the United States did not receive prenatal care during the first trimester of pregnancy (see Figure 8.3). The percentage of mothers who began care in the third trimester or received no care is about 6%.[6] The percentage of live births in which the woman received early prenatal care can be broken down by race and ethnicity of the mother. White Americans (79.2%) and Asian Americans (75.1%) had the highest rates of early prenatal care, while Americans of Hispanic origin (60.2%), black Americans (60.6%), and Native Americans (57.9%) had the lowest.[2]

Factors associated with the failure to receive prenatal care include poverty, lack of education, and lack of experience with the health care system. Also, language problems and concerns about documentation of citizenship may have inhibited Mexican-American women from seeking prenatal care.[7, 8] Approximately 14 million women of reproductive years in the United States have no health insurance to cover maternity care.[9]

Young women are among the least likely to receive prenatal care, while women past 35 years of age tend to delay early prenatal care. Married women are more likely to receive prenatal care than single women, regardless of educational level or race. If a woman already has children, she is less likely to receive prenatal care, regardless of race. Well-educated women are more likely to receive prenatal care than less-educated women.[8]

Reasons given for not seeking or obtaining prenatal care are sometimes referred to as *barriers*. Barriers to prenatal care include both personal barriers and system barriers. Personal barriers include inadequate finances, lack of transportation, tendency not to value prenatal care or understand its importance, failure to realize one is pregnant, ambivalence or fear of pregnancy, and dislike or fear of the health care provider. System barriers include such things as negative institutional practices, limited availability of providers, and lack of child care.[8]

Teenage Pregnancies

Teenage pregnancies are a significant community health problem in the United States, which boasts the highest teenage pregnancy rate of any developed country in the world. More than 1 million teenage pregnancies occur in this country every year. About 2,740 teen pregnancies begin every day, and almost every one of us knows a teenager who has become pregnant unexpectedly.

The United States provides over $25 billion annually for programs such as Aid to

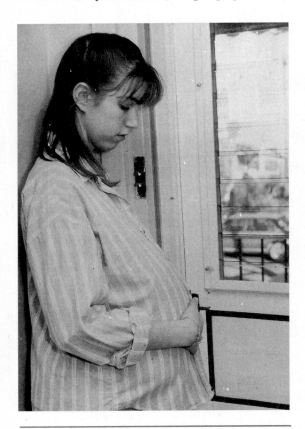

FIGURE 8.3

One in four pregnant women in America receives no prenatal care during the first three months of her pregnancy.

Families with Dependent Children (AFDC), Medicaid, and Food Stamps—programs that support families, many of which began with a birth to a teenage mother. Estimates suggest that if all teen pregnancies could be delayed until the mother was in her twenties, the United States would save $10.2 billion a year.[10, 11]

The rate of teenage pregnancies declined in the 1970s until about 1986, when this trend reversed. Teenage pregnancy rates for 15- to 17-year-olds increased 19% between 1986 and 1991.[10] Because most sexually active teens do not routinely use effective contraception, about 10% percent of all teenage females in the United States conceive every year. Furthermore, the average age of first intercourse has declined from age 19 in 1971 to approximately 16.5 in 1988. More than 75% of young women and 85% of young men have had sexual intercourse before age 20.[10]

A teenage pregnancy means greater health risks for both mother and child and represents a significant burden to the community. The teenage mother is more likely to experience an early divorce if she marries and is less likely to attain an adequate education than her nonpregnant counterpart. Moreover, these young mothers are at increased risk for having additional unwanted pregnancies.

Teenage mothers are more likely to be single parents and economically disadvantaged. Estimates suggest that as many as 53% of all Aid to Families with Dependent Children cases involve a mother who had her first child as a teenager.[12] Babies born to teenage mothers have a greater incidence of low birth weight and prematurity, lower IQ scores, and higher mortality rates. Due to lack of money and family support, many pregnant teens do not receive proper maternal health care. The lack of proper nutrition and prenatal care leads to a death rate that is nearly twice that for infants born to mothers in their twenties.

Black American teenage girls are much more likely to become pregnant than white American teenage girls and are more likely to keep their babies. It has been estimated that 40% of all women in this country have been pregnant at least once before their twentieth birthday; approximately 63% of these women are black Americans.[7]

INFANT HEALTH

An infant's health depends upon many factors including the mother's health and her health behavior prior to and during pregnancy, her level of prenatal care, the quality of her delivery, and the infant's environment after birth. The infant's environment includes not only the home and family environment but also the availability of essential medical services such as a postnatal physical examination by a **neonatologist,** a medical doctor who specializes in the care of newborn children up to two months of age, regular visits to a physician, and receiving appropriate immunizations. The infant's health also depends on proper nutrition and other nurturing care in the home. Shortcomings in these areas can result in illness and even death of the child.

Infant Mortality Rates

An **infant death (infant mortality)** is the death of a child under one year of age. The **infant mortality rate** is expressed as the number of deaths of children under one year of age per 1,000 live births. The infant mortality rate in the United States has declined from 29.2 per 1,000 live births in 1950 to 8.9 in 1991 (see Table 8.1 and Figure 8.4). This decrease can be attributed

Table 8.1

Infant Mortality Rates, Fetal Death Rates, and Perinatal Mortality Rates, According to Race: United States, Selected Years 1950–1991

[Data are based on the National Vital Statistics System.]

Race and Year	Infant Mortality Rate[1] Neonatal				Fetal Death Rate[2]	Late Fetal Death Rate[3]	Perinatal Mortality Rate[4]
	Total	Under 28 Days	Under 7 Days	Postneonatal			
All Races	*Deaths per 1,000 Live Births*						
1950[5]	29.2	20.5	17.8	8.7	18.4	14.9	32.5
1960[5]	26.0	18.7	16.7	7.3	15.8	12.1	28.6
1970	20.0	15.1	13.6	4.9	14.0	9.5	23.0
1975	16.1	11.6	10.0	4.5	10.6	7.8	17.7
1980	12.6	8.5	7.1	4.1	9.1	6.2	13.2
1985	10.6	7.0	5.8	3.7	7.8	4.9	10.7
1990	9.2	5.8	4.8	3.4	7.5	4.3	9.1
Provisional Data:							
1990[5]	9.1	5.7	–	3.3	–	–	–
1991	8.9	5.5	–	3.4	–	–	–
Race of Child:[6] White							
1950[5]	26.8	19.4	17.1	7.4	16.6	13.3	30.1
1960[5]	22.9	17.2	15.6	5.7	13.9	10.8	26.2
1970	17.8	13.8	12.5	4.0	12.3	8.6	21.0
1975	14.2	10.4	9.0	3.8	9.4	7.1	16.0
1980	11.0	7.5	6.2	3.5	8.1	5.7	11.9
1985	9.3	6.1	5.0	3.2	7.0	4.5	9.6
1990	7.7	4.9	4.0	2.8	6.4	3.8	7.8

(continued)

to improvements in overall socioeconomic status, housing, nutrition, levels of immunization, and the availability of clean water, pasteurized milk, and antibiotics. There has also been an improvement in the availability of prenatal and postnatal care and modern technology to assist in the care of deliveries with complications.[13]

Infant deaths, or infant mortality, can be divided into neonatal mortality and postneonatal mortality. **Neonatal deaths (neonatal mortality)** are deaths that occur during the first 28 days after birth. These deaths are most often attributed to prenatal events and events occurring just after birth. Adequate prenatal care, with assessment and management of risks, and ad-

vances in technology of newborn intensive care can help reduce neonatal mortality. **Postneonatal deaths (postneonatal mortality)** are deaths that occur between 28 days and 365 days after birth. The health of the infant during the post-neonatal period is more dependent on the infant's environment, including parenting skills and the availability and use of pediatric services. **Fetal deaths** are deaths in utero with a gestational age of at least 20 weeks.

A comparison of infant mortality rates among developed nations reveals that the United States must find a better way to protect the health of its youngest members. Japan leads the world with the lowest infant mortality rate, 4.6 per 1,000 live births; Swe-

Table 8.1 (continued)

Race and Year	Total	Infant Mortality Rate[1] Neonatal Under 28 Days	Under 7 Days	Postneonatal	Fetal Death Rate[2]	Late Fetal Death Rate[3]	Perinatal Mortality Rate[4]
Race of Child:[6] Black							
1950[5]	43.9	27.8	23.0	16.1	32.1	–	–
1960[5]	44.3	27.8	23.7	16.5	–	–	–
1970	32.6	22.8	20.3	9.9	23.2	–	34.5
1975	26.2	18.3	15.7	7.9	16.8	11.4	26.9
1980	21.4	14.1	11.9	7.3	14.4	8.9	20.7
1985	18.2	12.1	10.3	6.1	12.6	7.1	17.4
1990	17.0	10.9	9.2	6.1	12.9	6.6	15.7
Race of Mother:[7] White							
1980	10.9	7.4	6.1	3.5	8.1	5.7	11.8
1985	9.2	6.0	5.0	3.2	6.9	4.5	9.5
1990	7.6	4.8	3.9	2.8	6.4	3.8	7.7
Race of Mother:[7] Black							
1980	22.2	14.6	12.3	7.6	14.7	9.1	21.3
1985	19.0	12.6	10.8	6.4	12.8	7.2	17.9
1990	18.0	11.6	9.7	6.4	13.3	6.7	16.4

[1]Infant mortality rate is deaths under 1 year of age per 1,000 live births. Neonatal deaths occur within 28 days and early neonatal deaths within 7 days of birth; postneonatal deaths occur 28–365 days after birth.

[2]Number of fetal deaths of 20 weeks or more gestation per 1,000 live births plus fetal deaths.

[3]Number of fetal deaths of 28 weeks or more gestation per 1,000 live births plus late fetal deaths.

[4]Number of late fetal deaths plus infant deaths within 7 days of birth per 1,000 live births plus late fetal deaths.

[5]Includes births and deaths of nonresidents of the United States.

[6]Infant deaths and fetal deaths are tabulated by race of decedent; live births are tabulated by race of child.

[7]Infant deaths are tabulated by race of decedent; fetal deaths and live births are tabulated by race of mother.

From: U.S. Dept. of Health and Human Services (1993). *Health United States, 1992 and Healthy People 2000 Review.* Washington, D.C.: U.S. Government Printing Office, pp. 35–36.

den is second with a rate of 5.8 per 1,000 live births. Despite our considerable investment in neonatal intensive care and our higher-than-average per capita income, America ranked twenty-fourth in infant mortality in 1989 (see Table 8.2). Japan and Sweden have standards of living comparable to that of the United States, but Ireland, Spain, and Hong Kong do not. Yet, these countries also have lower infant mortality rates.

Critics of America's health care system point to the vast expenditures in the United States for the expensive technology and highly trained personnel needed to save premature babies and the insufficient invest-ments in prenatal care that would prevent many premature births from occurring in the first place. Another reason for high infant mortality rates in the United States is the social and cultural diversity of our population, a diversity that does not exist in Japan or Sweden. Declines in infant mortality rates among black Americans, for example, have always lagged behind those of white Americans (see Table 8.1). One reason may be that many minorities in the United States are in the lowest socioeconomic groups and, because of this, may lack appropriate health care. Americans living in southern states that have high percentages

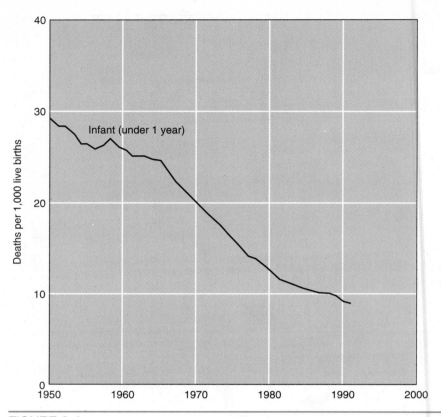

FIGURE 8.4

Infant mortality rates, United States, 1950–1991.

From: Monthly Vital Statistics Report *40, no. 13 (Sept. 30, 1992): 8.*

of minorities generally have higher infant mortality rates than those living in northern states. In 1985, 10 of the 12 states with the highest infant mortality rates were located in the South.[14]

Causes of Infant Mortality

The leading causes of infant mortality are prematurity and low birth weight, birth defects, and sudden infant death syndrome.

Prematurity and Low Birth Weight

A **premature infant** is one born following a gestation period of 38 weeks or less or one born at a low birth weight. A premature infant is 40 times more likely to die than a normal infant. Nearly two-thirds of the infant deaths occur in low-birth-weight babies. Low-birth-weight infants are also more likely to have health problems later in life (see Figure 8.5 and Table 8.3). Internationally, the United States is tied with eight other nations for thirty-first in the rate of low-birth-weight infants (see Table 8.4). The United States' black population fairs worse than most developing countries in this regard (see Box 8.1).

In addition to race, there are a number of other maternal risk factors associated with giving birth to low-birth-weight infants. These include smoking; alcohol and other drug abuse; inadequate nutrition; giving birth prior to 17 years of age or after 40; exposure to environmental hazards like viruses, chemicals, and radiation; marital status; educational status; lack of social support; and poverty. Babies born to mothers with several of these risk factors are at proportionately greater risk for illness or death in their first year.[14]

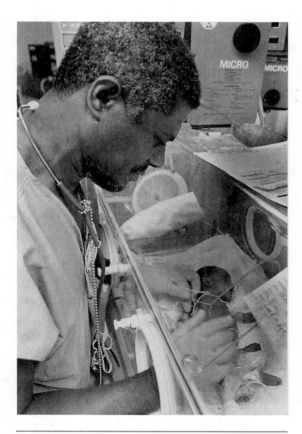

FIGURE 8.5

A low-birth-weight baby (less than 2500 g) is 40 times more likely to die than a normal infant.

Smoking

Maternal smoking during pregnancy increases the risk of prenatal and postnatal health conditions in infants. Possible consequences of smoking during pregnancy include: intrauterine growth retardation, low birth weight, prematurity, and other complications. Nonsmoking mothers who are exposed to environmental tobacco smoke (ETS) are also at greater risk for low-birth-weight babies than those who are not. One study found that pregnant women exposed to ETS for at least two hours a day had an increased relative risk of 2.17 for delivery of a low-birth-weight infant.[15]

Alcohol and Other Drugs

Heavy maternal alcohol consumption can lead to a condition known as Fetal Alcohol Syndrome (FAS), discussed later in this chapter. A safe level of alcohol consumption during pregnancy has not been determined, but adverse effects are known to be associated with heavy consumption during the first few months of pregnancy.[7] Recent data indicate illicit drug use during pregnancy has a number of deleterious effects on the developing fetus, including impaired fetal growth. The study showed infants born to women using marijuana and/or cocaine were significantly smaller than infants of nonusers. Marijuana's effect of increasing maternal heart rate, blood pressure, and carbon monoxide levels may be responsible for impairing the growth of the fetus. Maternal use of cocaine results in lower fetal oxygen levels by inducing uterine contractions.[16]

Poverty and Minority Status

Because the number of maternal risk factors for low-birth-weight infants may be higher for members of racial minorities or those in poverty, women in these groups are more likely to give birth to low-birth-weight babies. For example, black Americans are

Table 8.2
Infant Mortality Rates, and Average Annual Percent Change: Selected Countries, 1984 and 1989

[Data are based on reporting by countries.]

| | Infant Mortality Rate* | | |
Country[†]	1984	Average Annual 1989[‡]	Percent Change
Japan	5.99	4.59	−5.2
Sweden	6.40	5.77	−2.1
Finland	6.62	6.03	−1.8
Singapore	8.76	6.61	−5.5
Netherlands	8.36	6.78	−4.1
Northern Ireland	10.51	6.90	−8.1
Canada	8.11	7.13	−2.5
Switzerland	7.13	7.34	0.6
Hong Kong	9.17	7.43	−4.1
Federal Republic of Germany	9.64	7.44	−5.0
France	8.29	7.54	−1.9
Ireland	9.63	7.55	−4.8
German Democratic Republic	10.05	7.56	−5.5
Norway	8.33	7.72	−1.5
Denmark	7.66	7.95	0.7
Australia	9.25	7.99	−2.9
Spain	10.02	8.07	−5.3
Austria	11.41	8.31	−6.1
England and Wales	9.48	8.45	−2.3
Belgium	9.84	8.64	−2.6

(continued)

almost twice as likely to give birth to low-birth-weight infants as are white Americans. Many of these babies are also born prematurely or are small for their gestational age. The incidence of low birth weight is even higher among certain Hispanic groups, such as Puerto Ricans and Cubans, than it is for black Americans. The high incidence of low birth weight among black Americans may be related to the higher incidence of prematurity as well as a higher proportion of black babies who are small for their gestational age.

Birth Defects

Birth defects, deleterious medical conditions present at birth, constitute the second leading cause of infant deaths. Birth defects account for about 20% of infant mortality in the United States and 30% of the admissions to pediatric hospitals.[17, 18] The most frequent types of birth defect are those affecting the cardiovascular system. The second leading type of birth defects are those involving the nervous system, such as spina bifida. Defects of the respiratory system rank third.

Approximately 75% of all birth defects are caused by environmental hazards and behavior of the mother during pregnancy.[19] Environmental hazards include exposure to biological disease agents, toxic chemicals, or radiation. An example of a biological disease agent that can cause birth defects is the rubella (German measles) virus. Exposure of a pregnant woman to this virus can result

Table 8.2 (continued)

	Infant Mortality Rate*		
		Average Annual	
Country†	1984	1989‡	Percent Change
Scotland	10.32	8.73	−3.3
Italy	11.44	8.80	−5.1
Greece	14.34	9.78	−7.4
United States	10.79	9.81	−1.9
Israel	12.80	9.94	−4.9
New Zealand	11.70	10.19	−2.7
Cuba	15.01	11.08	−5.9
Czechoslovakia	15.32	11.31	−5.9
Portugal	16.73	12.18	−6.2
Costa Rica	20.25	13.90	−7.2
Puerto Rico	15.61	14.27	−1.8
Bulgaria	16.09	14.37	−2.2
Hungary	20.41	15.74	−5.1
Poland	19.23	15.96	−3.7
Chile	19.55	17.06	−2.7
Kuwait	18.55	17.33	−2.2
Yugoslavia	27.67	22.21	−4.3
U.S.S.R.	25.92	22.97	−2.4
Romania	23.41	26.90	2.8

*Number of deaths of infants under 1 year per 1,000 live births.

†Refers to countries, territories, cities, or geographic areas.

‡Data for Spain are for 1988 and data for Kuwait are for 1987.

Notes: Rankings are from lowest to highest infant mortality rates based on the latest data available for countries or geographic areas with at least 1 million population and with "complete" counts of live births and infant deaths as indicated in the *United Nations Demographic Yearbook,* 1990. Some of the international variation in infant mortality rates (IMR) is due to variation among countries in distinctions between fetal and infant deaths. The feto-infant mortality rate (FIMR) attempts to reduce international variation due to clinical distinctions between fetal and infant deaths. The United States ranks 24th on the IMR and 21st on the FIMR and 22nd on the postneonatal mortality rate.

From: U.S. Dept. of Health and Human Services (1993). *Health United States, 1992 and Healthy People 2000 Review.* Washington, D.C.: U.S. Government Printing Office, p. 41.

Table 8.3
Birth Weight and Health Conditions at School Age*

	Birth Weight		
Health Condition	<1000 gm	1501–2500 gm	>2500 gm
Asthma	17.1%†	11.7	11.1
Learning problems	24.8	13.0	10.5
(IQ < 70)	13.3	4.8	0.0
Behavior problems	29.2	29.4	21.2
Other conditions	23.6	16.3	9.8

*Data from McCormick et al. (1992).

†Percent of children for whom conditions were reported; in these conditions, there was a significant difference across birth-weight groups.

From: Silbergeld, E. K. (1993). *Investing in Prevention.* Washington, D.C.: Environmental Defense Fund, p. 14.

Table 8.4
Percentage of Infants Born at Low Birth Weight, Selected Countries, 1990

Rank	Nation	Percent	Rank	Nation	Percent
1	Spain	1	40	Uruguay	8
2	Norway	4	40	Tunisia	8
2	Sweden	4	40	Botswana	8
2	Ireland	4	40	Benin	8
2	Finland	4	40	Colombia	8
6	Kuwait	5	40	Ethiopia	8
6	Jordan	5	40	Cuba	8
6	New Zealand	5	50	Peru	9
6	Switzerland	5	50	Mauritius	9
6	Portugal	5	50	Venezuela	9
6	Japan	5	50	South Korea	9
6	Belgium	5	50	Burundi	9
6	Hong Kong	5	50	Algeria	9
6	Egypt	5	50	Iraq	9
6	Iran	5	50	China	9
6	France	5	58	Malaysia	10
17	Romania	6	58	Mongolia	10
17	Greece	6	58	Madagascar	10
17	Germany	6	58	Hungary	10
17	Saudi Arabia	6	58	Lebanon	10
17	United Arab Emirates	6	63	Senegal	11
17	Soviet Union	6	63	Syria	11
17	Singapore	6	63	Lesotho	11
17	Bulgaria	6	63	Mauratania	11
17	Austria	6	67	South Africa	12
17	Australia	6	67	Thailand	12
17	Canada	6	67	Bolivia	12
17	Denmark	6	67	Mexico	12
17	Czechoslovakia	6	71	Zaire	13
17	Costa Rica	6	71	Guinea-Bissau	13
31	United Kingdom	7	71	Cameroon	13
31	Turkey	7	74	Guatemala	14
31	Yugoslavia	7	74	Tanzania	14
31	**United States**	**7**	74	Indonesia	14
31	Paraguay	7	74	Cote d'Ivoire	14
31	Chile	7		**U.S. black**	**14**
31	Albania	7	78	Niger	15
31	Oman	7	78	Sudan	15
31	Israel	7	78	Kenya	15
40	Panama	8	78	Central African Rep.	15
40	Jamaica	8	78	El Salvador	15
40	Poland	8	83	Sri Lanka	25

Source: UNICEF, *State of the World's Children, 1992.*

in permanent damage to the developing fetus. A chemical agent that can produce birth defects is the drug thalidomide, which was first introduced in 1956 in Europe to treat nausea and vomiting during pregnancy. The drug was found to cause the absence or malformation of limbs in the developing fetus. Fortunately, the FDA did not allow the drug to be used in the United States. Thus, it is important that women avoid any unnecessary drug use during pregnancy. It is also important that pregnant woman avoid un-

BOX 8.1
Healthy People 2000—Objective

14.5   Reduce low birth weight to an incidence of no more than 5% of live births and very low birth weight to no more than 1% of live births. (Baseline: 6.9% and 1.2%, respectively, in 1987)

Special Population Target

		1987 Baseline	*2000 Target*	*Percent Decrease*
14.5a	*Low Birth Weight* Blacks	12.7%	9%	
	Very Low Birth Weight Blacks	2.7	2	

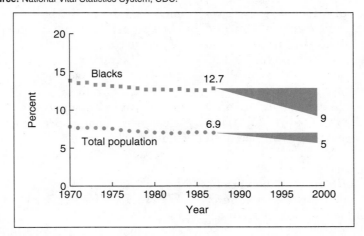

Note: *Low birth weight is weight at birth of less than 2,500 grams; very low birth weight is weight at birth of less than 1,500 grams.*

Baseline data source: National Vital Statistics System, CDC.

Incidence of low birth weight

For Further Thought

If you had to cast the deciding vote on whether to provide prenatal care for all or spend an equivalent amount of money on a new piece of machinery to help the survival rate of premature infants, how would you vote? Why? Do you think all women in the United States should be entitled to prenatal care?

necessary medical X-rays because the radiation could adversely affect the developing fetus.

Researchers are currently looking into whether exposure of the parents to certain harmful substances before conception can cause birth defects. It is not known whether exposure to certain chemicals, such as lead, or to radiation, can damage either sperm or egg and thereby produce birth defects.[7]

Behavioral factors such as nutritional patterns and substance abuse by the mother during pregnancy can also lead to increased risk of abnormal fetal development. **Fetal alcohol syndrome (FAS)** is a term used to describe a group of defects in babies born to some mothers who have consumed high levels of alcohol during their pregnancies. These abnormalities may include growth retardation, abnormal appearance of face and head, and evidence of central-nervous-system abnormalities including mental retardation. Other drug use can also result in congenital defects. Crack cocaine use during pregnancy can result in genital and urinary tract malformations in the baby. Marijuana use has also been associated with increased risk of birth defects.[7]

The remaining 25% of all birth defects are caused by genetic factors, conditions that were present before or at the time of conception.[19] If a couple is aware of birth defects that occurred in previous generations of their families, they should seriously consider preconception genetic counseling.

Sudden Infant Death Syndrome (SIDS)

The third leading cause of infant death is **sudden infant death syndrome (SIDS).** A SIDS death is defined as sudden unanticipated death of an infant in whom, after examination, there is no recognized cause of death. SIDS usually occurs in infants between the ages of two and four months. The occurrence of SIDS after the child has reached six months of age is rare. Some reports indicate that between 1% and 3% of SIDS cases occur during the first two weeks of life. However, most researchers exclude this age group from SIDS classification based on the presumption that death was due to some undetected prenatal cause.[20]

The exact cause of SIDS deaths is unknown, although there are numerous studies indicating associations between various factors and SIDS. Maternal factors such as smoking or other drug use during pregnancy, teenage status of the mother, or the mother's acquisition of an infection late in pregnancy have all been associated with an increased risk of SIDS. SIDS is more common in infants in the lower socioeconomic classes, perhaps due to the lower frequency of adequate prenatal care received by this group. Likewise, there is a greater risk of SIDS among black American and Native-American infants than among white American infants; and there is also a higher incidence among premature infants and twins.[20]

CHILD HEALTH

Good health during the childhood years is essential to each child's optimal development and achievement. America cannot hope for every child to become a productive member of society if children in this country are allowed to grow up unimmunized and without such basic needs as treatment for strep throat, dental care, hospital care, home health care, medicines, or eyeglasses. Failure to provide timely and remedial care leads to unnecessary illness, disability, and death—events associated with much greater costs than the timely care itself. The example of

Table 8.5
Child Mortality Rates, Selected Countries, 1990

Rank	Nation	Rate*	Rank	Nation	Rate*
1	Japan	6	5	Switzerland	9
2	Finland	7	5	United Kingdom	9
2	Hong Kong	7	16	Australia	10
2	Sweden	7	16	Italy	10
5	Austria	9	16	Norway	10
5	Belgium	9	16	Spain	10
5	Canada	9	20	Greece	11
5	Denmark	9	20	Israel	11
5	France	9	**20**	**United States**	**11**
5	Germany	9	23	New Zealand	12
5	Ireland	9	24	Czechoslovakia	13
5	Netherlands	9	25	Cuba	14
5	Singapore	9	26	Hungary	16

*Deaths among children younger than five per 1,000 live births.

From: Children's Defense Fund (1992). "Child Care and Early Childhood Development." *The State of America's Children, 1992.* Washington, D.C.: Author, p. 5.

BOX 8.2
Is This the Best America Can Do?

- Every 12 seconds of the school day, an American child drops out (380,000 a year).
- Every 13 seconds, an American child is reported abused or neglected (2.9 million a year).
- Every 26 seconds, an American child runs away from home (1.5 million a year).
- Every 61 seconds, an American teenager has a baby.
- Every 9 minutes, an American child is arrested for a drug offense.
- Every 40 minutes, an American child is arrested for drunk driving.
- Every 53 minutes in our rich land, an American child dies from poverty.
- Every 3 hours, a child is murdered.
- Every day, one child is killed by a family member; 90% of these children are under five years of age.

Sources: Children's Defense Fund and National Committee for the Prevention of Child Abuse (1992).

the cost of not providing prenatal care, given earlier in this chapter, presents a vivid illustration. For those who believe that "access to basic health care is a hallmark of equity and fairness in any civilized society," America lags sadly behind many of her sister nations in the health of her children (Box 8.2).[21]

Childhood Mortality Rates

In 1990, the United States ranked twentieth in childhood mortality (see Table 8.5). The leading cause of death in children that year was unintentional injuries, which accounted for 43% of all deaths of children (1–14 years). Of these, 48% resulted from motor vehicle crashes, 16% from drownings, 15% from fires and burns, 4% from choking and suffocation, and 3% from firearms.[22] Other major causes were cancer (10%) and problems present at birth (9%).

Statistics that divide childhood into two periods of development, 1–4 years and 5–14 years, reveal that the 1990 mortality rate for 1- to 4-year-olds (46.8/100,000) was nearly twice that for 5- to 14-year-olds

Table 8.6

Vaccinations of Children 1–4 Years of Age for Selected Diseases, According to Race and Residence in Metropolitan Statistical Area (MSA): United States, 1970, 1976, 1983–1985, and 1991

[Data are based on household interviews of a sample of the civilian noninstitutionalized population.]

Vaccination and Year	Total	Race		Inside MSA		Outside MSA
		White	All Other	Central City	Remaining Areas	
All Respondents		*Percent of Population*				
DTP[1,2]:						
1970	76.1	79.7	58.8	68.9	80.7	77.1
1976	71.4	75.3	53.2	64.1	75.7	72.9
1983	65.7	70.1	47.7	55.4	69.4	69.4
1984	65.7	69.1	51.3	57.9	66.6	69.8
1985	64.9	68.7	48.7	55.5	68.4	67.9
1991	65.8	68.6	54.6	60.1	68.7	68.2
Polio[2]:						
1970	65.9	69.2	50.1	61.0	70.8	64.7
1976	61.6	66.2	39.9	53.8	65.3	63.9
1983	57.0	61.9	36.7	47.7	60.3	60.3
1984	54.8	58.4	39.9	48.7	55.2	58.5
1985	55.3	58.9	40.1	47.1	58.4	58.0
1991	50.6	52.7	42.1	47.3	52.2	52.1
MMR[3]:						
Measles:						
1970	57.2	60.4	41.9	55.2	61.7	54.3
1976	65.9	68.3	54.8	62.5	67.2	67.3
1983	64.9	66.8	57.2	60.4	66.3	66.7
1984	62.8	65.4	52.0	56.6	63.3	66.4
1985	60.8	63.6	48.8	55.5	63.3	61.9

(continued)

(24.0/100,000).[1] Children aged 1–4 were almost twice as likely to die from a problem that was present at birth than were children ages 5–14.[1,3]

Childhood Morbidity Rates

While childhood morbidity rates, particularly in the 5- to 14-year-old age group, are much improved over those of earlier years, significant room for improvement remains. The United States needs to do a better job of protecting its children from infectious diseases, unintentional injuries, and domestic violence and neglect. It must do more to encourage good health behaviors and to improve access to dental (oral) health care and health care in general.

Unintentional Injuries

While unintentional injuries are the leading cause of childhood deaths, many survive their injuries (see Figure 8.6). The causes of unintentional childhood injuries include falls, car crashes, firearm discharges, poisonings, fires/burns, drownings, and recreational/sports. It is estimated that more than 14 million children under the age of 14 years were injured in 1985 and some of these became permanently disabled.[23] Unintentional injuries are discussed in more detail in Chapter 17.

Table 8.6 (continued)

Vaccination and Year	Total	Race		Inside MSA		Outside MSA
		White	All Other	Central City	Remaining Areas	
Mumps:						
1970	—	—	—	—	—	—
1976	48.3	50.3	38.7	45.6	50.7	47.9
1983	59.5	61.8	50.0	52.6	60.2	63.6
1984	58.7	61.3	47.7	51.8	58.3	63.6
1985	58.9	61.8	47.0	52.4	61.0	61.4
Rubella:						
1970	37.2	38.3	31.8	38.3	39.2	34.3
1976	61.7	63.8	51.5	59.5	63.5	61.5
1983	64.0	66.3	54.7	59.5	65.2	66.0
1984	60.9	63.9	48.3	56.1	60.4	64.6
1985	58.9	61.6	47.7	53.9	61.0	60.3
MMR[3]:						
1991	77.6	77.9	76.4	75.6	78.8	77.9
Respondents Consulting Vaccination Records, 1991[4]						
DTP[1,2]	84.2	86.2	74.1	78.9	86.3	86.7
Polio[2]	68.9	70.6	60.3	65.5	70.9	69.2
MMR[3]	79.5	80.2	75.7	76.6	80.9	80.3

[1]Diphtheria-tetanus-pertussis.

[2]Three doses or more.

[3]Measles-mumps-rubella.

[4]The data in this panel are based only on 49.3% of white respondents and 40.7% of all other respondents who either consulted records for all of the vaccination questions or reported no vaccinations.

Notes: Beginning in 1976, the category "don't know" was added to response categories. In 1970, the lack of this option resulted in some forced positive answers, particularly for vaccinations requiring multiple dose schedules, that is, polio and DTP. In 1991, refusals and unknowns (2% of sample) were coded as not vaccinated.

From: U.S. Dept. of Health and Human Services (1993). *Health United States, 1992 and Healthy People 2000 Review*. Washington, D.C.: U.S. Government Printing Office, p. 87

Infectious Diseases

Infectious diseases affecting children include not only the so-called childhood diseases, such as diphtheria, pertussis (whooping cough), tetanus (lock jaw), chicken pox, polio, measles, mumps, Haemophilus influenzae type b, and rubella, but also other infectious diseases including AIDS, gonorrhea, streptococcal infections, hepatitis B, syphilis, and tuberculosis. The United States lags behind other nations in protecting its children from communicable childhood diseases. While the incidence of polio (paralytic poliomyelitis) has remained very low since 1984, below ten cases per year, the incidence of measles has not. For example, in 1990,

27,786 cases of measles were reported in the United States;[24] 8,633 of these were in children 1–14 years of age. Tables 8.6 and 8.7 provide an indication of how well the United States is doing to protect its children against childhood disease. As noted in Table 8.7, there has been a fivefold increase in cases of two diseases from the earlier "best year" of reporting. These figures for entirely preventable childhood diseases document the fact that the current system for immunizing infants and toddlers in this country is not working. The United States ranks fifteenth in the percentage of one-year-old children fully immunized against polio. Note, in Table 8.8, that immunization rates for nonwhite

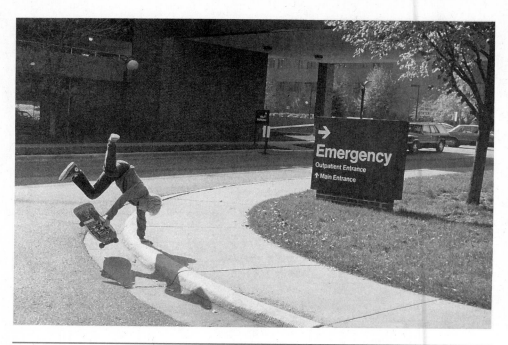

FIGURE 8.6
Unintentional injuries are the leading cause of childhood morbidity.

American children rank next-to-last among the countries reporting rates.

Unfortunately, diseases other than the childhood diseases just discussed also affect children. For example, in 1990, HIV infections were the eighth leading cause of death in 1- to 4-year-old children and the tenth leading cause of death in 5- to 14-year-old children.[3] Two other diseases that have affected children are gonorrhea and tuberculosis. In 1990, there were more than 12,000 cases of gonorrhea in children 5–14 years of age (most of them the result of sexual child abuse) and more than 1,100 cases of tuberculosis in children 1–14.[21]

Oral Health

Oral health, like infant mortality and immunizations status, is an indicator not only of child health but also of the availability of child health care services. Poor oral health during childhood increases the risk for poor nutrition and other health problems. Some 27% of all 6- to 8-year-olds (43%

Table 8.7
Trends in Preventable Childhood Diseases in the United States

	Lowest Number of Cases (Year)	Number of Cases in 1991*	Increase from Best Year to 1991
Measles	1,497 (1983)	9,488	533.8%
Mumps	2,982 (1985)	4,031	35.2
Pertussis	1,248 (1981)	2,575	106.3
Rubella	225 (1988)	1,372	509.8

*Provisional data.

From: Children's Defense Fund (1992). "Child Care and Early Childhood Development." *The State of America's Children, 1992.* Washington, D.C.: Author, p. 6.

Table 8.8
Percentage of One-Year-Old Children
Fully Immunized Against Polio, Selected Countries, 1990

Rank	Nation	Rate	Rank	Nation	Rate
1	Denmark	100	38	Iran	91
2	Bulgaria	99	40	Austria	90
2	Chile	99	40	Dominican Republic	90
2	Czechoslovakia	99	40	Finland	90
2	Hungary	99	40	Malaysia	90
2	North Korea	99	40	Mauritius	90
7	China	98	40	Sri Lanka	90
7	Sweden	98	40	Syria	90
7	Switzerland	98	40	Tunisia	90
10	Greece	97	48	Algeria	89
11	Albania	96	48	Argentina	89
11	Hong Kong	96	50	Phillipines	88
11	Mexico	96	50	Uruguay	88
11	Oman	96	52	Egypt	87
11	Pakistan	96	52	Honduras	87
11	Poland	96	52	Jamaica	87
17	Australia	95	52	Trinidad & Tobago	87
17	Belgium	95	52	United Kingdom	87
17	Bhutan	95	52	Vietnam	87
17	Costa Rica	95	58	Burundi	86
17	France	95	58	Nicaragua	86
17	Germany	95	58	Panama	86
17	Romania	95	61	Canada	85
17	**United States**	**95**	61	Italy	85
25	Cuba	94	61	Mongolia	85
25	Kuwait	94	61	Singapore	85
25	Netherlands	94	61	United Arab Emirates	85
25	Saudi Arabia	94	66	Morocco	84
29	Brazil	93	66	Norway	84
29	Colombia	93	68	Rwanda	83
29	India	93	68	Sierra Leone	83
29	Israel	93	70	Botswana	82
29	Japan	93	70	Central Africa Rep.	82
34	Jordan	92	70	Lebanon	82
34	Portugal	92	70	Tanzania	82
34	Thailand	92		**U.S., Nonwhite**	**82**
34	Yugoslavia	92	74	Libya	81
38	Indonesia	91			

From: Children's Defense Fund (1992). "Child Care and Early Childhood Development." *The State of America's Children, 1992.* Washington, D.C.: Author, p. 4.

of children in low-income families) had untreated dental decay in 1987.[21] These problems accumulate so that, by age 15, 78% of youth have experienced cavities in permanent teeth. Data show that 23% of the general population, 44% of those with low incomes, and 84% of Native Americans aged 15 years had untreated cavities.[21]

Domestic Problems

Domestic problems such as child abuse and neglect, broken homes, and runaway youth jeopardize the health of children. In 1992, 2.9 million children in the United States were reportedly abused, neglected, or both. While this figure represents more than a 50% increase over the 1982 figure, there is little doubt that it still underrepresents the problem. Many children develop severe emotional problems that prevent them from being successful in school and perhaps in society. It has been estimated that 1.5 million children run away from home each year, many to escape abusive and neglectful domestic situations. (See Chapter 17 for more detailed information on child abuse and neglect.)

Pregnancies in Childhood

In 1990, there were 11,657 babies born to girls younger than 15 and another 521,826 born to girls and young women 15 to 19 years old.[6] While the health risks of teenage pregnancies (discussed above) are considerable, the social ramifications of children having children are enormous. For example, in fiscal year 1990, an estimated 360,000 children in the United States were under state supervision and in foster care. This figure increased 29% in just three years.[21] Many other children live in families denied support services that would help these families stay together. In many states, there seem to be inadequate numbers of trained personnel and financial resources to serve all the children in need of assistance.

HEALTH INSURANCE AND HEALTH CARE FOR WOMEN, INFANTS, AND CHILDREN

There is a clear association between family income level and health care coverage. Because the number of children living in poverty increased by more than 2 million during the 1980s, the number of families and children without health care coverage also increased. The cost of routine pediatric care can consume 10% of a poor family's annual income, while the cost of maternal care can exceed the annual income of many low-income, working families.[21]

Approximately two-thirds of the 35 million Americans who live in medically underserved communities are children and women of childbearing age. About 800 counties in the United States have neither a prenatal care provider nor a public health department clinic. In 1989, 85% of pediatricians in private practice had limited the number of Medicaid-insured children they would see, while 23% refused to treat any at all.

Exacerbating the problem is the fact that three federal programs designed to increase the number of medical care providers in underserved areas lost ground during the 1980s. Real-dollar funding for community and migrant health centers fell by 33% and for maternal and child health programs by 39%, while funding for the National Health Service Corp was all but eliminated.[21] (See Chapter 14 for a more detailed discussion about health insurance.)

SOLUTIONS AND PROGRAMS

In the preceding pages, many problems associated with maternal, infant, and child health have been identified. Solutions to many of these problems have been proposed, and in some cases, programs are already in place. Some of these programs are aimed at preventing or reducing the levels of maternal and infant morbidity and mortality, while others are aimed at preventing or reducing childhood morbidity and mortality.

Prevention of Maternal and Infant Morbidity and Mortality

Programs that are designed to prevent or reduce the level of maternal and infant illnesses, injuries, and deaths include family planning programs, a program aimed at reducing teen pregnancy rates, and universal prenatal care. Similarly, programs aimed at reducing birth defects and preventing SIDS hold promise for lowering infant deaths. Lastly, nutrition programs such as the federally funded Women, Infants, and Children (WIC) nutrition program help to insure healthy infants and healthy mothers.

Planning Families

Estimates suggest more than 10% of infant deaths could be prevented by effective family planning. Family planning is an important element in reducing adverse pregnancy outcomes. **Family planning** can be defined as determining the preferred number and spacing of children and choosing the appropriate means to achieve this preference. Effective family planning requires careful decision making and personal responsibility to carry out these decisions. Such decisions include choices such as childbearing, adoption, abstinence from sexual activity, monogamy, use of contraception, and treatment for infertility. The National Family Planning Program (P.L. 91–572), created under Title X of the Public Health Service Act, provides funding for family planning services. Facilities receiving funding under the Title X program must offer a broad range of acceptable family planning methods (oral contraceptives, condoms, sterilization, abstinence); they must encourage family participation; they must give priority to low-income families; and they must not use abortion as a method of family planning.[25]

The inability to conceive a child can be just as difficult to deal with as an unplanned pregnancy. Counseling and instruction concerning infertility is available in some family planning clinics. When most people think of government-supported family planning clinics they think of a place to go for a pregnancy or STD test. Many centers do provide pregnancy screening, but services in family planning centers extend beyond testing. For the pregnant woman, a family planning clinic can provide prenatal care or a referral to a prenatal care provider. For women who are not pregnant, counseling in effective contraception and STD risk reduction may be appropriate. In 1981, family planning clinics that received federal funds were required to provide counseling on all options open to a pregnant woman, including abortion, as outlined in Title X. However, these facilities were not allowed to perform abortions. In 1988, the **"gag rule"** regulations were enacted. These regulations barred physicians and nurses in clinics receiving federal funds from counseling clients about abortions. Family planning providers challenged this legislation on the grounds that it denied women their rights to information that was needed to make an informed decision. Many health care providers felt that the 'gag rule' restricted their rights to counsel a client, even when childbirth could be detrimental to her health.[25]

Supporters of the gag rule regulation felt that the Title X (Family Planning Act) program was created to help prevent unwanted pregnancy by providing educa-

---

family planning Determining the preferred number and spacing of children and choosing the appropriate means to accomplish it.

gag rule Regulations that barred physicians and nurses in clinics receiving federal funds from counseling clients about abortions.

tion and contraception services and was not intended to provide services related to pregnancy options. **Title X** of the Public Health Service Act was established in 1970 to provide family planning services to low-income people. The approximately 3,800 government-funded clinics serve about 4.1 million women each year. Almost 30% of these women are under the age of 20, and 31% are living in poverty. A disproportionate number of the Title X facilities clients are minority-group members.[25]

In 1992, congressional action loosened the gag rule and allowed for abortion options to be discussed between a client and her physician at Title X facilities. While this may appear to be a reasonable compromise, in reality most women who visit family planning clinics are served by a nurse or nurse-practitioner and never see a physician. Therefore, this change in the gag rule still did not permit the free exchange of information between client and all professionals in the clinic. In January 1993, President Clinton signed a presidential memorandum reversing the gag rule regulations. This change allows Title X facilities to discuss abortion as an option to the pregnancy. The presidential memorandum also allows abortions to be performed on U.S. military bases in foreign countries, provided that private funds pay for the abortion.

Legalized Abortion

The fate of legalized abortion itself is as unclear as the right of a client to discuss abortion options in federally funded clinics. The Hyde Amendment of 1976 made it illegal to use federal funds to perform an abortion except in cases where the woman's life was in danger.

In 1992, the Supreme Court was asked to rule on the constitutionality of the landmark court decision of **Roe vs. Wade.** This 1973 Supreme Court ruling made it unconstitutional for state laws to prohibit abortions. In effect, this decision concluded that an unborn child is not a person, and as such, has no rights under the law. The decision to have an abortion or not was left up to the woman until she was 12 weeks pregnant. After the twelfth week, an abortion was permissible only when the health of the mother was in question. In 1989, the Supreme Court appeared to reverse this decision. It ruled that the individual states could place restrictions on a woman's right to obtain an abortion. Some states now have a 24-hour waiting period after counseling before permitting an abortion. The issue of abortion has become a hotly debated topic. Political appointments can be won or lost depending upon a candidate's stance as "pro-life" or "pro-choice," vis-à-vis the abortion issue (see Figure 8.7).

Pro-life groups argue that performing an abortion is an act of murder. Generally, they believe that life begins at conception and that an embryo is a person. The **pro-choice** position is that women have a right to reproductive freedom. Pro-choice advocates feel that the government should not be allowed to force a woman to carry to term and give birth to an unwanted child. They support this argument by raising issues of child abuse and neglect against unwanted children. To counter this argument, pro-life advocates support adoption as an alternative.

Roe vs. Wade A 1973 Supreme Court decision that made it unconstitutional for state laws to prohibit abortions.
pro-life A medical/ethical position that holds that performing an abortion is an act of murder.
pro-choice A medical/ethical position that holds that women have a right to reproductive freedom.

Title X A portion of the Public Health Service Act of 1970 that provides funds for family planning services for low-income people.

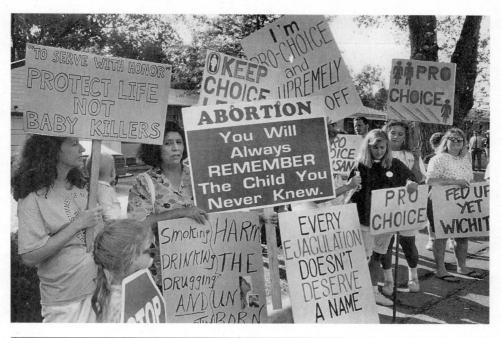

FIGURE 8.7

Political appointments and elections can be won or lost on the issue of abortion.

Approximately 1.5 million abortions are performed each year in this country. According to CDC, in 1990 the ratio of abortions to live births was 34.4 abortions per 100 live births. For white Americans, the ratio was 25.3/100; for Americans of all other races, the ratio was 47.5/100.[2, 26] Abortion among teenagers in this country far exceeds the rate in any other developed country. Of all induced abortions in this country, 26% are performed on teenagers. The majority of women who receive abortions are single, childless, white, 15 to 24 years old, live in urban areas, and qualify for welfare.[11, 27] As a result of the Roe vs. Wade decision, the number of women dying from illegal abortions diminished sharply during the 1980s, as did the number of white babies available for adoption. Clearly, there is no easy solution to the question of abortion. The question of when life begins can only be decided by each individual, based upon his or her own values and beliefs.[11]

Reducing Teenage Pregnancies

The objectives for the nation to improve family planning by the year 2000 include the following objective: to reduce teenage pregnancies to no more than 50 per 1,000 girls aged 17 and younger. Such an objective would decrease the present teenage pregnancy rate by 30% (see Box 8.3).

Many programs that aim to reduce teenage pregnancy in this country do exist. The Children's Defense Fund supports the Adolescent Pregnancy Prevention Clearinghouse to help prevent teen pregnancy. Vincent, Lepro, Baker, and Garvey[28] demon-

BOX 8.3
Healthy People 2000—Objective

5.1   Reduce pregnancies among girls aged 17 and younger to no more than 50 per 1,000 adolescents. (Baseline: 71.1 pregnancies per 1,000 girls aged 15–17 in 1985)

Special Population Target

		1987 Baseline	*2000 Target*	*Percent Decrease*
5.1a	Black adolescent girls aged 15–19	186*	120	
5.1b	Hispanic adolescent girls aged 15–19	158	105	

*Non-white adolescents

Note: For black and Hispanic adolescent girls, baseline data are unavailable for those aged 15–17. The targets for these two populations are based on data for women aged 15–19. If more complete data become available, a 35% reduction from baseline figures should be used as the target.

Baseline data source: The Alan Guttmacher Institute, calculated using birth data from the National Vital Statistics System, characteristics of abortion patients compiled by the Centers for Disease Control, and abortion data collected by the Alan Guttmacher Institute.

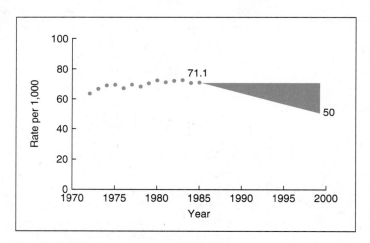

Pregancy rate among adolescent girls aged 15–17.

For Further Thought

Create a list of lifelong consequences that result from teenagers becoming pregnant and having babies.

strated the effectiveness of a community-based approach to reduce the risk of teen pregnancy. The adolescent pregnancy risk reduction program, based in a rural community in South Carolina, targeted teachers, parents, school-aged children, ministers, and community representatives. The interventions focused on developing adolescent decision-making skills and enhancing their self-esteem and their knowledge of human reproduction. The intervention used peer counseling as well as parent education classes to develop positive communication between the adolescents, their parents, and the community. It is projected that this program will save over $600,000 in a 20-year period.

Another program, called the "Teen Outreach Program," is "a nationwide school-based teen pregnancy and dropout prevention program. The program discovered that academically disadvantaged teens who participated in after-school discussion groups and community volunteer activities experienced lower pregnancy and dropout rates and more grade promotions than their non-participating counterparts.[21]

In an attempt to counteract the message that television is sending American teens—namely that sex is romantic, exciting, and everyone is doing it—California has spent $5.7 million to try to prevent teenage pregnancy. In 1993, youth-targeted television shows began carrying state-sponsored commercials that relay the message: If you are not ready for sex, you are not alone.

Expanding Prenatal Care

As mentioned earlier, nearly 25% of all mothers received either no prenatal care or only late prenatal care. For unmarried and teenage mothers, this figure is 47%. These low rates of prenatal care are a major contributing factor to the poor health status of our infants. The 1989 Federal Office of Budget Reconciliation Act expanded the Medicaid eligibility for pregnant women to include a segment of the women who had previously been slightly above the poverty line and therefore ineligible for prenatal care. While this act did increase the number of women eligible for prenatal care, the number of physicians accepting Medicaid patients declined during this period so that, in reality, fewer women received care.

A possible solution to the problem of the lack of prenatal care has been demonstrated in a new program developed in south-central Idaho. This program combined services into a "one-stop shopping" clinic that included an expanded Women, Infants, and Children program. The core of the program is a public health nurse who coordinates the medical and support services. In the first year of operation, three times the number of pregnant women in this health district received prenatal care as in the previous year. It is too early to tell how effective this program is on preventing infant mortality. However, early data show a 1% drop in low-birth-weight and very-low-birth-weight deliveries from 1988 to 1990. There has been a decline in drop-in deliveries (those who have had no prenatal care) at the regional medical center and a decrease of 1,000 newborn intensive-care-unit days for an estimated savings of $300,000.[29]

Maintaining Records of Birth Defects

The federal government and 22 states maintain surveillance systems to amass data on birth defects. These systems can be used to assess the effectiveness of intervention programs in preventing birth defects and can serve to establish a basis for the epidemiological research needed to understand the cause of birth defects.[30]

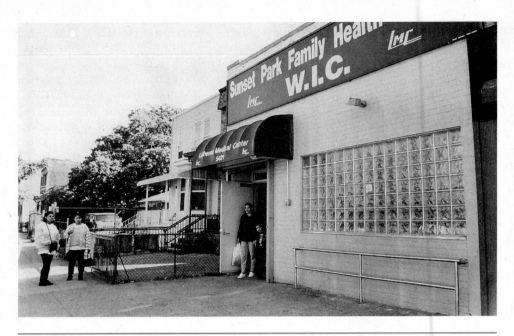

FIGURE 8.8
The WIC program, which serves more than 4 million women and children, saves $3 for each tax dollar spent.

Supporting Parents of SIDS Victims

Treating those who have suffered the trauma of losing an infant to SIDS largely consists of family counseling. Due to the nature of the condition, striking seemingly healthy infants in their sleep, family members experience severe psychological trauma. The local branch of an organization such as the National Foundation for Sudden Infant Death Syndrome (8240 Professional Pl., Landover, MD 20785) can be helpful to family members. Participating in such an organization which is made up of other SIDS surviving parents can be excellent therapy.[31]

Providing Supplemental Nutrition

The Special Supplemental Food Program for Women, Infants, and Children,

known as the **WIC Program** and sponsored by the United States Department of Agriculture, serves more than 4 million women and children including 20%–25% of women giving birth in the United States (see Figure 8.8). The program was designed to complement traditional medical and public health services. The WIC Program provides free nutritious foods, nutrition education and counseling, and access to health care to low-income pregnant, breastfeeding, or postpartum women and to infants and children under the age of five years. More specifically, these individuals must meet the following three criteria to be eligible for WIC: (1) reside in the state in which they are applying for the WIC program, (2) meet the income

---

WIC program A special supplemental food program for women, infants, and children, sponsored by the USDA.

guidelines (these guidelines are reviewed yearly and posted in the *Federal Register*), and (3) meet the nutritional risk criteria as determined by a medical and/or nutritional assessment.[32] WIC programs are offered most often through local health departments, but they can be housed in other social service agencies.

Research indicates that women who participate in the WIC program during pregnancy give birth to babies with higher birth weights, have fewer fetal deaths, and help to reduce Medicaid expenses.[29] It has been estimated that $3 are saved for each $1 spent on the WIC Program. For this reason, the WIC Program has enjoyed strong bipartisan support in Congress.

In addition to WIC, the federal government has over 35 health programs in 16 different agencies to serve the needs of our nation's children. Some of these programs are well respected and help meet the needs of many children. However, many others are **categorical programs,** meaning that they are only available to people who can be categorized into a specific group based on disease, age, family means, geography, or other variables. This means that many children fall through the cracks and are not served. The Department of Health and Human Services houses the Office of Adolescent Programming, the Office of Maternal and Child Health, and the Adolescent and School Health Division. The Departments of Education, Agriculture, and Justice all administer programs involving child health. Some children require services from multiple programs, which complicates the eligibility determination of each child. The result is a wasteful and inefficient system of child health care.

---

categorical programs Programs available only to people who can be categorized into a group based on specific variables.

Prevention of Childhood Morbidity and Mortality

Much can be done to reduce the incidence of disease, injury and death among this nation's children. Among the most important actions are those to reduce the number of unintentional injuries, to increase the percentage of children who complete their immunizations, and to improve education levels and parenting skills for all (see Box 8.4).

Reducing Unintentional Injuries

Chapter 17 contains a discussion about the actions that can be taken to reduce the number of unintentional injuries. Those of particular importance to children include the use of child safety seats, flame retardant sleepwear, and smoke detectors; use of life jackets and safe boating practices; and use of bicycle helmets and appropriate safety equipment for recreation and sporting activities.

Immunizing Children

Recent statistics indicate a serious problem with the United States' immunization system. As mentioned earlier, the Centers for Disease Control and Prevention reported 27,672 cases of measles in 1990. This outbreak occurred in the face of a 1979 forecast by public health officials that the United States would have childhood diseases under control by the end of the 1980s and that there would be no more than 500 cases of measles in 1990. The incidence of mumps, rubella, and whooping cough also exceeded desired levels (see Table 8.7).

All 50 states require evidence of vaccination before a child may enter school. In fact, approximately 98% percent of United States children are fully immunized against five childhood diseases by the time they begin school.[33] So what has caused these cases of disease? First, some children (approxi-

BOX 8.4
Health Diary for Mothers and Children

The Department of Health and Human Services (HHS) has launched "Health Diary," an interactive handbook that educates pregnant women and new mothers about such topics as when to schedule physician visits and vaccines, what to avoid during pregnancy, and what to look for in their newborn infants.

The publication, with spaces to record appointments, milestones, and advice, was developed within HHS by the Health Resources and Services Administration's Maternal and Child Health Bureau. It is designed to encourage early and continual prenatal care, plus regular physician visits and early immunization, typically at 2, 4, 6, and 15 months, for infants and toddlers.

The diary also provides advice on diet, exercise and other health behaviors during pregnancy, information on fetal development, and tells what to expect at each prenatal care visit. It also covers child development, effective parenting, and the immunization and health care supervision babies need during the first 2 years of life.

A health diary is not a new idea; more than 100 other countries provide maternal and child handbooks for their citizens. In Japan when a mother registers a pregnancy, she receives a letter from the government congratulating her, and a handbook detailing what she must do to help ensure that she has a healthy baby. The letter and handbook may seem like gimmicks to a jaded American public, but they symbolize Japan's deep commitment to overcoming the tragedy of infant mortality—a commitment that has established Japan as the world leader in preventing infant mortality.

Copies of the "Health Diary" are being sent to state and local maternal and child health agencies and other organizations for free distribution to publicly supported centers and clinics. Secretary Donna E. Shalala said the Dept. of Health and Human Services will work further with Congress, States, and outside groups to ensure wide distribution to women across the country. Professional groups, corporations, state and local government agencies, and voluntary organizations are encouraged to purchase bulk copies at a reduced rate or to reprint the handbook for distribution to employees, health care providers, and patients, or through community organizations.

From: No author (1993). "HHS Issues 'Health Diary' for Mothers and Children." *Public Health Reports* 108(4): back cover.

---

mately 2%) enter school without being properly immunized. Second, even when properly administered, immunizations have a failure rate of 2%–5%. Third, about 5% of students are given exemptions from immunization requirements for religious or medical reasons. These unprotected individuals lower the overall immunity of the population (**herd immunity)** and serve as reservoirs of infection for other unprotected individuals. Still, these few people represent only a small part of the problem. The Centers for Disease Control and Prevention estimates that as many as one-third of the preschoolers in the United States are not properly vaccinated against childhood diseases. The frequency of inadequately or improperly immunized preschoolers may be over 50% in inner-city populations (see Table 8.6). Many parents no longer believe that childhood illnesses are a problem in

---

herd immunity The overall immunity of a population against a particular disease

this country; hence, they do not vigorously pursue immunizations for their children.

More stringent measures by the medical community are needed to ensure that all children are immunized. Opportunities to vaccinate are frequently missed by health care practitioners in primary care settings who do not routinely inquire about the immunization status of the child. Parents and health practitioners need to work together to ensure that youth are protected from communicable diseases. Timely immunization of children must be accepted as a national obligation, because America cannot afford the waste that results from unnecessary illness, disability, and death.[33] The currently recommended immunization schedule is provided in Table 8.9 (see Box 8.5).

Formerly, one problem with making sure that children were immunized in a timely manner was the total number of immunizations required. However, on March 30, 1993, the Food and Drug Adminstration licensed a combination vaccine that requires only four injections instead of the eight required before. The new vaccine, Tetramune, is recommended for use at 2, 4, 6, and 15 months of age to immunize against diptheria, tetanus, pertussis, and *Haemophilus influenzae* type B.[34]

While there is certainly a need for a new national initiative on immunization—one that includes education of the public about the importance of completing each child's immunizations—a national initiation may not be enough. We may need to rethink the way we produce and sell vaccines. More than half of the nation's children are immunized in public health clinics. Recently, these clinics have been experiencing shortages of vaccines that are supplied by the government, which purchases them from the pharmaceutical industry. But industry concern over liability for rare but serious complications that can occur, even with our safest immunizations, has caused some pharmaceutical com-

Table 8.9
Recommended Schedule of Vaccinations for All Children, 1993

Age	DTP	DTaP	OPV	MMR	Hib Option 1[1]	Hib Option 2[1]	HBV Option 1	HBV Option 2
Birth	...	...	...	...	...	...	X	...
2 months	X	...	X	...	X	X	X[2]	X[2]
4 months	X	...	X	...	X	X	...	X[2]
6 months	X	...	...	...	X	...	...	...
12 months	...	...	...	...	...	X	...	...
15 months	X[3]	X[3]	X[3]	X[4]	X	...	...	...
6–18 months	...	...	...	...	...	...	X[2]	X[2]
4–6 years (before school)	X	X	...	X[5]	...	...	...	...

[1]Vaccine is given in either a 4-dose schedule in option 1 or a 3-dose schedule in option 2, depending the type of vaccine used.

[2]Hepatitis B vaccine can be given simultaneously with DTP, OPV, MMR, and Hib at the same visit.

[3]Many experts recommend these vaccines at 18 months.

[4]In some areas, this dose of MMR may be given at 12 months.

[5]American Academy of Pediatrics recommends that this dose be given at entry to middle school or junior high school.

Note: DTP = Diphtheria, tetanus, and pertussis vaccine; DTaP = Diphtheria, tetanus, and acellular pertussis vaccine; OPV = Live oral polio vaccine; MMR = Measles, mumps, and rubella vaccine; Hib = Haemophilus b conjugate vaccine; HBV = Hepatitis B vaccine.

From: Robinson, C. A., S. J. Sepe, and K. F. Y. Lin (1993). "The President's Child Immunization Initiative—A Summary of the Problem and the Response." *Public Health Reports* 108(4): 420.

BOX 8.5
A New Vaccine

A bacterium, *Haemophilus influenzae* type b disease, also called Haemophilus b or "Hib" disease, can be a very serious disease, especially among children under 5 years of age. Hib causes about 12,000 cases of meningitis (inflammation of the covering of the brain) in the United States each year, mostly in the under-5 age group. Of these 12,000 children, about 3000 suffer permanent brain damage and about 600 die. Hib can also cause pneumonia and infections of the blood, joints, bones, soft tissues, throat, and the covering of the heart.

In the United States, Hib disease strikes about 1 child out of 200 before the fifth birthday. Most serious Hib disease occurs in children between 6 months and 1 year of age. Despite its name, Hib does not cause the flu (influenza).

Hib Immunization

There are several vaccines available at this time for protection against Hib disease, but only two are approved for use in children under 15 months of age. These are the vaccines that are recommended because they provide protection during the time children are most susceptible to Hib disease. Depending on the type of vaccine, it is given either at 2, 4, and 6 months with a booster dose at 15

months, or at 2 and 4 months with a booster dose at 12 months. For children who are late in getting their first dose, the total number of doses they receive may be different. Hib vaccine is usually not recommended for children after their 5th birthday.

Possible Side Effects and Adverse Reactions to Hib Immunization

Hib vaccine is among the safest of all vaccine products. The vaccine cannot cause meningitis and has not been associated with any other serious reactions. About 2 in every 100 children who receive the current Hib vaccine will have some slight redness in the area where the shot is given, and about 1 in 100 will have swelling or warmth in that area. About 2 in every 100 will develop a moderate fever (higher than 101°F). These reactions begin within 24 hours after the shot and usually go away within 48 to 72 hours.

State Immunization Requirements

No states have laws requiring schoolchildren to be immunized against Hib disease, because children are no longer at high risk by the time they reach school age.

From: U.S. Dept. of Health and Human Services (1991). *Parents' Guide to Childhood Immunization.* Washington, D.C.: U.S. Government Printing Office.

panies to discontinue manufacturing vaccines; those remaining in business have had to increase vaccine prices.[35] Figure 8.9 shows price increases for selected vaccines for the period 1981–1991. In 1982, the average cost to completely immunize a child was $6.69. By 1990, the cost to immunize a child against the same diseases had risen to an astounding $91.20. While Medicaid should be able to assist low-income families to pay

for immunizations, one study found that in a single office visit for immunizations for a 15-month-old, Medicaid typically underpays doctors by nearly $40.00.[36]

The Public Health Service is requesting additional money to purchase the vaccines and deliver them to clinics and private physicians at no charge. Although this approach will be expensive to the American public, estimates suggest a higher vaccination rate of America's children could save between $10 and $14 for every dollar the government spends.[35, 37]

President Clinton, recognizing the efficacy and need for childhood immunizations, announced a comprehensive childhood immunization initiative after only 24 days in office. This initiative was designed to assure that all children in the United States were immunized against the preventable childhood diseases through funding for communities to extend clinic hours, provide more staff, and increase information and education efforts and for the planning and implementation of a national immunization tracking system.[38] At the time of this writing, the legislative portion of the initiative had been acted on by the House of Representatives on May 27, 1993, and by the Senate on June 25, 1993. A House-Senate conference committee reconciled the differences between the two bills, and President Clinton's Vaccines for Children was slated to begin October 1, 1994.[33, 39]

Listening to Children's Advocates

There are numerous groups that advocate for children's health and welfare. Included are UNICEF, the Children's Defense Fund, and the American Academy of Pediatrics.

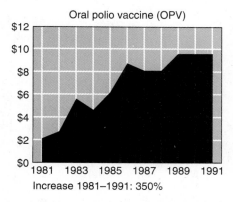

Oral polio vaccine (OPV)

Increase 1981–1991: 350%

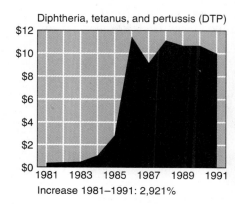

Diphtheria, tetanus, and pertussis (DTP)

Increase 1981–1991: 2,921%

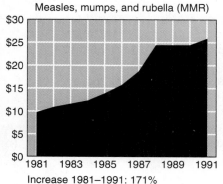

Measles, mumps, and rubella (MMR)

Increase 1981–1991: 171%

FIGURE 8.9

Prices for selected vaccines per dose 1981–1991.

From: Children's Defense Fund. The State of America's Children *(1992): 9.*

United Nations Children's Fund (UNICEF)

The United Nations Children's Fund (UNICEF) gathers data on the health of children throughout the world and has joined the World Health Organization in its goal of "Health for all by the year 2000." UNICEF has assisted in mass vaccinations and been involved in other international health efforts to protect children.

Children's Defense Fund (CDF)

The Children's Defense Fund (CDF) is a private, nonprofit organization headquartered in Washington, D.C., dedicated to providing a voice for the children of America. The CDF focuses on the needs of poor, minority, and handicapped children and their families. The aim of the CDF is to provide support and education about the need for primary care and prevention of risk among America's youth.

American Academy of Pediatrics

To help serve all our nation's children, the American Academy of Pediatrics has developed a plan to provide care for all children through the age of 21 years and for all pregnant women.[40] Mandated benefits would be provided either through employer-based insurance or through private insurance contracted for by states. State funding would come from three sources: continuation of currently budgeted state and federal Medicaid expenditures, insurance premiums, and—for those employers who choose not to cover pregnant women and children—an employer payroll tax. The plan includes methods to assure adequate provider reimbursement. The Academy intends to introduce the proposed legislation soon.

Providing Child Care

In the near future, two of three new employees will be women. By 1995, 75% of all mothers will be working outside of the home.

These demographic changes have altered American family life. Two issues that are important to the health and welfare of America's children are family care leave and availability of quality day care (Figure 8.10). On August 5, 1993, the **Family and Medical Leave Act** proposed by President Clinton went into effect. The act grants a 12-week unpaid leave to men or women after the birth of a child, an adoption, or in the event of illness in the immediate family. The act only affects businesses with 50 or more employees. Those employees covered in the law include those who have worked 1,250 hours for an employer over a 12-month period (an average of 25 hours per week). This excludes about 40% of American employees who work in small businesses that do not fall under the law's guidelines. Also, employers covered by the act can exempt key salaried employees who are among their highest paid 10%, if they are needed to prevent "substantial and grievous" economic harm to the employer. Some experts feel the law divides the people by class, helping those who can afford the 3 months without pay, and bypassing those who cannot. Experts have recommended a 6- to 12-month family care leave program with partial pay for at least 3 months. America is the only industrialized nation that has not enacted a paid infant care leave.

The children least likely to receive adequate child care are the children of working lower- and middle-class families. Wealthy families can pay for excellent care while the poor can take advantage of government-sponsored programs.[41]

In 1988, Congress passed the Family Support Act, which provided funding for

---

Family and Medical Leave Act Federal law that provides up to a 12-week unpaid leave to men and women after the birth of a child, an adoption, or an event of illness in the immediate family.

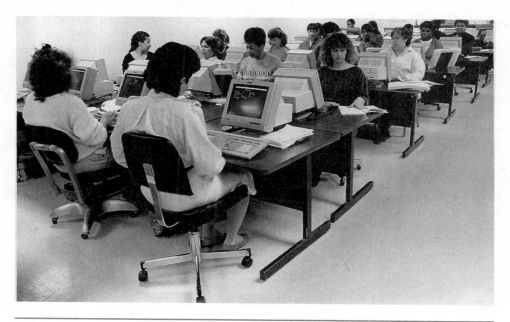

FIGURE 8.10

With nearly 75% of mothers working outside the home, infant-care leave and quality day care have become national concerns.

child care assistance to welfare parents who are employed or participating in an approved training program. Unfortunately, states must match federal funds for this program, which makes meeting the needs of eligible participants difficult for poor states. In 1990, Congress passed the Child Care and Development Block Grant, which provides child care subsidies for low-income children and funding to improve the quality of child care services. Funding for the Child Care Block Grant for the 1992 fiscal year was $825 million. The "At Risk" Child Care Program, also passed in 1990, provided $1.5 billion over a five-year period to support child care assistance to low-income families at risk of going on welfare. With the initiation of the "At Risk" Child Care Program and the Child Care and Development Block Grant, states can pro-vide assistance to many more low-income families.

Another concern of child health advocates is child day care. Too many children, they point out, spend their days in unsafe and disease-ridden child care. Far too often, the quality of the care a child receives is not good enough to meet the child's developmental and emotional needs. The average number of children per staff in day care centers has risen by 25% since the late 1970s. The low salary of a child care worker (the average salary in 1988 was $9,363) makes it difficult to attract and retain qualified teachers. As a country, we cannot afford not to invest in the early childhood care of millions of children. We must examine our priorities and allocate the resources to provide comprehensive, high-quality care for America's children.[36]

CHAPTER SUMMARY

Maternal and child health encompasses the health of women of childbearing age from prepregnancy through pregnancy, labor and delivery, and in the postpartum period. It also includes the health of infants and children through 14 years of age. Maternal and child health are important indicators of a community's overall health.

Maternal mortality rates have declined over the past 20 years but have remained much too high for minority women. Infant mortality rates have also declined, but rates for the United States remain higher than those of most other industrial nations. The major contributing factors to maternal and infant mortality are the teenage status of a large number of mothers and inadequate prenatal care. These factors result in too many low-birth-weight babies and in birth defects. Other contributing factors are heredity, poverty, low educational achievement, and substance abuse.

Childhood mortality rates for the United States are higher than those in many other countries. The leading causes of childhood mortality are unintentional injuries, cancer, and birth defects. Childhood health is jeopardized by infectious diseases, poor oral health, child abuse and neglect, inadequate health care and health insurance, and, for girls, pregnancy.

The health of mothers, infants, and children can be protected and improved by better efforts at family planning, preventing teenage pregnancies, extending prenatal care to more women, reducing birth defects, and providing adequate nutrition and immunization to all infants and children. We must also listen to advocates of maternal and child health who propose greater support for families with infants and children, including liberal family leave laws and better day care opportunities.

SCENARIO: ANALYSIS AND RESPONSE

We have learned that a lack of prenatal care increases the risk of premature delivery and possible health problems for the infant.

1. If Susan had received prenatal care, how could it have helped in the normal development of the infant? How could the doctor have counseled Susan?

2. How could Susan have found out about opportunities for prenatal care that she could afford?

3. The cost of treating Susan's infant could run into the hundreds of thousands of dollars and there is no guarantee that the child will survive. Do you think it would be more cost effective to assure prenatal care to all women or to continue under the system that is in place now? How would you suggest that the United States approach this problem?

4. What programs mentioned in this chapter could have helped Susan?

REVIEW QUESTIONS

1. What has been the trend in infant mortality rates in the United States since 1960? What is the current rate? How does this rate compare with that of other industrial countries?

2. Americans are a heterogeneous society. What are the differences in the infant mortality rates among geographical regions and among races?

3. What are some of the factors that contribute to infant mortality? What is the relationship between infant mortality and prenatal care?

4. What types of services are included in prenatal care?

5. What is sudden infant death syndrome (SIDS), and what are some of the factors that may increase risk of SIDS?

6. What are the consequences of teen pregnancy to the mother? To the infant?

7. What are the leading causes of death in children 1–14 years of age?

8. What are the nine childhood diseases for which immunizations are now available? What are some other communicable diseases that affect children as well as adults?

9. What are some of the factors that have led to the failure to better control the preventable childhood diseases?

10. What are the major programs in this country that help promote maternal, infant, and child health?

11. What is included in family planning?

12. Discuss the pro-life and pro-choice positions on the abortion issue.

13. Why was the Roe vs. Wade court decision so important?

14. What is the WIC Program?

15. Name three groups that are advocates for the health of children and what they have done to show their support.

16. What is the Family and Medical Leave Act? What are its keys elements?

17. What are the major problems associated with day care for children in the United States?

ACTIVITIES

Write a two-page paper summarizing the results/information you gain from one of the activities below.

1. Survey 10 classmates and friends and ask them what leads to teen pregnancy. What prompts adolescents to risk pregnancy if they have adequate knowledge of contraception? Ask if they know anyone who became pregnant as an adolescent. Are the reasons they give different from your own? Divide your list into categories of personal beliefs, barriers to action, and social pressure. For example, a comment that might fit under beliefs is, "They don't think they can get pregnant the first time"; under barriers, "They are too embarrassed to buy contraception"; under social pressure, "All the messages in society push sex." Which of the three categories had the most responses? Does this surprise you? What implications does this have for programs trying to reduce the incidence of teen pregnancy?

2. Call your local health department and ask for information about the local WIC program. Ask permission to visit and talk to a representative about the program and its clientele.

3. Contact your state health department and find out how many cases of childhood communicable diseases were reported in your state during the past year. What are your state's laws about childhood immunizations? What qualifications must a person meet to receive these immunizations free?

4. Call your local obstetricians' offices and ask if they take Medicaid patients. What is their normal fee for prenatal care and delivery? If they do not take Medicaid patients, ask them to whom they would refer a pregnant woman with no insurance.

5. Create a record of your own or a family member's immunizations. Find out when and where you were immunized for each of the immunizations listed in Figure 8.4. Are there any immunizations you need to get? When are you scheduled to get your next tetanus/toxoid immunization?

REFERENCES

1. Pillitteri, A. (1992). *Maternal and Child Health Nursing: Care of the Childbearing and Childrearing Family.* Philadelphia: J. B. Lippincott.

2. U.S. Dept. of Health and Human Services, National Center for Health Statistics (1993). *Health, United States, 1992 and Healthy People 2000 Review* (DHHS pub. no. PHS-93-1232). Washington, D.C.: U.S. Government Printing Office.

3. U.S. Dept. of Health and Human Services (1993). "Advance Report of Final Mortality Statistics, 1990." *Monthly Vital Statistics Report* 41(7).

4. No Author (1993). "HHS Issues 'Health Diary' for Mothers and Children." *Public Health Reports* 108(4): back cover.

5. Silbergeld, E. K. (1993). *Investing in Prevention: Opportunities to Reduce Disease and Health Care Costs Through Identifying and Reducing Environmental Contributions to Preventable Disease.* Washington, D.C.: Environmental Defense Fund.

6. U.S. Dept. of Health and Human Services (1993). "Advance Report of Final Natality Statistics, 1990." *Monthly Vital Statistics Report* 41(9): 1–14.

7. U.S. Dept. of Health and Human Services (1990). *Healthy People 2000* [short version] (DHHS pub. no. 91-50213). Washington, D.C.: U.S. Government Printing Office.

8. Currey, M. (1990). "Factors Associated with Inadequate Prenatal Care." *Journal of Community Health Nursing* 7(4): 245–252.

9. The Alan Guttmacher Institute (1987). *Blessed Events and the Bottom Line: The Financing of Maternity Care in the U.S.* New York: Author.

10. Center for Population Options (1992). *Teenage Pregnancy and Too-Early Childbearing: Public Costs, Personal Consequences.* Washington, D.C.: Author.

11. Kelley, K., and D. Bryne (1992). *Birth Control: Exploring Human Sexuality.* Englewood Cliffs, N.J.: Prentice-Hall, pp. 123–129.

12. Southern Regional Project Report on Infant Mortality (1988). *Adolescent Pregnancy in the South.* Washington, D.C.: Author.

13. Nersesian, W. S. (1988). "Infant Mortality in Socially Vulnerable Populations." *Annual Review of Public Health* 9: 361–377.

14. Swartz, M. (1990). "Infant Mortality: Agenda for the 1990's." *Journal of Pediatric Health Care* 4: 169–174.

15. Overpeck, M., and A. Moss (1991). "Children's Exposure to Environmental Cigarette Smoke Before and After Birth." *Advance Data* 202 (June 18, 1991).

16. Goldsmith, S. (1990). "Prosecution to Enhance Treatment." *Children Today* July–Aug.: 13–15.

17. Centers for Disease Control (1988). "Leading Major Congenital Malformations Among Minority Groups in the United States, 1982–1986." *Morbidity and Mortality Weekly Report* 37(ss-3): 17–24.

18. U.S. Dept. of Health and Human Services (1991). *Health Status of Minorities and Low-Income Groups,* 3rd ed. Washington, D.C.: U.S. Government Printing Office.

19. U.S. Dept. of Health and Human Services (1991). *Healthy People 2000: National Health Promotion and Disease Prevention Objectives* [Full report, with commentary] (DHHS pub. no. PHS-91-50212). Washington, D.C.: U.S. Government Printing Office.

20. Editors (1992). "Editorial," *American Family Physician* 45(2): 921.

21. Children's Defense Fund (1990). *S.O.S. America: A Children's Defense Budget.* Washington, D.C.: Author.

22. National Safety Council (1991). *Accident Facts, 1991 Edition.* Chicago: Author.

23. Rice, D. P., E. J. McKenzie, et al. (1989). *Cost of Injury in the United States: A Report to Congress.* San Francisco: Institute for Health and Aging, Univ. of California, and Injury Prevention Center, The Johns Hopkins Univ.

24. Centers for Disease Control (1992). "Summary of Notifiable Diseases, United States, 1991." *Morbidity and Mortality Weekly Report 1991* 40(53): 1–63.

25. *Congressional Digest* (1991). "Title X Pregnancy Counseling Act." 70(8,9) 195–224.

26. U.S. Dept. of Commerce (1992). *Statistical Abstract of the United States: 1992,* 112th ed. Washington, D.C.: U.S. Government Printing Office.

27. Henshaw, S. K., and J. Van Vort (1992). "Abortion Service in the United States, 1987 and 1988." *Family Planning Perspectives* 24(2): 85–87.

28. Vincent, M., E. Lepro, S. Baker, and D. Garvey (1991). "Projected Public Sector Savings in a Teen Pregnancy Prevention Project." *Journal of Health Education* 22(4): 208–213.

29. Machala, M., and M. Miner (1991). "Piecing Together the Crazy Quilt of Prenatal Care." *Public Health Reports* 106(4): 353–360.

30. Centers for Disease Control (1989). "Contribution of Birth Defects to Infant Mortality—United States, 1986." *Journal of the American Medical Association* 262(14): 1923–1927.

31. Guntheroth, W. (1986). "SIDS and Near-Miss SIDS." *Current Pediatric Therapy* vol. 12. Philadelphia: W.B. Saunders, pp. 752–754.

32. U.S. Dept. of Agriculture (1993). *Code of Federal Regulations 7, (parts 210–299).* Washington, D.C.: U.S. Government Printing Office.

33. Robinson, C. A., and K. J. Bart (1993). "Editorial: Disease Prevention Through Immunization; The Beginning of Health Care Reform." *Public Health Reports* 108(4): 417.

34. No author (June 1993). "FDA Licenses Combination Childhood Vaccine. *FDA Consumer,* p. 2.

35. Harrington-Lueker, D. (1991). "A Shot in the Arm for Child Health." *The American School Board Journal* 178(8): 37–38.

36. Children's Defense Fund (1992). "Child Care and Early Childhood Development." *The State of America's Children 1992.* Washington, D.C.: Children's Defense Fund.

37. No Author (1991). "A Shot in the Arm." *U.S. News and World Report* 110(21): 16.

38. Robinson, C. A., S. J. Sepe, and K. F. Y. Lin (1993). "The President's Child Immunization Initiative—A Summary of the Problem and the Response." *Public Health Reports* 108(4): 419–425.

39. Lee, P. R., and B. C. Vladeck (1994). "Childhood Immunization Initiative." *Journal of the American Medical Association* 271(16): 1230.

40. Harvey, B. (1990). "Toward a National Child Health Policy." *Journal of the American Medical Association* 264(2): 252–253.

41. Ziegler, E., and E. Gilman (1993). "Day Care in America! What Is Needed?" *Pediatrics* 91(1): 175–178.

Chapter 9

COMMUNITY HEALTH
AND MINORITIES

Chapter Outline

Chapter Objectives

After studying this chapter, you should be able to:

1. Explain the concept of diversity as it describes the American people, and identify minority and majority groups.
2. Explain why the racial/ethnic mix in the United States will continue to change well into the twenty-first century.
3. List the racial and ethnic groups used by the United States government for collecting census data.
4. Identify the limitations of racial/ethnic health data.
5. Explain the difference between race and ethnicity.
6. Describe the socioeconomic characteristics of Americans of Hispanic origin.
7. Identify the major health problems of Americans of Hispanic origin.
8. Provide an overview of the Asian/Pacific Islander culture.
9. Explain how slavery has given rise to poor health care for black Americans.
10. Describe the socioeconomic characteristics of black Americans.
11. List and briefly describe the major community health problems of black Americans.
12. Define sickle cell disease, sickle cell anemia, and sickle cell trait.
13. List some of the beliefs and values of Native American culture.
14. Trace the evolution of the Indian Health Service from its establishment to the present.
15. Identify the three major theories for excessive alcohol use among Native Americans.
16. Define *cultural sensitivity*.
17. List and briefly describe three solutions to community health problems faced by racial/ethnic minorities.

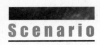
Tom just returned from a cross-country business trip that took him from New York City to Miami, to San Antonio, to Los Angeles, and back to his hometown, Middletown, U.S.A. When his curious teenagers asked him to tell them about the people who live in the "big cities," he began by saying, "There seem to be more minorities and foreigners in the cities than before. I heard at least five or six different languages spoken. Signs in the hotels and in the storefronts are written in at least two, and sometimes three or four, languages."

"Another thing that always amazes me is the number of ethnic restaurants. Here, we have just one Mexican, one Italian, and one Chinese restaurant, but in New York City and other big cities there are hundreds of restaurants serving foreign foods. I get the feeling that the United States is more culturally diverse than at anytime in its past, even when it was considered the "melting pot" for the world's populations."

INTRODUCTION

The strength and greatness of America lies in the diversity of its people. Over the centuries, wave after wave of immigrants have come to America to start new lives. They have brought with them many of their traditions and cultures. In 1990, one American in seven (31.8 million) spoke a language other than English at home, a striking 34% increase in the ratio of speakers of another language from just a decade before.[1] As we approach the twenty-first century, immigration continues, and the diversity it provides continues to be an important element in our society (see Figure 9.1).

One reflection of our diversity is skin color. According to the 1990 census,[2] the population of the United States continues to be predominantly white. In that year, the **majority** (80.3%) of the almost 249 million people living in the United States were white. The remaining 19.7% of the population, by definition, comprises **minority groups.** In contrast, the 1980 Census reported minority groups accounting for only 16.9% of the population (see Table 9.1). This trend toward population diversity is expected to continue so that by the middle of the twenty-first century, the size of the majority will be significantly smaller. There are three primary reasons for this. The first is that both the birth and fertility rates of minorities living in this country are higher than those of the majority. Second, immigration into the United States is expected to continue. In 1990, former president Bush signed a law raising the ceiling on legal immigration by 25% to 675,000 a year. It is anticipated that many of those who will be immigrating will be of Asian and Hispanic descent and of childbearing age. Third, the number of interracial marriages is increasing. In 1980, 1 out of 100 marriages was interracial. By 1992 that number increased to 1 in 50. These marriages will yield biracial children, many of whom will associate with minority groups. The combined effects of

---

majority Those with characteristics found in over 50% of a population.

minority groups Subgroups of the population making up less than 50% of the population..

immigration, births of minorities, and off-spring of interracial marriages is expected to swell the total population in the United States to 383 million by 2050, by which time the number of persons considered as being members of a minority group will have doubled and nearly half of the entire United States population will belong to either a racial or ethnic minority.[3]

The impact of a more diverse population in the United States on community health issues will be significant. "While great strides have been made in improving the health of the American people, there is still a marked disparity in the burden of death and illness borne by ethnic and minority populations compared with the majority white population."[4] The nature of this disparity is the subject of this chapter. If you recall from Chapter 1, one of the three broad health goals of the nation for the year 2000 is to "reduce health disparities among Americans."

It should be pointed out that the link between minority status and health status may be indirect. Research suggests that minority status is often linked with socioeconomic status and other social factors, which in turn impact morbidity and mortality (see Figure 9.2). This chapter surveys the health status of various racial/ethnic groups in the United States and reviews some of the major community health issues that they face. A group's social and economic characteristics are often linked to their health status. As health statistics for racial/ethnic minority groups are presented, we will identify some of the social and economic characteristics of that group that contribute to these health statistics. Among the most common are level of education, status of employment, family type, and level of income.

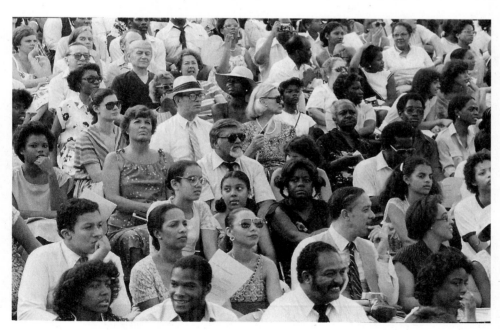

FIGURE 9.1

The strength and greatness of America lie in the diversity of its people.

Table 9.1

Resident Population, by Race and Hispanic Origin: 1980 and 1990

[As of April 1, 1991]

Race and Hispanic Origin	Number (1,000)		Percent Distribution		Change 1980–1990	
	1980	1990	1980	1990	Number (1,000)	Percent
All persons	**226,546**	**248,710**	**100.0**	**100.0**	**22,164**	**9.8**
Race						
White	188,372	199,686	83.1	80.3	11,314	6.0
Black	26,495	29,986	11.7	12.1	3,491	13.2
American Indian, Eskimo, or Aleut	1,420	1,959	0.6	0.8	539	37.9
American Indian	1,364	1,878	0.6	0.8	514	37.7
Eskimo	42	57	(Z)	(Z)	15	35.6
Aleut	14	24	(Z)	(Z)	10	67.5
Asian or Pacific Islander	*3,500	7,274	1.5	2.9	3,773	107.8
Chinese	806	1,645	0.4	0.7	839	104.1
Filipino	775	1,407	0.3	0.6	632	81.6
Japanese	701	848	0.3	0.3	147	20.9
Asian Indian	362	815	0.2	0.3	454	125.6
Korean	355	799	0.2	0.3	444	125.3
Vietnamese	262	615	0.1	0.2	353	134.8
Hawaiian	167	211	0.1	0.1	44	26.5
Samoan	42	63	(Z)	(Z)	21	50.1
Guamanian	32	49	(Z)	(Z)	17	53.4
Other Asian or Pacific Islander	(NA)	822	(NA)	0.3	(NA)	(NA)
Other race	6,758	9,805	3.0	3.9	3,047	45.1
Hispanic origin						
Hispanic origin†	14,609	22,354	6.4	9.0	7,745	53.0
Mexican	8,740	13,496	3.9	5.4	4,755	54.4
Puerto Rican	2,014	2,728	0.9	1.1	714	35.4
Cuban	803	1,044	0.4	0.4	241	30.0
Other Hispanic	3,051	5,086	1.3	2.0	2,035	66.7
Not of Hispanic origin	211,937	226,356	93.6	91.0	14,419	6.8

NA Not available. Z Less than .05%.

*Not entirely comparable with 1990 counts. The 1980 count shown here which is based on 100% tabulations includes only the nine specific Asian or Pacific Islander groups listed separately in the 1980 race item. The 1980 total Asian or Pacific Islander population of 3,726,440 from sample tabulations is comparable to the 1990 count; these figures include groups not listed separately in the race item on the 1980 census form.

†Persons of Hispanic origin may be of any race.

From: U.S. Dept. of Commerce (1992). *Statistical Abstract of the United States 1992: The National Data Book.* Washington, D.C.: U.S. Government Printing Office, p. 17.

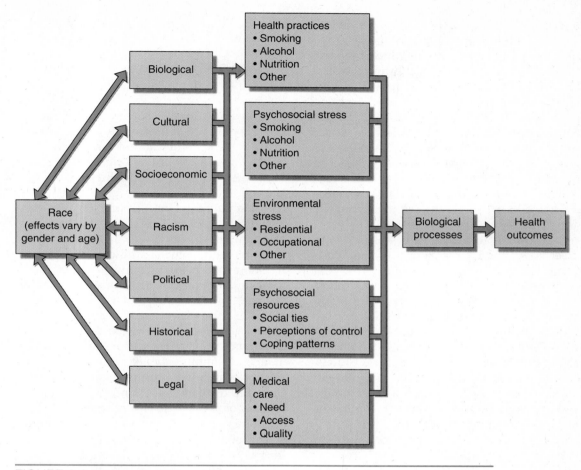

FIGURE 9.2

A framework for understanding the relationship between race and health.

From: Williams, D. R. (1993). "Race in the Health of America: Problems, Issues, and Directions." MMWR *42 (RR-10): 9.*

DATA SOURCES AND THEIR LIMITATIONS

In order to collect accurate data about different subgroups within the population, researchers have struggled to identify common variables that can be used to classify individuals. With regard to minorities, race and ethnic origin have been the identifying commonalities. In the 1960s, the United Nations recommended using the term *ethnic group* rather than *race* to identify subgroups.[5] The United States government uses a classification system that includes both race and ethnicity, perhaps because this system works best for enumerating and describing our diverse population. The current regulations used for the statistical classification of racial and ethnic groups by federal agencies were published in 1978 in the Office of Management and Budget's *Directive 15* entitled "Race and Ethnic Standards for Federal Statistics and Administrative Reporting."[6] The directive presents brief rules for classifying persons into four racial categories (American Indian or Alaskan Native, Asian or Pacific Islander, black, and white) and two ethnic categories (Hispanic origin or not of Hispanic origin). It also requires the categorization of blacks and whites into one of the two ethnic categories. *Directive 15* was not intended to be scientific or anthropological in nature but rather a way to **operationalize** race and ethnicity. (See Appendix 5 for a listing of the operational definitions used to collect the 1990 census data.)

Several authors[7-10] have warned of the dangers of lumping individuals into so few categories, because there exists much diversity. For example, race and ethnicity categories do not take into consideration **nativity.** Epidemiological data have repeatedly shown that mortality rates of foreign-born and native-born within the same minority category are much different. Yu and Liu[10] provide a vivid example of this point (see Table 9.2). They state:

> The term 'Asian/Pacific Islanders' covers a great number of cultures and at least 32 linguistic groups whose ancestral origins can be traced to places that include Mongolia to the north, the islands near Australia to the south, India and Pakistan to the west, and Hawaii to the east. The inhabitants of these vast land masses differ immensely in terms of racial stock, language, religion, life-style, diet and health behaviors, and other characteristics. Just as one would not merge statis-

tical data files that display widely differing characteristics or distributions, so too it makes little sense to aggregate extremely diverse groups into a single category.

Similar statements could be made of the difference within the other racial/ethnic groups. For example, people of Hispanic origin who live in California and New Mexico are different from those who live in New York. The same could be said for blacks and Native Americans living in different parts of the country.

Recognizing the limitations of the racial/ethnic classification system used in the United States, we can conclude that most epidemiological studies using minority subjects concentrate on broad racial/ethnic comparisons rather than on careful investigation of social and other ecological factors.[11] Knowing that the available data are not as precise as we would like, we present what we feel is the best information about the community health issues faced by the major minority groups. However, as you continue to read this chapter, please be reminded of the limitations of the data.

Please note throughout the remainder of the chapter we have chosen to use the terms *Americans of Hispanic origin, Asian/Pacific Islanders, black Americans, Native Americans* (instead of *American Indian* or *Alaskan Native*), and *white Americans,* unless there is a direct quotation or extrapolation from data or documents which use other terminology (e.g., *American Indians* in lieu of *Native Americans*). "Insofar as possible, negative descriptors (e.g., non-white, non-poor) have not been used, unless the source data were classified in this manner. The term *African American,* which is increasingly used in lieu of *black Americans,* has not been used because none of the available data are reported using this terminology."[12]

---

operationalize (operational definition) Provide working definitions.
nativity Birthplace.

Table 9.2
Asian or Pacific Islander Groups Reported in the 1990 Census

Asian	Pacific Islander
Chinese	Hawaiian
Filipino	Samoan
Japanese	Guamanian
Asian Indian	Other Pacific Islander*
Korean	Carolinian
Vietnamese	Fijian
Cambodian	Kosraean
Hmong	Melanesian‡
Laotian	Micronesian‡
Thai	Northern Mariana Islander
Other Asian*	Palauan
Bangladeshi	Papua New Guinean
Bhutanese	Ponapean (Pohnpeian)
Borneo	Polynesian‡
Burmese	Solomon Islander
Celebesian	Tahitian
Ceram	Tarawa Islander
Indochinese	Tokelauan
Indonesian	Tongan
Iwo-Jiman	Trukese (Chuukese)
Javanese	Yapese
Malayan	Pacific Islander, not specified
Maldivian	
Nepali	
Okinawan	
Pakistani	
Sikkim	
Singaporean	
Sri Lankan	
Sumatran	
Asian, not specified†	

*In some data products, specific groups listed under "Other Asian" or "Other Pacific Islander" are shown separately. Groups not shown are tabulated as "All other Asian" or "All other Pacific Islander," respectively.

†Includes entries such as Asian American, Asian, Asiatic, Amerasian, and Eurasian.

‡Polynesian, Micronesian, and Melanesian are Pacific Islander cultural groups.

From: U.S. Dept. of Commerce (1992). *1990 Census of Population and Housing, Summary Population and Housing, Characteristics, United States.* Washington D.C.: U.S. Government Printing Office, p. B-13.

Finally, specific health-related problems are presented for each racial/ethnic group discussed in this chapter. The health problems are not discussed in order to stereotype any group, for it is known that each of the problems cut across all racial and ethnic groups, but to show that the groups identified have been disproportionately affected by the problem.

AMERICANS OF HISPANIC ORIGIN

As we begin our discussion of Americans of Hispanic origin, readers are reminded that Hispanic origin is an ethnicity classification, not a race. For the purposes of census data, the only ethnic distinctions the United States government makes are "Hispanic" or "non-Hispanic." Therefore, all Americans of Hispanic origin are also classified by a race. Most are either white Hispanic or black Hispanic.

In 1990, Americans of Hispanic origin were officially counted at 22,354,059.[13] This number accounted for almost 9% of the total U.S. population (see Figure 9.3). In contrast, the 1980 census counted 14,608,673 (6.4%) Americans of Hispanic origin (see Table 9.1). Geographically, in 1990, almost 87% of Hispanic Americans lived in just ten states (mostly western and southern states). California was home to almost 7.7 million or about 34% of all Hispanic Americans.[14] The fewest Americans of Hispanic origin are found in the Midwest.

Socioeconomic Characteristics

A positive relationship between educational achievement and positive health status has been shown over and over; simply stated, better-educated people are healthier. The educational level of Americans of Hispanic origin is below that for the general population and may contribute to this group's poorer health status. In 1991, 78.4% of all Americans over 25 years of age had four years of high school or more. For white Americans, that number was 79.9%, for non-Hispanics it was 77.2%, and for Americans of Hispanic origin the figure was 51.3%. Similar disparity exists with regard

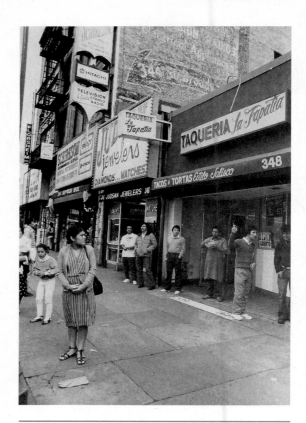

FIGURE 9.3

Americans of Hispanic origin represent one of the fastest-growing minority groups in the United States.

to four years of college or more. Also in 1991, about 21.4% of all Americans, and 22.2% of white Americans, had graduated from college, versus 9.7% of Americans of Hispanic origin.[14,15]

Unemployment rates are also higher in the Hispanic community. In 1991, the unemployment rates for males over 16 years of age were 7.3% for white Americans and 10.6% for Americans of Hispanic origin.[15]

Data on family type reveal that in 1990 a greater proportion of households in the Hispanic community (22.0%) were headed by women, as compared with only 17% of the overall population in the United States and 16% of non-Hispanics. For white Americans, the proportion was much lower (13.2%).[14, 15]

On average, Hispanics earn less and have a greater proportion of their population living in poverty than non-Hispanic Americans. In 1991, the median family income for non-Hispanics was $37,013 as compared to $23,895 for Americans of Hispanic origin. When adjustments were made for differences in educational levels, the median income of white Americans was still higher at all educational levels.[13, 14]

Americans of Hispanic origin are 2.7 times more likely to live below the poverty level than white Americans and 2.5 times more likely than non-Hispanics.[13, 14] In 1990, 25% of Americans of Hispanic origin lived in poverty as compared to 10.7% for the general population.[15]

In examining the relationship between health, poverty, and education, it is important to note that 52.8% of women of Hispanic origin who give birth have less than a high school education, almost 17% are 19 years of age or younger, and over a third (35.5%) are unmarried. All three of these figures exceed those for the general United States population (see Table 9.3).

Vital Statistics

Vital statistics data that specifically list Americans of Hispanic origin are limited, because these data are, as a rule, recorded by race not ethnic origin. Life expectancy data, for example, while available for different racial groups and populations in foreign countries, are not available on Americans of Hispanic origin. The vital statistics that are available for Americans of Hispanic origin include birth and fertility rates, years of potential life lost, mortality rates, and infant mortality rates.

Birth and Fertility Rates

As noted earlier in the chapter, the birth rates of all minority groups in the United States are higher than those of white Americans. Table 9.4 provides data that show both the birth rate and the fertility rate (the number of births per 1,000 women of childbearing age) for Americans of Hispanic origin and several subgroups as compared to those of all origins. The rates in this table are all higher than the 1987 data and would indicate that the percentage of Americans of Hispanic origin will continue to climb.

Table 9.3
Socioeconomic Characteristics of Mothers in 1989

| | Percent of live births | | | | | |
	All Mothers	Asian/ Pacific Islanders	Black Americans	Americans of Hispanic Origin	Native Americans	White Americans
Education of mother <12 years	23.2%	19.5%	30.4%	52.8%	37.2%	21.6%
Education of mother >16 years	17.4	31.2	7.2	5.1	4.3	19.2
Age of mother <18 years	4.8	2.0	10.5	6.7	7.5	3.6
Age of mother 18–19 years	8.1	3.7	12.9	10.0	12.1	7.2
Unmarried mothers	27.1	12.4	65.7	35.5	52.7	19.2

From: U.S. Dept of Commerce (1992). *Statistical Abstract of the United States 1992: The National Data Book* Washington, D.C.: U.S. Government Printing Office.

Table 9.4

Birth and Fertility Rates, Total Fertility Rates, and Birth Rates by Age of Mother, by Hispanic Origin of Mother, and by Race of Mother for Mothers of non-Hispanic Origin (total of 48 reporting states and the District of Columbia, 1990)

[Birth rates by age of mother are live births per 1,000 women in specified group]

| Measure | All origins[1] | Origin of Mother | | | | | | | |
| | | Hispanic | | | | | Non-Hispanic[1] | | |
		Total	Mexican	Puerto Rican	Cuban	Other Hispanic[2]	Total[3]	White	Black
Birth rate[4]	16.7	26.7	28.7	21.6	10.9	27.5	15.7	14.4	23.0
Fertility rate[5]	71.0	107.7	118.9	82.9	52.6	102.7	67.1	62.8	89.0
Total fertility rate[6]	2,083.0	2,959.5	3,214.0	2,301.0	1,459.5	2,877.0	1,979.5	1,850.5	2,547.5
Birth Rates by Age of Mother[7]									
10–14 years	1.4	2.4	2.5	2.9	*	2.1	1.3	0.5	5.0
15–19 years	59.9	100.3	108.0	101.6	30.3	86.0	54.8	42.5	116.2
20–24 years	116.4	181.0	200.3	150.1	64.6	162.9	108.1	97.5	165.1
25–29 years	120.3	153.0	165.3	109.9	95.4	155.8	116.5	115.3	118.4
30–34 years	81.0	98.3	104.4	62.8	67.6	106.9	79.2	79.4	70.2
35–39 years	31.9	45.3	49.1	26.2	28.2	49.4	30.7	30.0	28.7
40–44 years	5.5	10.9	12.4	6.2	4.9	11.6	5.1	4.7	5.6
45–49 years	0.2	0.7	0.8	0.5	*	0.7	0.2	0.2	0.3

*Data not available.

[1]Includes origin not stated.

[2]Includes Central and South American and other and unknown Hispanic.

[3]Includes races other than white and black.

[4]Rate per 1,000 total population.

[5]Rate per 1,000 women aged 15–44 years.

[6]Rates are sums of birth rates for 5-year age groups multiplied by 5.

[7]Rates per 1,000 women in specified group.

Note: Excludes New Hampshire and Oklahoma, which did not report Hispanic origin of mother on the birth certificate.

From: U.S. Dept. of Health and Human Services (1993). Advance Report of Final Natality Statistics, 1990. *Monthly Vital Statistics Report* 41(a): 40.

Years of Potential Life Lost

Years of potential life lost before the age of 65 (YPLL <65) is a common measure of premature mortality (refer to Chapter 7). In a recent study comparing YPLL <65 by race, ethnicity, and gender on the 1986–1988 death cohort, Americans of Hispanic origin were found to be the median subgroup (see Figure 9.4).[16] The rate of YPLL <65 for both males and females were lower than or similar to rates among non-Hispanic white Americans for all chronic diseases except cirrhosis. Most of the excess YPLL <65 (all causes) for male Americans of Hispanic origin, compared to non-Hispanic white American counterparts, occurred as a

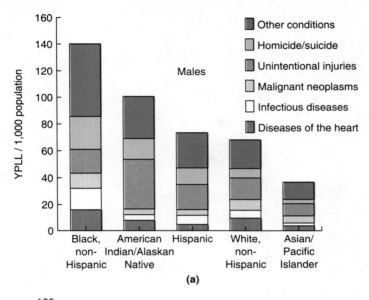

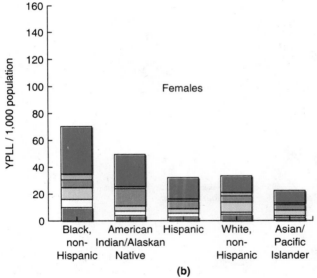

FIGURE 9.4

Rate of years of potential life lost (YPLL) before age 65, for males and females by race, Hispanic origin, and sex—United States, 1986–1988.

From: Desenclos, J. C. A., and R. A. Hahn (1992). "Years of Potential Life Lost Before Age 65 by Race, Hispanic Origin, and Sex—United States 1986–1988." MMWR 41(SS-6): 17.

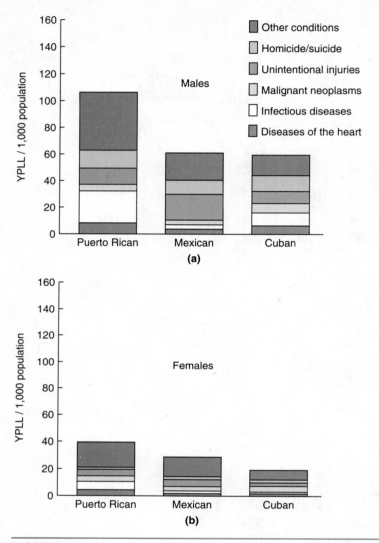

FIGURE 9.5

Rate of years of potential life lost (YPLL) before age 65, by Hispanic origin and sex—United States, 1986–1988.

From: Desenclos, J. C. A., and R. A. Hahn (1992). "Years of Potential Life Lost Before Age 65 by Race, Hispanic Origin, and Sex—United States, 1986–1988." MMWR 41 (no. SS-6): 20.

result of homicides, unintentional injuries, cirrhosis, and infectious diseases. These four causes alone accounted for 46% of all YPLL <65 for male Americans of Hispanic origin.

The lower rate of YPLL <65 for female Americans of Hispanic origin, compared to non-Hispanic white American females, was due to their lower rates of suicide and unintentional injuries.

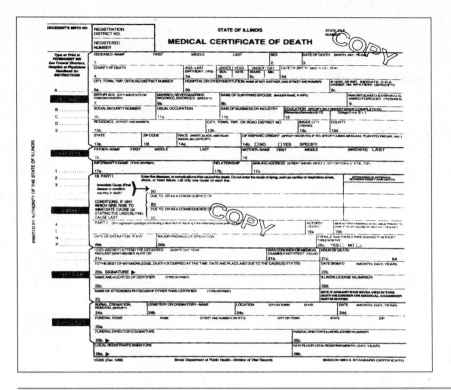

FIGURE 9.6

Even today not all states include a Hispanic origin item on their death certificates.

As noted earlier, one must be cautious of the heterogeneity within major ethnic and racial subgroups. This is particularly true with YPLL <65 for Americans of Hispanic origin. Figure 9.5 shows that premature mortality varied significantly among those of Hispanic origin, Cubans having the lowest rates, followed by Mexicans and Puerto Ricans.

Mortality Rates

Mortality data for Americans of Hispanic origin are limited because until recently, most states did not include a Hispanic-origin item on their death certificates (see Figure 9.6). For example, in 1987,

only 18 states and the District of Columbia recorded this information on death certificates. In 1990, however, 45 states (and the District of Columbia) included it, accounting for about 97% of the Hispanic population in the United States. The five states still without Hispanic mortality data in 1990 were Connecticut, Louisiana, New Hampshire, Oklahoma, and Virginia.[13, 17]

Crude mortality data for Americans of Hispanic origin in the 1988–1990 mortality cohort compare very favorably with that for the general population and also to that of white Americans. For this three-year period of time, the age-adjusted mortality rate for

Table 9.5
Death Rates for Selected Causes of Death,
According to Race, Gender, and Ethnic Origin, 1988–1990

	Deaths per 100,000 Resident Population		
Cause of Death, Race, and Age	Both Sexes	Males	Females
Homicide and legal intervention			
All races			
15–24 years	17.2	27.9	6.0
25–44 years	14.3	22.6	6.0
45–64 years	6.4	10.2	2.8
White Americans			
15–24 years	8.6	13.0	3.9
25–44 years	8.3	12.6	3.9
45–64 years	4.6	7.1	2.2
Black Americans			
15–24 years	67.6	117.9	17.9
25–44 years	57.9	100.6	20.5
45–64 years	22.4	40.8	7.5
Asian/Pacific Islander			
15–24 years	7.4	12.3	2.3
25–44 years	6.8	9.8	4.1
45–64 years	4.8	7.3	2.6
Native Americans			
15–24 years	19.0	27.7	9.8
25–44 years	18.1	29.0	7.6
45–64 years	8.4	12.5	4.5
Americans of Hispanic origin			
15–24 years	27.5	45.7	6.2
25–44 years	24.4	41.5	6.0
45–64 years	11.2	20.0	3.1
AIDS			
All races			
25–44 years	19.8	35.6	4.2
45–64 years	9.3	18.0	1.2
White Americans			
25–44 years	15.9	29.6	1.9
45–64 years	7.9	15.6	0.7
Black Americans			
25–44 years	52.8	90.4	19.8
45–64 years	23.1	44.6	5.7
Asian/Pacific Islander			
25–44 years	3.8	7.3	0.6
45–64 years	2.9	5.6	0.6
Native Americans			
25–44 years	4.0	7.2	0.8
45–64 years	1.8	3.2	0.5
Americans of Hispanic origin			
25–44 years	28.7	48.9	6.9
45–64 years	16.3	31.3	2.5

From: U.S. Dept. of Health and Human Services, (1993). *Health United States, 1992 and Healthy People 2000 Review.* Washington, D.C.: U.S. Government Printing Office.

Table 9.6
Prenatal Care and Low Birth Weights in 1989

	Percent of live births					
	All Mothers	Asian/ Pacific Islanders	Black Americans	Americans of Hispanic Origin	Native Americans	White Americans
Prenatal care begun in first trimester	75.5%	74.8%	60.0%	59.5%	57.9%	78.9%
Prenatal care begun in third trimester or no prenatal care	6.4	6.1	11.9	13.0	13.4	5.2
Low birth weight (<2500 grams)	7.05	6.51	13.51	6.18	6.26	5.72
Very low birth weight (<1500 grams)	1.28	0.90	2.95	1.05	1.00	0.95

From: U.S. Dept. of Commerce (1992). *Statistical Abstract of the United States 1992: The National Data Book.* Washington, D.C.: U.S. Government Printing Office.

Americans of Hispanic origin was 405.1/100,000 resident population, compared to 528.6/100,000 for all races and 501.1/100,000 for white Americans. Even when the data were examined by gender, Americans of Hispanic origin compared well. Using the same cohort years, the mortality rate for Hispanic females was 289.2/100,000 versus 397.4/100,000 for all races and 376.6/100,000 for white females. For males, the figures were 536.6/100,000 for Americans of Hispanic origin, 690.7/100,000 for all races, and 655.0/100,000 for white Americans.[18] The reasons for these differences are not clear, but one explanation may be the lower rates of death from chronic disease.

An examination of cause-specific mortality rates reveals that Americans of Hispanic origin fare better than other races in per capita deaths from heart disease, stroke, cancer, motor vehicle crashes, and suicides. However, mortality rates are higher in this group for homicides, legal intervention, and AIDS. These higher mortality rates can be accounted for almost entirely by the males (see Table 9.5). Only black American males have higher figures.

Infant Mortality Rates

The infant mortality rate of 7.8/1,000 live births for Americans of Hispanic origin reported in 1990 is remarkably low when compared to the general population rate of 9.1/1000 and the white population rate of 7.4/1,000 during that same year.[17] It is so low that some have questioned its validity. Because of the unfavorable socioeconomic characteristics reported earlier and the fact that many Hispanic women lack prenatal care (see Table 9.6), it is difficult to believe the infant mortality rate could be this favorable. It has been suggested that undocumented out-of-hospital births and deaths are a likely cause of the underestimation of Hispanic infant mortality rates.[12] On the other hand, others feel that the data are a good indicator of the true infant mortality. The reason they give for this is the excellent social support traditionally provided by Hispanic families to other family members. The extended family is still very much a part of the Hispanic culture. Thus, those in need of health care or other things can count on the support of family members to help them.

Acquired Immunodeficiency Syndrome (AIDS) and Human Immunodeficiency Virus (HIV): A Community Health Concern for Americans of Hispanic Origin

Acquired Immunodeficiency Syndrome (AIDS) is a deadly disease caused by the human immunodeficiency virus (HIV). The disease kills by attacking one's immune system so that otherwise nonthreatening diseases become fatal.[19] By midyear 1993, it was estimated that between 2 million and 5 million people (1 in 250) in the United States were infected with HIV, most between 25 and 49 years of age. Also by that time, over 315,000 had been diagnosed with AIDS and about 65% of them had died—making AIDS and re-

lated infections the leading killer of 25- to 44-year-old men in five states and 64 cities.[20, 21]

Two of the minority groups in the United States that have been hardest hit by AIDS/HIV are Hispanic and black Americans. A vivid example of this is the data presented in Figures 9.7 and 9.8, showing how Hispanic and Black American children and women of childbearing age have accounted for a disproportionate share of AIDS cases compared with the proportion of the U.S. population they represent.[22]

The excessive cases of AIDS and HIV in Americans of Hispanic origin have been attributed to unsafe or high-risk behaviors (e.g., intravenous [IV] drug use and unprotected sexual intercourse), the existence of co-conditions (e.g., genital ulcer disease), and the lack of access to health care that

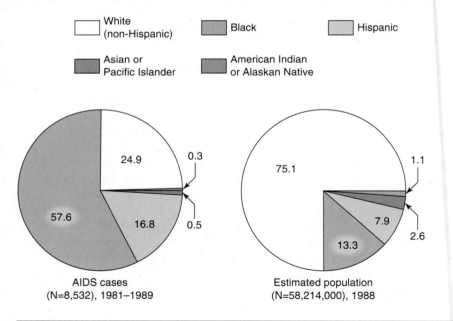

AIDS cases
(N=8,532), 1981–1989

Estimated population
(N=58,214,000), 1988

FIGURE 9.7

Percentage distribution of AIDS cases among women 15–44 years of age reported 1981–1989, compared with estimated population of women 15–44 years of age in 1988, by race/ethnicity—United States.

From: Gayle, J. A., R. M. Selik, and S. Y. Chu (1990). "Surveillance for AIDS and HIV Infection Among Black and Hispanic Children and Women of Childbearing Age, 1981–1989." MMWR 39(SS-3): 25.

would provide early diagnosis and treatment.[23] Specifically, many AIDS cases in women have been traced to IV drug use (either directly, by sharing needles or syringes, or indirectly, by sexual contact with an IV drug user). Cases among children can be traced to indirect perinatal transmission from their infected mothers.[24]

The factors that contribute to the incidence of AIDS in Americans of Hispanic origin are the same ones that increase AIDS in all races. With no cure for AIDS/HIV in sight, better health education (to reduce and eliminate unsafe behaviors) and increased access to medical resources for existing cases are essential (see Box 9.1).

BOX 9.1
Healthy People 2000—Objective

18.1 Confine annual incidence of diagnosed AIDS cases to no more than 98,000 cases. (Baseline: An estimated 44,000 to 50,000 diagnosed cases in 1989)

Special Population Target

	Diagnosed AIDS cases	1989 Baseline	2000 Target
18.1a	Gay and bisexual men	26,000–28,000	48,000
18.1b	Blacks	14,000–15,000	37,000
18.1c	Hispanics	7,000–8,000	18,000

Note: Targets for this objective are equal to upper bound estimates of the incidence of diagnosed AIDS cases projected for 1993.
Baseline data source: Center for Infectious Diseases, CDC.

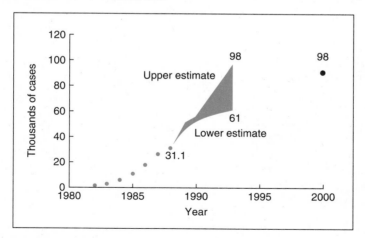

Incidence of AIDS cases

For Further Thought

What is the key to stopping the spread of AIDS?

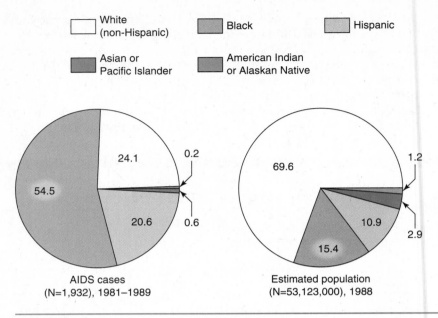

FIGURE 9.8

Percentage distribution of AIDS cases among children <15 years of age, reported 1981–1989, compared with estimated population of children <15 years of age in 1988, by race/ethnicity—United States.

From: Gayle, J. A., R. M. Selik, and S. Y. Chu (1990). "Surveillance for AIDS and HIV Infection Among Black and Hispanic Children and Women of Childbearing Age, 1981–1989." MMWR 39(SS-3): 25.

ASIAN/PACIFIC ISLANDERS

Numbering almost 7.3 million in the 1990 United States Census (see Table 9.1), Asian Americans and Pacific Islanders (or Asian/Pacific Islanders) are the fastest-growing minority in America, increasing 108% in the ten-year period from 1980 to 1990.[8, 9] If growth continues at this rate, it is projected that this minority group will comprise 3.7% of the total projected U.S. population (268 million) in the year 2000.[25] As noted in Table 9.7, the single largest Asian/Pacific Islander subgroup will be Filipinos and the smallest will be the Japanese.

Table 9.7
Projected Numbers and Percentages of Asian Americans in the United States by Group in the Year 2000

Group Population	Number	Percentage of Total As
Filipino	2,070,571	21.0
Chinese	1,683,537	17.1
Vietnamese	1,574,385	16.0
Korean	1,320,759	13.4
Asian Indian	1,006,305	10.2
Japanese	856,619	8.7
Other Asian	1,338,188	13.6
Total	9,850,364	

From: U.S. Dept. of Health and Human Services (1990). Health States of the Disadvantaged: Chartbook 1990 (DHHS pub. no. HRSA-HRS-P-DV 90-1). Washington, D.C.: U.S. Government

Asian/Pacific Islander Culture

Perhaps more than any other group, the Asian/Pacific Islanders represent a vast diversity of cultures, nations, and histories. Even among those who have come from the same country, immigration to America may have occurred at different times, producing generational differences. For example, some families may have immigrated well over a hundred years ago as laborers, while those coming today carry with them professional degrees.[24]

While there are a great many differences among the Asian/Pacific Islander subgroups, they share certain values that distinguish them from the other Americans. These values include:

1. More dependence and reliance on members of their group, especially the family.
2. More formalized family roles, especially in regard to male-female and sibling relationships.
3. Great sense of obligation to one's family, and accompanying feelings of shame and guilt if the obligations are ignored.
4. Greater respect for age, rank, status, and power.
5. Obedience.
6. Modesty.

Vital Statistics

While vital statistic data for Asian/Pacific Islanders are somewhat limited, data indicate that the health status of this minority group compares favorably with that of the other minority groups, white Americans, and the general population.

Birth and Fertility Rates

As with other minority groups, the birth rate for Asian/Pacific Islanders is higher than the rates for white Americans and the total United States population. However, unlike the other minority groups, the fertility rate for Asian/Pacific Islanders is comparable to those for white Americans and the total population.[26] (See Tables 9.4 and 9.8.)

Years of Potential Life Lost

Of all the racial and ethnic minorities, Asian/Pacific Islanders have the lowest rates of premature mortality (YPLL <65 years). This statistic holds for both males and females (see Figure 9.4). While no single cause of death stands out as remarkable, several causes do contribute to premature deaths. In males there are motor vehicle injuries, unintentional injuries, heart disease, suicides, and infections. In females the greatest contributors to premature mortality are motor vehicle injuries, infections, breast cancer, and homicides.[16]

No one knows for sure why premature mortality in Asian/Pacific Islanders is so low. Evidence seems to indicate that this minority group characteristically shares fewer unsafe and unhealthy behaviors.[16]

Mortality Rates and the Leading Causes of Death

When mortality rates for the 1988–1990 Asian/Pacific Islander cohort are examined and compared to similar data for other races and ethnic groups, the rates for this group are among the lowest. This is true whether one compares mortality rates for all causes (295.4/100,000 resident population) or for most specific causes, including heart disease, motor vehicle accidents, suicide, and homicide and legal intervention. Mortality rates for several other causes, such as stroke, cancer, and HIV infection, in this group—while lower than those for white Americans and for the general population—are not the lowest of all minority groups. Native Americans and Americans of Hispanic origin have lower rates of stroke mortality, and Native Americans have lower rates of mortality from cancer and HIV infection.[18]

The leading causes of death for Asian/Pacific Islanders are similar to those for the general population, with the exception of the fifth leading cause (see Table 9.9). In Asian/Pacific Islanders, the fifth leading cause of death is pneumonia and influenza instead of chronic obstructive pulmonary diseases. There is also a slight difference between male and female Asian/Pacific Islanders. In females, the leading killer is malignant neoplasms, in males, it is diseases of the heart. These differences may be the result of the great stress experienced by males of this race.

Infant Mortality Rates, Prenatal Care, and Related Maternal Characteristics

According to comparative data on the birth cohort of 1985—1987, the Asian/Pacific Islanders have the lowest infant mortality rates of any minority in the United States (7.6/1000 live births). This compares to 8.5/1000 for white American mothers and 10.1/1000 for the United States population in general. Among the subgroups of Asian/Pacific Islanders, the lowest rates occur in Chinese Americans (6.0/1000), followed by Japanese Americans (6.6/1000), Filipino Americans (7.2/1000), and all other Asian/Pacific Islanders (8.3/1000).[18] These low infant mortality rates can probably be attributed to more widespread prenatal care and higher levels of education. As noted in Table 9.6, almost 75% of the women of this subpopulation receive prenatal care that begins in the first trimester. Almost one-third (31.2%) of Asian/Pacific Islander mothers have a college education, and only 12.4% are unmarried when they give birth (see Table 9.3).

Table 9.8

Birth Rates by Age and Specified Race of Mother: United States, 1990

[Birth rates by age of mother are live births per 1,000 women in specified group]

Measure	All Races*	White	Black	American Indian[†]	Asian or Pacific Islander
Birth rate[‡]	16.7	15.8	22.4	18.9	19.0
Fertility rate[§]	70.9	68.3	86.8	76.2	69.6
Birth Rates by Age of Mother					
10–14 years	1.4	0.7	4.9	1.6	0.7
15–19 years	59.9	50.8	112.8	81.1	26.4
15–17 years	37.5	29.5	82.3	48.5	16.0
18–19 years	88.6	78.0	152.9	129.3	40.2
20–24 years	116.5	109.8	160.2	148.7	79.2
25–29 years	120.2	120.7	115.5	110.3	126.3
30–34 years	80.8	81.7	68.7	61.5	106.5
35–39 years	31.7	31.5	28.1	27.5	49.6
40–44 years	5.5	5.2	5.5	5.9	10.7
45–49 years	0.2	0.2	0.3	0.3	1.1

*Includes births of other races not shown separately.

[†]Includes births to Aleuts and Eskimos.

[‡]Rate per 1,000 total population.

[§]Rate per 1,000 women aged 15–44 years.

From: U.S. Dept. of Health and Human Services (1993). *Monthly Vital Statistics Report* 41(9-5): 42.

Table 9.9
Leading Causes of Deaths According to Gender and Race; U.S., 1989

	Asian/ Pacific Islander		All Races	Black Americans		Native Americans		White Americans	
	Female	Male	Male and Female	Female	Male	Female	Male	Female	Male
Diseases of the heart	2	1	1	1	1	1	1	1	1
Cerebrovascular diseases	3	3	3	3	5	4	—	3	4
Malignant neoplasms	1	2	2	2	2	2	3	2	2
Chronic obstructive pulmonary diseases	—	—	5	—	—	—	—	5	5
Pneumonia and influenza	5	5	—	—	—	—	—	4	—
Chronic liver disease and cirrhosis	—	—	—	—	—	—	4	—	—
Diabetes mellitus	—	—	—	4	—	5	—	—	—
Accidents and adverse effects	4	4	4	5	3	3	2	—	3
Suicide	—	—	—	—	—	—	5	—	—
Homicide and legal intervention	—	—	—	—	4	—	—	—	—

From: Data tables in U.S. Dept. of Health and Human Services (1992). *Health United States 1991 and Prevention Profile* (DHHS pub. no. PHS-92-1232). Washington, D.C.: U.S. Government Printing Office.

Community Health Problems of Asian/Pacific Islanders

In comparison with other racial/ethnic minority groups in the United States, the Asian/Pacific Islanders are faced with relatively few community health problems. However, there are some problems that seem to plague this subgroup more than others.

Tuberculosis

In the nineteenth century, tuberculosis (TB), an infectious disease caused by a bacteria called *Mycobacterium tuberculosis,* was the leading cause of death in the United States, and it remained so well into the twentieth century. Improved living conditions, including better housing, and specific public health measures reduced the number of deaths so that by 1984 many felt the disease might be eliminated.[27] However, TB is on the rise again. In 1953, the number of re-

ported TB cases in the United States was 84,304 (53/100,000). By 1984, that number dropped to 22,255 (9.4/100,000). However, in 1990, 25,701 (10.3/100,000) cases were reported; this represents a 9.4% increase over the cases reported in 1989 and is 15.5% higher than the 1984 figures (see Figure 9.9). Factors associated with the upswing in the number of cases include adverse social and economic factors, the HIV epidemic, immigration of persons with TB infection, physician nonadherence in prescribing recommended treatment regimens, and patient noncompliance to treatment regimens.[28] Such factors place minority populations at high risk.

For example, in 1990, almost 70% of all reported TB cases and almost 86% of reported cases in children under 15 years occurred among racial/ethnic minorities (see Figures 9.10 and 9.11). During that year, the risk of TB was 9.9 times higher for Asian/Pacific Islanders, 7.9 times for black

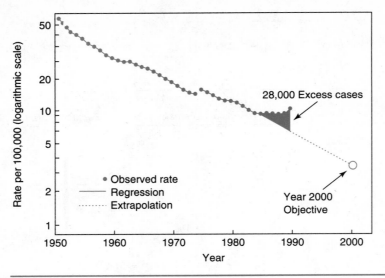

FIGURE 9.9

Actual and expected tuberculosis cases, United States.

From: Centers for Disease Control (1992). "Prevention and Control of Tuberculosis in U.S. Communities with At-Risk Minority Populations." MMWR 41 (RR-5): 3.

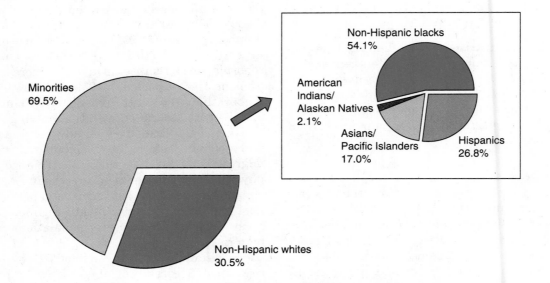

FIGURE 9.10

Total tuberculosis cases United States, 1990.

From: Centers for Disease Control (1992). "Prevention and Control of Tuberculosis in U.S. Communities with At-Risk Minority Populations." MMWR 41 (RR-5): 2.

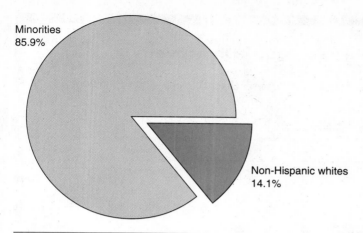

Minorities
85.9%

Non-Hispanic whites
14.1%

FIGURE 9.11

Reported tuberculosis cases among children, United States, 1990.

From: Centers for Disease Control (1992). "Prevention and Control of Tuberculosis in U.S. Communities with At-Risk Minority Populations." MMWR 41 (RR-5):2.

Americans, 5.1 times for Americans of Hispanic origin, and 4.5 times higher for Native Americans. Furthermore, most of the minority cases are localized. Almost 80% of these cases were reported by only 106 counties, each of which reported ten or more cases. These counties are located primarily in the Southeastern states, along the East and West Coasts, and in Texas.[28]

As mentioned above, the resurgence of TB is linked to a variety of social conditions, among them poverty, substance abuse, substandard housing, homelessness, and limited public health clinics. Until these conditions can be altered, a comprehensive public health effort must be implemented to limit the spread of TB in the high-risk minority populations.[28] Such an effort should include public awareness campaigns, training and education of public and private health care providers, coalition building, screening and prevention, case reporting, appropriate treatment, and adherence to recommended treatment regimens. The latter often involves **directly observed therapy (DOT),** a procedure in which a public health out-

reach worker watches while the TB patient takes prescribed medication. DOT is essential because a large proportion of TB cases occur in people who, for a variety of reasons, fail to complete their medication regimens (see Box 9.2).

BLACK AMERICANS

In 1990, black Americans were officially counted at almost 30 million and constituted 12.1% of the population, the single largest minority group. Those figures accounted for a 13.2% gain over the 1980 census data (see Table 9.1).

Understanding the Past

Much of the disparity that exists today between the health of and the health care provided for black Americans, as compared

---

directly observed therapy (DOT) Visual verification of an individual taking a prescribed therapy.

BOX 9.2
Healthy People 2000—Objective

20.4 Reduce tuberculosis to an incidence of no more than 3.5 cases per 100,000 people. (Baseline: 9.1 per 100,000 in 1988)

Special Population Target

	Tuberculosis Cases (per 100,000)	1988 Baseline	2000 Target	
20.4a	Asians/Pacific Islanders	36.3	15	
20.4b	Blacks	28.3	10	
20.4c	Hispanics	18.3	5	
20.4d	American Indians/Alaska Natives	18.1	5	

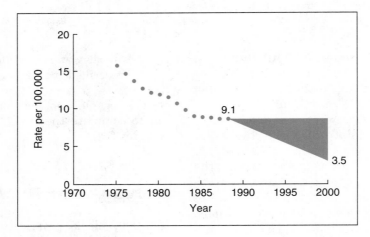

Baseline data source: Center for Prevention Services, CDC.

Incidence of tuberculosis

For Further Thought

Each of the special target populations noted has an incidence rate for tuberculosis higher than the national average. If you had to write a hypothesis to explain these high rates, what would it be? Why?

to that of white Americans, can be traced to the period when slavery was practiced in the United States. Slaveowners provided health care to their slaves for several reasons. "One was that slaves not be allowed to malinger; another concern was for the owner's property; a third concern was preventing disease from spreading; and the fourth was an actual concern for the health of the slaves."[30] These concerns plus the law that forbade slaves from providing health care to each other, upon penalty of death, led to an underground system of health care by mostly untrained providers.

After the Civil War, poverty, discrimination, and poor living conditions led to high prevalences of disease, disability, and death among black Americans.[29] Racial discrimination limited this group's access to adequate health care through the middle of this century, much as it limited access to education and voting rights. This discrimination continues to have an impact on the health status of black Americans. Many black Americans still find it difficult to gain access to health care because of discrimination.

Socioeconomic Characteristics

Disparities in health statistics among black Americans, white Americans, and the general population (all Americans) can be traced to differences in education or employment status. In 1991, of all Americans age 25 and over, 78.4% had completed high school. The completion rate for white Americans was slightly higher (79.9%) but much lower for black Americans (66.7%). Slightly over one-fifth (21.4%) of all Americans have four or more years of college (22.2% of white Americans), but just over one-tenth (11.5%) of black Americans are similarly well educated.[15]

In 1991, the unemployment rate for white male civilians 16 years and older was 7.3%, and 14.6% for a similar black population.[15]

Another important social economic characteristic is family type—specifically, the proportion of females who are heads of families with no male spouse present and with children under 18 years of age. In 1991, 17.0% of American females were in this situation. While only 13.2% of white females were sole heads of households with dependents, 45.9% of black females were.

Thus during this year, close to one-half of all black American families were headed by women with no spouses present and with children under the age of 18.[15]

Table 9.3 provides other socioeconomic data for American women. Of the black American women who gave birth in 1989, almost one-third (30.4%) had less than a high school education, few (7.2%) have a college education, over a fifth (23.4%) were teenagers, and almost two-thirds (65.7%) were unmarried.[13]

There is also a disparity in reported income between blacks and other Americans and in the proportion of population living below the poverty level. In 1987, the median family income for the general population was $29,458, for white Americans $30,809, and for black Americans, $17,604.[13] Poverty level by race shows that 10.7% of the all races' population lived in poverty in 1990, 8.1% of white Americans, and nearly one-third (29.4%) of black Americans.[15]

Vital Statistics

Health status of black Americans, as evidenced by vital statistics data, has improved significantly in the past 40 years. However, it continues to lag behind that of other racial/ethnic subgroups and that of the population as a whole. In the sections below, these differences will be evident.

Birth and Fertility Rates

The birth and fertility rates for black American women are higher than similar rates for all Americans, white Americans, and other racial minority groups (see Table 9.8). They are, however, lower than those for Americans of Hispanic origin.[30]

Life Expectancy

The life expectancy of black Americans has remained below that of both the general population and that of white Americans throughout the twentieth century (see Table 7.4 in Chapter 7). Alarmingly, since the mid-1980s, the gap has widened. In 1984, life expectancy for black Americans at birth was 69.5 years, while it was 74.7 years for the general population and 75.3 for whites. In 1990, the life expectancy of black Americans dropped to 69.1 years, compared to 75.4 years for the general population and 76.1 years for whites. The discrepancy is also apparent when comparing data by gender. In 1990, life expectancy of black males was 64.5 years as compared to 71.8 years for males in general and 72.7 years for white males. Black females could expect to live an average of 73.6 years in 1990, as compared to 78.8 years for all females and 79.4 years for white females.[17]

Years of Potential Life Lost

In a recent study,[16] it was shown that black Americans have the highest rate of YPLL <65 per 1,000 population of any of the racial or ethnic groups identified in the United States (see Figure 9.4). The high total YPLL <65 rate for black Americans reflects high YPLL <65 rates compared to other subgroups for most causes of death, particularly homicide. Homicide accounted for 14% of total YPLL <65 in black American males and 6% of black American females.

There seem to be two major reasons for the large differences in YPLL <65 rates for black Americans compared to other subgroups. These include: (1) the higher incidence of disease and (2) a higher case fatality rate at young ages. These higher rates are reflective of the greater prevalence of preventable risk factors early in life (e.g., smoking, alcohol use, poor diet, and lack of exercise) and the fact that screenings and adequate treatment are less accessible to, or less utilized by, black Americans.[16]

Mortality Rates and the Leading Causes of Death

Age-adjusted mortality rates for black Americans are and always have been significantly higher than those for the general population and for white Americans. The 1988–1990 mortality cohort of black Americans had an age-adjusted mortality rate from all causes of death of 800.0/ 100,000 resident population, compared to 528.6/100,000 for the general population, and 501.1/100,000 for white Americans. Cause-specific death rates revealed that black Americans had the highest mortality rates for all of the following: heart disease, stroke, cancer, homicide and legal intervention, and HIV infection. Similar discrepancies held true when comparing gender mortality data of these groups. The two causes of death for which black Americans' death rates are lower than those for the general and white populations are motor vehicle crashes and suicide. In fact, the black American suicide rate is the lowest of any group except that of the Asian/Pacific Islanders.[18]

The two leading killers of black Americans and of the general population are diseases of the heart and malignant neoplasms (see Table 9.9). Beginning with the third leading cause of death, the comparisons differ. For black American women, the third to fifth leading causes of death are cerebrovascular disease, diabetes mellitus, and accidents. More black American males die violent deaths than males in general. The third through fifth leading causes of death are accidents, homicide, and cerebrovascular disease.

Infant Mortality Rates

The mortality rate for black American infants, as well as for infants of all races, has dropped significantly since 1950. In 1950, the infant mortality rate for black

Americans was 43.9/1,000 live births. That figure dropped to 17.0/1,000 in 1990. However, the infant mortality rate for black Americans has consistently been 75 to 125% greater than for those of all races and white Americans. In 1990, the infant mortality rate for all races' population in the United States was 9.2/1,000 live births and 7.7/1,000 for white American infants.[17, 18]

Though there are many reasons for a high infant mortality rate in this subpopulation, maternal health and low birth weight play significant roles (see Chapter 8). Only 60% of black American mothers receive prenatal care in their first trimester of pregnancy. The rate of low-birth-weight babies among blacks (13.5%) is more than twice that of whites (5.72%).

Community Health Problems of Black Americans

As noted in the previous sections of this chapter, there is much disparity between the health of black Americans and the majority. Identifying all community health problems of black Americans in this chapter is not possible. We have, however, identified four of particular concern.

Infant Mortality

The infant mortality crisis in black Americans reflects the complex quality-of-life issues such as social, economic, and cultural factors that converge and consequently cause children to die.[31] Black American infants die at a rate of about twice that of their white counterparts. A majority of these deaths could be prevented. The causes of infant mortality are known. The knowledge and programs to significantly reduce it are in place—it remains for black Americans to gain access to the services.

A primary prevention approach to reducing infant mortality among black Americans

is the provision of family planning services to all who wish to use them. Unintended pregnancies put both child and mother at greater risk than when pregnancies are planned. A part of family planning is the preparation for pregnancy. Primary to having a healthy infant is to start with a healthy mother. Issues such as nutrition, substance use/abuse, and sexually transmitted diseases must be addressed.[31]

As a secondary approach, appropriate prenatal care must be available to expectant mothers. Statistics reveal that many black women receive either no prenatal care or receive care only late in pregnancy. Floyd[31] has noted that prenatal care should not be limited to the traditional medical care but should also include other social components: transportation, child care, parenting education, and literacy-skill building if it is going to reach those in greatest need. This group of people is often referred to as the **hard-to-reach population.**

Preparation for pregnancy and care during pregnancy are important components of any program aimed at reducing infant mortality in black Americans. There are also two other issues of importance: the availability of medical services during delivery of the infant and the provision of appropriate postpartum services for both mother and child. Finally, there is need for well-baby care as the child grows. (See Box 9.3.)

Sickle Cell Disease

Sickle cell disease was recognized as early as the late seventeenth century, but it was not named until 1904. The disease gains its name from the sickle-shaped red

---

hard-to-reach population Those in a target population who are not easily reached by normal means.

sickle cell disease A genetic disease most common in black Americans and those of Mediterranean, Caribbean, South and Central American, Arabian, and East Indian ancestry.

blood cells that can be observed in the blood of people with the disease. These cells carry a defective type of hemoglobin designated as *sickle hemoglobin*. The sickle cells are harder and less pliable than normal red blood cells; thus, they do not pass through the blood vessels as easily as normal red blood cells and sometimes obstruct the flow of blood. The restriction of blood flow restricts the distribution of oxygen to the cells, which in turn results in tissue and organ damage. Sickle cell disease

---

BOX 9.3
Healthy People 2000—Objective

14.1 Reduce the infant mortality rate to no more than 7 per 1,000 live births. (Baseline: 10.1 per 1,000 live births in 1987)

Special Population Target

	Infant Mortality (per 100,000 live births)	1987 Baseline	2000 Target	Percent Decrease
14.1a	Blacks	17.9	11	
14.1b	American Indians/Alaska Natives	12.5	8.5	
14.1c	Puerto Ricans	12.9	8	

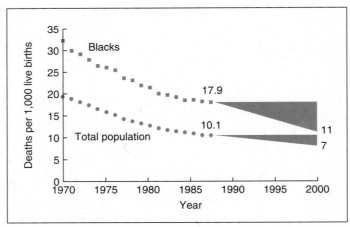

Baseline data sources: National Vital Statistics System, CDC; Linked Birth and Infant Death Data Set, CDC.

Infant mortality rates

For Further Thought

If you could institute one national policy to reduce infant mortality in special target populations, what would it be? Why?

greatly increases morbidity and mortality in infants and children who are so afflicted.[32, 33]

Sickle cell disease is a genetic disease. Parents carry two genes for hemoglobin. If children inherit a sickle cell gene from each parent, they will have sickle cell anemia (SCA), a disease characterized by anemia, pain, susceptibility to pneumococcal infections, leg ulcers, growth retardation, delayed onset of puberty, gallstones, strokes, and even death.[32]

Inheritance of a sickle cell gene from only one parent will result in sickle cell trait (SCT), a condition in which only about half of the hemoglobin is sickled. This is not enough to cause sickling of the red blood cells, but it does make the child with SCT a carrier of the gene and able to pass it on to the next generation.[32]

In the United States sickle cell conditions are found disproportionately in black Americans (see Figure 9.12)—1 in 12 is born with SCT and 1 in 375 with SCA. It is also present, at a somewhat lower frequency, in those of Mediterranean, Caribbean, South and Central American, Arabian, and East Indian ancestry.[32, 33]

Efforts to control sickle cell disease have been slow in developing. It was not until 1971 that provisions for research and services made significant progress. Two of the more promising research areas are bone marrow transplants (replacing the bone marrow that produces the red blood with sickled hemoglobin with bone marrow that produces a normal cell) and gene therapy (removing the sickle cell gene and replacing it with a gene that produces normal hemoglobin). Efforts to produce a drug to keep red blood cells from sickling have not been successful.[32] In 1986, a clinical trial revealed that twice-daily doses of oral penicillin reduced mortality and morbidity from pneumococcal infections in children

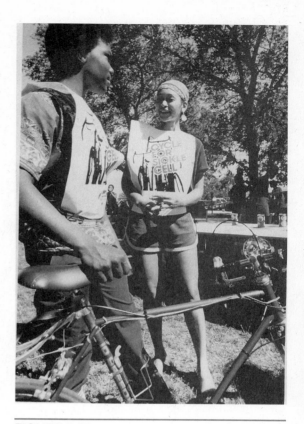

FIGURE 9.12

Sickle cell conditions are found disproportionately in black Americans.

under five years of age with sickle cell disease.

Until these research efforts bear fruit, education and screening programs provide the best hope for alleviating suffering from this disease. Educating target populations about the disease itself and the importance of being tested for SCT and SCA should be followed by counseling for those with positive tests. Early education efforts were funded by both private sector and federal government money, but a reduction in federal dollars led to the formation of the National Association for Sickle Cell Disease

(NASCD) in 1971. NASCD is a voluntary health agency that emphasizes the importance of education and testing. Unfortunately, activities of NASCD have been curtailed because of inadequate funding.

The most recent support for dealing with sickle cell disease came in 1993. That year the Sickle Cell Disease Guideline Panel, convened by the agency for Health Care Policy and Research, recommended that all newborns, regardless of racial or ethnic background, be screened for sickle cell. This recommendation was based on the facts that: (1) even though sickle cell disease is more prevalent in certain racial and ethnic groups, it is not possible to define accurately an individual's heritage by physical appearance or surname, (2) oral penicillin can reduce morbidity and mortality in those affected, and (3) screening should benefit all babies equally, as state-sponsored newborn screening programs in the United States are supported at least in part by public funds and are often mandated by law. At the time of this writing, sickle cell screening existed in more than 40 states.[33]

Other Noncommunicable Health Problems

Morbidity and mortality rates are higher in black Americans for a variety of noncommunicable diseases including cancer, heart disease, stroke, and hypertension.[34, 35] Of the estimated 60 million Americans with hypertension, approximately 28% are black Americans.[36] The disparity between black and white Americans for cancer incidence, mortality, and survival rates are all increasing.[37]

Though there is some evidence that the genetic, hormonal, and physiological differences may contribute to differing rates of hypertension between black and white Americans,[35] the preponderance of evidence indicates that these differences are associated with health behavior, knowledge and attitudes toward health promotion and disease prevention, health care resources, and socioeconomic status. For example, black Americans have a higher prevalence of smoking, greater exposure to environmental carcinogens, and consume diets higher in fat and lower in fiber. Also, black Americans have less knowledge of health promotion and disease prevention than the general population.[34] Finally, Black Americans' access to health care and socioeconomic status greatly influences their health.

Acquired Immunodeficiency Syndrome (AIDS) and Human Immunodeficiency Virus (HIV)

Black Americans have the highest prevalence rates of AIDS and HIV of any racial/ethnic group in the United States. Through 1991, almost 30% of all AIDS cases were among black Americans. Black men are more than three times as likely to contract AIDS than white men.[19] Black women of childbearing age and black children are also overrepresented (see Figures 9.7, 9.8).

The reasons for the disproportionate numbers of AIDS and HIV cases in black Americans are identical to those mentioned for Americans of Hispanic origin: risky health behaviors, existing co-conditions (e.g., genital ulcer disease), and diminished access to health care. The solutions to the problem are better education and improved access to health care.

NATIVE AMERICANS

Native Americans, the original inhabitants of America, numbered almost 2 million in 1990 (see Table 9.1). It has been estimated that prior to the arrival of European explorers, 12 million Indians lived and flourished throughout what is now the United States. Exposure to diseases and ecological changes introduced by explorers and colonists decimated the Native American population. While many of the descendants were assimilated by intermarriages or successfully adapted to the new culture, as a group, the Native Americans became economically and socially disadvantaged, and this situation is reflected in their relatively poor health status.[38, 39]

Native American Culture

Native Americans comprise many different American Indian tribal groups and Alaskan villages. Each of these tribes/villages has distinct customs, languages, and beliefs. The majority, however, share the same cultural values that have been identified by Edwards and Egbert-Edwards:[40]

1. Appreciation of individuality with emphasis upon an individual's right to freedom, autonomy, and respect.
2. Group consensus in tribal/village decision making.
3. Respect for all living things.
4. Appreciation, respect, and reverence for the land.
5. Feelings of hospitality toward friends, family, clanspeople, tribesmen, and respectful visitors.
6. An expectation that tribal/village members will bring honor and respect to their families, clans, and tribes. Bringing shame or dishonor to self or tribe is negatively reinforced.
7. A belief in a supreme being and life after death. Indian religion is the dominant influence for traditional Indian people.

Central to Native American culture is that they "strive for a close integration within the family, clan and tribe and live in harmony with their environment. This occurs simultaneously on physical, mental, and spiritual levels; thus, individual well-ness is considered as harmony and balance among mind, body, spirit and the environment."[39] This concept is not congruent with the medical model approach or public health approach generally accepted by the majority of Americans. As a result, in many Native American communities, there is conflict between the medical/public health approach and the approaches used by Native American healers[39] (see Table 9.10). Providing appropriate health care for Native Americans usually involves resolving conflicts between the two approaches in such a way that they complement each other.

Demographic Characteristics of Native Americans

In recent years, the Native American population has been growing rapidly at a rate of 2.7% per year.[39] This recent increase, which can be traced to increased fertility and birth rates, has altered the demographic characteristics of this minority group. Native Americans are younger, come from larger families, and have smaller family and individual incomes (see Table 9.11). Also, they are more likely to be below the

Table 9.10
A Comparison of Indian Medicine and Modern Medicine

Indian Medicine	Modern Medicine
Behavior-oriented	Complaint-oriented
Whole-specific	Organ-specific
Imbalance	Caused
Visionary diagnosis	Technical diagnosis
Wellness-oriented	Illness-oriented

From: Garrett, J. T. (1990). "Indian Health: Values, Beliefs, and Practices." In M. S. Harper, ed. *Minority Aging: Essential Curricula Content for Selected Health and Allied Health Professionals* (DHHS pub. no. HRS-P-DV90-4). Washington, D.C. US Government Printing Office.

Table 9.11

Social and Economic Characteristics of American Indians in 33 Reservation States, 1980

	American Indians, Eskimos, and Aleuts	United States, All Races
Median age	22.6	30.0
Percent female	50.7%	51.4%
Percent male	49.3%	48.6%
Average number of persons per family	4.6	3.8
Median family income	$13,700	$19,900
Average family income	$16,500	$23,100
Per capita income	$3,600	$7,300
Percent of all persons, below poverty level	28.2%	12.4%
Percent high school graduates	55.4%	66.5%
Percent college graduates	7.4%	16.2%
Percent in labor force, 16 years old and over	57.8%	62.0%
Female, 16 years old and over	47.7%	49.9%
Male, 16 years old and over	68.6%	75.1%
Percent of civilian labor force unemployed	13.3%	6.5%
Female, 16 years old and over	11.9%	6.5%
Male, 16 years old and over	14.5%	6.5%

Note: There were 28 reservation states in 1980, 31 in 1983, 32 in 1984, and 33 in 1988.

From: U.S. Dept. of Health and Human Services (1991). *Health Status of Minorities and Low-Income Groups,* 3rd ed. Washington, D.C.: U.S. Government Printing Office, p. 21.

poverty level, have less education, and have greater unemployment.[40] While a rapid increase in the population growth rate of Native Americans is a sign of strength, there remains clear evidence that many in the population are disadvantaged.

Vital Statistics

The vital statistics of Native Americans are considerably different than those of all other races. Some of these statistics are noted below.

Birth Rates

The most recently published birth rate data for Native Americans is for the 1985–1987 cohort living on reservation states. The rate for that group was 27.9 per 1,000 population. That figure is 79% greater than the 1986 birth rate of 15.6 for the United States' all-races population.[42]

Life Expectancy

The life expectancy of Native Americans has risen in the last 40 years, but as with other minorities, it lags behind that of the general population. From 1955 to 1989 the life expectancy rose 19% to an average life expectancy of 67.9 years for males and 75.1 years for females. These figures are lower than those for white Americans (72.7 years for males and 79.2 years for females in 1989) and Americans in general (71.8 years for males and 78.5 years for females in 1989).[39,43]

Years of Potential Life Lost

Native Americans have the second highest rate of YPLL <65, surpassed only by black Americans (Figure 9.4). Several causes of death account for a significant portion of the total YPLL <65 in Native Americans, according to a study conducted on the 1986–1988 death cohort.[16] Deaths from motor vehicle injuries, other unintentional injuries, suicides, cirrhosis, and diabetes accounted for 48% and 34% of the total YPLL <65 for Native American males and females respectively. The vast majority of these premature deaths can be considered preventable, because they are attributable to preventable risk factors present early in life and to less-than-adequate health care services.[16]

Mortality Rates and the Leading Causes of Death

The 1988–1990 mortality cohort of Native Americans had an age-adjusted mortality rate of 457.6/100,000 resident population as compared with a rate of 528.6/100,000 for the all-races' population, and 501.1/100,000 for white Americans. This lower mortality rate enjoyed by Native Americans is probably attributable to this group's lower mortality rates for several very prevalent chronic diseases, including heart disease, stroke, cancer, and HIV infection. Their mortality rates for stroke and cancer are the lowest of any race of ethnic group. However, Native Americans have the highest age-adjusted mortality rate for motor vehicle crashes (34.5/100,000 resident population), the highest for suicide, and the third highest for homicide and legal intervention.[18] Many die from violent causes.

The five leading causes of death for Native Americans residing in reservation states in 1990 were similar to those of the general population (Table 9.12). However, within the Native American population, there are significant differences in cause-specific mortality rates between genders. A leading cause of death among Native American females is diabetes mellitus, whereas leading causes of death among males are accidents, chronic liver disease and cirrhosis, and suicide (Table 9.9). These differences are even more apparent when the age-adjusted specific cause mortality rates of Native Americans and the total U.S. all-races' population are compared.[43]

Infant Mortality Rates

The infant mortality rate for Native Americans living in reservation states dropped an amazing 85% in 32 years from 62.7/100,000, for the 1954–1956 birth cohort, to 9.7/100,000, for the 1986–1988 birth cohort. By comparison, the infant mortality rate for the overall population in the United States in 1987 was 10.1/1,000.[43]

It is interesting to note that this low infant mortality rate was achieved even though less than 60% of Native American mothers receive standard prenatal medical care in their first trimester. This prenatal

---

Table 9.12

Comparison of Five Leading Causes of Death, Native Americans in Reservation States vs. General U.S. Population (all ages 1990)

Indians in Reservation States	General U.S. Population
1. Diseases of the heart	1. Diseases of the heart
2. Accidents	2. Malignant neoplasms
3. Malignant neoplasms	3. Cerebrovascular diseases
4. Cerebrovascular diseases	4. Accidents
5. Chronic liver disease and cirrhosis	5. Chronic obstructive pulmonary diseases

From: U.S. Dept. of Health and Human Services (1992). *Comprehensive Health Care Program for American Indians and Alaska Natives.* Washington, D.C.: U.S. Government Printing Office, p. 4.

care rate is a lower rate than that for the general population (75.5%) and the white population (78.9%) but very comparable to black populations' (60.0%) and Americans' of Hispanic origin (Table 9.6). It is also interesting that the proportion of babies born at low and very low birth weight is also low, comparing very favorably with the best of the other races. While some have suggested that this could be a reporting phenomenon, more believe that low infant mortality rates occur because Native Americans have a very strong social support system, which embraces the expectant mother to ensure support and positive birth outcomes (see Figure 9.13).

U.S. Government, Its Relationship to Native Americans, and the Provision for Health Care

Though classified by definition and for statistical purposes as a minority group, Native Americans are unlike any other subgroup in the United States. Some (but not all) tribes are sovereign nations, based in part upon their treaties with the United States government. Tribal sovereignty, which is perhaps the most important Indian issue, creates a distinct and special relationship between various tribes and the U.S. government. This sovereignty came about when the tribes transferred virtually all the land in the United States to the federal government in return for the provision of certain services. The U.S. government agreed to manage the land, water, agriculture, and mineral and timber resources, and to provide education and health services to members of the tribe. In the eyes of these Native Americans, each of these services is owed to them, and they become rightfully indignant when people suggest they are getting them for free.[41]

Provisions of education for Native Americans date to the Civilization Act of 1819, while provisions for health services began in 1832.[38] The first medical efforts were carried out by Army physicians who vaccinated against smallpox and applied sanitary procedures to curb other communicable diseases among tribes living in the vicinity of military posts. The health services provided for Native Americans after the signing of the early treaties were limited. It was common for the U.S. government, via the treaties, to impose time limits of 5–20 years on the provisions of health care.[39]

The original government agency overseeing the welfare of Native Americans was the **Bureau of Indian Affairs (BIA).** When this bureau was transferred from the War Department to the Department of the Interior in 1849, physician services were extended to Native Americans. Over the next seventy-plus years, health care services were continually improved, with the first Indian hospital built in 1882, but comprehensive health services were still lacking. It was not until 1921, when the Snyder Act created the BIA Health Division, that more emphasis was given to providing health services to Native Americans. In 1954 with the passage of Public Law 83-568, known as the Transfer Act, the responsibility of health care for Native Americans was transferred from the Department of Interior's BIA to the Public Health Service (PHS). It was at this time that the Indian Health Service (IHS) was created. With this act, the health needs of Native Americans were finally met in a comprehensive way.

In keeping with the concept of tribal sovereignty, the Indian Self-Determination and Education Assistance Act (P.L.93-63) of

---

Bureau of Indian Affairs (BIA) The original federal government agency charged with the responsibility for the welfare of Native Americans.

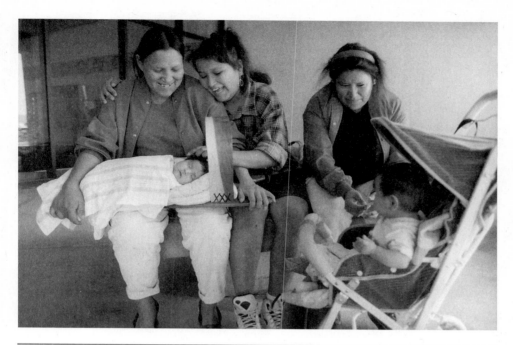

FIGURE 9.13

A strong social support system among Native Americans ensures positive birth outcomes.

1975 authorized the IHS to involve tribes in the administration and operation of all or certain programs under a special contract. It authorized the IHS to provide grants to tribes on request for planning, development, and operation of health programs.[38, 41] Today, a number of programs are managed and operated under contract by individual tribes.[39]

Indian Health Service

As was noted in Chapter 2, the **Indian Health Service (IHS),** with its headquarters in Rockville, Maryland, is one of seven agencies within the Public Health Service. It is organized into 12 areas throughout the United States (see Table 9.13) and operates

Indian Health Service (IHS) The division of the PHS that provides health services for Native Americans.

43 hospitals, ranging in size from 11 to 170 beds per hospital, several hundred clinics and health stations, and a variety of other programs.[39, 41] The goal of the IHS is to raise the health status of American Indians and Alaskan Natives to the highest possible level. To attain this goal, the IHS:

1. assists Indian tribes in developing their health programs through activities such as health management training, technical assistance and human resource development;
2. facilitates and assists Indian tribes in coordinating health resources available through Federal, state, and local programs, in operating comprehensive health care services and in health program evaluation;
3. provides comprehensive health care services, including hospital and ambulatory medical care, preventive and rehabilitative services, and development of community sanitation facilities; and

---

Table 9.13

Locations of Indian Health Service Administration Offices

IHS Headquarters
Rockville, MD 20852
(301) 443-4242

Area Offices

Aberdeen Area IHS
Federal Office Bldg.
115 4th Ave., SE
Aberdeen, SD 57401
(605) 226-7581

Alaska Area Native
Health Service
Box 107741
250 Gambell St.
Anchorage, AK 99501-7741
(907) 257-1153

Albuquerque Area IHS
Western Bank Bldg.
Marquette, N.W., Suite 1502
Albuquerque, NM 87102-2163
(505) 766-2151

Bemidji Area IHS
203 Federal Bldg.
Bemidji, MN 56601
(218) 759-3412

Billings Area IHS
P.O. Box 2143
711 Central Ave.
Billings, MT 59103
(406) 657-6403

California Area IHS
1825 Bell St., Suite 200
Sacramento, CA 95825-1097
(916) 978-4202

Nashville Area IHS
Oaks Tower Bldg.
3310 Perimeter Hill Dr.
Nashville, TN 37211-4139
(615) 781-5550

Navajo Area IHS
NAIHS Complex
P.O. Box G
Hwy. 264 (St. Michaels)
Window Rock, AZ 86515-5004
(602) 871-4811

Oklahoma City Area IHS
5 Corporate Plaza
3625 N.W. 56th
Oklahoma City, OK 73112
(405) 945-6820

Phoenix Area IHS
3738 North 16th St.
Suite A
Phoenix, AZ 85016-5981
(602) 640-2119

Portland Area IHS
1220 SW 3rd Ave., Rm. 476
Portland, OR 97204-2892
(503) 326-3900

Tuscon Area IHS
7900 S.J. Stock Rd.
Tuscon, AZ 85746-9352
(602) 670-6600

From: U.S. Department of Health and Human Services (1992). *Comprehensive Health Care Program for American Indians and Alaska Natives.* Washington, D.C.: U.S. Government Printing Office, p. 31.

4. serves as the principal Federal advocate for Indians in the health field to ensure comprehensive health services for American Indian and Alaska Native people."[39]

In carrying out these tasks, the IHS has developed a program of clinical public health with emphasis on the community, the promotion of health, and the prevention of disease. This approach has yielded, perhaps, the best example of a health care system that integrates preventive, community, and clinical aspects.[41]

Community Health Problems of Native Americans

Just as other minority groups experience certain debilitating health problems at higher rates than the general population, so do Native Americans. Two of the most important of their health problems are alcohol abuse and injuries.

Alcohol

It is indeed unfortunate that Native Americans have experienced and continue to experience substantial health problems as a result of alcohol consumption. It is noteworthy that alcohol use among Native Americans was nonexistent prior to the arrival of early European settlers, who introduced its use to them. Unscrupulous settlers soon learned to use alcohol and its effects to secure greater advantages in business negotiations.[44] By the beginning of the nineteenth century, many astute Native

American leaders recognized the serious problems caused by the unrestricted use of alcohol by their people and so petitioned Congress to prohibit the sale of alcohol to Indians. Such a law was passed in 1832, putting in place an "Indian prohibition" which lasted until 1953.[45]

Even though the alcohol prohibition for Native Americans lasted for well over a hundred years, the impact of alcohol on these Americans continues to be overwhelming. Recent studies[46, 47] have shown that Native American adolescents, on average, report greater use of alcohol and other drugs than any other racial/ethnic subgroup. While the percentage of Native American adults who consume alcohol is relatively low (50%) compared with the general United States population (70%) and other minority groups, the proportion of alcoholics is very high. Mortality and morbidity data for Native Americans reflects the magnitude of the alcohol abuse problem in this population. Conservative reports indicate that Native American deaths resulting from alcoholism are anywhere from four to eight times higher than the national average.[48, 49] Approximately 70% of all health care provided to Native Americans is alcohol related.[50] And a 1992 study[51] by the IHS and tribally operated hospitals revealed that almost one-fifth (17.9%) of patients who were hospitalized were in for an alcohol-related problem.

There is no clear explanation for the alcohol use and alcoholism rates for Native Americans. There are, however, some theories why the problems exist. Lamarine[44] reviewed the three leading theories: historical theory, physiological factors, and social factors.

Historical Theory

This theory includes two major components. First, the Native American culture had no exposure to alcohol until European settlers introduced it; thus, they were not socially prepared for its devastating effects. Second, Native Americans have failed to set acceptable standards of behavior for those under the influence of alcohol. That is, there has been a lack of tribal laws to deter individuals from committing crimes while intoxicated.[44]

Physiological Factors

Several researchers have tried to prove that Native Americans have a peculiar physiological response to alcohol. For each study that has indicated such, there are others to show that there is no relationship. Many Native Americans have shown that they are able to drink responsibly.[44]

Social Factors

There are many social factors and conditions that could encourage Native Americans to abuse alcohol. Those most often cited include, but are not limited to, emulation of white Americans; defiance against prohibition; disintegration of traditional Native American customs and culture; an escape from the reality of socioeconomic conditions like poverty, unemployment, inadequate education, prejudice, and lack of opportunity; peer pressure to join a social drinking group; and acculturation into a dominant white society, which contributes to significant stress and low self-esteem.[44]

To date, the treatment of alcohol abuse and alcoholism in Native Americans has not been overwhelmingly successful. Because of the difference between the culture and customs of Native Americans and the white majority, treatment modalities found to be helpful in the white culture are frequently not useful in Native American populations. The treatments that seem to be most promising for Native Americans are those that include community members in planning, implementing, and organizing programs at the community level. Suggestions for more effective treatment programs include the use of traditional native healing methods and practitioners, the inclusion of Native Americans as members of the treat- ment staff, the creation of linkages with Native American organizations, and the provision for maximum participation in the programs by those Native Americans who are treated.[44] (See Box 9.4.)

BOX 9.4
Healthy People 2000—Objective

4.1   Reduce deaths caused by alcohol-related motor vehicle crashes to no more than 8.5 per 100,000 people. (Age-adjusted baseline: 9.8 per 100,000 in 1987)

Special Population Target

	Alcohol-Related Motor Vehicle Crash Deaths (per 100,000)	1987 Baseline	2000 Target	Percent Decrease
4.1a	American Indian/Alaska Native men	52.2	44.8	
4.1b	People aged 15–24	21.5	18	

Baseline data source: Fatal Accident Reporting System, U.S. Dept. of Transportation.

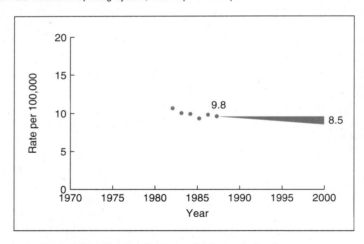

Age-adjusted alcohol-related motor vehicle crash death rate.

For Further Thought

Based upon the theories presented in this chapter on alcohol abuse and Native Americans, how would you respond to the statement "The problem of alcohol abuse by Native Americans is not solveable?"

Intentional and Unintentional Injuries

Compared with the general population, Native Americans are disproportionately affected both by intentional and unintentional injuries and by injury deaths. Unintentional injuries are the second leading cause of death for Native American males and the third leading cause for Native America females (see Table 9.9). Homicide and suicide rates are nearly twice those for the general population or for white Americans.

While not the sole cause, alcohol is a primary contributing factor in many of these deaths. Approximately 75% of all unintentional deaths, 80% of all suicides, and 90% of all homicides among Native Americans are alcohol related.[48, 52, 53] These data reflect the urgency of the need to prevent and treat alcohol abuse problems among this population.

REFUGEES: THE NEW IMMIGRANTS

In this section, we introduce several new terms that describe people who have arrived in the United States relatively recently. Because of their status as new arrivals, these people sometimes share similar health problems. The first term, **refugees,** means people who flee one area, usually their home country, to seek shelter or protection from danger. Refugees arriving in the United States may be seeking political asylum, refuge from war, or escape from famine or other environmental disaster. The second term, **immigrants,** describes individuals who migrate here from another country for the purpose of seeking permanent residence and hopefully a better life. **Aliens** are people born in and owing allegiance to a country other than the one in which they live. Thus, these individuals are not citizens and are only allowed to stay in a foreign country for a specified period of time defined by law or policy. Many aliens, while in the United States legally, are not permitted to work. Sometimes, however, they violate this provision and find employment illegally. Shortly after President Clinton was elected, this practice was brought to the public's attention when two of his cabinet nominees withdrew their names from consideration because they had hired, as domestic help, aliens who entered this country without permission to work. Lastly, **illegal aliens** are those who enter this country without any permission whatsoever. Most of these illegal aliens have entered from Mexico, simply by crossing the Rio Grande at night.

Although all refugees who enter this country can be classified into one of the existing racial/ethnic categories used by our government, as a single group they present many special concerns not seen in minorities who are born and raised in the United States. Most of the refugees currently entering the United States, arrive from **Third World countries,** countries with meager economic resources. These refugees usually settle in urban areas, even though they may have a rural orientation. Many refugees are poor and have low levels of formal education and few marketable work skills. Many arrive with serious health problems, including undernourishment or starvation, physical and emotional injuries from hostile action,

---

refugee A person who flees one area or country to seek shelter or protection from danger in another.

immigrant Individuals who migrate from one country to another for the purpose of seeking permanent residence.

alien A person born in and owing allegiance to a country other than the one in which he or she lives.

illegal alien An individual who entered this country without permission.

confinement in refugee camps, poor health care, and overcrowdedness[54] (see Box 9.5). A majority of the refugees are young, many of the women are of childbearing age, and most come from Latin American and Southeast Asian countries.

The arrival of such refugees places new strains on both the private workplaces and the governmental social services (see Figure 9.14). Here are some of the problems that have surfaced.[54, 55]

• Lack of jobs to fit the skills of the refugees.
• New competition for the lower socioeconomic groups in the United States for work and housing.
• Strain on the budgets of the public education systems to meet the needs of the non-English-speaking refugee children.

• Further burden on the human, health, and mental health services provided mostly by minority communities.
• Cultural barriers to using the United States health care system include lack of financial resources, cultural ignorance of health care providers, lack of bilingual health care workers, distrust and unfamiliarity with Western medicine, poor understanding of the etiology of certain diseases, difficulties of accessing services, and ignorance of available services.
• Growing backlash movements against refugees in some areas of the country such as by the "Only English Movement," and the Immigration Reform and Control Act of 1986, which requires employers to prove the identity and work authorization of every prospective employee. The logic of this section of the law is based on the per-

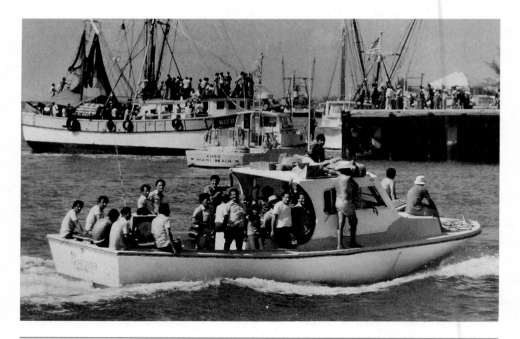

FIGURE 9.14

Arrival of refugees places additional burdens on both private workplaces and public social services.

BOX 9.5
Health Status of Haitian Migrants

Following the military coup in Haiti in the early 1990s, thousands of Haitians fled their country in small, open boats to seek a new home in the United States. Most of these migrants were intercepted by the U.S. Coast Guard cutters and transported to the United States Naval Base in Guantanamo Bay, Cuba. While at the base, the Haitians were provided with medical care and given the necessary medical screenings required for entry into the United States. During the period from November 1991 through April 1992, approximately 18,000 migrants received medical care at the naval base. Among the chief health problems for which care was needed were dermatologic problems, respiratory infections, malaria, active tuberculosis (TB), measles, and sexually transmitted diseases. A total of 7,315 of the Haitians were more than 15 years of age and were thus required by the Immigration Act of 1990 to be screened for syphilis, HIV, and TB. Approximately 5% (366) had serologic evidence of past or present syphilis infection, and 7% (479) were positive for HIV.[55] Originally, it was believed that those who tested positive for HIV would not be allowed to enter the United States. However, in 1993 a federal judge ruled that these individuals could be admitted.

nificant barriers to the social integration of refugees into American society. Will the official U.S. policy toward refugees create a new at-risk population? Like most of the other minority groups in the United States, refugees may become a part of those disadvantaged in this country.[56]

There is, however, one bright note to the increase in refugees in this country, and that is the enrichment of the U.S. culture. Until 1970, the United States was primarily composed of only black and white Americans. In the last 25 years, this country has been significantly enriched by the cultures of those coming from other countries.[56]

SOLUTIONS TO THE COMMUNITY HEALTH PROBLEMS OF THE RACIAL/ETHNIC MINORITIES

As noted throughout this chapter, the community health problems faced by the racial/ethnic minorities of this country are many. These health problems are inextricable from a variety of other social problems, making simple solutions unlikely. We know that many health problems faced by minorities are attributable not to race of ethnic origin but to social or economic conditions or to disenfranchisement. We also know that multiple resources will be required to resolve these social and economic problems. Solutions to these problems for one group may not work for another. Americans of Hispanic origin, Asian/Pacific Islanders, black Americans, and Native Americans each have unique cultural traditions that must be respected if solutions are to be successful. In other words, they must opera-

ception of work as a privilege associated with citizenship, and by extension, with legal residence.

The combination of difficulties facing refugees in the United States—including finding employment and obtaining access to education and appropriate human, health, and mental health services—represent sig-

tionally integrate an understanding of the culture of the target population—solutions must be **culturally sensitive**. In a more general sense, however, significant strides in the improvement of health in minority groups can be achieved by reducing poverty, increasing access to health care, and empowering local communities.

Addressing the Poverty Problem

Throughout this chapter, we have discussed the differences in health status among races and ethnic groups; and on several occasions, we have stressed that socioeconomic status is actually a better predictor of health status than race or ethnic origin. That is, the lower one's socioeconomic status, the worse one's health status. In a recent study,[57] researchers hypothesized that when socioeconomic status was adequately considered, different mortality rates due to coronary heart disease between black Americans and white Americans were insignificant. After following a cohort of men for 28 years, they found that their hypothesis was indeed true.

In 1990, 10.7% of Americans were living below the poverty level, including 8.1% of white Americans, 29.4% of black Americans, and 25.0% of Americans of Hispanic origin (see Table 9.14).[15] Social and economic programs that reduce the number of persons living in poverty would reduce the discrepancies in health statistics among groups of Americans.

Programs to reduce poverty are not easily developed, because poverty is not an independent state; it is closely tied to education, opportunity, health, motivation, and a number of other variables. Until now,

---

culturally sensitive Having respect for cultures other than one's own.

Table 9.14 Families Below Poverty Level in 1990 by Race and Ethnicity: March 1991 *(numbers in thousands)*		
Characteristic	Estimate	Percentage
Below poverty level	7,098	10.7%
White	4,622	8.1
White, not Hispanic	3,442	6.6
Black	2,193	29.4
Black, not Hispanic	2,153	29.3
Hispanic	1,244	25.0
White Hispanic	1,180	24.8
Black Hispanic	40	35.4
Non-Hispanic	5,854	9.5

From: U.S. Dept. of Commerce (1992). *Exploring Alternative Race-Ethnic Comparison Groups in Current Population Surveys.* (Series P23-182). Washington, D.C.: U.S. Government Printing

poverty has been treated as a welfare issue, but few believe that welfare payments represent a long-term solution to the poverty problem. The Clinton administration is looking for new programs that would help those in poverty to become independent from the welfare system. Only time will tell whether these new programs will work. One measure of success will be improvement in the health statistics of minorities.

Providing Universal Access to Health Care Services

If one sweeping change could be made to improve the disparity between the health of minorities and the rest of the nation, it would be the provision of universal access to health care services, especially preventive health care services. Today, many of those in the United States who are either medically unserved or underserved belong to racial or ethnic minorities. Many lack health insurance altogether, while others who are insured live in areas where health care workers are scarce or access to health care services are nonexistent, limited, or sporadic in nature.[58] To achieve universal health care, we know that, "Services must be where people are, at a time that is convenient and delivered in a specific manner that is culturally sensitive."[31] To meet this goal will require that the present health care system in the United States be radically changed. The concept of such a system is discussed in Chapter 14, and only time will tell if the United States will move in that direction. (See Box 9.6.)

Empowering Self and Community

One reason why minority groups lack the resources to eliminate community health problems is their lack of empowerment. To **empower** means to give power or authority; to enable or permit. With reference to our discussion, it means to enable people to work to solve community health problems. Simply put, to acquire better health and health care services, a community must be empowered to do so.

Friedman[59] identified three kinds of power associated with empowerment: social, political, and psychological. An increase in social power brings with it access to "bases" of production such as information, knowledge and skills, participation in social organizations, and financial resources. An increase in productivity allows for greater influence on markets, which in turn can influence change.

A social power base is needed to gain political power. Political power is more than just being able to vote; it is also the power of voice and of collective action. In a democracy, seldom does a single voice effect change. It is the collective voice that can make things happen. The early labor movement in this country which led to unions is a good example.

Psychological power is best described as an individual sense of potency demonstrated in self-confident behavior. It is often the result of successful action in the social and political domains. With the investiture of all three types of power, empowerment can take place. Empowerment replaces hopelessness with a sense of being in control and a sense that one can make a difference. Once people are empowered, then the power needs to be transferred to the communities. When communities are empowered, they can affect change and solve problems. (See Chapter 6 for a discussion of community organization as a means of empowering a community.)

The process of empowerment may seem abstract because of the theoretical concepts that are involved, but it is not. Follow the process in this example. A group of people, a community, lacks access to appropriate health care. For this group to be empowered, they must build a foundation with social power. To do this, the group must gain access to the bases of production. They must acquire information about available health care programs and obtain the knowledge and skills to access care. Some in the group need to become members of social organizations concerned with health care, such as health departments or voluntary agencies; and the group has to obtain the necessary financial resources to make them noticed in the marketplace as a consumer group. To gain such social power, it is imperative that the group be literate and have the appropriate education. Many groups never gain social power because they do not possess the education to access the bases of production.

When the group has attained social power, a subgroup is able to work toward political power. They can be heard in the marketplace with vote and voice. They can organize to present a united front for collec-

BOX 9.6
Selected International Comparisons

Indicators		Canada	France	Germany*	Japan	United Kingdom	United States
Percentage of low-birth-weight babies	1990	6	5	6	6	7	7
Infant mortality rate (per 1,000 live births)	1990	6.8	7.4	7	4.6	7.9	9.1
Teen birth rate (per 1,000 teens) (1988)	Selected years	23.1 (1988)	9.5 (1988)	10.3 (1988)	3.5 (1989)	31.8 (1989)	54.8
Percentage of appropriate age group enrolled in secondary education	1988–1989	93	83	85	96	79	88
Percentage of all deaths that are violent deaths, ages 15–24 (1986)	Selected years	76.2 (1986)	70 (1986)	68.7 (1987)	66.5 (1987)	62.3 (1987)	77.8
Percentage of children in poverty (1987)	Selected years	9.6 (1987)	4.6 (1984)	2.8 (1984)	—	7.4 (1986)	20.4
Percentage of all households that are married couples with children (1988)	Selected years	32.3 (1986)	30.2 (1988)	21.8 (1988)	39.2 (1985)	28 (1987)	27
Percentage of all households that are single-parent households	Selected years	5.6 (1986)	3.7 (1988)	3.4 (1988)	2.5 (1985)	4 (1987)	8

tive action. Minority groups have the potential to have a loud voice if united. Once united, they are in a position to influence decision makers at various levels of government. In the specific case, in which the goal is greater access to health care, this could mean getting the local health department to expand the types and numbers of clinics available.

Increased political power can lead to psychological power. Such power would make this particular group confident that the expansion of health department clinics is just the first of many achievements. Through this same process, other community improvements can be made.

CHAPTER SUMMARY

One of the great strengths of the United States has been and remains the diversity of its people. One of the results of this diversity is the disparity in the health status among various racial and ethnic minority groups.

The federal government has categorized the U.S. population into five racial groups (Asian/Pacific Islanders, black Americans, Native Americans, white Americans, and others) and two ethnic groups (Americans of Hispanic origin and non-Hispanics). With the exception of Asian/Pacific Islanders, on almost every measure of health status, minority groups rank lower than the white American majority. Glaring differences exist with regard to life expectancy, years of potential life lost, mortality statistics, infant mortality statistics, and with specific health problems such as HIV/AIDS, tuberculosis, violence, alcohol and other drug abuse, and sickle cell disease.

If the health status of the nation as a whole is to improve, concentrated efforts must aim at solving both health and social problems facing these racial/ethnic minority groups. Specifically, poverty must be reduced, access to education and health services improved, and specific health problems addressed. Lastly, minority groups must be enabled, through the processes of social, political, and psychological empowerment, to solve their own problems.

SCENARIO:
ANALYSIS AND RESPONSE

1. Do you agree with Tom when he says the United States is more culturally diverse than at any time in the past? Why or why not? Do you see this as a strength or weakness for the country?

2. What signs are there in your community that the United States is becoming more internationalized and that minority groups are growing?

3. What rewards do you see as a result of an increasingly diverse population in the United States? What liabilities?

4. What do you see as the major health problems associated with the growth of minority groups in the United States?

REVIEW QUESTIONS

1. Why is it said that the United States was built on diversity?

2. What are the reasons that minority groups in the United States continue to grow as a proportion of the overall population?

3. What is the Office of Management and Budget's *Directive 15*?

4. Why do some researchers feel that the classification of racial/ethnic groups used by our federal government does not accurately represent the people of those groups?

5. How do the birth and fertility rates of Hispanic Americans compare with those of other races and the general population?

6. What is so unusual about the reported infant mortality rates for Americans of Hispanic origin? Explain.

7. What is the difference between having a seropositive test result for HIV and having AIDS?

8. Compared with other racial/ethnic minorities, what is so unusual about mortality rates of Asian/Pacific Islanders?

9. What are the causes for the resurgence of tuberculosis in this country? What solutions have been proposed?

10. In general, how do the health status indicators for black Americans compare with those of white Americans? With the overall population?

11. What actions can be taken to reduce the infant mortality rate in black Americans?

12. Why is sickle cell disease such a threat to black Americans?

13. How would you describe, demographically, today's Native Americans?

14. How do the leading causes of death in Native Americans differ from those of other minorities? From the general population?

15. What are the major goals of the Indian Health Service?

16. Which of the three theories about why Native Americans abuse alcohol do you believe is most accurate? Why?

17. What reasons can you give for the high rates of intentional and unintentional injuries and injury deaths in Native Americans?

18. What steps can be taken to help reduce/eliminate the community health problems faced by racial/ethnic minorities?

ACTIVITIES

1. Using the 1990 Census Report (available in your library), create a demographic profile of the state and county in which you live. Locate the following information: population, racial/ethnic composition, percentage of people represented by the different age groups, gender breakdown, martial status, and percentage of people living in poverty.

2. Make an appointment with an employee of the health department in your hometown. Find out the differences in health status between the racial/ethnic groups in the community by obtaining the race/ethnicity specific morbidity and mortality data. Discuss these differences with the health department employee, then summarize your findings in a one-page paper.

3. In a two- to three-page paper, present the proposal you would recommend to the President of the United States for closing the health status gap between the races and ethnic groups.

4. Identify a health problem that is specific to a racial/ethnic minority group. Research the topic and present in a three-page paper, the present status of the problem, the future outlook for the problem, and what could be done to reduce or eliminate the problem.

5. Write a two-page position paper on "Why racial/ethnic minority groups have a lower health status than the majority white Americans."

REFERENCES

1. Bovee, T. (April 28, 1993). "One in Seven Americans Doesn't Speak English at Home." *The Muncie Star,* p. 1D.

2. U.S. Dept. of Commerce (1992). *1990 Census of Population and Housing, Summary Population and Housing, Characteristics, United States.* Washington, D.C.: U.S. Government Printing Office.

3. Bovee, T. (Dec. 4, 1992). "Immigrants to Fuel Population Boom." *The Muncie Star,* p. 1D.

4. Houk, V. N., and R. C. Warren (1991). "Foreword to the Proceedings." *Public Health Reports* 106(3): 226.

5. Polednak, A. P. (1989). *Racial and Ethnic Differences in Disease.* New York: Oxford Univ. Press.

6. Office of Management and Budget (1978). "Directive 15: Race and Ethnic Standards for Federal Statistics and Administrative Reporting." In *Statistical Policy Handbook,* pp. 37–38. Washington, D.C.: Office of Federal Statistical Policy and Standards, U.S. Dept. of Commerce.

7. Hahn, R. A. (1992). "The State of Federal Health Statistics on Racial and Ethnic Groups." *Journal of the American Medical Association* 267(2): 268–271.

8. Lacey, E. P. (1992). "U.S. Census Procedures: A Backdrop for Consideration of Ethnic and Racial Issues in Health Education Programming." *Journal of Health Education* 23(1): 14–21.

9. Yu, E. S. H. (1991). "The Health Risks of Asian Americans." *American Journal of Public Health* 81(11): 1391–1393.

10. Yu, E. S. H., and W. T. Liu (1992). "U.S. National Health Data on Asian Americans and Pacific Islanders: A Research Agenda for the 1990s." *American Journal of Public Health* 82(12): 1645–1652.

11. Harper, M. S. (1990). "Introduction." In M. S. Harper, ed. *Minority Aging: Essential Curricula Content for Selected Health and Allied Health Professions* (DHHS pub. No. HRS-P-DV90-4), pp. 3–22. Washington, D.C.: U.S. Government Printing Office.

12. U.S. Dept. of Health and Human Services (1991). *Health Status of Minorities and Low-Income Groups,* 3rd ed. Washington, D.C.: U.S. Government Printing Office.

13. U.S. Dept. of Commerce (1992). *Statistical Abstract of the United States 1992: The National Data Book.* Washington, D.C.: U.S. Government Printing Office.

14. U.S. Dept. of Commerce (1993). *Hispanic Americans Today* (series p23–183). Washington, D.C.: U.S. Government Printing Office.

15. U.S. Dept. of Commerce (1992). *Exploring Alternative Race-Ethnic Comparison Groups in Current Population Surveys* (series p23–182). Washington, D.C.: U.S. Government Printing Office.

16. Desenclos, J. C. A., and R. A. Hahn (1992). "Years of Potential Life Lost Before Age 65 by Race, Hispanic Origin, and Sex—United States, 1986–1988." *Morbidity and Mortality Weekly Report* 41(SS-6): 13–23.

17. U.S. Dept. of Health and Human Services (1993). "Advance Report of Final Mortality Statistics, 1990." *Monthly Vital Statistics Report* 41(7): 50.

18. U.S. Dept. of Health and Human Services, Center for Health Statistics (1993). "*Health, United States, 1992* and *Healthly People 2000 Review*" (DHHS pub. no. PHS-93-1232). Washington, D.C.: U.S. Government Printing Office.

19. Jenkins, B. (1992). "AIDS/HIV Epidemics in the Black Community." In R. L. Braithwaite and S. E.

Taylor, eds. *Health Issues in the Black Community,* pp. 55–63. San Francisco: Jossey-Bass.

20. American National Red Cross (1992). *HIV and AIDS.* Washington, D.C.: Author.

21. Associated Press (June 6, 1993). "AIDS Adds More Notches to Deadly Belt." *Bellingham (WA) Herald.*

22. Centers for Disease Control (1990). "Surveillance for AIDS and HIV Infection Among Black and Hispanic Children and Women of Childbearing Age, 1981–1989." *Morbidity and Mortality Weekly Report* 39(ss-3): 23–30.

23. National Research Council (1989). *AIDS: The Second Decade.* Washington, D.C.: National Academy Press.

24. Gayle, J. A., R. M. Selik, and S. Y. Chu (1990). "Surveillance for AIDS and HIV Infection Among Black and Hispanic Children and Women of Childbearing Age, 1981–1989." *Morbidity and Mortality Weekly Report* 39(ss-3): 23–30.

25. U.S. Dept. of Health and Human Services (1990). *Health Status of the Disadvantaged: Chartbook 1990* (DHHS pub. no. [HRSA] HRS-P-DV 90-1). Washington, D.C.: U.S. Government Printing Office.

26. Kitano, H. H. L. (1990). "Values, Beliefs, and Practices of Asian-American Elderly: Implications for Geriatric Education." In M. S. Harper, ed. *Minority Aging: Essential Curricula Content for Selected Health and Allied Health Professions* (DHHS pub. no: HRS-P-DV 90-4), pp. 341–348. Washington, D.C.: U.S. Government Printing Office.

27. AIDS Working Group (1992). *Tuberculosis and HIV Disease: A Report of the Special Initiative on AIDS of the American Public Health Association.* Washington, D.C.: American Public Health Association.

28. Center for Disease Control (1992). "Prevention and Control of Tuberculosis in U.S. Communities with At-Risk Minority Populations." *Morbidity and Mortality Weekly Report* 41(RR-5): 1–11.

29. Satcher, D., and D. J. Thomas (1990). "Dimensions of Minority Aging: Implications for Curriculum Development for Selected Health Professions." In M. S. Harper, ed. *Minority Aging: Essential Curricula Content for Selected Health and Allied Health Professions* (DHHS pub. no. HRS-P-DV 90-4), pp. 23–32. Washington, D.C.: U.S. Government Printing Office.

30. U.S. Dept. of Health and Human Services (1993). Advance Report of Final Mortality Statistics, 1990." *Monthly Vital Statistics Report* 41(9): 42.

31. Floyd, V. D. (1992). "Too Soon, Too Small, Too Sick: Black Infant Mortality." In R. L. Braithwaite and S. E. Taylor, eds. *Health Issues in the Black Community,* pp. 165–177. San Francisco: Jossey-Bass.

32. Whitten, C. F. (1992). "Sickle Cell Anemia and African Americans." In R. L. Braithwaite and S. E. Taylor, eds. *Health Issues in the Black Community,* pp. 192–205. San Francisco: Jossey-Bass.

33. U.S. Dept. of Health and Human Services (1993). *Sickle Cell Disease: Screening, Diagnosis, Management, and Counseling in Newborns and Infants. Clinical Practice Guideline No. 6* (AHCPR pub. no. 93-0562). Washington, D.C.: U.S. Government Printing Office.

34. Baquet, C. R., and T. Gibbs (1992). "Cancer and Black Americans." In R. L. Braithwaite and S. E. Taylor eds. *Health Issues in the Black Community,* pp. 106–120. San Francisco: Jossey-Bass.

35. Hildreth, C. J., and E. Saunders (1992). "Heart Disease, Stroke and Hypertension in Blacks." In R. L. Braithwaite and S. E. Taylor, eds. *Health Issues in the Black Community,* pp. 90–105. San Francisco: Jossey-Bass.

36. Saunders, E. (1985). "Special Techniques for Management of Hypertension in Blacks." In W. D. Hall, E. Saunders, and N. B. Shulman, eds. *Hypertension in Blacks: Epidemiology, Pathophysiology, and Treatment,* pp. 209–236. Chicago: Year Book.

37. Baquet, C. R., J. W. Horm, T. Gibbs, and P. Greenwald (1991). "Socioeconomic Factors and Cancer Incidence Among Blacks and Whites." *Journal of the National Cancer Institute* 83(8): 551–557.

38. Garrett, J. T. (1990). "Indian Health: Values, Beliefs and Practices." In M. S. Harper, ed. *Minority Aging: Essential Curricula Content for Selected Health and Allied Health Professionals* (DHHS pub. no. HRS-P-DV90-4), pp. 179–191. Washington, D.C.: U.S. Government Printing Office.

39. U.S. Dept. of Health and Human Services (1992). *Comprehensive Health Care Program for American Indians and Alaska Natives.* Washington, D.C.: U.S. Government Printing Office.

40. Edwards, E. D., and M. Egbert-Edwards (1990). "Family Care and Native American Elderly." In M. S. Harper, ed. *Minority Aging: Essential Curricula Content for Selected Health and Allied Health Professions* (DHHS pub. no. HRS-P-DV90-4), pp. 145–163. Washington, D.C.: Government Printing Office.

41. Rhoades, E. R. (1990). "Profile of American Indians and Alaska Natives." In M. S. Harper, ed. *Minority Aging: Essential Curricula Content for Selected Health and Allied Health Professions* (DHHS pub. no. HRS-P-DV 90-4), pp. 45–62. Washington, D.C.: U.S. Government Printing Office.

42. U.S. Dept. of Health and Human Services (1990). *Trends in Indian Health, 1990.* Washington, D.C.: U.S. Government Printing Office.

43. U.S. Dept. of Health and Human Services, Center for Health Statistics (1992). *Health, United States, 1991* (DHHS pub. no. PHS-92-1232). Washington, D.C.: U.S. Government Printing Office.

44. Lamarine, R. J. (1988). "Alcohol Abuse Among Native Americans." *Journal of Community Health* 13(3): 143–155.

45. Lookout, M. (1975). "Alcohol and the Native American." *Alcohol: Technical Reports* 4: 30–37.

46. Bachman, J. G., J. M. Wallace, P. M. O'Malley , L. D. Johnston, C. L. Kurth, and H. W. Neighbors (1991). "Racial/Ethnic Differences in Smoking, Drinking, and Illicit Drug Use Among American High School Seniors, 1976–1989." *American Journal of Public Health* 81(3): 372–377.

47. Beauvais, F., E. R. Oetting, W. Wolf, and R. W. Edwards (1989). "American Indian Youth and Drugs, 1976–87: A Continuing Problem." *American Journal of Public Health* 79(5): 634–636.

48. Andre, J. M. (1979). *The Epidemiology of Alcoholism Among American Indians and Alaskan Natives.* Albuquerque: Indian Health Service.

49. National Institute on Alcohol Abuse and Alcoholism (1980). *Alcohol and American Indians.* Rockville, Md.: National Clearinghouse for Alcohol Information.

50. Indian Health Service (1977). *Alcoholism: A High Priority Health Problem.* Washington, D.C.: Dept. of Health and Human Services.

51. Center for Disease Control (1992). "Alcohol-related Hospitalizations—Indian Health Service and Tribal Hospitals, United States, May, 1992." *Morbidity and Mortality Weekly Report* 41(41): 757–760.

52. Rhoades, E. R., J. Hammond, T. K. Welty, A. O. Handler, and R. W. Amler (1987). "The Indian Burden of Illness and Future Health Interventions." *Public Health Reports* 102: 361–368.

53. Levy, J. E., and S. J. Kunitz (1974). *Indian Drinking: Navajo Practices and Anglo-American Theories.* New York: John Wiley & Sons.

54. Uba, L. (1992). "Cultural Barriers to Health Care for Southeast Asian Refugees." *Public Health Reports* 107(5): 544–548.

55. Centers for Disease Control (1993). "Health Status of Haitian Migrants—U.S. Naval Base, Guantanamo Bay, Cuba, Nov. 1991–April 1992." *Morbidity and Mortality Weekly Report* 42(7): 138–140.

56. Sotomayor, M. (1990). "The New Immigrants: The Undocumented and Refugees." In M. S. Harper, ed. *Minority Aging: Essential Curricula Content for Selected Health and Allied Health Professions* (DHHS pub. no. HRS-P-DV 90-4), pp. 627–637. Washington, D.C.: U.S. Government Printing Office.

57. Keil, J. E., S. E. Sutherland, R. G. Knapp, and H. A. Tyroler (1992). "Does Equal Socioeconomic Status in Black and White Men Mean Equal Risk of Mortality?" *American Journal of Public Health"* 82(8): 1133–1136.

58. Sundwall, D. N., and C. Tavani (1991). "The Role of Public Health in Providing Primary Care for the Medically Underserved." *Public Health Reports* 106(1): 2–5.

59. Friedmann, J. (1992). *Empowerment: The Politics of Alternative Development.* Cambridge, Mass.: Blackwell.

Chapter 10
SENIORS

Chapter Outline

Chapter Objectives

After studying this chapter you will be able to:

1. Identify signs of an aging population.
2. Define the following groups: old, young old, old old, and oldest old.
3. Define the terms *aged, aging, elderly, seniors, gerontology,* and *geriatrics.*
4. State several commonly held myths about the senior population.
5. Explain the meaning of an age-pyramid.
6. List the factors that affect the size and age of a population.
7. Define fertility and mortality rates and explain how they impact life expectancy.
8. Explain the difference between dependency and labor force ratios.
9. Describe the typical senior, with regard to marital status, living arrangements, racial and ethnic background, economic status, and geographic location.
10. Identify the six special needs of seniors.
11. Briefly summarize the Older Americans Act of 1965.
12. List the services provided for seniors in most communities.
13. Explain the difference between respite care and adult day care.
14. Identify the four different levels of tasks with which elderly need assistance.

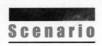
Carl and Sarah have now been retired for about five years. Carl retired in good health after 35 years as an insurance agent, and Sarah stopped working outside the home after their children were grown and had families of their own. Upon retirement, they sold their home and paid cash for a condominium that had about half the square footage of their home. They now live on a fixed income (Social Security and investment income) and are eligible for Medicare. Though they continue to enjoy their lives, they are now faced with an increasing number of health problems while they seem to have less interaction with their friends, some of whom have moved to Sun Belt states or other retirement areas; others have died or are dying. They find that they must ask others for help with things they used to do routinely for themselves and that they have to watch their spending very closely. They are now beginning to worry more about their future. What if their property taxes increase so much that they have to sell their condominium? Will they have enough money to enjoy the independent life-style they have become used to for the rest of their lives? What if one of them has to enter a nursing home? What if one of them becomes an Alzheimer's patient? Their physician, old Doc Wilson, might retire this year. What if they cannot find a new doctor who will accept Medicare patients? So many questions with only guesses for answers! Who knows what the future will hold for Carl and Sarah, and for that matter, for any of us?

INTRODUCTION

The American populace is growing older. For the first time in U.S. history, a significant majority of Americans will achieve senior citizen status and, in doing so, live long enough to assume some responsibilities for the care of their aging parents.[1] We only need to look around us to see the change that is taking place (see Figure 10.1). The number of gray heads in restaurants, malls, and movie theaters is increasing. Senior centers, retirement villages, and nursing homes are being built in record numbers. And today, more than ever before, many people belong to multigenerational families, where there are opportunities to develop long-lasting relationships with parents, grandparents, and even great-grandparents.[1] There are now many families in which members of three different generations receive monthly Social Security checks. As we approach the twenty-first century, the economic, social, and health issues associated with the growing proportion of seniors in America have become major political concerns as well. In this chapter, we will define terminology, describe the demographics, and discuss the special needs of and community service for the aging.

DEFINITIONS

How old is old? The ageless baseball pitcher Satchel Paige once said "How old would you be if you didn't know how old you was [sic]?" While his English might be found wanting, Paige's point is important (see

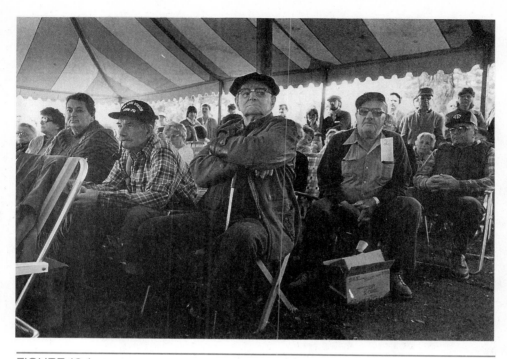

FIGURE 10.1

The number of senior citizens in the United States is on the rise.

Figure 10.2). A person's age might depend upon who measures it and how they define it. For example, while demographers might define **old** according to chronological years, clinicians might define it by stages of physiological development, psychologists by developmental stages. Children might see their 35-year-old teacher as old, while the 35-year-old teacher might regard her 61-year-old principal as old. Age is and always will be a relative concept.

Bould, Sanborn, and Reif have stated that people are old once they reach the age of 65.[2] But because there are a number of people who are very active and healthy at age 65 and will live a number of productive years after 65, they have subdivided old into the **young old** (65–74), the **old old** (75 and over), and the **oldest old** (85 and over). Also for the purposes of our discussion in this chapter we will use terms associated with aging as they have been defined in *Age Words*.[3]

aged The state of being old. A person may be defined as aged on the basis of having reached a specific age; for example, 65 is often used for social or legislative policies, while 75 is used for physiological evaluations.

aging The changes that occur normally in plants and animals as they grow older. Some age changes begin at birth and continue until death; other changes begin at maturity and end at death.

elderly or elder Generally referring to individuals over age 60.

gerontology The study of aging from the broadest perspective. Gerontologists examine not only the chemical and biological aspects of aging but also psychosocial, eco-

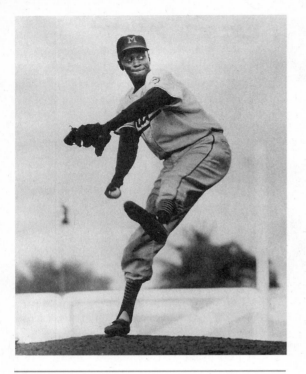

FIGURE 10.2

Some would say you are only as old as you think you are. (Satchel Paige remained active in professional baseball long after reaching the age at which others retired.)

nomic, and historical conditions. Elie Merchmkoff, of the Pasteur Institute in Paris, first used the term in 1903 to describe the biological study of senescence (aging).

geriatrics The branch of medicine that deals with the structural changes, physiology, diseases, and hygiene of old age. (Note: There are only 400 board certified MDs who specialize in geriatrics in the United States, while there are 40,000 board certified pediatricians. Yet the senior population is growing while the childhood population is in decline.)

In the United States, the term **seniors** has gained popularity. It implies having

achieved a certain status as a citizen. Indeed, many seniors do not define themselves as being elderly until they begin to experience functional decline. We have chosen the term *seniors* to designate those who have reached their sixty-fifth birthday.

MYTHS SURROUNDING AGING

Like other forms of prejudice and discrimination, **ageism** is the result of ignorance, misconceptions and half-truths about aging and the elderly. Since most people do not interact with older people on a daily basis, it is easy to create a stereotypical image of seniors based upon the atypical actions of a few.

When you think of older people, what comes to mind? Do you immediately think of a lonely man with a disheveled appearance sitting on a park bench or an older person lying in bed in a nursing home making incomprehensible noises? Or, do you think of Bob Hope and George Burns (each past 80) singing and dancing across a stage before thousands of people?

Ferrini and Ferrini[4] and Dychtwald and Flower[5] have identified a number of myths that many people hold about seniors. They are presented here to remind all that seniors are not run down, worn out members of our society, but for the most part are independent, capable, and valuable resources for our communities. Do not forget that both Ronald Reagan and George Bush were eligible for Social Security and Medicare when they served as presidents of the United States. Here are the myths and the reasons why they are only myths:

---

seniors   Those 65 years of age or older.

ageism   Prejudice and discrimination against the aged.

1. *Myth:* "After age 65, life goes steadily downhill."

   Truth: There is no magic age that defines the boundary between healthy middle age and total decrepitude.

2. *Myth:* "Old people are all alike."

   Truth: There are more differences among seniors than any other segment of the U.S. population.

3. *Myth:* "Old people are lonely and ignored by their families."

   Truth: Seniors are the least likely to be lonely of any age group; and those who live alone are likely to be in close contact, either in person or by telephone, with close friends and/or their children.

4. *Myth:* "Old people are senile."

   Truth: Senility is the result of disease and only affects about 5% of seniors living in noninstitutional settings.

5. *Myth:* "Old people have a good life."

   Truth: Though seniors do gain certain advantages when they retire and when their children leave home, they still face a number of concerns such as loss of loved ones, loss of health, and loss of value in society.

6. *Myth:* "Most old people are sickly."

   Truth: Most older people do have at least one chronic health problem, but the majority of seniors are able to live active life-styles.

7. *Myth:* "Old people no longer have any sexual interest or ability."

   Truth: Sexual interest does not diminish with age, but there is a slight alteration in sexual response. Nonetheless, many seniors in reasonably good health have active and satisfying sex lives.

8. *Myth:* "Most old people end up in nursing homes."

   Truth: Only approximately 6% of those above the age of 65 live in nursing homes. While that percentage jumps to 25% for the oldest old (those 85 and older), it is still well below half.

9. *Myth:* "Older people are unproductive."

   Truth: There is no consistent pattern to show superior productivity in any age group.

Though a number of issues and concerns facing seniors are presented later in this chapter, the majority of seniors in the United States today are active and well (see Figure 10.3). In all parts of the country,

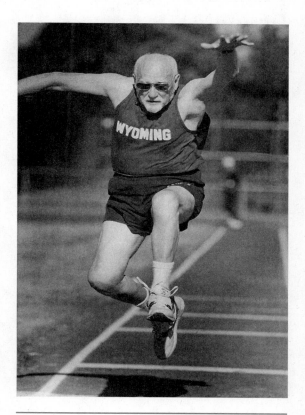

FIGURE 10.3

This 81-year-old long-jumper is one of many seniors who remain active well after retirement age.

seniors are: (1) attending **elderhostel** programs, (2) remaining politically active (the American Association of Retired Persons [AARP] is one of the most active lobbying groups in the United States), and (3) volunteering countless hours as tutors at schools, workers for hospices and hospitals, advocates and companions for the mentally ill, intake personnel at crisis centers, members of community agency boards, and churches, to name a few. Seniors are an important part of society and play active roles in making communities work.

DEMOGRAPHY OF AGING

Demography has been defined as "the study of a population (an aggregate of individuals) and those variables bringing about change in that population."[3] The demography of aging is the study of those who have reached their sixty-fifth birthday and of the variables that bring about change in their lives. In the paragraphs that follow, we review some of the demographic features of the senior population, including size, rate of growth, and the factors that contribute to this growth. We also discuss other demographic characteristics of this population, such as living arrangements, racial and ethnic composition, geographic distribution, economic status, and housing.

Size and Growth of the Senior Population

The aging of any population can be graphically illustrated with a theoretical **age pyramid**[6] (see Figure 10.4). The base

of this pyramid represents the youngest and largest number of people in the population. The sloping sides indicate high mortality rates and limited life expectancy. Until the mid-1950s, the population pyramid for the United States was not so very different from the traditional age-pyramid (see Figure 10.5).

Since the mid-1950s, however, the shape of America's population pyramid has changed (see Figure 10.6). Both the number of elderly and the proportion of the total population have grown significantly. This trend toward aging exists not only in this country, but in many countries throughout the world (see Box 10.1). The aging of many of the world's populations is projected to continue well into the twenty-first century (see Figures 10.7 and 10.8).

In the United States, the proportion of the population who are 65 years old and older (seniors) has increased steadily throughout most of this century, and the proportion of those over 85 has increased more dramatically than any other age group within the population. At the beginning of the twentieth

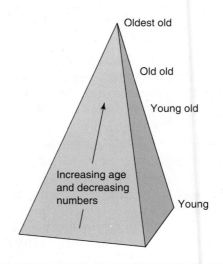

FIGURE 10.4

Theoretical age pyramid.

---

elderhostel Education programs specifically for seniors, held on college campuses.
demography The study of a population and those variables bringing about change in that population.

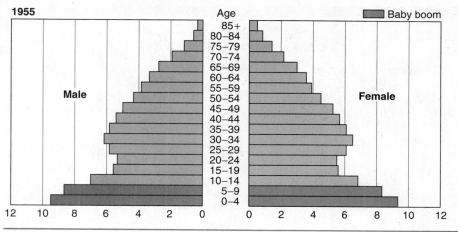

FIGURE 10.5

Population by age and sex, United States: 1955 (in millions).

From: U.S. Bur. of the Census (1965). "Estimates of the Population of the United States by Single Years of Age, Color, and Sex: 1900 to 1959." Current Population Reports, series P-25, no. 311. Washington, D.C.: U.S. Government Printing Office, p. 2–5.

century, only 1 in 25 Americans was over the age of 65 years. In 1992, that number had increased to 1 in 8. By 2030, the segment of the population over 65 is expected to double, and there will be almost as many seniors (20.2%) as people under the age of 18 (23.4%).[7,8]

As one might guess, the projected growth of the senior population is expected to raise

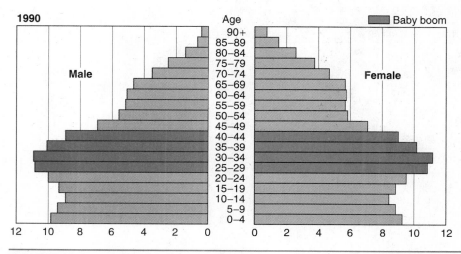

FIGURE 10.6

Population by age and sex, United States: 1990 (in millions).

From: Spencer, Gregory. U.S. Bur. of the Census (Jan. 1989). "Projections of the Population of the United States by Age, Sex, and Race: 1988 to 2080." Current Population Reports, series p.25, no. 1018. Washington, D.C.: U.S. Government Printing Office (middle series projections).

BOX 10.1
The World Is Growing Older

The United States is not alone when it comes to an aging population. The impact of lower fertility, infant mortality, and maternal mortality rates; the reduction of infections and parasitic diseases; and improved education is being felt worldwide. By the year 2020, every major region in the world will show an increased proportion of the population over 65 years of age.

Countries with More than 2 Million Elderly Persons in 1991

(In thousands)

Country	Population Aged 65 and Over	Country	Population Aged 65 and Over	Country	Population Aged 65 and Over
China, mainland	67,967	Indonesia	5,962	Turkey	2,789
India	32,780	Spain	5,378	Nigeria	2,676
United States	**32,045**	Pakistan	4,734	Romania	2,489
Japan	15,253	Poland	3,851	Philippines	2,380
Germany	12,010	Mexico	3,522	Thailand	2,350
United Kingdom	9,025	Bangladesh	3,492	Yugoslavia	2,328
Italy	8,665	Vietnam	3,196	South Korea	2,135
France	8,074	Canada	3,140	Egypt	2,077
Brazil	6,680	Argentina	3,012	Iran	2,052

Source: U.S. Bur. of the Census, Kevin Kinsella, Center for International Research, International Data Base.

Countries with More than 2 Million Elderly Persons in 2020

(In thousands)

Country	Population Aged 65 and Over	Country	Population Aged 65 and Over	Country	Population Aged 65 and Over
China, mainland	179,561	Poland	7,243	Burma	3,425
India	88,495	Vietnam	6,707	Czechoslovakia	3,149
United States	**52,067**	Philippines	6,646	Morocco	2,972
Japan	33,421	South Korea	6,550	Venezuela	2,912
Indonesia	22,183	Canada	6,404	Saudi Arabia	2,867
Brazil	18,800	Egypt	5,680	North Korea	2,734
Germany	18,396	Iran	5,235	Zaire	2,643
Italy	13,078	Yugoslavia	4,933	Peru	2,580
France	12,119	Argentina	4,862	Sri Lanka	2,527
United Kingdom	12,108	Romania	4,588	Algeria	2,450
Mexico	10,857	Colombia	4,464	Greece	2,237
Pakistan	9,678	South Africa	4,084	Hungary	2,186
Nigeria	9,152	Australia	3,956	Malaysia	2,139
Bangladesh	9,057	Ethiopia	3,920	Chile	2,133
Spain	8,162	China, Taiwan	3,500	Belgium	2,071
Turkey	7,990	Netherlands	3,461	Portugal	2,053
Thailand	7,828				

Source: U.S. Bur. of the Census, Kevin Kinsella, Center for International Research, International Data Base.

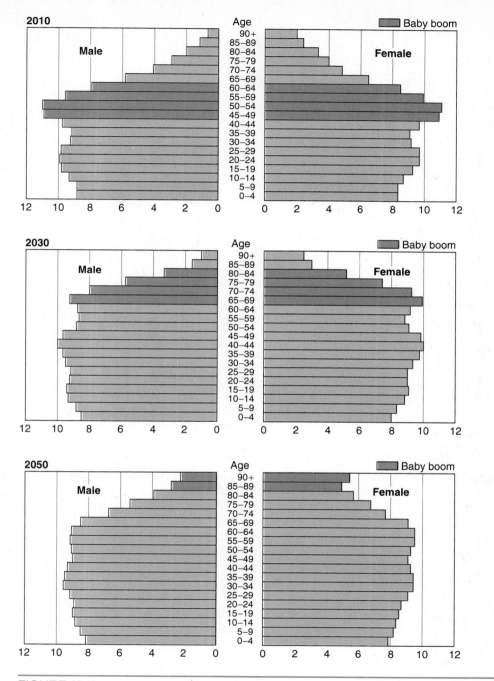

FIGURE 10.7

The aging population of the twenty-first century. Population by age and sex (in millions).

From: Spencer, Gregory. U.S. Bur. of the Census (Jan. 1989). "Projections of the Population of the United States by Age, Sex, and Race: 1988 to 2080." Current Population Reports, *series p.25, no. 1018. Washington, D.C.: U.S. Government Printing Office (middle series projections).*

the **median age** of the United States population. In 1990, the median age was 33 years. This is expected to climb to 39 by the year 2010 and to 43 by the year 2050[7,9] (see Figure 10.9).

Factors That Affect Population Size and Age

There are three factors that affect the size and age of a population: its fertility rates, its mortality rates, and gain or loss from migration of individuals into or out of that population.[1] Though one might assume that all populations will age with time, that is not necessarily true. In fact, a population could get younger with time.[1] If fertility rates and mortality rates are both high, life expectancy would be low and the age of a population could grow younger. However, this has not been the case in the United States.

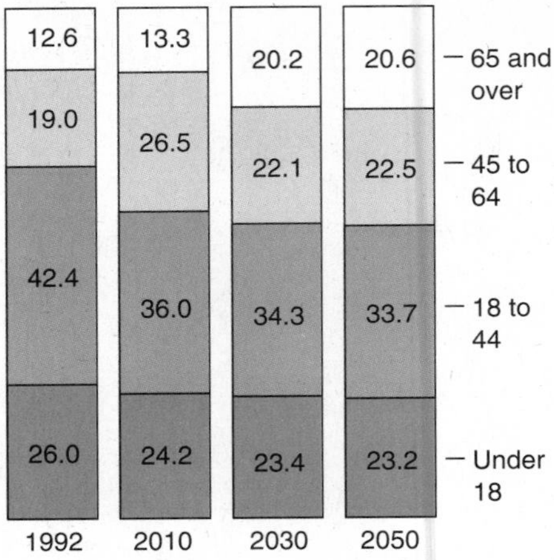

Fertility Rates

The **fertility, or natality, rate** is an expression of the number of births per 1,000 women of childbearing age (15–44) in the population during a specific time period. Fertility rates in the United States were at their highest at the beginning of this century. Those rates dipped during the Depression years but rebounded after World War II. The period of consistently high fertility rates immediately following World War II has become known as the "baby boom years," hence the name *baby boomers* for those born from 1946 through 1964. Since the end of the baby boom years, the fertility rate has steadily declined and is projected to continue to decline through the year 2000 (see Table 10.1). As the baby

---

median age   The age at which half of the population is older and half is younger.

FIGURE 10.8

Percent distribution of the population by age: 1992–2050 (middle series projections).

From: U.S. Bur. of the Census (1993). "How We're Changing: Demographic State of the Nation, 1993." Current Population Reports, *series p-23, no. 184. Washington, D.C.: U.S. Government Printing Office.*

boomers continue to age, a bulge can be seen ascending in the United States age pyramid (see Figure 10.7). A declining fertility rate means that there will be fewer and fewer young people in the United States relative to total population. This has significance for the future economic prospects of Social Security and Medicare, as we shall see, since there will be fewer young persons working to pay taxes.

Mortality Rates

The mortality, or death, rates (usually expressed in deaths per 1,000 population) also have an impact on the aging population. As can be seen in Table 10.2 the annual mortality rate in 1900 was 17.2 (per 1,000). That figure dropped to about 8.6 in 1990 and is projected to stay close to that lower figure through the year 2000. The decrease in annual mortality rate achieved over the first 75 years of this century was

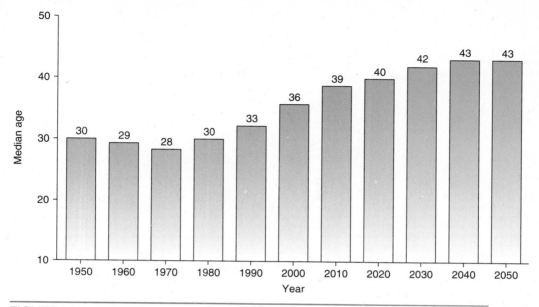

FIGURE 10.9

Median age of the population: 1950–2050.

From: U.S. Dept. of Health and Human Services (1991). Aging America: Trends and Projections (DHHS pub. no. FCOA-91-28001). Washington, D.C.: U.S. Government Printing Office, p. 6.

the result of triumphs in medical science and public health practice.[1]

Another demographic variable that interacts with the mortality rates is life expectancy. While the mortality rates in the United States have been fairly constant for more than twenty years, life expectancy has continued to increase. During this century, there has been an overall jump in life expectancy from 47.3 years in 1900 to 75.7 years in 1991. The life expectancies of men and blacks have always trailed those for women and whites, respectively (see Tables 7.4 and 10.3). While increases in life expectancy in the first half of the century can be attributed to the decrease in infant and early childhood deaths, increases in life expectancy since 1970 can be traced to the postponement of deaths among the middle-aged and senior populations.[7, 9, 10]

Migration

The movement of people from one country to another, **migration,** has also contributed to the aging of the population. **Net migration** is the population gain or loss from the movement of migrants in (immigration) and out (emigration) of a country. Historically, in the United States, net migration has resulted in population gain; more people immigrate than emigrate. The greatest immigration in the United States occurred between the end of the Civil War and the beginning of the Great Depression. Most of the immigrants were between the ages of 18 and 35 years, childbearing age. As these immigrants had children, the population of the United States remained young. However, the decline in immigration

net migration   The population gain or loss resulting from migration.

Table 10.1

Live Births, Birth Rates, and Fertility Rates, by Race: United States, Specified Years 1940–90

[Birth rates are live births per 1,000 population in specified group. Fertility rates per 1,000 women aged 15–44 years in specified group. Population enumerated as of April 1 for census years and estimated as of July 1 for all other years. Beginning with 1970, excludes births to nonresidents of the United States.]

Year	Number				Birth Rate				Fertility Rate			
	All Races	White	All Other Total	Black	All Races	White	All Other Total	Black	All Races	White	All Other Total	Black
Registered Births												
Race of mother:												
1990	4,158,212	3,290,273	867,939	684,336	16.7	15.8	21.7	22.4	70.9	68.3	83.2	86.8
1989	4,040,958	3,192,355	848,603	673,124	16.4	15.4	21.6	22.3	69.2	66.4	82.7	86.2
Race of child:												
1990	4,158,212	3,225,343	932,869	724,576	16.7	15.5	23.3	23.8	70.9	66.9	89.4	91.9
1985	3,760,561	2,991,373	769,188	608,193	15.8	14.8	21.4	21.3	66.3	63.1	82.3	82.4
1980*	3,612,258	2,898,732	713,526	589,616	15.9	14.9	22.5	22.1	68.4	64.7	88.6	88.1
1975*	3,144,198	2,551,996	592,202	511,581	14.6	13.6	21.0	20.7	66.0	62.5	87.7	87.9
1970†	3,731,386	3,091,264	640,122	572,362	18.4	17.4	25.1	25.3	87.9	84.1	113.0	115.4
1965†	3,760,358	3,123,860	636,498	581,126	19.4	18.3	27.6	27.7	96.3	91.3	131.9	133.2
1960†	4,257,850	3,600,744	657,106	602,264	23.7	22.7	32.1	31.9	118.0	113.2	153.6	153.5
Births Adjusted for Underregistration												
Race of child:												
1955	4,097,000	3,485,000	613,000	—	25.0	23.8	34.5	—	118.3	113.7	154.3	—
1950	3,632,000	3,108,000	524,000	—	24.1	23.0	33.3	—	106.2	102.3	137.3	—
1945	2,858,000	2,471,000	388,000	—	20.4	19.7	26.5	—	85.9	83.4	106.0	—
1940	2,559,000	2,199,000	360,000	—	19.4	18.6	26.7	—	79.9	77.1	102.4	—

*Based on 100% of births in selected states and on a 50% sample of births in all other states.

†Based on a 50% sample of births.

Note: Rates for 1981–1989 have been revised.

From: U.S. Dept. of Health and Human Services (1993). *Monthly Vital Statistics Report 41*(9-S): 17.

Table 10.2
Death Rates per 1,000 Population: 1900–2000

Year	Deaths per 1,000 Population
2000*	8.8
1995*	8.7
1990	8.6
1987	8.7
1985	8.7
1980	8.8
1975	8.8
1970	9.5
1965	9.4
1960	9.5
1955	9.3
1950	9.6
1945	10.6
1940	10.7
1935	10.9
1930	11.3
1925	11.7
1920	13.0
1915	13.2
1910	14.7
1905	15.9
1900	17.2

*Projected.

From: U.S. Bur. of the Census, *Statistical Abstract of the United States: 1990,* 110th ed. Washington, D.C., 1990.

U.S. Bur. of the Census, *Statistical Abstract of the United States: 1955,* 76th ed. Washington, D.C., 1955.

U.S. Bur. of the Census, *Statistical Abstract of the United States: 1946,* 67th ed. Washington, D.C., 1946.

Table 10.3
Life Expectancy at Specified Ages, by Race and Sex: United States, Selected Years 1960–1989

Age, Sex, and Race	Remaining Life Expectancy in Years			
	1960*	1970	1980	1990
White male				
At 65 years	12.9	13.1	14.2	15.2
At 85 years	4.4	5.2	5.0	5.0
Black male				
At 65 years	12.7	12.5	13.0	14.0
At 85 years	5.7	5.9	4.5	5.8
White female				
At 65 years	15.9	17.1	18.4	19.2
At 85 years	4.9	5.9	6.3	6.6
Black female				
At 65 years	15.1	15.7	16.8	17.3
At 85 years	6.2	7.0	6.1	7.0

*Includes deaths of nonresidents of the United States.

From: National Center for Health Statistics. *Vital Statistics of the United States,* vol. 2, part A, selected years.

following the Depression led to the aging of the American populace as the early immigrants grew old and were not replaced by younger immigrants.[1, 11]

Dependency (Support) and Labor-Force Ratios

Other demographic signs of an aging population are changes in dependency and labor-force ratios. The **dependency ratio** or **support ratio** is a comparison between those individuals whom society considers economically productive (the working population) and those it considers economically unproductive (the nonworking or dependent population).[1, 3, 12] Traditionally, the productive and nonproductive populations have been defined by age; the productive population includes those who are 15–59 years old,[12] 18–64,[3, 7] or 20–64.[1] The unproductive population includes both youth (0–14, 0–17, or 0–19 years old) and the elderly (60+ or 65+ years). When the dependency ratio includes both youth and elderly, it is referred

---

dependency (support) ratio A ratio that compares the number of individuals whom society considers economically productive to the number it considers economically unproductive.

to as **total dependency ratio.** When only the youth are compared to the productive group, the term used is **youth dependency (support) ratio,** and when only the elderly are compared, it is called **elderly dependency (support) ratio.**[1]

Communities can refer to dependency ratio data as a guide to the best social policy decisions and as a way to allocate resources. For example, leaders in a community with a relatively high youth dependency ratio compared to elderly dependency ratio may want to concentrate community resources on programs like education for the young, health promotion programs for children, special programs for working parents, and other youth-associated concerns. Communities with high elderly dependency ratios might increase programs for seniors.

As can be seen in Figure 10.10, the total dependency ratio in the United States is currently close to its lowest point in this century, and it is projected to stay low for the next 25–30 years Also, the current youth dependency ratio is greater than the elderly dependency ratio. The two ratios are expected to even out by 2030, after which time the elderly dependency ratio will be greater.

Such an increase in the elderly dependence ratio provides an interesting political scenario because the costs to support youth and the elderly are not the same.[12] Parents pay directly for most of the expenditures to support their children, with the primary exception being public education, which is paid for by taxes. In contrast, much of the support for seniors comes from tax-supported programs such as Social Security and Medicare and Medicaid. In order to meet the impending burden of the elderly, taxes will most certainly need to be raised. Therefore, the question for the future is, "Will the productive population be willing to pay increased taxes to support seniors?"

While dependency ratio data clearly show one trend, they are merely an estimate and should not be the only accepted estimate. Actually the dependency ratios presented in Figure 10.10 are not all that accurate.[9] These ratios are based on the assumption that everyone of productive age supports all members of the nonproductive age group. This is not true. A number of those in the productive age group (like homemakers, the unemployed, and some disabled persons) do not participate in the paid labor force. Conversely, many teenagers and older persons do. Thus, dependency ratios may provide misleading figures for decision makers.

Schulz et al.[12] believe that **labor-force dependency ratios** also need to be considered. Labor-force dependency ratios differ from dependency (support) ratios in that they are based on the number of people who are actually working and those who are not, independent of their ages. When labor force participation rates are used to calculate the labor-force dependency ratios, it is projected that the burden of support for the labor force in the future will be somewhat lighter than that projected through dependency ratios. Nonetheless, under either method of calculation, the ratio of workers to dependents will be lower in the future than it is today.

---

total dependency (support) ratio   The dependency ratio that includes both youth and elderly.
youth dependency (support) ratio   The dependency ratio that includes only youth.
elderly dependency (support) ratio   The dependency ratio that includes only the elderly.

labor-force dependency ratio   A ratio of the total number of those individuals who are working to the number of those who are not.

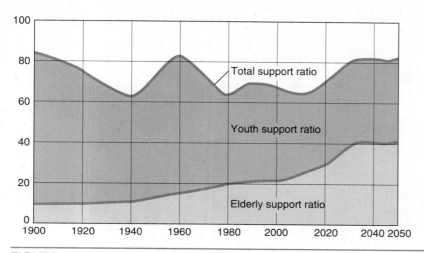

FIGURE 10.10

Trends in total support ratios, 1990–2050.

Note: Total Support Ratio is the sum of the Youth Support Ratio and the Elderly Support Ratio. Youth Support Ratio is the number of persons under age 20 divided by the number of persons aged 20–64 times 100. Elderly Support Ratio is the number of persons age 65 years and over divided by the number of persons aged 20–64 times 100.

Sources: Taeuber, Cynthia. U.S. Bur. of the Census (Sept. 1983). "America in Transition: An Aging Society."
Current Population Reports, series p. 23, no. 128. Spencer, Gregory. U.S. Bur. of the Census (Jan. 1989).
"Projections of the Population of the United States by Age, Sex, and Race: 1988 to 2080." Current Population
Reports, series p-25, no. 1018. Washington, D.C.: U.S. Government Printing Office (middle series projections).
U.S. Bur. of the Census. "Modified and Actual Age, Sex, Race, and Hispanic Origin Data." 1990 Census of
Population and Housing, series CPH.L-74, p. 1–2. Projections for certain years are from unpublished tables
consistent with p-25, no. 1018.

Other Demographic Variables of the Aging

There are a number of other demographic variables that will impact the community health programs of older Americans. Each of these is briefly described below.

Marital Status

Most senior men remain married until they die. In 1990, 74% of all senior men were married and living with their spouses, as compared to only 40% of senior women. In addition, senior women were three times more likely as men to be widowed (49% vs. 14%). There are three primary reasons for these differences. The first is that men have shorter average life expectancy and thus tend to precede their wives in death (see

Figure 10.11). Second, men tend to marry women who are younger than themselves. Finally, men who lose a spouse through death or divorce are more likely to remarry than women in the same situation.[7,9] These statistics imply that most elderly men have a spouse for assistance, especially when health fails, but most women do not.[9]

There also seems to be a new trend occurring with increasing frequency among seniors—divorce. In 1990, about 5% both of senior men and women were divorced. Thirty years ago, in 1960, less than 2% of elderly persons were divorced.[9] For the first time, a new type of senior is appearing in significant numbers—the divorced senior. These divorced seniors represent a new type of need group—those who lack the retirement bene-

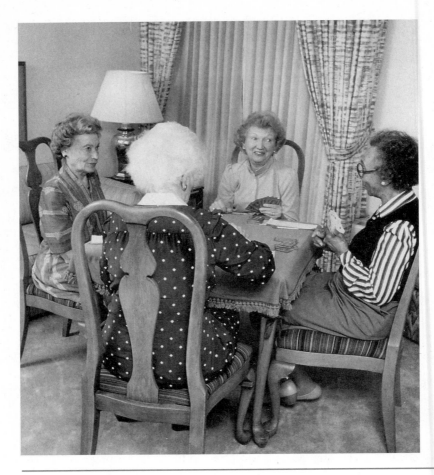

FIGURE 10.11

Senior women are three times more likely to be widowed than senior men.

fits, insurance, and net worth assets associated with being married.

Living Arrangements

In 1990, the majority (69%, 20.4 million) of noninstitutionalized seniors were living with someone else (spouse, relative, or other seniors), while the remainder (31%, 9.2 million) were living alone.[9] Of those living alone, nearly four in five are women (78.8%, 7.2 million), while just over one in five are men (21.2%, 1.9 million).[9]

Seniors who live alone constitute one of the most vulnerable and impoverished segments of American society. Of those who lived alone in 1990, 25% (2.3 million) were poor, the majority have a chronic illness, and they rely heavily on family, friends, and community services (senior centers, special transportation, meals, visiting nurses or health aides, and adult day care) for help. The proportion of those living alone is projected to remain about the same, but the numbers are expected to increase dramatically, from 9.2 million in 1990 to 10.9 million in 2005 to 15.2 million in 2020.[7, 9]

Racial and Ethnic Composition

The senior population in the United States is predominately white. Of the total senior population in 1990, about 28 million were white; 2.5 million black; 116,000 Native American; 450,000 Asian/Pacific Islanders; and 1.1 million were of Hispanic origin. The senior Asian/Pacific Islanders, Native Americans, and Americans of Hispanic origin populations had relatively large gains (75–220%) between 1980 and 1990.[9] These proportions are expected to remain relatively stable through the end of the century. However, beginning in the early part of the next century, the senior population will be much more racially and ethnically diverse than in 1990. Of the nearly 69 million seniors projected in 2050, nearly 10 million will be black, 5 million will belong to races other than white or black, and possibly 8 to 12 million will be Hispanic.[9] This growth will be the result of continued immigration and the higher fertility rates in nonwhites over the past 50 years.[7, 9]

Geographic Distribution

In 1990, about one-third of America's seniors lived in Southern states, and just over half lived in nine states: California, Florida, Illinois, Michigan, New Jersey, New York, Ohio, Pennsylvania, and Texas (see Figure 10.12). Each of these states had over 1 million seniors. California had the greatest

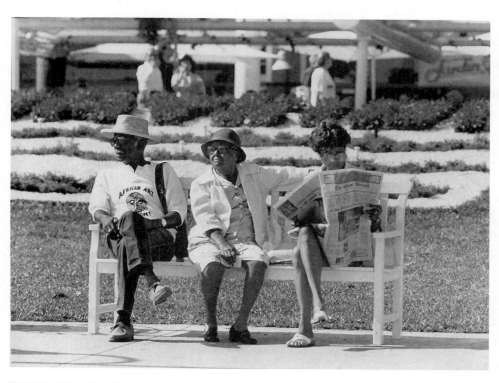

FIGURE 10.12

Many seniors choose to spend their retirement years in states with warm weather.

number, with 3.1 million; while Florida had the greatest proportion, with 18% (2.3 million people). The national average was about 12.5%.[7, 9] Some states (Midwestern) have a small total number of older adults but have a large percentage of their total population classified as older.

Populations of some states (such as Florida) "age" because of the inward migration of seniors, others (like the Farm Belt states) "age" because young people leave. Still other states "age" because of low fertility or some combination of factors.[9]

From an ethnic and racial standpoint, the largest percentage of minority-group seniors live in the southern and western parts of the country (see Table 10.4).

Economic Status

The overall economic position of seniors has improved significantly since the 1970s.[9] Nevertheless, seniors have a lower economic status than adults in the 25–64 age group. The annual median income of families with senior heads of households in 1989 was $22,806, as compared with $36,058 for fami-

Table 10.4
Persons 65 Years and Over for Regions, by Age, Sex, Race, and Hispanic Origin: 1990

Age, Race, and Hispanic Origin	United States	Northeast	Midwest	South	West
All persons					
65 years and over	31,241,831	6,995,156	7,749,130	10,724,182	5,773,363
65 to 84 years	28,161,666	6,285,347	6,909,267	9,732,160	5,234,892
85 years and over	3,080,165	709,809	839,863	992,022	538,471
White					
65 years and over	27,851,973	6,409,025	7,205,491	9,172,048	5,065,409
65 to 84 years	25,063,921	5,744,880	6,412,420	8,326,660	4,579,961
85 years and over	2,788,052	664,145	793,071	845,388	485,448
Black					
65 years and over	2,508,551	454,809	474,957	1,386,175	192,610
65 to 84 years	2,278,368	417,408	432,595	1,251,232	177,133
85 years and over	230,183	37,401	42,362	134,943	15,477
American Indian, Eskimo, and Aleut					
65 years and over	114,453	8,575	17,461	40,379	48,038
65 to 84 years	105,248	7,872	16,258	37,167	43,951
85 years and over	9,205	703	1,203	3,212	4,087
Asian and Pacific Islander					
65 years and over	454,458	64,960	30,427	39,525	319,546
65 to 84 years	424,720	61,132	28,681	37,491	297,416
85 years and over	29,738	3,828	1,746	2,034	22,130
Other races					
65 years and over	312,396	57,787	20,794	86,055	147,760
65 to 84 years	289,409	54,055	19,313	79,610	136,431
85 years and over	22,987	3,732	1,481	6,445	11,329
*Hispanic origin**					
65 years and over	1,161,283	199,502	71,169	446,984	443,628
65 to 84 years	1,066,719	183,808	65,525	409,681	407,705
85 years and over	94,564	15,694	5,644	37,303	35,923

*Hispanic origin may be of any race.

From: U.S. Bureau of the Census, 1990 Census of Population and Housing, Summary Tape File 1A.

Table 10.5

Poverty Thresholds in 1990, by Size of Family and Number of Related Children Under 18 Years

Size of Family Unit	Weighted Average Thresholds	Related Children Under 18 Years								
		None	One	Two	Three	Four	Five	Six	Seven	Eight or More
One person (unrelated individual)	$6,652									
Under 65 years	6,800	$6,800								
65 years and over	6,268	6,268								
Two persons	8,509									
Householder under 65 years	8,794	8,752	$9,009							
Householder 65 years and over	7,905	7,900	8,975							
Three persons	10,419	10,223	10,520	$10,530						
Four persons	13,359	13,481	13,701	13,254	$13,301					
Five persons	15,792	16,257	16,494	15,989	15,598	$15,359				
Six persons	17,839	18,693	18,773	18,386	18,015	17,464	$17,137			
Seven persons	20,241	21,515	21,650	21,187	20,864	20,262	19,561	$18,791		
Eight persons	22,582	24,063	24,276	23,839	23,456	23,913	22,223	21,505	$21,323	
Nine persons or more	26,848	28,946	29,087	28,700	28,375	27,842	27,108	26,445	26,280	$25,268

From: U.S. Bur. of the Census (1991). "Poverty in the United States 1990." *Current Population Reports* (series P-60, no. 175). Washington, D.C.: U.S. Government Printing Office, p. 195.

BOX 10.2
Determining the Poverty Level

The poverty level, developed by the Social Security Administration in 1964 and revised in 1969 and 1981 by interagency committees, is often used as an index of income need. The definition was established as the official definition of poverty for statistical use in all Executive departments by the Bureau of the Budget (in *Circular No. A-46*) and later by the Office of Management and Budget (in *Statistical Directive No. 14*).

The original poverty index provided a range of income cutoffs adjusted by such factors as family size, sex of the family head, number of children under 18 years old, and farm-nonfarm residence. At the core of this definition of poverty was the economy food plan, the least costly of four nutritionally adequate food plans designed by the Department of Agriculture. It was determined from the Department of Agriculture's 1955 survey of food consumption that families of three or more persons spent approximately one-third of their income on food; the poverty level for these families was, therefore, set at three times the cost of the economy food plan. For smaller families and persons living alone, the cost of the economy food plan was multiplied by factors that were slightly higher in order to compensate for the relatively larger fixed expenses of these smaller households. Annual revisions of these SSA poverty cutoffs were based on price changes of the items in the economy food budget.

As a result of deliberations of a federal interagency committee in 1969, the following two modifications to the original SSA definition of poverty were recommended: (1) that the SSA thresholds for nonfarm families be retained for the base year 1963, but that annual adjustments in the levels be based on changes in the Consumer Price Index (CPI) rather than on changes in the cost of food included in the economy food plan; and (2) that

the farm thresholds be raised from 70% to 85% of the corresponding nonfarm levels. The combined impact of these two modifications resulted in an increase of 360,000 poor families and 1.6 million poor persons in 1967.

In 1980, another interagency committee recommended three additional modifications that were implemented in the March 1982 CPS as well as the 1980 census: (1) elimination of separate thresholds for farm families, (2) averaging of thresholds for female-householder and "all other" families, and (3) extension of the poverty matrix to families with nine or more members. For further details, see the section, "Changes in the Definition of Poverty," in *Current Population Reports,* Series P-60, No. 133.

The poverty thresholds rise each year by the same percentage as the annual average Consumer Price Index. The table 1 shows the CPI and the corresponding thresholds for a family of four for the 1959–1990 period.

Consumer Price Index and Average Poverty Threshold for a Family of Four: 1959–1990

Year	Consumer Price Index (1967 = 100)	Average Threshold for a Family of Four Persons*
1990	391.3	$13,359
1989	371.3	$12,674
1988	354.3	12,092
1987	340.4	11,611
1986	328.4	11,203
1985	322.2	10,989
1984	311.1	10,609
1983	298.4	10,178
1982	289.1	9,862
1981	272.4	9,287
1980	246.8	8,414
1979	217.4	7,412
1978	195.4	6,662
1977	181.5	6,191
1976	170.5	5,815

			BOX 10.2 (continued)			
Year	Consumer Price Index (1967 = 100)	Average Threshold for a Family of Four Persons*	Year	Consumer Price Index (1967 = 100)	Average Threshold for a Family of Four Persons*
1975	161.2	5,500	1966	97.2	3,317
1974	147.7	5,038	1965	94.5	3,223
1973	133.1	4,540	1964	92.9	3,169
1972	125.3	4,275	1963	91.7	3,128
1971	121.3	4,137	1962	90.6	3,089
1970	116.3	3,968	1961	89.6	3,054
1969	109.8	3,743	1960	88.7	3,022
1968	104.2	3,553	1959	87.3	2,973
1967	100.0	3,410			

*For years prior to 1981, average threshold for a nonfarm family of four is shown.

From: U.S. Bur. of the Census (1991). "Poverty in the United States, 1990." *Current Population Reports* (series P-60, no. 175). Washington, D.C.: U.S. Government Printing Office, pp. 194–195.

lies with heads whose ages were 25–64 years. However, the median income for seniors not living in families was $9,422, less than half that of comparable people under 65 ($20,277). One-fourth of seniors have incomes and other economic resources below or just barely above the poverty level—a measure of adequacy of financial income in relation to a minimal level of consumption (see Box 10.2). The poverty levels for 1990 are presented in Table 10.5. Since most seniors do not work, they are economically more vulnerable to circumstances beyond their control, such as the loss of a spouse; deteriorating health and self-sufficiency; changes in Social Security, Medicare, and Medicaid legislation; and inflation.[7]

Housing

Of all the households in the United States in 1990, 22% (20.2 million) were headed by seniors. Of this number, approximately 76% were owner-occupied and 24% were rental units. Characteristic of the households of seniors are: (1) homes of lower values than homes of younger people, (2) homes in need of repair (7% of seniors' homes have physical problems), and (3)

homes without telephones (9% versus 3% of households headed by younger people).[7]

Geographically, most senior householders live in the suburbs (42% versus 31% in metropolitan areas and 27% outside metropolitan areas). Regionally, about one-third of the senior householders live in the South, about one-fourth each in the Northeast and Midwest, and about one-fifth in the West.[13]

For most seniors, housing represents an asset because they have no mortgage or rental payments or they can sell their home for a profit. But for others with low incomes, housing becomes a heavy burden. The cost of utilities, real estate taxes, insurance, repair, and maintenance have forced many to sell their property or live in a less-desirable residence.

SPECIAL NEEDS OF SENIORS

Atchley[14] lists five essential needs that determine life-styles for people of all ages. They are: income, housing, health care, transportation, and community facilities and services. However, the aging process can alter these needs in unpredictable ways. While younger seniors usually do not experience appreciable changes in their lifestyles relative to these five needs, seniors in the old old group (75–84) and the oldest old group (85 and older) eventually do. The remaining portions of this chapter will explore these five needs, discuss their implications for seniors, and describe community services for seniors. In addition, we will identify and discuss a sixth need that is specific to seniors—personal care.

Income

Though the need for income continues throughout one's life, achieving senior status often reduces income needs. Perhaps the major reduction occurs with one's retirement. Retirees need not purchase job-related items such as special clothing or tools, pay union dues, or join professional associa-

tions. Expenses are further reduced because retirees no longer commute every day, buy meals away from home, or spend money on business travel. Reaching senior status also usually means that children are grown and no longer dependent, and the home mortgage is often paid off. Taxes are usually lower because income is lower. Many community services are offered at reduced prices for seniors.

But aging usually means increased expenses for health care and for home maintenance and repairs that aging homeowners can no longer do themselves. In spite of these increased costs, the overall need for income seems to decrease slightly for people after retirement.

There are five sources of income for seniors: retirement benefits (Social Security, government employee pensions, and private pensions or annuities), earnings from jobs, income from assets (e.g., savings accounts, stocks, bonds, real estate, etc.), public assis-

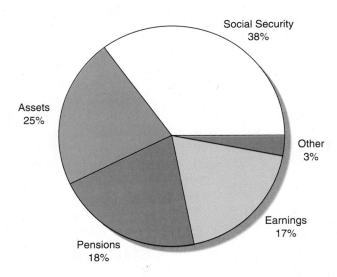

FIGURE 10.13

Income sources of people 65 years of age and older.

From: Grad, Susan (June 1990). Income of the Population 65 or Over, 1988. *Pub. no. 13-11871. Washington, D.C.: U.S. Social Security Administration.*

Table 10.6

Elderly and Nonelderly People, by Ratio of Income to Poverty: 1989

Ratio of Income to Poverty Level	Number (in thousands)		Percent	
	Under 65	65+	Under 65	65+
Below poverty	28,165	3,369	13.0	11.4
100–124% of poverty level	8,845	2,280	4.1	7.7
125–149% of poverty level	8,979	2,404	4.1	8.1
Total below 150% of poverty level	45,989	8,053	21.2	27.2

From: U.S. Bur. of the Census (Sept. 1990). "Money Income and Poverty Status in the United States: 1989." *Current Population Reports* (series P-60, no. 168). Washington, D.C.: U.S. Government Printing Office, p. 41.

tance for the poor seniors, and miscellaneous sources. Seniors depend more heavily on Social Security for their income than on any other single source (see Figure 10.13). During 1988, 90% of seniors received some income from Social Security, 13% received all their income from Social Security, and 30% depended on Social Security for 80% or more of their income.[7] It should be noted that the benefits received from Social Security are very modest. The average Social Security payments to retired couples and to individuals are only slightly higher than their respective poverty levels.

In recent years, the income of seniors has improved significantly. When income and other assets of seniors are combined, the economic status of seniors and nonseniors is not that far apart. However, the fact remains that 27% of seniors have incomes at or below 149% of the poverty level (see Table 10.6). This group of seniors consists predominately of widows, retirees with no private pensions, lifelong poor, women, and minorities. Many seniors are financially unable to live a comfortable life-style. At the present time, the only way for seniors to increase their incomes is by getting a job, applying for public assistance (e.g., low rent housing, food stamps, Supplemental Security Income), or requesting help from their families.

Housing

Housing is an important source of continuity for seniors. A home is more than just a place to live. It is a symbol of independence; a place for family gatherings; a source of pleasant memories; and a link to friends, the neighborhood, and the community.[14]

Probably the single biggest change in the housing needs of seniors is the need for special modifications because of physical disabilities. Such modifications can be very simple, such as handrails for support in bathrooms, or more complex, such as chair lifts for stairs. Sometimes there is need for live-in help, while at other times, disabilities may force seniors to leave their homes and seek specialized housing. Table 10.7 provides a listing of levels of housing by degree of independence.

The decision to remove seniors from their long-term residences is not easily made. Because of the psychological and social value of the home, changing a senior's place of residence has negative effects for both the senior and the family members who help make the arrangements for the move. Recognizing the importance of a home and independence, families often feel tremendous conflict and guilt in deciding to move a senior relative. If the senior does not adjust to the new situa-

Table 10.7
Levels of Housing, by Degree of Independence

Housing Type	Significant Criteria
Independent household:	
Fully independent	Household is self-contained, self-sufficient; residents do 90% or more of cooking and household chores.
Semi-independent	Household is self-contained but not entirely self-sufficient; may require some assistance with cooking and household chores (e.g., an independent household augmented by meals-on-wheels, homemaker services, or adult foster care).
Group housing:	
Congregate housing	Household may still be self-contained but is less self-sufficient; cooking and household tasks are often incorporated into the housing unit. (A common example is the full-service retirement community.)
Personal care home	Resident unit is neither self-contained nor self-sufficient; help given in getting about, personal care, grooming, and so forth. Cooking and household tasks are usually done by paid staff. (A common type is the group home.)
Nursing home	Resident units are neither self-contained nor self-sufficient; total care, including health, personal, and household functions. (A common example is the skilled nursing facility.)

From: Atchley, R.C. (1991). *Social Forces and Aging,* 6th ed. Belmont, Calif.: Wadsworth.

tion, the guilt continues. Sometimes family members continue to question their decision even after the senior dies. Though moving a senior is very difficult, it is usually best for all involved. For example, moving a frail person from a two-story to a one-story home makes good sense. Or moving a senior from a very large home to a smaller home or an apartment is logical.[1]

One of the biggest fears associated with relocating a senior is the move to group housing, especially a nursing home. The stereotype that many people have about group housing is not very positive, and most know it can be very expensive: $2,200–4,000 per month for a total care nursing home. However, just like any other consumer product, good group homes are available. Today, only 6% of those age 65+ live in group housing, but that figure jumps to 25% at age 85+. And it is estimated that 43% of persons over 65 will spend some time in a nursing home during their life.[15]

To ease the stress and anxiety of relocating a senior, Borup[16] has noted the following:

1. Relocation stress is usually temporary.
2. Those unwilling to move are most likely to experience stress.
3. Making the new environment predictable to the senior can help to reduce stress.
4. Keeping those being moved and their families informed can help to reduce stress.

The relocation of seniors is not always traumatic or against their will. Many seniors are finding housing in communities that have been planned as **retirement communities.** Though these communities are available in all areas of the country,

---

retirement communities Residential communities that have been specifically developed for those in their retirement years.

they are most popular in areas with temperate climates (see Figure 10.14). Some of the communities are built as private associations, while others are developed as special areas within larger, already established communities. Legally, the private associations are able to adopt by-laws that put restrictions on the residents, such as a minimum age to move into the area, no children under a certain age living in the residence, and no pets. Retirement communities usually offer a variety of housing alternatives, ranging from home or condominium owner-

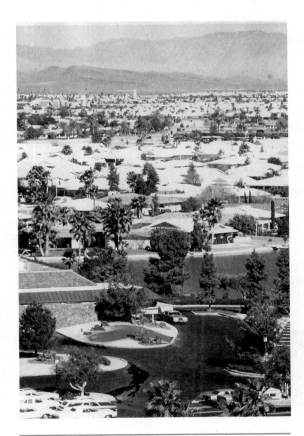

FIGURE 10.14
Sun City, Arizona, is one of the largest and most popular totally planned retirement communities in the United States.

ship to apartment living. Since these communities are developed to meet the needs of seniors, special accommodations are usually made for socializing, recreation, shopping, transportation, and selected educational programs.

Among the most recent innovations in the retirement community industry are the **continuing-care retirement communities** (CCRCs). Such communities guarantee the residents a lifelong residence and health care. They work in the following way: the retirees either purchase or term lease (sometimes lifelong) a living unit on a campuslike setting. The living unit could be a single-family dwelling; an apartment; or a room, as in a nursing home. In addition to the living units, the campus usually includes a health clinic and often has either a nursing home or health care center. These other facilities are available to the residents for an additional fee. Residents of the CCRCs can live as independently as they wish but have available to them a variety of services, including housekeeping, meals, transportation, organized recreational and social activities, health care, and security. Many living units are equipped with emergency call buttons.

CCRCs are a housing alternative for well-to-do seniors.[1, 17, 18] Unfortunately, CCRCs are beyond the reach of many seniors. The purchase or lifelong lease is more than $100,000, and the fee for each service is extra. Obviously, seniors who enter into contractual agreements for CCRCs should read their contracts carefully before signing them.

Of all the housing problems that confront seniors, the availability of affordable housing is the biggest. Unfortunately, those

continuing-care retirement communities (CCRCs) Planned communities for seniors which guarantee a lifelong residence and health care.

seniors who are most in need of such housing are often frail and disabled, have low incomes, and live in rural areas. There is no federal program to help finance low-cost nonmedical housing programs, even though there is a shortage of low-rent, private housing and public housing. New public policy is needed to change this situation. Housing seems to be less of a problem for the chronically ill, because Medicaid and, to a far lesser extent, Medicare help pay the cost.[14]

Health Care

Health care is a major issue for all segments of our society but particularly for seniors. While significant progress has been made in extending life expectancy, a longer life does not necessarily mean a healthier life. Health problems naturally increase with age. More than four out of five seniors live with at least one chronic condition, and many, especially women, have multiple chronic conditions. The ten most frequently occurring conditions for seniors in 1989 were: arthritis (48.3%), hypertension (38.0%), hearing impairment (28.6%), heart disease (27.9%), cataracts (15.7%), orthopedic impairments (15.5%), chronic sinusitis (15.3%), diabetes (8.8%), visual impairments (8.2%), and varicose veins (7.8%).[7] With these conditions comes a need for increased health care services (see Box 10.3).

Seniors are the heaviest users of health care services. On the average, seniors visit a physician eight times per year compared with only five visits by the general population. They are hospitalized more than three times as often as younger people, stay in the hospital 50% longer, and use twice as many prescription drugs.[7] In addition, seniors have higher usage rates for professional dental care (3.2 versus 2.8 visits per year), vision aids (93% versus 46% with corrective lenses), and medical equipment and supplies, than people under age 65. Usage of

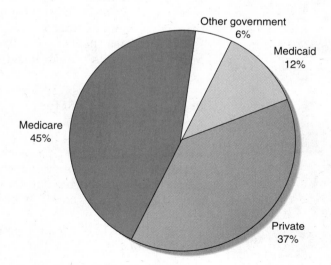

FIGURE 10.15

Personal health care expenditures for the elderly, by source of payment: 1987.

From: Waldo, Daniel R., Sally T. Sonnefeld, David R. McKusick, and Ross H. Arnett III. "Health Expenditures by Age Group, 1977 and 1987." Health Care Financing Review *10, no. 4 (Summer 1989).*

BOX 10.3
Healthy People 2000—Objective

17.6 Reduce significant hearing impairment to a prevalence of no more than 82 per 1,000 people. (Baseline: Average of 88.9 per 1,000 during 1986–1988)

Special Population Target

Hearing Impairment (per 1,000)	1986–88 Baseline	2000 Target	Percent Decrease
17.6a People aged 45 and older	203	180	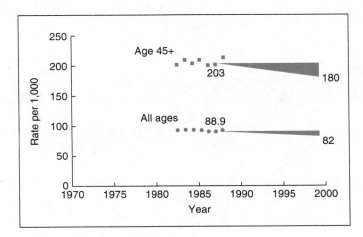

Note: Hearing impairment covers the range of hearing deficits from mild loss in one ear to profound loss in both ears. Generally, inability to hear sounds at levels softer (less intense) than 20 decibels (dB) constitutes abnormal hearing. Significant hearing impairment is defined as having hearing thresholds for speech poorer than 25 dB. However, for this objective, self-reported hearing impairment (i.e., deafness in one or both ears or any trouble hearing in one or both ears) will be used as a proxy measure for significant hearing impairment.

Baseline data source: National Health Interview Survey, CDC.

Prevalence of hearing impairment.

For Further Thought

Most people either have a grandparent or know another senior who has a hearing impairment. As a younger person, what is your reaction to seniors when they ask you to repeat a sentence one or more times? How do you think the seniors feel when they have to ask you to repeat it?

health care services increases with age, and much of the money spent in health care is spent in the last year of life.

While private sources, such as employer-paid insurance, are the major sources of health care payment for people under age 65, public funds are used to pay for the majority (63%) of the health care expenses for seniors (see Figure 10.15). Medicare, which was enacted in 1965 and became effective July 1, 1966, provides almost universal health insurance coverage for seniors (in 1989, only 5.2% of people over age 65 were not covered). Medicare, which covered about 45% of all personal health care expenditures of seniors in 1987, has a primary role of financing acute care services (see Figures 10.16 and 10.17). It covered about 67% of all hospital care, 61% of physician costs, and only 1% of seniors' nursing home costs in 1987.[7] As concerns about the

federal budget deficit grow, the percentage of medical expense covered by Medicare may decline.

In addition to Medicare, approximately three-fourths of seniors have private health insurance to supplement their Medicare coverage. This private insurance is referred to as *Medigap,* because it helps to fill the gaps in health care cost that Medicare leaves. Also Medicaid, a federal-state program, helps to cover the health care costs of poor seniors, primarily for nursing home care (continuing care), home health care, and prescription drugs (see Figure 10.18). (See Chapter 14 for a complete discussion of Medicare, Medicaid, and Medigap.)

All indications are that the health care costs for seniors will continue to escalate because of the aging population and rising health care costs. Future legislators will be forced to choose from among the following

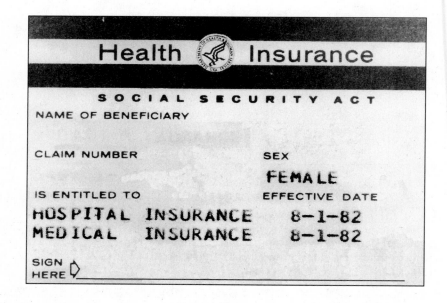

FIGURE 10.16

Medicare provides almost universal health insurance for seniors.

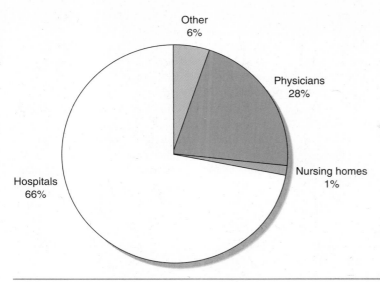

FIGURE 10.17

Where the Medicare dollar for the elderly went: 1987.

Note: Total exceeds 100% due to rounding.

From: Waldo, Daniel R., Sally T. Sonnefeld, David R. McKusick, and Ross H. Arnett III. "Health Expenditures by Age Group, 1977 and 1987." Health Care Financing Review 10, no. 4 (Summer 1989).

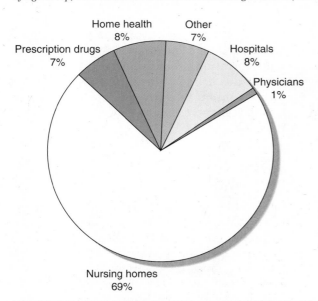

FIGURE 10.18

Where the Medicaid dollar for the elderly went: 1989.

From: Reilly, Thomas W., Steven B. Clauser, and David K. Baugh. "Trends in Medicaid Payment and Utilization, 1975–1989." Health Care Financing Review (1990 Annual Supplement).

alternatives: (1) raising taxes to pay for the care, (2) cutting back on coverage presently offered, or (3) completely revamping the present system under which care is funded.

In the meantime, the importance of instilling in Americans the value of preventing the onset of chronic diseases through healthy living cannot be overstated. While it is not possible to prevent all chronic health problems, encouraging healthy behaviors is a step in the right direction.

Transportation

Transportation is of prime importance to seniors because it enables them to remain independent. The two factors that have the greatest effect on the transportation needs of seniors are income and health status. Some seniors who have always driven their own automobiles eventually find that they are no longer able to do so. The ever-increasing costs of purchasing and maintaining an automobile sometimes become prohibitive on a fixed income. Also, with age come physical problems such as visual impairments or other disabilities that restrict one's ability to operate an automobile safely. Those with extreme disabilities may find that they will need a modified automobile (to accommodate their disability) or specialized transportation (e.g., a vehicle that can accommodate a wheelchair) in order to be transported.

With regard to transportation needs, seniors can be categorized into three different groups: (1) those who can use the present forms of transportation, whether it be their own vehicle or public transportation, (2) those who could use public transportation if the barriers of cost and access (no service available) were removed, and (3) those who need special services beyond those available through public transportation.[14]

Approximately 10 million senior Americans *cannot* afford a car, bus fare, or a taxi ride. Another 8 million live in areas (mostly rural and suburban) that are without public transportation service.[14] The unavailability of transportation greatly restricts the activities and curtails the independence of these people.

The unavailability of transportation services has stimulated a number of private and public organizations that serve seniors (e.g., churches, community services and facilities) to provide these services. Some communities even subsidize the cost of public transportation by offering reduced rates for seniors. While these services have been helpful to seniors, mobility is still more difficult for seniors than for other adults. Try to imagine what it would be like if you had to depend constantly on someone else for all your transportation needs.

The ideal solution to the transportation needs of seniors according to Atchley[14] would include four components: (1) fare reductions or discounts for all public transportation, including that for interstate travel, (2) subsidies to insure adequate scheduling and routing of present public transportation, (3) subsidized taxi fares for the disabled and infirm, and (4) funds for senior centers to purchase and equip vehicles to transport seniors properly, especially in rural areas.

Community Facilities and Services

As has been mentioned several times within this chapter, one of the most common occurrences of the aging process is loss of independence. Even some of the most basic activities of nonseniors become major tasks for seniors because of lack of income, ill health, and lack of transportation. Because of the limitations of seniors and the barriers they must face, they have special needs with regard to community facilities and services. If these needs are met, the life-styles of seniors are greatly enhanced. If not, they are confronted with anything from a slight inconvenience to a very poor quality of life.

With a view toward improving the lives of seniors, Congress enacted the **Older Americans Act of 1965** and has amended it several times since. Among the programs created by key amendments are the national nutrition program for seniors (1972), the Area Agencies on Aging (1973), and Title programs (I, II, III, IV, V, VI) to increase the services and protect the rights of seniors (1981, 1987).

Though the act and all its amendments are important, the services and facilities available to seniors were greatly improved after the passage of the 1973 amendments, which established the Area Agencies on Aging (AAsA). Each agency is responsible for "developing plans for a comprehensive and coordinated network of services to older people and offering services in the areas of information and referral, escort, transportation, and outreach."[14] The amendments were written to provide the AAsA with the flexibility to develop plans that allow for local variations. In 1992, there were approximately 700 AAsA in the United States.

With each part of the country—and for that matter each community—having its own peculiarities, the services available to seniors can vary greatly from one community to another. "It is important to keep in mind, however, that the growth in our nation's senior population, combined with this population's financial ability to pay for service, has created an entrepreneurial atmosphere surrounding adult care services. In some larger communities, or in those communities with a large number of senior residents, the range of services can be astonish-

ing."[1] Presented below is a list with brief descriptions of facilities and services available in many communities. To inquire about eligibility for and availability of these services, seniors should contact their local Area Agency on Aging.

Meal Service

The 1972 amendments to the Older Americans Act outlined a national nutrition program for seniors and provided funds for communities to take on such a task. Today's meal services are provided through delivered meal and congregate meal programs. The concept of the home-delivered meal programs (often known as **Meals-on-Wheels**) is the regular delivery of meals, usually once a day, five to seven days per week, to seniors in their homes. The meals are prepared in a central location, sometimes a health care facility or senior center, and delivered by community volunteers (see Box 10.4).

Congregate meal programs are provided for individuals who can travel to a central site, often within publicly funded housing units. Usually, it is the noon meal that is provided. Generally, these meals are funded by federal and state monies and make use of commodity food services.[1] In recent years, congregate meal programs seem to be gaining favor over home-delivered meal programs because they also provide social interaction (see Figure 10.19) and the opportunity to tie in with other social services.[14] However, there will always be a segment of the population requiring home-delivered meals because of their homebound status.

Older Americans Act of 1965 Federal legislation to improve the lives of seniors.

Meals-on-Wheels program A community-supported nutrition program in which prepared meals are delivered to seniors in their homes, usually by volunteers.

congregate meal programs Community-sponsored nutrition programs that provide meals at a central site, such as a senior center.

Both types of meal programs are strictly
regulated by federal and state guidelines to
ensure that the meals meet standard nutritional requirements. The cost of the meals
varies by site and client income level.
Seniors may pay full price, pay a portion of
the cost, or just make a contribution. When
the program is fully supported by federal,
state, or local funding (e.g., United Way),
the meals are free.

Homemaker Service

For a number of seniors, periodic home-
maker services can be the critical factor en-
abling them to remain in their own homes.
For these seniors, physical impairment restricts their ability to carry out normal
housekeeping activities such as houseclean-
ing, laundry, and meal preparation. The
availability of these services allows many

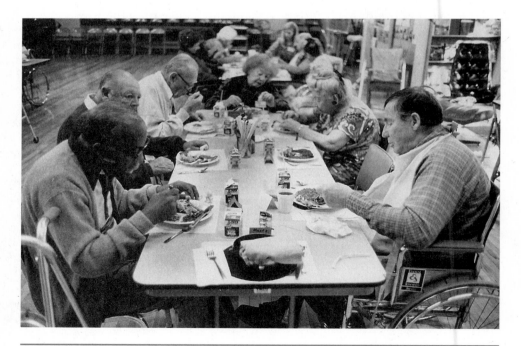

FIGURE 10.19

Congregate meals programs are gaining favor over Meals-on-Wheels programs because of the social interaction.

seniors to live semi-independently and delays their moving in with relatives or into group housing.

Chore and Home Maintenance Service

Chore and home maintenance service includes such services as yard work, cleaning gutters and windows, installing screens and storms, making minor plumbing and electrical repairs, maintaining the furnace and air conditioners, and helping to adapt a home to any impairments seniors might have. This adaptation may include provisions for wheelchairs and installing ramps or special railings to assist seniors to move from one area to another. Chore and home maintenance service, which is most often used by senior single women, is usually available through referrals from Area Agencies on Aging.

Visitor Service

Social interaction and social contacts are an important need for every human being, regardless of age. **Visitor services** amount to one individual taking time to visit with another person who is **homebound,** unable to leave his or her residence. This service is usually done on a voluntary basis, many times with seniors doing the visiting, and serves both homebound and those who are institutionalized. It is not uncommon for church or social organizations to conduct a visitor program for homebound members.

Adult Day Care Service

Adult day care programs provide care during the daytime hours for seniors who are unable to be left alone. These relatively new services are modeled after child day care services. Most programs offer meals, snacks, and social activities for the clients. Some either provide or make arrangements for the clients to receive therapy, counseling, education, or other services. Other day care programs are designed for seniors with special needs like Alzheimer clients, the blind, or veterans. Adult day care programs allow families to continue with daytime activities while still providing the primary care for a senior family member.

Respite Care Service

Respite care is planned, short-term care. Such care allows families who provide primary care for a senior family member to leave their senior in a supervised care setting for anywhere from a day to a few weeks. Respite services provide full care, including sleeping quarters, meals, bathing facilities, social activities, and the monitoring of medications.[1] This is the service most frequently requested by informal caregivers.[19] (See the section on personal care later in chapter.) Such a program allows primary caregivers to take a vacation, visit other relatives, or to be otherwise relieved from constant caregiving responsibilities.

Home Health Care Service

For seniors who do not need to be hospitalized but are unable, because of transportation, cost, or impairment, to go to health care providers, there are **home health care services.** These programs, run by official health agencies, like the local

---

homebound A person unable to leave home for normal activities.
visitor services One individual taking time to visit with another who is unable to leave his or her residence.
adult day care programs Daytime care provided to seniors who are unable to be left alone.

respite care Planned short-term care, usually for the purpose of relieving a full-time informal caregiver.
home health care services Health care services provided in the patient's place of residence.

health department, hospitals, and private companies, provide a full range of services including preventive, primary, rehabilitative, and therapeutic services in the client's home. The care is often provided by nurses, home health aides, and personal care workers (licensed health care workers), and may be paid for by Medicare or reimbursed by Medigap insurance policies. Unfortunately, Medicaid, which pays for nursing home care, will not pay for home health care, which is less expensive.

Senior Centers

The enactment of the Older Americans Act of 1965 provided funds to develop multipurpose **senior centers,** facilities where seniors can congregate for fellowship, meals, education, and recreation. Today, most larger communities throughout the United States have senior centers, which may represent the community's sole attempt to provide recreational and educational programs for seniors. Nationwide, the centers are not used extensively (usually by less than 10% of the eligible population).[14] This may be because the centers seem unattractive to healthy seniors and inaccessible to the ill and poor. In some communities, senior centers serve as sites for congregate meals and provide a central location for offering a variety of other senior services including legal assistance, income counseling, income tax return assistance, program referrals, employment services, and other appropriate services and information.

Other Services

There are many other services available to seniors in some communities. Usually, the larger the community and the number of seniors living in the community, the greater the variety of available services. The types of services provided in any one community is limited only by the creativity

of those providing service. Conner[1] even reports that in some communities, "service packages" are being offered. Such packages allow seniors to pick several services they need and pay for them as if they were a single service.

Personal Care

While most seniors are able to care for themselves, there is a significant minority of seniors who require personal assistance for an optimal or even adequate existence. The size of this minority increases as the seniors attain old old (75–84) and oldest old (85+) status.

Several authors[1, 9, 20–22] have identified four different levels of tasks with which seniors may need assistance:

1. Instrumental tasks—such as housekeeping, transportation, maintenance on the automobile or yard, and assistance with business affairs.
2. Expressive tasks—including emotional support, socializing and inclusion in social gatherings, and trying to prevent feelings of loneliness and isolation.
3. Cognitive tasks—assistance that involves scheduling appointments, monitoring health conditions, reminding seniors of the need to take medications, and in general, acting as a backup memory.
4. Tasks of daily living—such as eating, bathing, dressing, toileting, walking, getting in and out of bed or a chair, and getting outside. (Note: This last group of tasks, in addition to being a part of this listing, has special significance. These items have been used to develop a scale, called **Activities of Daily Living**

Activities of Daily Living (ADLs) Eating, toileting, dressing, bathing, walking, getting in and out of a bed or chair, and getting outside.

Table 10.8
Functional Limitations

*(Percent distribution of persons 65 years of age and over by activities of daily living
for which difficulty was reported and percent of persons who received the help
of another person in performing activities of daily living,
according to sex and age: United States, 1986)*

Age and Sex	Number of ADLs		
	None	*With Difficulty One or More*	*Help Received One or More*
Sex			
Male	81.9	18.2	6.7
Female	74.2	25.8	12.1
Age			
65–74 years	83.2	16.9	5.9
75–84 years	71.1	29.0	13.5
85 years and over	55.5	44.4	28.8
Male			
65–74 years	84.8	15.3	5.2
75–84 years	78.5	21.6	8.0
85 years and over	64.9	35.1	18.9
Female			
65–74 years	81.9	18.2	6.4
75–84 years	66.6	33.4	16.8
85 years and over	51.5	48.6	32.9

Note: Activities of daily living (ADLs) include eating, toileting, dressing, bathing, walking, getting in and out of a bed or chair, and getting outside.

From: National Center for Health Statistics: Data from the National Health Interview Survey.

[ADLs], to measure **functional limitations.** *Functional limitation* refers to a difficulty in performing personal care and home management tasks. See Table 10.8.)

When seniors begin to need help with one or more of these tasks, it is usually adult children or other family members who first provide the help, thus assuming the role of informal caregivers. An **informal caregiver** has been defined as one who pro-

vides unpaid care or assistance to one who has some physical, mental, emotional, or financial need that limits his or her independence.[1, 22, 23] An informal caregiver can be either a care-provider or care-manager.[24] The **care-provider** helps identify the needs of the individual and personally performs the caregiving service. Obviously, this can only be done if the person-in-need and the caregiver live in close proximity to each other. The **care-manager** also helps to identify

---

functional limitations Difficulty in performing personal care and home management tasks.
informal caregiver One who provides unpaid assistance to one who has some physical, mental, emotional, or financial need limiting his or her independence.

care-provider One who helps identify the health care needs of an individual and also personally performs the caregiving service.
care-manager One who helps identify the health care needs of an individual but does not actually provide the health care services.

the needs, but because of living some distance away or for other reasons, does not provide the service. The care-manager makes arrangements for someone else (volunteer or paid) to provide the services.

With the aging of the population, it is now most probable that many, if not most, adults can expect to have some responsibility as caregivers for their parents (see Figure 10.20). Their role may be as care-provider, care-manager, or in making the decision to relocate their parents by bringing them into their home, moving them to a smaller home or apartment, or moving them into a group home. This is a relatively new task since many of the seniors of today did not have to care for their parents. Life expectancy was much shorter, and most did not live long enough to be cared for by their adult children.

Caregivers for seniors face a number of problems including decreased personal free-dom, lack of privacy, constant demands on their time and energy, resentment that siblings do not share in the caregiving, and an increased financial burden. Many experience feelings of guilt for asking a spouse to help with the care of an in-law, or in knowing that the end of caregiving responsibilities usually means either the elder person's death or placement in a group home. Caregivers often experience a change in lifestyle, especially associated with time for leisure and recreation.[1, 20, 24, 25]

The need for personal care for seniors is projected to increase in the coming years. The primary responsibility for providing and financing this care will fall on the family. Because of the financial burden, more families will begin purchasing long-term health care insurance policies. These policies are very expensive but do provide seniors with sufficient income protection against the depletion of assets.[14] Medicaid

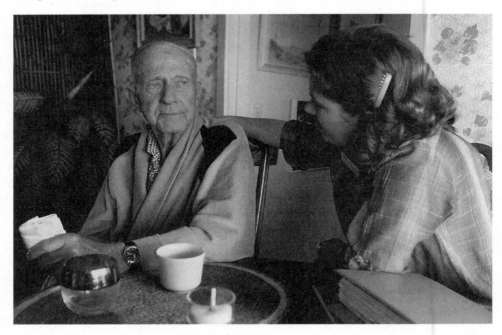

FIGURE 10.20

Adult children are gaining greater responsibility as caregivers.

will continue to be able to help those with incomes low enough to qualify.

CHAPTER SUMMARY

The median age of the United States population is at an all-time high, and will continue to rise well into the next century. The reasons for the rise are decreasing fertility rates, declining mortality rates, and the decline in immigration. We are now at a point in history when a high proportion of Americans will live long enough to assume some responsibility for the care of their aging parents.

An aging population presents the community with several concerns. One is the shrinking dependency ratio. For the next 30–40 years, the dependency ratio will change slightly, but the number of dependent seniors will increase more rapidly than the number of dependent youth. This means legislators and taxpayers will be faced with decisions about how best to afford the costs (Social Security, government employee pensions, Medicare, etc.) of an ever-decreasing elderly dependency ratio. A second concern for the future is the response communities will need to make to the special needs of income, housing, health care, transportation, community facilities and services, and personal care for seniors. All projections indicate that seniors' incomes will remain lower than those of the general population, that the need for affordable and accessible housing will increase, that health care needs and costs will increase, that the demand for barrier-free transportation will increase, and that there will be increased needs for personal services and care for seniors. The demographic and dependency ratio data presented in this chapter suggest that community leaders will need to pay more attention to resources and services for the senior population in the future.

SCENARIO:
ANALYSIS AND RESPONSE

1. Based upon what you read in this chapter, how would you predict that Carl's and Sarah's lives might turn out? Consider the six special needs presented in the chapter.

2. What could Carl and Sarah have done when they were working to better plan for their retirement?

3. If you had to give Carl and Sarah two pieces of health care advice, what would they be?

REVIEW QUESTIONS

1. What are some signs, visible to the average person, that the United States population is aging?

2. What are the differences among old, young old, old old, and oldest old?

3. What is meant by the terms *aged, aging, elderly, senior, gerontology,* and *geriatrics?*

4. Why is it that there is a myth that old people are sickly?

5. What are demographers? What do they do?

6. Why does a pyramid represent the age characteristics of the United States population of the 1950s?

7. What are the three factors that affect the size and age of a population?

8. How have life expectancy figures changed over the years in the United States? What were the major reasons for the change in the first half of the twentieth century? The second half?

9. Why are dependency and labor-force ratios so important?

10. How are dependency ratios calculated?

11. Are all seniors the same with regard to demographic variables? If not, how do they differ?

12. How do the income needs of people change in retirement?

13. Why do adults feel so guilty when they have to relocate their aged parents?

14. Why are continuing-care retirement communities so attractive to seniors?

15. What are the most frequently occurring health problems of seniors?

16. From what financial sources do seniors normally pay for health care?

17. What does the term *Medigap* mean?

18. How do income and health status impact the transportation needs of seniors?

19. What is the ideal solution to the transportation needs of seniors?

20. What are Area Agencies on Aging (AAsA)?

21. Why is a visitor service so important for homebound and institutionalized persons?

22. What is the difference between adult day care and respite care?

23. What is the difference between a care-provider and a care-manager?

24. What are some of the major problems care-givers face?

ACTIVITIES

1. Make arrangements with a local long-term care facility to visit one of their residents. Make at least three one-hour visits to a resident over a six-week period of time. Upon completion of the visits, write a paper that answers the following questions:

   What were your feelings when you first walked into the facility? What were your feelings when you first met the resident?

   What did you learn about the elderly that you didn't know before?

   What did you learn about yourself because of this experience?

   Did your feeling about the resident change during the course of your visits? If so, how?

   Would you like to live in a long-term care facility? Why or why not?

2. Interview a retired person over the age of 65. In your interview, include the following questions. Write a two-page paper about this interview.

   What are your greatest needs as a senior?

   What are your greatest fears connected with aging?

   What are your greatest joys at this stage in your life?

   If you could have done anything differently when you were younger to impact your life now, what would it have been?

   Have you had any problems getting health care with Medicare? If so, what were they? Do you have a Medigap policy?

   In what ways are you able to contribute to your community?

3. Spend a half-day at a local senior center; then write a paper that: (a) summarizes your experience, (b) identifies your reaction (personal feelings) to the experience, and (c) shares what you have learned from the experience.

4. Review a newspaper obituary column for fourteen days straight. Using the information provided in the obituaries: (1) demographically describe those who died, (2) keep track of what community services are noted, and (3) consider what generalizations can be made from the group as a whole.

REFERENCES

1. Conner, K. A. (1992). *Aging America: Issues Facing an Aging Society*. Englewood Cliffs, N.J.: Prentice Hall.

2. Bould, S., B. Sanborn, and L. Reif (1989). *Eighty-five Plus: The Oldest Old*. Belmont, Calif.: Wadsworth.

3. U.S. Dept. of Health and Human Services (1986). *Age Words: A Glossary on Health and Aging* (NIH pub. no. 86-1849). Washington, D.C.: U.S. Government Printing Office.

4. Ferrini, A. F., and R. L. Ferrini (1989). *Health in the Later Years*. Dubuque, Ia.: Wm. C. Brown.

5. Dychtwald, K., and J. Flower (1989). *Age Wave: The Challenges and Opportunities of an Aging America*. Los Angeles: Jeremy P. Tarcher.

6. Thomlinson, R. (1976). *Population Dynamics: Causes and Consequences of World Demographic Change*. New York: Random House.

7. U.S. Dept. of Health and Human Services (1991). *Aging America: Trends and Projections, 1991 Edition* (DHHS pub. no. FCoA-91-28001) Washington, D.C.: U.S. Government Printing Office.

8. U.S. Dept. of Commerce (1993). *How We're Changing*. Current Population Reports, Series p-23, no. 184. Washington, D.C.: U.S. Government Printing Office.

9. U.S. Dept. of Commerce (1992). *Sixty-five Plus in America*. Current Population Reports, Special Studies,

series P-23, no. 178. Washington, D.C.: U.S. Government Printing Office.

10. U.S. Dept. of Health and Human Services (1993). "Advance Report of Final Mortality Statistics, 1990." *Monthly Vital Statistics Report* 41(7): 16.

11. Rosenwaike, I. (1985). *The Extreme Aged in America: A Portrait of an Expanding Population.* London: Greenwood Press.

12. Schulz, J. H., A. Borowski, and W. H. Crown (1991). *Economics of Population Aging: The "Graying" of Australia, Japan, and the United States.* New York: Auburn House.

13. U.S. Dept. of Housing and Urban Development (April 1992). *Housing in America: 1989/90* (pub. no. H123/91-1). Washington, D.C.: U.S. Government Printing Office.

14. Atchley, R. C. (1991). *Social Forces and Aging: An Introduction to Social Gerontology,* 6th ed. Belmont, Calif.: Wadsworth.

15. Boyd, B. (Aug. 20, 1993). "Smart Choices." National Public Radio.

16. Borup, J. H. (1981). "Relocation: Attitudes, Information Network and Problems Encountered." *The Gerontologist* 21: 501–511.

17. Branch, L. G. (1987). "Continuing Care Retirement Communities: Self-Insuring for Long-Term Care." *The Gerontologist* 27: 4–8.

18. No Author (1990) "Communities for the Elderly." *Consumer Reports* (Feb.): 123–131.

19. Chappell, N. L. (1990) "Aging and Social Care." In R. H. Binstock and L. K. George, eds. *Handbook of Aging and the Social Sciences,* 3rd ed., pp. 438–454. San Diego: Academic Press.

20. Brody, E. M., and Schooner, C. B. (1986). "Patterns of Parent-Care When Adult Daughters Work and When They Do Not." *The Gerontologist* 26: 372–381.

21. Finley, N. J. (1989). "Theories of Family Labor as Applied to Gender Differences in Caregiving for Elderly Parents." *Journal of Marriage and the Family* 51: 79–86.

22. U.S. House of Representatives, Select Committee on Aging (Oct. 1987) *Long-Term Care and Personal Impoverishment: Seven in Ten Elderly Living Alone Are at Risk.* Washington, D.C.: U.S. Government Printing Office.

23. Horowitz, A. (1985). "Sons and Daughters as Caregivers to Older Parents: Differences in Role Performance and Consequences." *The Gerontologist,* 25: 612–617.

24. Archbold, P. G. (1983) "Impact of Parent-Caring on Women." *Family Relations* 32: 39–45.

25. Kleban, M. H., E. M. Brody, C. B. Schoonover, and C. Hoffman (1989). "Family Help to the Elderly: Perceptions of Sons-in-Law Regarding Parent Care." *Journal of Marriage and the Family* 51: 303-312.

Chapter 11

COMMUNITY
MENTAL HEALTH

Chapter Outline

Chapter Objectives

After studying this chapter, you should be able to:

1. Define *mental health* and *mental disorders*.
2. Explain what is meant by *DSM-III-R.*
3. Identify the major causes of mental disorders.
4. Explain why mental health is one of the major public health problems in the United States.
5. Define *stress* and explain its relationship to physical and mental health.
6. Briefly trace the history of mental health care in America, highlighting the major changes both before and after World War II.
7. Define the term *deinstitutionalization.*
8. Explain the movement toward community mental health centers.
9. Explain what is meant by *Community Support Program.*
10. Summarize mental health care in America in the 1990s.
11. Identify the major mental and physical problems of the homeless.
12. Describe the primary and secondary prevention services for mental illness available to communities today.
13. List and briefly describe the three basic approaches to treatment for mental disorders.
14. List the types of social services needed by mentally ill persons trying to live independently in local communities.
15. Explain the purpose of the Substance Abuse and Mental Health Services Administration.

Jen was 20 and in her second year at college when Laura, her roommate, began to notice a change in her behavior. Jen had begun to spend more time by herself reading, sometimes in the library, but increasingly in their room. She seldom went to classes and took less and less interest in her appearance. Laura began spending nights bunking with friends because Jen would often be up all night reading and talking to herself. One day, when Laura went to her room to get some clothes, she found Jen hiding in the closet. The room was a mess, and there was a partially packed suitcase. Jen confided to Laura that someone had been spying on her and that she might have to get away— to another country! As Laura gathered up some of her clothes, she realized that Jen was in urgent need of help. She knew she had to call someone, but who?

INTRODUCTION

Mental illness is one of the major health issues facing every community. It has been estimated that as many as one in five persons will need hospitalization for mental illness in his or her lifetime. Some of these people will need only minimal counseling, followed perhaps by support group meetings, while others will suffer repeated episodes requiring intervention. Still others may not be able to live independently at all and, therefore, will require permanent institutionalization.

Because the needs of the mentally ill are many and diverse, the services required to meet these needs are likewise diverse and, as we will explain, include not only therapeutic services but social services too. Because many mental disorders are chronic in nature, significant community resources are continually needed to meet the demands for care.

Definitions

Mental health can be defined as the emotional and social well-being of an individual, including one's psychological resources for dealing with the day-to-day problems of life (see Figure 11.1). Characteristics of people with good mental health include possessing a good self-image, feeling right about other people and being able to meet the demands of everyday life.[1]

Good mental health can be expressed as emotional maturity. In this regard, adults who have good mental health are able to:

1. Function under adversity.
2. Change or adapt to changes around them.
3. Maintain control over their tension and anxiety.
4. Find more satisfaction in giving than receiving.
5. Show consideration for others.
6. Curb hate and guilt.
7. Love others.

Unfortunately, there are many in the community who do not have good mental health or who have poor mental health. Some of these people have insufficient psychological resources for dealing with everyday life, which may cause them to behave in ways that are destructive to themselves or

---

mental health Emotional and social well-being, including one's psychological resources for dealing with the day-to-day problems of life.

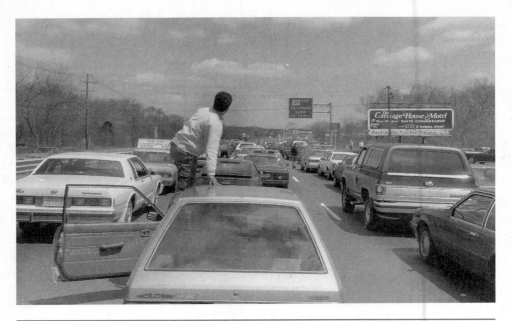

FIGURE 11.1

Ability to cope with the stresses of everyday living are a sign of good mental health.

to society. Others have organic or metabolic deficiencies that prevent them from functioning effectively and happily in society. Still others are mentally retarded.

The origins of these **mental disorders,** while not always fully understood, can frequently be traced to either hereditary or environmental factors or sometimes to a combination of both.

Classification of Mental Disorders

It is always important to keep in mind that classification systems of human origin are imperfect attempts to arrange natural

---

mental disorder Deficiency of psychological resources for dealing with everyday life, usually characterized by distress or impairment of one or more areas of functioning.

phenomena into artificial, and sometimes arbitrary, categories. Such is the case with the classification of mental disorders, which are for the most part based on descriptions of behavioral signs and symptoms. The most often cited reference for the classification of mental disorders is the *Diagnostic and Statistical Manual of Mental Disorders, third edition, revised*—abbreviated simply as ***DSM-III-R.***[2] The *DSM-III-R,* published by the American Psychiatric Association, represents the best current thinking on the diagnosis and classification of mental disorders but does not in all cases describe the causes of these disorders. The onset of some disorders occurs in infancy, others in adulthood. Examples of mental disorders that are first evident at an early age include developmental disorders, like mental retardation, behavioral disruptive disorders, like attention-deficit hyperactivity, and gender-identity disorders of childhood. Disorders of adolescence and adulthood include psychoactive substance abuse disorder, schizophrenia, and mood disorders. Each of these disorders can be mild, moderate, or severe, and each may result in mild to severe impairments of social functioning. A list of the disorders classified in the *DSM-III-R* are listed in Table 11.1.

Causes of Mental Disorders

There are several causes of mental disorders including mental deficiency at birth, physical (or physiological) impairment, and psychological causes. Mental deficiency at birth can be inherited (genetic causes), have an idiopathic (unknown) origin, or be the result of maternal exposure to physical, chemical, or biological agents. Two-thirds of mental retardation cases are traceable to environmental factors such as poor prenatal care, poor maternal nutrition, or maternal exposure to alcohol, tobacco, or other drugs; as such, they are preventable. For example, fetal alcohol syndrome, a condition that includes mental deficiency, is the result of maternal (and fetal) exposure to excessive amounts of alcohol during gestation.

Inherited causes of mental disorders can be present at birth or appear later in life. For example, an imbalance in the levels of neurotransmitters in the brain could appear during adolescence or young adulthood. Abnormal neurotransmitter levels, which often have a genetic origin, can result

Table 11.1
Diagnostic Categories of Mental Disorders

Category	Example
Disorders usually first evident in infancy, childhood, or adolescence	Mental retardation; attention-deficit hyperactivity disorder
Organic mental disorders	Alzheimer's disease; dementia associated with alcoholism or chronic drug use
Psychoactive substance use disorders	Alcohol, nicotine, cocaine, or other drug dependence
Schizophrenia	Paranoid schizophrenia
Delusional (paranoid) disorder	Persecutory delusional (paranoid) disorder
Miscellaneous psychotic disorders	Brief reactive psychosis
Mood disorders	Major depression; bipolar disorder
Anxiety disorders	Panic disorder; obsessive compulsive disorder; post-traumatic stress disorder
Somatoform disorders	Conversion disorder; hypochondriasis
Dissociative disorders	Multiple personality disorder
Sexual disorders	Paraphilias (exhibitionism, fetishisms); sexual dysfunctions
Sleep disorders	Insomnia disorder; dream anxiety disorder
Factitious disorders	Pathologic lying
Impulse control disorders	Kleptomania; pathological gambling
Adjustment disorders	Anxious mood; withdrawal
Personality disorders	Avoidant; dependent; obsessive

BOX 11.1
Recognizing Signs and Symptoms of Major Depression

Recognizing signs and symptoms of depression is a key to helping someone get help. People with major depression usually have a "down" mood for weeks and are unable to derive pleasure from almost anything. They also have at least four of the following eight symptoms:

1. Sleep problems—sleeping too little or too much
2. Loss of interest
3. Feelings of guilt
4. Low energy
5. Inability to concentrate
6. Loss of appetite (or eating too much)
7. Agitation (pacing) or slowing of activity (lethargic)
8. Thoughts of suicide

in such **affective (mood) disorders** as **bipolar disorder** and **major depression** (see Box 11.1).

Mental disorders can also occur from postnatal exposure to physical, chemical, and biological agents. Brain function impairment can occur from trauma, such as a car crash or bullet wound, or from disease, such as syphilis, cancer, or stroke. Mental impairment can also be caused by such envi-

ronmental factors as chronic nutritional deficiency or by lead poisoning.[3]

Psychological sources of mental disorders include dysfunctional family environments. Children reared in abusive, neglectful, or violent family environments can develop mental disorders (see Figure 11.2). The prevalence of child abuse and neglect has reached epidemic proportions in America. An estimated 2.7 million children were reported to child protection agencies as victims of maltreatment in 1991. In 1989, 12% of all children younger than 18 years of age suffered mental disorders.[3]

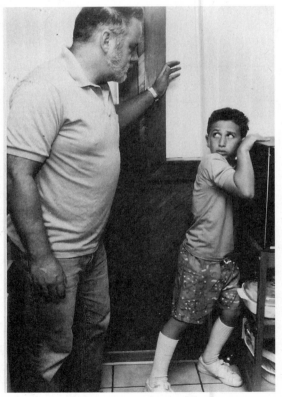

FIGURE 11.2

A dysfunctional family environment can increase one's risk for mental illness.

affective disorder   A mental disorder characterized by a disturbance of mood, either depression or elation (mania); examples: bipolar disorder, major depression.

bipolar disorder   An affective disorder characterized by distinct periods of elevated mood alternating with periods of depression.

major depression   An affective disorder characterized by a dysphoric mood, usually depression, or loss of interest or pleasure in almost all usual activities or pastimes.

The negative influences of unhealthy neighborhoods and deviant peer groups, such as gangs, on those who have been reared in dysfunctional families may further increase the risk that these young people will develop mental disorders. Challenging economic conditions make it more difficult for families to survive. The resulting broken families add to the burden on our nation's mental health services, leading children's advocates to question the priorities of federal programs that provide more money to the states for foster care than for programs designed to strengthen families.[3]

MENTAL ILLNESS IN AMERICA

Mental illness constitutes one of the major public health problems in America in the 1990s. The following statistics reflect the fact that mental illness is widespread in this country.

Statistical Indicators of Mental Illness

Currently, the **National Institute of Mental Health (NIMH),** the nation's leading mental health agency, estimates that there are 4–5 million adults with serious mental illness (SMI) in the United States. It has been estimated that 15.4% of the U.S. population 18 years of age and older have had at least one incident that would meet the criteria of a mental health or substance abuse disorder within the past 30 days.[4] Frequently, these mental disorders are chronic in nature; approximately half of those admitted to mental institutions have had previous admissions.

Results of a household survey conducted in 1989 revealed that 18.2 adults per 1,000 had experienced an episode of SMI in the 12 months immediately prior to the survey. Approximately 1.4 million Americans between the ages of 18 and 69 years old were either unable to work or limited in their ability to work because of mental illness.[5]

Social Indicators of Mental Illness

The social statistics that reflect the depth and breadth of the mental illness problem in our society are staggering. There are approximately 30,000 suicides each year in the United States.[6,7] In 1991, the Number 2 and Number 3 leading causes of death in youth aged 15–24 were homicide (including legal intervention) and suicide[6] (see Box 11.2).

Mental illness is perhaps both a cause and an effect of many of this country's domestic problems. In 1990, the divorce rate (4.7/1,000) was nearly half the marriage rate (9.8/1,000 population).[8] That same year, an estimated 4.5 million women of childbearing age were current users of illegal substances.[3] Perhaps it is not a totally unrelated fact that a reported 1,383 children died from abuse or neglect in 1991. The widespread abuse of alcohol, tobacco, and other drugs in America (discussed in Chapter 12) is further evidence that many in this county lack the necessary psychological resources for coping with life's problems.

Stress: A Contemporary Mental Health Problem

Stress can be defined as one's psychological and physiological response to **stressors,** stimuli in the physical and social environment that produce feelings of tension and strain. Stress, as a contributor to mental health problems, is likely to remain important in the 1990s as life becomes increasingly more complex. Even Americans who

BOX 11.2
BOX 11.2
Healthy People 2000—Objective

6.1   Reduce suicides to no more than 10.5 per 100,000 people. (Age-adjusted baseline: 11.7 per 100,000 in 1987)

Special Population Targets

	Suicides (per 100,000)	1987 Baseline	2000 Target	Percent Decrease
6.1a	Youth aged 15–19	10.3	8.2%	
6.1b	Men aged 20–34	25.2	39.2	
6.1c	White men aged 65 and older	46.1	39.2	
6.1d	American Indian/Alaska Native men in reservation states	15	12.8	

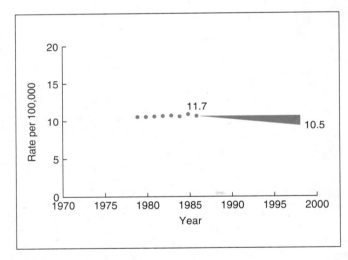

Baseline data sources: National Vital Statistics System, CDC; Indian Health Service Administrative Statistics IHS.

Age-adjusted suicide rate.

For Further Thought

The overall suicide rate in the United State has changed relatively little since 1950. However, there has been a steady increase in suicide among all youth aged 15–19 since the 1950s. How can this change be explained?

consider themselves to be in good mental health carry out their everyday activities under considerable stress. Stressors can be subtle, such as having to wait in line, getting stuck in traffic, or having to keep an appointment, or they can be major life events such as getting married or divorced or losing a loved one. While some exposure to stressors is good, perhaps even essential to a satisfying life, chronic exposure to stressors that exceed one's coping resources—biological, psychological, and social—can undermine one's health. One well-known study[9] actually classified and ranked various stressors and found a relationship between these stressors and physical health.

The process through which exposure to stressors results in health deficits has been described by Selye[10] and Sarafino.[11] According to Selye's model, which he called the **General Adaptation Syndrome (GAS),** confrontation with a stressor results in a three-stage physiological response: (1) an alarm reaction stage, (2) a stage of resistance, and finally (3) a stage of exhaustion (see Figure 11.3). In the alarm reaction stage, the body prepares to strongly resist the stressor. Various hormonal changes in the body increase the individual's heart rate, respiration, and blood pressure. This is the **fight or flight reaction,** a response that the body cannot maintain for very long. Continued presence of the stressor produces a stage of resistance. In this stage, the body tries to adapt to the stressor. The level of physiological arousal declines somewhat but still remains above normal. During the stage of resistance, the body begins to replenish the hormones released in the alarm

reaction stage, but the body's ability to resist new stressors is impaired. As a result, according to Selye, the person is increasingly vulnerable to certain health problems which he calls **diseases of adaptation.** Such diseases include ulcers, high blood pressure, coronary heart disease, asthma, and other diseases related to impaired immune function.[11]

The third stage of GAS is the stage of exhaustion. Prolonged physiological arousal produced by continual or repeated stress can deplete energy stores until one's physical ability to resist is very limited. During this stage, physiological damage, physical diseases, mental health problems, and even death can occur.

Evidence suggests that stress can affect health either directly via physiologic changes in the body or indirectly via a change in a person's behavior. The clearest connection between stress and ill health is demonstrated by the release of hormones by the endocrine system during the alarm reaction stage of the GAS. Both the cardiovascular and immune systems of the body are affected. Hormones produce fast or erratic beating of the heart, which can be fatal. The same hormones have been associated with increases in levels of blood lipids. High blood lipids cause a buildup of plaque on the blood vessel walls and greatly increase the likelihood of hypertension, stroke, and heart attack.[12, 13] The release of certain hormones also impairs the functioning of the immune system.[14, 15] These hormones reduce the activity of T-cells and B-cells, making it more difficult for the immune system to fight cancer and other

---

General Adaptation Syndrome (GAS) The complex physiological responses resulting from exposure to stressors.

fight or flight reaction An alarm reaction that prepares one physiologically for sudden action.

diseases of adaptation Diseases that result from chronic exposure to excess levels of stressors which produce a general adaptation syndrome response.

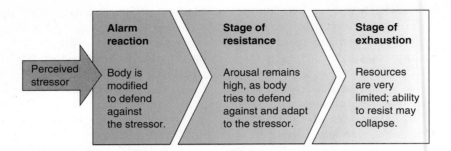

FIGURE 11.3

General adaptation syndrome.

From: Sarafino, E. P. (1990). Healthy Psychology: Biopsychosocial Interactions. New York: John Wiley & Sons, p. 84.

diseases. Table 11.2 provides a list of psychophysiological disorders that have been found to be associated with stress.

The indirect effects of stress on health occur when those who experience high levels of stress respond with unhealthy behaviors. For example, it has been shown that individuals under more stress consume more alcohol, smoke more cigarettes, and drink more coffee than those under less

stress.[16, 17] Use of these substances has been associated with higher risks for heart disease and cancer, as well as trauma and death from unintentional injuries.

The relationship between stress and mental illness is not a simple one. Severe stress such as that experienced under military combat conditions or by children who are sexually and physically abused has been well documented. It stands to reason that even exposure to less intense stressors would likewise result in stress and impact one's health adversely (see Box 11.3).

One might also infer that the stress upon an entire community would result in a decline in a community's health. Do the religious and political tensions endured by those in Sarajevo, the capital of Bosnia and Herzegovina in the former Yugoslavia, exemplify a community under stress? Do communities struggling for civil rights, human rights, and freedom of expression likewise exhibit the signs of stress? Were the Los Angeles riots which followed the Rodney King verdict a sign of a community's response to stressors that exceeded the community's resources for dealing with them?

Table 11.2

Psychophysiological Disorders Associated with Stress

Asthma

Cancer

Coronary heart disease

Depression

Dysmenorrhea (painful menstruation)

Exhaustion

Gastrointestinal problems (colitis, stomach pain, ulcers)

Headaches (muscle-contraction and migraine)

Hypertension

Inflammatory bowel disease

Skin disorders (eczema, hives, psoriasis)

BOX 11.3
Healthy People 2000—Objective

6.5   Reduce to less than 35% the proportion of people aged 18 and older who experienced adverse health effects from stress within the past year. (Baseline: 42.6% in 1985)

Baseline data source: Prevention Index, Rodale Press, Inc.

Special Population Target

	1985 Baseline	2000 Target Percent Decrease	
6.5a People with disabilities	53.5%	40%	All, a

Note: For this objective, people with disabilities are people who report any limitation in activity due to chronic conditions.

Baseline data source: National Health Interview Survey, CDC.

6.9   Decrease to no more than 5% the proportion of people aged 18 and older who report experiencing significant levels of stress and who do not take steps to reduce or control their stress. (Baseline: 21% in 1985)

For Further Thought

Most adult Americans report a great deal of stress in their lives. However, it is known that not all stress is bad; in fact, some stress is good. But it is the inability to control stress that causes health-related problems. Can you identify at least five different ways to prevent, reduce, or manage stress?

HISTORY OF MENTAL HEALTH CARE IN AMERICA

Before discussing our nation's response to mental illness, we present a brief history of past efforts to confront this issue. Collective response to mental illness in America has been a cyclic phenomenon, marked by enthusiastic reform movements followed by periods of national ambivalence toward those suffering from mental disorders. The reform movements we discuss below began when an existing system for caring for the mentally ill became intolerable for society and ended when their economic burden became unbearable.

Mental Health Care Before World War II

In Colonial America, when communities were sparsely populated, people experiencing mental illness were cared for by their families or private caretakers. Those who were not cared for this way usually ended up in local poorhouses or almshouses, along with "the mentally retarded, the physically handicapped, the homeless, and the otherwise deviant." This group was collectively referred to as "the poor."[18]

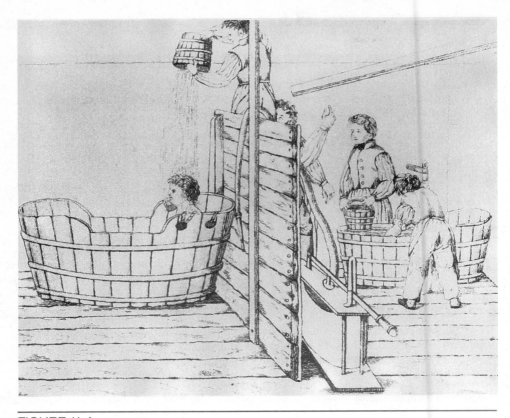

FIGURE 11.4

Treatment for mental illness in the eighteenth and nineteenth centuries was often inhumane and unsuccessful.

As America's population grew in the late eighteenth and early nineteenth centuries, so did the number of people who were unable to live independently. Gradually, as the situation in the poorhouses and almshouses worsened, efforts were made to separate people by type of disability. One of the first efforts was that of Dr. Thomas Bond, who had been to England and visited the famous Bedlam Hospital, in which the mentally ill were housed. In 1851, he built Pennsylvania Hospital, a public hospital for the mentally ill indigents in Philadelphia.[18] Pennsylvania Hospital was the first institution in America specifically designed to care for the mentally ill. Conditions in the hospital were harsh (see Figure 11.4), and treatments, which consisted of "blood letting, blistering, emetics, and warm and cold baths," were unpleasant.[19]

The Moral Treatment Era

While care for the indigent mentally ill in the nineteenth century was gruesome, care for the well-to-do was much better. William Tuke, an English Quaker, established a therapy known as **moral treat-**

moral treatment Treatment for mental illness based on belief that mental illness was caused by moral decay.

ment and put it into practice beginning in 1792 at York Retreat. This treatment was based on his belief that the causes of mental illnesses were moral deterioration, exemplified by "infidelity, overwork, envy, gluttony, drinking, sexual excesses, and the like."[19] In a peaceful rural setting, mentally ill people were removed from the everyday-life stressors of their home environments and given "asylum" in a quiet country environment. They received a regimen of rest, light food, exercise, fresh air, and amusements. They were cared for by a caring and respectful staff. It was supposed that the environment of the asylum would result in the spontaneous recovery of patients who had come to their state through immoral behavior. While actual recovery rates are debatable, this approach, at the time, was deemed successful and became widely accepted as the ideal form of treatment for the mentally ill in small, relatively homogeneous, New England Protestant communities of that era.[20]

The apparent successes of the moral treatment approach in the private sector led to attempts to adapt this model of mental health care to the public sector. However, by the 1840s, because of massive immigration and rapid urbanization, there was such a heterogeneous mass of mentally ill people that the capacity of the public asylums was soon overrun. The majority of those who were mentally and socially unfit again ended up in the urban almshouses, which were chronically underfunded and overpopulated. This was the state of affairs when Dorothea Lynde Dix undertook her campaign to close down county-run almshouses and establish state-run hospitals.

Dorothea Dix (1802–1897) (see Figure 11.5) was a Sunday-school teacher from Cambridge, Massachusetts, who worked tirelessly for 45 years advocating decent care for the indigent mentally ill. It was her

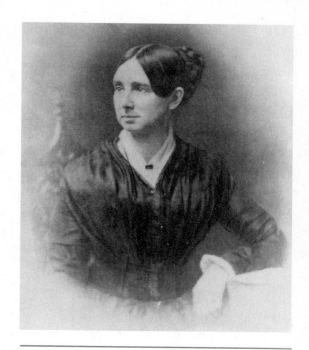

FIGURE 11.5

Dorothea Dix helped to establish public mental hospitals in many states.

belief that it was the responsibility of the state to care for the mentally ill. She publicized the deplorable conditions in the public almshouses, and over a period of seven years (1847–1854), she lobbied Congress for a bill granting the proceeds of a federal land sale for the building of public mental hospitals. Others, who felt that mental illness was a medical problem that could be made to yield before the advance of medical science, eventually joined in her cause; and Congress finally passed the bill she supported. President Franklin Pierce, however, vetoed it, citing his conviction that the treatment of the mentally ill was the province of the individual states, not the federal government. Following a brief rest, Dix resumed her lobbying, this time on a state-by-state basis. Her efforts were in most cases successful, and all in all, Dix was personally involved in the founding of 32 public mental hospitals.[21]

The State Hospitals

The institutional movement during this period was a general one that included the building of institutions for prisoners, orphans, and wayward youth, as well as for the mentally ill. There was widespread fear that the waves of immigrants included too many poor and insane people and that the social order in America was at risk. Also, a popular misinterpretation of Darwin's theories about evolution, called "social Darwinism," in which only those adapted to society's demands could be expected to survive, was used to justify the removal of misfits and

mad persons to state-run institutions where they could receive custodial care.[20] The state mental institutions were supposed to provide an environment in which medical care would be provided by professional staff, trained to work with each patient individually (see Figure 11.6). Initially, the upper limit of patients was set at 250 so that treatment could occur within the bonds of close personal relationships between caregiving staff members and patients, as prescribed in the methods of the moral treatment.

Unfortunately, even as new state hospitals continued to be built, the deterioration of those already in existence had begun. The chronic nature of mental illness was a large part of the problem. It became increasingly

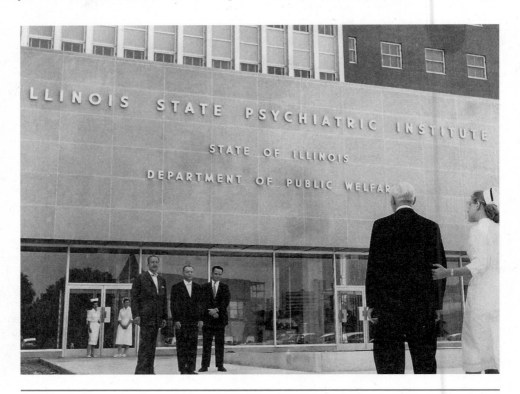

FIGURE 11.6

The state mental hospital was at one time viewed as the appropriate public response to the needs of the mentally ill.

apparent that long-term or even lifetime stays were the norm for many patients.[21] "Maximum capacities" were quickly reached, exceeded, and repeatedly revised upward. The ability to provide personalized care was lost, as was the promise of significant medical treatment. Staff members were unable to reward patients for efforts at self-control; and physical restraints became more practical, especially in large wards.[18] As funding for these institutions became increasingly susceptible to state budget cuts, the level of care also diminished until all that remained was custodial care. The institutions at that point had become little more than places to "warehouse" the mentally ill population. It became increasingly difficult to find dedicated staff to work at the unrewarding jobs in these institutions, and the turnover rate was high. Administration became more of a bureaucracy, so that treatment and cure were almost nonexistent.

The Mental Hygiene Movement

The next movement in mental health care in the United States was the **mental hygiene movement,** which occurred during the first decades of the twentieth century, a period known as the Progressive Era. The leaders of this movement believed that mental illness could be prevented if it was identified and treated early. They proposed attacking the problem of mental illness at the community level. They did not concern themselves so much with the problems of the state hospitals, and in this regard, they did not offer any solution to the problems existing in these institutions.

One of the figures in the reform movement was **Adolf Meyer** (1866–1950), a psychiatrist who felt that psychiatrists should

provide acute care for mentally ill patients in new psychopathic hospitals, after which the same patients would be remitted to community-based aftercare. The psychopathic hospitals would receive, diagnose, treat, and release patients, or in certain cases, remand them over to the state hospitals. Some of the receiving hospitals that were established during this period, such as Bellevue in New York and Boston Psychopathic Hospital, remain in operation today.[18]

Another name associated with the mental hygiene movement is that of **Clifford W. Beers** (1876–1943). Clifford Beers (see Figure 11.7) was a graduate of Yale University who

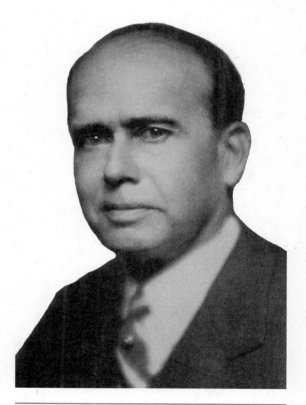

FIGURE 11.7

Clifford Beers, whose book described his treatment in mental hospitals, founded the National Committee on Mental Hygiene and led the fight for the mentally ill.

---

mental hygiene movement   A movement based on the belief that mental illness can be cured if identified and treated early.

suffered from a bipolar mood disorder that resulted in repeated hospitalizations throughout his life.[22] His book, *A Mind That Found Itself,* described his illness and experiences in mental hospitals. He was able to enlist the support of others in his cause to improve conditions and to promote research on the prevention and treatment of mental illness. He founded the National Committee on Mental Hygiene, which in 1950 became the **National Mental Health Association (NMHA).** While Meyer and Beers contributed to mental health education in many ways, the mental hygiene movement did little to advance institutional reform of state mental facilities.

During the first part of the twentieth century, conditions in the state mental hospitals continued to deteriorate. This period was also characterized by the struggle of psychiatry for acceptance as a legitimate form of medical practice. By associating itself with the popular and progressive prevention movement, rather than with the practice of housing the chronically ill in state institutions, psychiatry was able to gain stature. Public interest in mental hygiene also increased during this period, especially when it was reported that 20% of those discharged from the army in 1912 were found to have mental illness and that the mental illness rate of those discharged in 1916 was three times the national rate.[18]

In 1934, John Maurice Grimes, M.D., headed a study panel for the American Medical Association charged with surveying state mental institutions. Grimes's report provided suggestions for reducing the populations in these institutions and for developing community aftercare clinics staffed by social workers.[23] Grimes's suggestions were not acted upon, and conditions continued to deteriorate for another 25 years.

By 1940, the population in state mental institutions had grown to nearly a half-million, many of whom were elderly and senile. Budget cuts continued, and case loads per worker in the institutions became so large that only subsistence care was possible.

When World War II began, more than 1 million of the 15 million men who underwent military examinations were rejected for mental health reasons; about half of these were because of mental retardation and half because of mental illness.[18] The military's need for psychiatrists meant that even fewer trained professionals were available to manage state mental institutions.

One result of the war was that new crisis intervention methods were developed and the image of psychiatry improved. After the war, practicing psychiatrists were discharged from military service armed with new techniques and ready to attack the problem of mental disorders in American civilians.

Mental Health Care After World War II

Following World War II, the nation's attention was again directed toward the serious problems existing in the state mental institutions. A growing sense of urgency to respond to this problem was now joined by new feelings of optimism and a "can do" spirit that sprung from America's achievements in the war. There was a belief that any social problem could be solved with enough dedication and hard work.

In the post-war 1940s, a number of alliances formed to urge greater federal involvement in mental health care. One of these groups was the **National Mental Health Foundation (NMHF),** founded by a group of conscientious objectors (COs), people who objected to serving in the military on religious grounds. In place of military duty, many COs had spent their war years working in these mental institutions. Through the

NMHF, the COs publicized the deterioration of the state mental hospitals and lobbied for improvements. Other interest groups included influential private citizens and mental health professionals themselves. The mood of the country, together with testimony before Congress by both military and civilian experts, soon resulted in the passage of the **National Mental Health Act of 1946,** which established the **National Institute of Mental Health (NIMH).** Modeled after the National Cancer Institute, established in 1937, NIMH came under the umbrella of the National Institutes of Health. The purposes of NIMH were: (1) to foster and aid research related to the cause, diagnosis, and treatment of neuropsychiatric disorders, (2) to provide training and award fellowships and grants for work in mental health, and (3) to aid the states in the prevention, diagnosis, and treatment of neuropsychiatric disorders.[21] For the third responsibility, that of providing aid to states, a precedent had been set earlier with the federal venereal disease and tuberculosis control programs.

The National Institute of Mental Health enjoyed a great deal of support, not only from the public but also from some very influential private citizens, highly placed members of the psychiatric profession, and powerful Congressmen. Funding for NIMH, which had begun at $7.5 million in 1947, grew to $18 million by 1953 and to $315 million by 1967.[24]

Meanwhile, in the early 1950s, public distress about the conditions in state mental hospitals continued to grow, fed not only by the NMHF movement, but also by published articles and books, like *The Shame of the States,* by Albert Deutsch, and *The Snake Pit,* by Mary Jane Ward.[18] In 1950, a council of state governments came together to discuss the problem of mental health care costs. One of their conclusions was that, although there was an undeniable need for

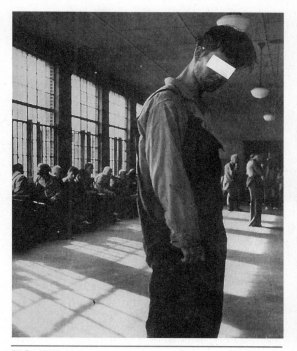

FIGURE 11.8

Before deinstitutionalization, populations in state mental hospitals reached a half-million patients.

greater revenues, there was an even greater need for fewer patients. They suggested more support for research into the etiology and treatment of the mentally ill so that they could be discharged.[18] The seeds of the next movements in mental health care—deinstitutionalization, the community mental health centers movement, and the community support movement—were now sown (see Figure 11.8).

Deinstitutionalization

The term **deinstitutionalization,** first suggested by Grimes in 1934, has been used

---

deinstitutionalization The process of discharging, on a large scale, patients from state mental hospitals to less-restrictive community settings.

to describe the discharging of thousands of patients from state-owned mental hospitals and the resettling and maintaining of these discharged persons in less restrictive community settings. The magnitude of the process can be told with the following statistics. In 1955, there were 558,922 resident patients in state and county mental institutions.[25] By 1970, the number had dropped to 337,619, by 1980, to 150,000, and by 1990, to 110,000–120,000.[25,26] Deinstitutionalization, which began in the 1950s and continued through the 1980s, was not a preplanned policy. Rather it occurred as a result of social and economic forces that had built up for more than half a century.

Deinstitutionalization was propelled by four forces: (1) economics, (2) idealism, (3) legal considerations, and (4) the development and marketing of antipsychotic drugs.[19] Economically, there was not only a push, there was also a pull. The push was the states' need to reduce expenditures for mental hospitals so that more could be spent on the other three major state budgetary items—education, roads, and welfare. Meanwhile, a pulling economic force began to germinate with the prospect of profits from providing outpatient and inpatient services to the mentally ill. This prospect became brighter with changes in legislation permitting these services to be paid for by public funds.

Examples of such legislation were the Social Security Amendments of 1962, known as **Aid to the Permanently and Totally Disabled (APTD)**.[19] Other federal legislation in the 1960s affected the direction of community mental health care services. A 1960 amendment to the old-age assistance program and regulatory changes permitting welfare payments to discharged psychiatric patients were two important actions. But the major changes came about as a result of the 1965 amendments to the Social Security

Act of 1935, known as Medicare and Medicaid, which took effect in 1966. Medicare provided hospital and physician services for the aged; Medicaid provided grants to the states for medical assistance to indigent persons. A remarkable feature of these amendments was the inclusion of psychiatric benefits.[25] With the passage of the social legislation of the Kennedy and Johnson years, patient populations in state and county hospitals decreased even faster.[25]

Another force propelling deinstitutionalization was idealism. Idealists felt that everything possible should be done to keep people out of mental hospitals and that perhaps it would be best if these institutions were shut down altogether.[19] They believed that life inside the state mental hospitals was destructive to human values, that therapies actually made patients' conditions worse, that patients held in these institutions were isolated and hard to visit, and that those who were discharged were often worse off than when they entered. Books, like Ken Kesey's *One Flew over the Cuckoo's Nest* (1962), and movies, like "Diary of a Mad Housewife" (1970), which depicted the unsavory conditions in state mental hospitals, helped to mold public opinion against public mental institutions.[25]

In the early 1960s, questions began to be raised about the legality of keeping people locked up, especially if no real effort was being made to treat them. The American Bar Association published a study in 1961 of the laws relating to this issue. One of the points raised in its review was that mental patients, even when institutionalized, had certain rights, including the right to treatment. That same year, Congressional hearings were held on the commitment procedures operating in Washington, D.C. The hearings focused on broad issues including the constitutional rights of patients. The fundamental issue discussed was, "whether society, which is unable or unwilling to provide treatment, has the right to deprive a patient of his liberty on the sole grounds that he is in need of care."[25]

Over the ensuing decade, there was a subtle change in how the courts viewed civil commitment. There was more concern for the rights of the mentally ill—who were viewed as needing the courts' protection from inappropriate involuntary commitment—and less concern for society's right to be protected from these individuals.[19] Eventually, the test for involuntary civil commitment became one of whether these individuals could be considered dangerous to themselves or others.

While economics, idealism, and legal considerations all helped to launch deinstitutionalization, another force expedited it—new antipsychotic drugs. The most widely used drug was **chlorpromazine,** introduced as **Thorazine** by Smith, Kline, and French in 1954. Chlorpromazine was termed **neuroleptic** because it appeared to reduce nervous activity. When used in the institutional setting, the purpose of Thorazine and the other phenothiazines introduced later was to make patients more amenable to other forms of therapy. The drug did produce a remarkably calming effect in psychotic patients, and as a result, patients became more cooperative and hospital psychopathic wards became much quieter. So unusual were the effects of chlorpromazine that the drug in many cases became the *only* form of treatment provided. In these situations, a "**chemical strait jacket**" was said to have been substituted for a physical one.

Prior to its appearance on the U.S. market as an antipsychotic, chlorpromazine had been tested as a cure for several other conditions. Thus, at the time of its introduction, only three research studies on its use for treating mental disorders had been published. These studies were not of the quality that would be required under today's more rigorous Food and Drug Administration guidelines; and, in the haste to put this drug into use, some of its long-term toxic effects on the central nervous system were not fully explored. Among the most significant and grave of these effects is **tardive dyskinesia,** the irreversible, involuntary, and abnormal movements of the tongue, mouth, arms, and legs.[18] In spite of these deleterious effects, Thorazine and the other phenothiazines are still used extensively to treat psychotic patients.

Community Mental Health Centers

In 1961, the report of the Joint Commission on Mental Illness and Health (JCMIH) was released. The JCMIH, established in the 1950s, was made up of representatives of both the American Medical Association and the American Psychiatric Association, along with members of several volunteer citizen groups. Among the JCMIH's recommendations was that acute mental illness be treated in community-based settings. Treatment in these settings was viewed as a form of secondary prevention, in which the development of more serious mental breakdowns would be prevented. There would still be a need for the hospitals to provide tertiary preven-

---

chlorpromazine The first and most famous antipsychotic drug, introduced in 1954 under the brand name Thorazine.

neuroleptic drugs Drugs that reduce nervous activity; another term for *antipsychotic drug.*

chemical strait jacket A drug that subdues a mental patient's behavior.

---

tardive dyskinesia Irreversible, involuntary, and abnormal movements of the tongue, mouth, arms, and legs, which can result from long-term use of certain antipsychotic drugs such as chlorpromazine.

tion when secondary prevention failed and to treat the chronically mentally ill. The goals of the voluntary citizen members—namely, the establishment of primary prevention programs in community mental health—were not prominent in the JCMIH report.[21]

President John Kennedy was said to have read the Commission's report at the insistence of his sister Eunice. In February 1963, he addressed the issue of mental health care in a speech to Congress.[20] The **Mental Retardation Facilities and Community Mental Health Centers (CMHC) Act** was passed later that year and signed on October 31, 1963. Funding legislation was not completed until 1965 and did not go into effect until 1966.

In funding the CMHC Act, the federal government did exactly what President Franklin Pierce refused to do in 1854. It made the federal government responsible, at least in part, for mental health care services in all the states. Even more remarkable was that the funding for this program bypassed the traditional federal to state, state to local funding route, by providing money directly to the localities themselves. In bypassing the state governments, the act created a situation in which the states had no ownership in the program or in the CMHCs. Furthermore, the act included a declining federal funding scheme but provided no incentive to states to gradually take over the financing of these centers. This situation was eventually addressed in President Carter's Mental Health Systems Act of 1980. However, before President Carter's act could take effect, it was repealed by President Reagan's Omnibus Budget Reconciliation Act of 1981. The Omnibus Budget Reconciliation Act restored the traditional federal state relationship in funding, at reduced levels, via block grants to states.[20]

The original goal of the CMHC Act was to provide to each community with a population of 50,000 or more one fully staffed, full-time **community mental health center.** By 1989, 750 of the originally planned 2,000 CMHCs were in operation across the United States (see Figure 11.9). About one-quarter of the U.S. population is now served by a CMHC. Each center is required to be comprehensive and to provide five services to its clients: inpatient, outpatient, emergency (24-hour) care, partial hospitalization, and consultation and education services. The centers were to be accessible and to coordinate their activities with other community agencies so as to provide a continuity of care and an emphasis on prevention.

While the CMHCs did provide mental health care services to residents in the communities in which they were built, they did not live up to their original expectations of serving the deinstitutionalized, chronically mentally ill. The latter arrived in communities that in most cases could not provide the type of comprehensive social service network they needed. The funds to do so were simply not there.

Meanwhile, many older, chronically mentally ill patients were never truly deinstitutionalized but **"transinstitutionalized"** to nursing homes, which in some cases cost more than state hospital care. The cost was now paid by the federal instead of the state governments. Many younger patients were also transinstitutionalized when they ended up in jails for minor offenses. Still other patients were actually reinstitutionalized after being repeatedly admitted to psychiatric wards of community hospitals.[19]

In the 1980s, which came to be known as the "Me Decade," federal spending for

---

transinstitutionalization Transferring patients from one type of public institution to another, usually as a result of policy change.

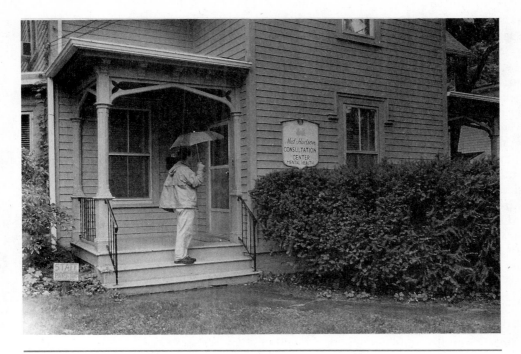

FIGURE 11.9

Between 1966 and 1989, 750 community mental health centers were established.

many health and social programs was reduced. For the deinstitutionalized chronically mentally ill, the cuts in social and welfare programming were more destructive than those in health programming. Many people who had been just managing to get by in their communities were no longer able to do so. Without other adequate social support services, many of these people became part of the growing homeless population.

It has been pointed out that concurrent demographic phenomena contributed growing numbers of those in need of mental health care in the 1970s and 1980s.[27] During the late 1970s, many of the baby boomers were reaching young adulthood, when schizophrenia has its highest incidence. Compounding this problem was the increasing prevalence of alcohol and cocaine abuse in the 1980s. Also, the fastest growing age

group of the population was the seniors, who are at greatest risk for developing dementia and other age-related mental disorders.

Despite all of the problems that have been attributed to deinstitutionalization, there have been some positive outcomes. One is that a majority of released mental patients surveyed have stated a preference for life in the community over life in an institution. Also, in some communities, halfway houses and support services were forthcoming once the need for these became clear. Finally, the quality of inpatient stays has improved and their duration shortened.

The Community Support Movement

The response of NIMH to the criticism that the CMHCs were not meeting the need of the deinstitutionalized chronically mentally ill was the **Community Support Program (CSP)** of 1977. The program offered grants to communities to develop needed social support systems to assist the chronically mentally ill. The ideal CSP includes crisis care services, psychosocial rehabilitation services, supportive living and working arrangements, medical and mental health care, and case management.[28]

Community Support Programs have been considered a novel approach in that they recognize for the first time that the problem of the chronically mentally ill is—first and foremost—a social welfare problem. In the CSPs, the focus is on services, not facilities as it was under the CMHCs movement. While federal support for CSP was reduced during the 1980s and its funding is always problematical, by 1989 there had been CSP grants to all 50 states.[20] Still, CSPs serve only a small number of clients, despite ever-increasing demand.

MENTAL HEALTH CARE IN AMERICA IN THE 1990S

Perhaps the most remarkable statement that can be made about community mental health in the 1990s is that America still does not have a national mental health program. President Reagan returned the responsibility for care of the indigent mentally ill back to the states, where President Franklin Pierce had left it in 1854. While some would say that in the 1990s mental health care has become more available and

acceptable in many communities, problems are still considerable. Among the most glaring problems are the large number of homeless mentally ill (a legacy of deinstitutionalization), the continued lack of a comprehensive, coordinated system of services for the mentally ill in most communities, the absence of national leadership in setting a mental health policy, and the need for better treatments.

Deinstitutionalization in the 1990s

Deinstitutionalization is now more than three decades old. While there have been some benefits, acknowledged earlier, there remain serious problems. One of the most consequential with regard to providing services is the enormous heterogeneity among patients. While most of these patients are able to live in their communities if provided appropriate levels of support, there is, indisputably, a small minority of deinstitutionalized chronically mentally ill who need highly structured, locked, 24-hour-a-day care. For them, the need remains for the tertiary care facility. For the rest, the challenge is before their communities to provide whatever assistance is required so that these people can achieve the highest degree of independence that is possible for them.

Homelessness

It is difficult to separate the social problem of homelessness from the problem of mental health care for the chronically mentally ill. One of the most often asked questions in this regard is, "What proportion of the homeless are mentally ill?" The difficulties encountered in providing an answer to this question have been recounted by Leona Bachrach.[29] Required for an accurate answer are: a definition of *homelessness,* including a delineation between the truly

---

Community Support Program (CSP) A federal program that provides funds to communities to develop a social support system for the mentally ill.

homeless and those choosing to roam streets, the so-called "urban nomads," and an assessment of the mental illness of the homeless population, or at least a sample of that population. Also, one must recall the enormous heterogeneity within the group we refer to as homeless. Some persons may be homeless only temporarily or seasonally, while others are homeless more or less permanently. While some may rotate between shelters in a single city, others migrate from city to city, being homeless in some cities and not in others, and so on.

In spite of the difficulty in answering the question, the General Accounting Office has estimated the proportion of homeless that are mentally ill to be at least one-third (see Figure 11.10). This range is not really meaningful for any particular location, however, because in some parts of the country 90% of the homeless are mentally ill while elsewhere only 5% of the homeless are mentally ill.[30]

While most of the chronically mentally ill patients who were discharged from mental institutions in the early days of deinstitutionalization are probably dead or in nursing homes by now, the current population of homeless mentally ill has been bolstered by the appearance of a considerable number of new, long-term, or young adult, chronic patients. Before deinstitutionalization, these patients would have been placed in long-term care institutions, if not after their first crisis or episode, at least after their second or third. Now, however, without the option of long-term care, these young, chronically ill persons are swelling the ranks of the homeless mentally ill.[29] Because these chronically ill young patients (patients under 30

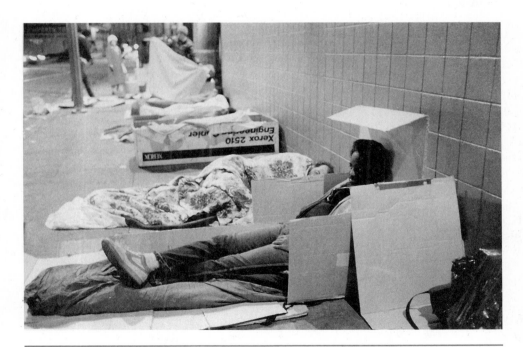

FIGURE 11.10
Between one-third and one-half of the homeless are mentally ill.

years of age) tend to suffer more crises and require more frequent hospitalization than older (over 30) patients, they utilize more of the community's resources.

Mental Health Problems Among Homeless Persons

Various studies have assessed the prevalence of mental health and substance abuse problems in the homeless population. Because of variations in designs and samples, the prevalence of mental health problems ranges from 2%–90%, alcohol problems from 4%–86%, and other drug problems from 1%–70%. As mentioned above, about one-third of adult homeless people have mental problems.[31] Severe and disabling disorders such as schizophrenia, dementia, mental retardation, antisocial personality disorder, and multiple coexisting disorders were higher in homeless persons than in persons included in a household population. However, conditions such as anxiety disorders, major affective disorders, and substance use disorders were more common in domiciled population.[31] In one study, homeless people were 38 times more likely to be schizophrenic, 22 times more likely to have antisocial personality disorder, and 5 times more likely to be cognitively impaired than those who were not homeless.

Mental deficits were also detected in homeless children, who were more likely to experience developmental delays, emotional problems, and abuse than those who are not homeless. Rates of psychiatric morbidity were much higher for both children and adolescents. While figures vary, one sample of New York City homeless youth found 70%–90% of the subjects suffering from mental problems.[31]

Physical Health Problems Among Homeless Persons

While the physical health problems of the homeless, including the homeless men-

tally ill, parallel those of the general population, a number of environmental factors influence the health status of this group in a particularly severe way. For example, this group is more exposed to extremes in temperature, moisture, burns, crowding, assaults, and vehicular accidents. These physical problems are worsened by the anxiety about where to find the next meal and safe shelter, and sometimes, by the effects of chronic alcohol or drug abuse.[32]

Among the clinical conditions that occur at a significantly higher rate in the homeless are communicable diseases, injuries, and nutritional deficiencies. Living in crowded shelters or single room occupancy (SRO) hotels is conducive to the transmission of respiratory and skin diseases. Homeless children are twice as likely to have upper respiratory or ear infections, and four times as likely to have gastrointestinal infections. Skin infections are the second most common acute physical disorder, and homeless children are much more likely to have lice or scabies.[33]

The incidence of tuberculosis (TB) is also higher in the homeless. One study found that in a large New York shelter 42.8% of the men had a positive TB skin test and 6% had active TB.[34] There was a correlation between the probability of a positive test and the length of time spent in the shelter. Those living in the shelter who were also intravenous drug users (IVDUs) were three times as likely to have active TB. Infection with TB is also correlated with HIV infections among shelter inhabitants. It is unusual for a TB-positive individual living in a shelter to test negative for HIV.

Trauma, resulting from both intentional and unintentional causes, occurs at a rate two to three times higher among the homeless than among domiciled persons. A life on the streets is not a safe life, particularly for women, children, and the elderly, who are perceived as weak and thus often become victims of assaults. But males, in at least some studies, were found to have the highest trauma rates and the most severe injuries, including stab wounds, fractures, head trauma, gunshot wounds, burns, and injuries from suicide attempts.[35]

Meeting the Needs of the Mentally Ill

Communities today are challenged with a difficult task in providing mental health care services for their members. These services need to be comprehensive, including primary, secondary, and tertiary prevention services.

The task of providing primary prevention services falls mainly on the private, voluntary agencies, such as the National Mental Health Association and its state and local affiliates. These agencies provide educational speakers, videos, books, and pamphlets about mental health, mental illness, and services. They may offer workshops on stress management, self-esteem development, and coping-skills development. Some sponsor support groups for parents of children who are emotionally handicapped or suffer from some other behavioral disorder. These agencies also act as referral agencies for those in crisis.

The needs of those in the community who require mental health care (secondary prevention) are met by an assortment of providers including treatment providers in private clinics, community mental health centers, and hospital emergency rooms; and social service providers in Social Security, welfare, veterans', and housing offices. For securing needed services, this hodgepodge of federal, state, and local offices and social programs is overwhelming even to someone in good mental health.

While some would say that community mental health services are improving by and large, significant problems remain. For example, a significant gap persists in the availability and quality of care for insured and uninsured patients. Continued federal and state budget constraints suggest that this gap will continue to widen. Many states and communities are making efforts to integrate funding and services for mental health care.[36] But successful integration of these services under a single authority that coordinates previously independent organizations has proven much more difficult than initially believed.[37] Among the problems encountered by managers of integrated systems are control over subordinate organizations that wish to maintain their independence, adequate resources to support all services, inadequate goal delineation, and inability to monitor results. Recalling the diversity of needs of the mentally ill, the value of a concerned and skilled case worker for each mental health care service consumer is inestimable.

Treatment Approaches

The NIMH has stated the goals of treatments for mental disorders. These are: (1) to reduce symptoms, (2) to improve personal and social functioning, (3) to develop and strengthen coping skills, and (4) to promote behaviors that make a person's life better. The three basic approaches to treatment of mental disorders are **biomedical, psychotherapeutic,** and **behavioral therapies.**[38]

Biomedical Therapy

Biomedical therapy involves treatment with medications. Since the introduction of chlorpromazine in 1954, a number of

---

biomedical therapy Treatment with psychotherapeutic drugs or electrical shock.

useful medications for the treatment of mental disorders have been developed. Among the conditions for which medications exist are schizophrenia, bipolar disorder, major depression, anxiety, panic disorder, and obsessive-compulsive disorder.

Another form of biomedical therapy is electroconvulsive treatment (ECT), formerly known as shock treatment. In ECT, alternating electric current passes through the brain to produce unconsciousness and a convulsive seizure. This form of treatment is sometimes used for major depression, selected cases of schizophrenia, or overwhelming suicide ideation, especially when the need for treatment is seen as urgent. Contemporary ECT methods employ low doses of electric shock to the brain. General anesthetics are provided to reduce the unpleasant side effects.

Psychotherapy

Psychotherapy involves face-to-face discussions with therapists who are trained to listen, interpret, define, and resolve troubling personal problems of the patient (see Figure 11.11). There are numerous approaches to psychotherapy including interpersonal, couple, group, and family approaches. Psychodynamic psychotherapy examines current problems as they relate to earlier experiences, even from childhood, while cognitive psychotherapy focuses on faulty or distorted thinking patterns. Psychotherapy is most likely to be successful in less severe cases of emotional distress or used in conjunction with other approaches.

Behavioral Therapy

In **behavioral therapy,** which involves the use of learning theory, a patient is en-couraged toward desired behaviors through rewards and satisfaction. Behavioral therapy usually involves the cooperation of persons important to the patient, such as other family members. Included in behavioral therapy are biofeedback, stress management, and relaxation training.

Social Services Intervention

In addition to specific treatments for their mental disorders, the mentally ill who are dependent upon publicly funded treatment usually require one or more social services. For example, patients may require assistance in locating housing in a **transitional care facility,** such as a personal care home, group home, foster home, shelter, or some type of independent living arrangement. The patient may need legal help with police matters or insurance problems, or to obtain welfare or veterans' benefits. Securing housing and warranted benefits or entitlements with minimal delay and patient stress may be critical to the successful outcome of therapy.

The Dilemma of Involuntary Commitment and Treatment

The dilemma of involuntary civil commitment still exists as a divisive issue in mental health care. Should a person be locked up if he or she is "acting crazy"? Should a doctor medicate someone who is having a psychotic episode as a result of not taking previously prescribed medication? Some feel that the law has now gone too far in protecting the rights of persons at high risk for injury to themselves and others and who are temporarily or perma-

---

psychotherapy A treatment methodology based on Freudian psychology.
behavioral therapy Treatment based on learning theory.

---

transitional care facility Residential housing that enables a mental patient to live in a community by providing some social support.

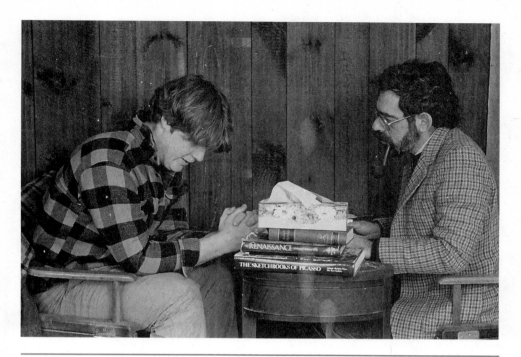

FIGURE 11.11

Psychotherapy is usually only one of the services needed by persons who are suffering from mental illness.

nently incapable of making reasonable decisions about their needs.[27] One solution, now being tried by many states, is **involuntary outpatient commitment.** Involuntary outpatient commitment, first used in the United States in the District of Columbia in 1972, involves a court order that a patient must conform to treatment in an outpatient setting.[39] In this regard, patient and provider alike are coerced into maintaining scheduled treatment—presumably, for the good of all. The advantages to involuntary outpatient commitment are the continuity of care, greater freedom for the patient, and prevention of rehospitalization. Involuntary outpatient commitment has been deemed a success in communities that have tried it. While it may not be the ultimate solution, it is, at least, a stop-gap measure that has been found useful until a more sensitive and caring procedure can be developed. The need for tertiary care for the chronically mental ill is no longer debatable. While the number of residents in state and county mental hospitals declined dramatically during the process of deinstitutionalization, the number of patients in private psychiatric hospitals and in general hospitals offering psychiatric services increased dramatically (see Figure 11.12).[40] What is debatable is *who* should be placed into long-term care facilities and what level of care or treatment should be provided.

involuntary outpatient commitment Court-ordered outpatient treatment.

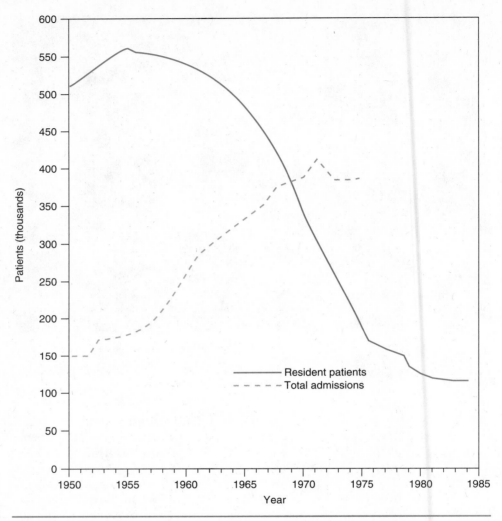

FIGURE 11.12

Resident patients and admissions, state and county mental hospitals, United States, 1950–1984.

From: Rochefort, D. A. (1989) ed. Handbook on Mental Health Policy in the United States. New York: Green-wood Press, p. 28.

FUTURE OUTLOOK

It is difficult to predict how the nation, states, and local communities will respond to the problems of the mentally ill in the future. It will depend on economics, on the degree to which taxpayers have been personally touched by mental illness, or on the degree to which they feel threatened by the growing legions of homeless mentally ill. It will also depend on the federal government's leadership and the success with which advocates for the mentally ill can rally support for their cause.

Federal Initiatives for Mental Health Care in the 1990s

President Clinton and Congress have declared the 1990s the "decade of the brain," because there is great anticipation that during this decade research will yield significant new knowledge about how the brain works.[38] Presumably, this new knowledge will bring with it important breakthroughs in the treatment of mental disorders.

In order to emphasize the research mission of NIMH, former president Bush signed the ADAMHA Reorganization act, which took effect on October 1, 1992. One of the provisions of the act was the return of the NIMH to the NIH. The act also established the **Substance Abuse and Mental Health Services Administration (SAMHSA),** to which it transferred the service components formerly under NIMH control.

Housed within the U.S. Public Health Service of the Department of Health and Human Services, SAMHSA has as its stated mission the reduction of the incidence and prevalence of alcohol and other drug use and mental disorders, the improvement of treatment outcomes for persons suffering from these disorders, and the curtailment of the consequences of these problems for families and communities.[39] Within SAMHSA are three centers: The Center for Substance Abuse Treatment (CSAT), the Center for Substance Abuse Prevention (CSAP), and the Center for Mental Health Services (CMHS). The mission of the CMHS is to assist the states in providing access to treatment, prevention, and rehabilitative services while reducing the impact of mental illness on families and communities.

The Center for Mental Health Services has, as one of the highest priorities, to respond to the growing crisis of mental, emotional, and behavioral problems among youth. The center hopes to accomplish this through two programs, the Child and Adolescent Service System Program (CASSP), charged with insuring the smooth delivery of child and adolescent mental health services, and the Child and Adolescent Research Demonstration Program, charged with supporting research and evaluation of these services.[40] Only time will tell whether the objectives of these programs will be reached.

Currently, all eyes in the mental health care field are on Congress as it debates on health care reform in America. Mental health care will receive a boost if mental health care services figure prominently in the new plan.

Advocacy for the Mentally Ill

The **National Alliance for the Mentally Ill (NAMI)** was founded in Madison, Wisconsin, in 1979. By 1989, the NAMI had 856 affiliates and more than 20,000 member families. The NAMI believes that major mental disorders are brain diseases and that these diseases are of genetic origin and biological in nature. Further, they believe that the family has no role in the production and maintenance of these diseases and that only biologically grounded treatment approaches are relevant.[20]

Based upon these beliefs, NAMI has developed a political platform and has been forceful in lobbying for policy changes. Among the planks in the NAMI platform are calls for an increase in research into the biological origin of mental disorders and an expediting of the development of neuroleptic drugs, drugs for treating mental illness. Members of NAMI call for the eradication of family therapy, because they do not believe that the family contributes in any way to major mental disorders. Some members even refer to family therapy as "family bashing." Instead, they encourage the education and training of medical and social workers in the biological basis of mental illness. Lastly, they welcome the return of the NIMH back into the NIH so that its research mission can be better supported.[20]

CHAPTER SUMMARY

Mental illness constitutes a major community health concern because of its prevalence and the demands it places on community resources. Americans are afflicted with a variety of mental disorders, caused by either genetic or environmental factors. These disorders, which can range from mild to severe, are often chronic and may limit the ability of those afflicted to live independently. Stress, resulting from social and environmental forces, can have a detrimental influence on both physical and mental health.

Over the years, society's response to the needs of the mentally ill has been characterized by long periods of apathy, interrupted by enthusiastic movements for new and enlightened approaches to care. Deinstitutionalization, in which thousands of mental patients housed in state and county hospitals were discharged and returned to their communities, was the most prominent movement of this century. The origins of many of the current problems in community mental health care can be traced to this movement. For example, significant numbers of individuals in today's homeless population suffer from severe mental disorders that prevent them from living independently. There are insufficient community resources to house and otherwise to provide for these people.

Historically, the quality of care for the mentally ill in America has depended to some degree upon the financial resources of the patient or his or her family. This situation, in which there is a disparity in the quality of care received by those with means and those without, can be seen today as a widening gap in the availability and quality of treatment for insured and uninsured mental patients. With the growing cost of health care and the shrinking availability of health care insurance, the outlook for community mental health care is rather grim.

SCENARIO: ANALYSIS AND RESPONSE

1. If you were Jen's roommate, would you have recognized the signals of mental illness before Laura did? What were some of those signals?

2. To whom should Laura report her observations and concerns? The girls across the hall? The R.A. (residence hall assistant)? The R.D. (residence hall director)? A professor she knows in the psychology department? The student health center? The university's counseling center? Jen's parents, who live about three hours away and whom she has met only once?

3. As she prepared to make the call, Laura remembered an incident that occurred the previous year in a nearby residence hall. A male student hanged himself during homecoming weekend. Soon after this incident occurred, the university's counseling center held some open discussions in which students were encouraged to share their feelings about this student's death. One of the primary feelings expressed was guilt. This feeling stemmed from the fact that everyone failed to recognize signals that pointed to the victim's mental problems and impending suicide. The implication was that if anyone had recognized the signals, he or she would have acted immediately. Is this true? What does it take for one human to decide to help another? Are we more likely to help someone with an obvious physical illness than someone with a mental one? Why or why not?

REVIEW QUESTIONS

1. What is meant by the term *mental health*?

2. What are the characteristics of a mentally healthy person?

3. What is the *DSM-III-R*?

4. Name and give examples of the different causes of mental disorders.

5. What evidence is there that mental health is one of the major public health problems in the United States?

6. What is stress? Give some examples of stressors.

7. How can stress result in physical illness?

8. What is the relationship between stress and mental health?

9. How were the mentally ill cared for in Colonial America?

10. What was included in Tuke's therapy, known as "moral treatment"?

11. What role did Dorothea Dix play in the treatment of the indigent mentally ill?

12. How would you characterize the treatment of the mentally ill in state hospitals prior to World War I?

13. When did the mental hygiene movement occur in the United States? What was the focus of this movement?

14. Who founded the National Committee on Mental Hygiene, which later became the National Mental Health Association?

15. What piece of legislation resulted in the establishment of the National Institute of Mental Health, and what were the purposes of the Institute?

16. Define the word *deinstitutionalization*. When did it start in the United States? What caused it?

17. Why was there a movement toward community mental health centers in the early 1960s?

18. What services are provided by community mental health centers?

19. Why is the Community Support Program considered a novel approach?

20. Approximately what percentage of the homeless are mentally ill? What physical health problems do these people face?

21. Who provides most of the primary preventive mental health services today in the United States?

22. How do each of the following therapies work: Biomedical? Psychotherapy? Behavioral?

23. What is involuntary outpatient commitment, and what are its benefits?

24. What is the purpose of the Center for Mental Health Services in the Substance Abuse and Mental Health Services Administration?

ACTIVITIES

1. Make a list of all the stressors you have experienced in the last two weeks. Select two of the items on the list and answer the following questions about them:

   Did you realize the stressor was a stressor when you first confronted it? Explain.

   What physiological responses did you notice when confronted with the stressor?

   Have you confronted the stressor before? Explain your answer.

   What stress mediators (coping responses) do you have to deal with each of the stressors?

   Do you feel you will some day fall victim to a disease of adaptation?

2. Using a local telephone book or one from your hometown, identify the organizations in the community that you believe would provide mental health services. Then create a list of the agencies/organizations. Divide the list into three sections based upon the type of service (primary, secondary, tertiary prevention) offered. If you are not sure what type of services are offered, call the agency/organization to find out. After you have completed your list, write a paragraph or two about what you feel to be the status of mental health care in your community.

3. Make an appointment with someone in the counseling and psychological service center on your campus for an orientation to the services offered by the center. Most mental

health services range from stress management to test anxiety to individual counseling. Find out what your school has to offer and write a one-page summary of available services.

4. Call agencies or service groups in your community to find out what services are needed for the homeless. Also find out how serious the homeless situation is in the community and what plans there are to deal with the problem. Summarize your findings in a two-page paper. Agencies or services to call include the American Red Cross, the local police department, the Salvation Army, the local soup kitchen, a community mental health center, local hospitals, local homeless shelters, and other shelters.

REFERENCES

1. National Mental Health Association (NMHA) (1992). Alexandria, Va.

2. American Psychiatric Association (1987). *Diagnostic and Statistical Manual of Mental Disorders,* 3rd ed., rev. Washington, D.C.: American Psychiatric Association.

3. Children's Defense Fund (1992). "Leave No Child Behind." *The State of America's Children, 1992.* Washington, D.C.: Author.

4. Regier, D. A., J. H. Boyd, J. D. Burke, D. S. Rae, J. K. Myers, M. Kramer, L. N. Robins, L. K. George, M. Karno, and B. Z. Locke (1988). "One-Month Prevalence of Mental Disorders in the United States." *Arch. Gen. Psychiatry* 45: 977–986.

5. Center for Mental Health Services and National Institute of Mental Health (1992). *Mental Health, United States, 1992.* R. W. Manderscheid, and M. A. Sonnenschein, eds. (DHHS pub. no. SMA-92-1942). Washington, D.C: U.S. Government Printing Office.

6. National Center for Health Statistics (1993). "Advance Report of Final Mortality Statistics, 1990." Monthly Vital Statistics Report 41(7), suppl. Hyattsville, Md.: Public Health Service.

7. U.S. Dept. of Health and Human Services (1991). *Healthy People 2000. National Health Promotion and Disease Prevention Objectives* (DHHS Pub. no. PHS-91-510212). Washington, D.C.: U.S. Government Printing Office.

8. National Center for Health Statistics (1991). "Annual Summary of Births, Marriages, Divorces and Deaths: United States, 1990." *Monthly Vital Statistics Report* 39 (13). Hyattsville, Md.: Public Health Service.

9. Holmes, T. H., and R. H. Rahe (1967). "The Social Readjustment Rating Scale." *Journal of Psychosomatic Research* 11: 213–218.

10. Selye, H. (1946). "The General Adaptation Syndrome and Disease of Adaptation." *Journal of Clinical Endocrinology and Metabolism* 6: 117–130.

11. Sarafino, E. P. (1990). *Health Psychology: Biopsychosocial Interactions.* New York: John Wiley & Sons.

12. McKinney, M. E., P. J. Hofschire, J. C. Buell, and R. S. Eliot (1984). "Hemodynamic and Biochemical Responses to Stress: The Necessary Link Between Type A Behavior and Cardiovascular Disease." *Behavioral Medicine Update* 6(4): 16–21.

13. Schneiderman, N. (1983). Animal Behavior Models of Coronary Heart Disease. In D. S. Krantz, A. Baum, and J. E. Singer, eds. *Handbook of Psychology and Health* (vol.3). Hillsdale, N.J.: Eilbaum.

14. Jemmott, J. B., and S. E. Locke, (1984). "Psychosocial Factors, Immunologic Mediation, and Human Susceptibility to Infectious Diseases. How Much Do We Know?" *Psychological Bulletin* 95: 78–108.

15. Schleifer, S. J., B. Scott, M. Stein, and S. E. Keller (1986). "Behavioral and Developmental Aspects of Immunity." *Journal of the American Academy of Child Psychiatry* 26: 751–763.

16. Baer, P. E., L. B. Garmezy, R. J. McLaughlin, A. D. Pokorny, and M. J. Wernick (1987). "Stress, Coping, Family Conflict, and Adolescent Alcohol Use." *Journal of Behavioral Medicine* 10: 449–466.

17. Conway, T. L., R. R. Vickers, H. W. Ward, and R. H. Rahe (1981). "Occupational Stress and Variation in Cigarette, Coffee, and Alcohol Consumption." *Journal of Health and Social Behavior* 22: 155–165.

18. Johnson, A. B. (1990). *Out of Bedlam: The Truth about Deinstitutionalization.* New York: BasicBooks, p. 306.

19. Gerhart, U. C. (1990). *Caring for the Chronic Mentally Ill.* Itasca, Ill.: F. E. Peacock, p. 5.

20. Mosher, L. R., and L. Burti, (1989). *Community Mental Health.* New York: W. W. Norton & Co.

21. Foley, H. A., and S. S. Sharfstein (1983). *Madness and Government.* Washington, D.C.: American Psychiatric Press.

22. Dain, N. (1980). *Clifford Beers—Advocate for the Insane.* Pittsburgh: Univ. of Pittsburgh Press.

23. Grimes, J. M. (1934). *Institutional Care of Mental Patients in the United States.* Chicago: J. M. Grimes. Reprint, New York: Arno, 1980, pp. viii–xii. As cited in Johnson, A. B. *Out of Bedlam: The truth about Deinstitutionalization.* New York: BasicBooks, 1990.

24. Chu, F. D., and S. Trotter (1974). *The Madness Establishment: Ralph Nader's Study Group on the National Institute of Mental Health.* New York: Grossman Publishers, p. 232.

25. Grob, Gerald N. (1991). *From Asylum to Community.* Princeton, N.J.: Princeton Univ. Press, 1991.

26. Peele, R. (1991). "Can a Public Psychiatric Administrator Be Ethical?" (In S. L. Keill, ed. *Administrative Issues in Public Mental Health.* San Francisco: Jossey-Bass, pp. 41–50.)

27. Mechanic, D. (1991). "Recent developments in Mental Health: Perspectives and Services." *Annual Review of Public Health* 12: 1–15.

28. Goldman, H. H., and J. P. Morrissey (1985). "The Alchemy of Mental Health Policy: Homelessness and the Fourth Cycle of Reform." *AJPH* 75(7): 727–730.

29. Lamb, R. H. (1992). "Deinstitutionalization in the Nineties," In R. H. Lamb, L. L. Bachrach, and F. I. Kass, eds. *Treating the Homeless Mentally Ill. A Report of the Task Force on the Homeless Mentally Ill.* Washington, D.C.: American Psychiatric Assn., pp. 41–73.

30. Bachrach, L. L. (1992). "What We Know About Homelessness Among Mentally Ill Persons: An Analytical Review and Commentary." In R. H. Lamb, L. L. Bachrach, and F. I. Kass, eds. *Treating the Homeless Mentally Ill: A Report of the Task Force on the Homeless Mentally Ill.* Washington, D.C.: American Psychiatric Assn., pp. 13–40.

31. Fischer, P. J., R. E. Drake, and W. R. Breakey (1992). "Mental Health Problems Among Homeless Persons: A Review of Epidemiological Research from 1980 to 1990." In R. H. Lamb, L. L. Bachrach, and F. I. Kass, eds. *Treating the Homeless Mentally Ill. A Report of the Task Force on the Homeless Mentally Ill.* Washington, D.C.: American Psychiatric Assn., pp. 75–93.

32. Brickner, P. W. (1992). "Medical Concerns of Homeless Patients." In R. H. Lamb, L. L. Bachrach, and F. I. Kass, eds. *Treating the Homeless Mentally Ill: A Report of the Task Force on the Homeless Mentally Ill.* Washington, D.C.: American Psychiatric Assn., pp. 249–261.

33. Lee, M. A., K. Haught, I. Redlener, et al. (1990). "Health Care for Homeless Families." In W. Brickner, L. K. Scharer, B. A. Conanan, M. Savarese, and B. C. Scanlan, eds. *Under the Safety Net: The Health and Social Welfare of the Homeless in the United States.* New York: W. W. Norton, pp. 119–138.

34. McAdam, J. M., P. W. Brickner, et al. (1990). "Tuberculosis in the Homeless: A National Perspective." In P. W. Brickner, L. K. Scharer, B. A. Conanan, M. Savarese, and B. C. Scanlan, eds. *Under the Safety Net: The Health and Social Welfare of the Homeless in the United States.* New York: W. W. Norton.

35. Scanlan, B. C., and P. W. Brickner (1990). "Clinical Concerns in the Care of Homeless Persons." In P. W. Brickner, L. K. Scharer, B. A. Conanan, M. Savarese, and B. C. Scanlan, eds. *Under the Safety Net: The Health and Social Welfare of the Homeless in the United States.* W. W. Norton.

36. Yank, G. R., D. S. Hargrove, and K. E. Davis, (1992). "Toward the Financial Integration of Public Mental Health Services." *Community Mental Health Journal* 26(2): 97–109.

37. Greenley, J. R. (1992). "Neglected Organization and Management Issues in Mental Health Systems Development." *Community Mental Health Journal* 28(5): 371.

38. U.S. Dept. of Health and Human Services, National Institute of Mental Health. (1992). *Mental Health/Mental Illness: A Consumer's Guide to Services.* (DHHS pub. no. ADA-92-0214). Washington, D.C.: U.S. Government Printing Office.

39. Armat, V. C., and R. Peele (1992). "The Need-for-Treatment Standard in Involuntary Civil Commitment." In R. H. Lamb, L. L. Bachrach, and F. I. Kass, eds. *Treating the Homeless Mentally Ill: A Report of the Task Force on the Homeless Mentally Ill.* Washington, D.C.: American Psychiatric Assn., pp. 183–202.

40. U.S. Dept. of Health and Human Services, Substance Abuse and Mental Health Services Admin., U.S. Public Health Service (1993). "CMHS Sponsors Initiative for Children with Mental Disorders." *SAMHSA News* 1(1): 14–15.

41. Teamer, F. G. (1989). "The Contemporary Mental Health System: Facilities, Services, Personnel, and Finances." In D. A. Rochefort, *Handbook on Mental Health Policy in the United States.* New York: Greenwood Press, pp. 21–42.

Chapter 12

ABUSE OF ALCOHOL
AND OTHER DRUGS

Chapter Outline

Chapter Objectives

After studying this chapter, you will be able to:

1. Identify personal and community consequences of the abuse of alcohol and other drugs.
2. Describe the trends of alcohol and other drug use by high school students.
3. Define *drug use, misuse,* and *abuse.*
4. Define *drug dependence,* both physical and psychological.
5. List and discuss the risk factors for the abuse of alcohol and other drugs.
6. List the types of abused drugs.
7. Explain why alcohol is considered the Number 1 drug abuse problem in America.
8. Describe the health risks of cigarette smoking.
9. Define the term *over-the-counter drugs* and explain the purpose of these drugs.
10. List the different types of illicit drugs.
11. Define the term *dangerous drugs*, and provide examples.
12. Describe the two major approaches to preventing and controlling drug abuse.
13. Summarize various programs that the U.S. federal government has in place to prevent and control drug abuse.
14. Summarize the role of state government in the prevention and control of drug abuse.
15. Describe the relationship between state and local governments in preventing and controlling drug abuse.
16. List and describe some community and school drug abuse prevention programs.

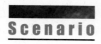
It was 10:30 P.M. on a Friday night; Glenda Bates had half an hour left on her shift. Glenda, 28, was an emergency room nurse at Clinton County Hospital. Glenda disliked working weekend nights, when most injuries are admitted to the ER. Some were victims of car crashes or falls; others had been injured in fistfights, shootings, and stabbings. Many of the victims were drunk or nearly so.

Glenda didn't like working late on this particular Friday night for another reason; it was "girls' night out" for her and her friends. Usually, she and her friends would go out for drinks and dancing about 8:30 or 9:00 P.M. Working the 3:00–11:00 P.M. shift meant Glenda would miss out on most of the fun.

At 11:00 P.M. sharp, Glenda changed clothes and left the hospital. She hurried to her car. She felt under the seat for the paper bag containing the half-pint bottle of gin that she had purchased on her way to work. She hurriedly gulped a couple of burning swallows and started her car. Glenda planned to arrive at the bar ready to party.

Although Glenda's drinking habits caused some of her friends to be concerned, they never told her. She drank quite a bit and usually was not ready to stop drinking when the rest of the group had decided to go home. Sometimes, a member of the group would have to drive her home, just to be sure she got there safely.

By 11:30 P.M. when she reached the bar, she had finished the gin. She felt warm, even though the night air was cold. She left the paper bag containing the empty bottle in the parking lot and hurried into the bar. As she joined her friends, Glenda noticed that some of them were already yawning. One of them said something about having to take her son to a soccer game at 8:30 the next morning; another announced that she had to be at work by 7:00 A.M.

By 11:45 P.M., four of her friends had said good night apologetically and departed. Glenda's loud and obnoxious complaints at their leaving "just when the party is getting started" drew looks and laughs from people at other tables. Glenda didn't care; she had had three more drinks since arriving. Now she and the last member of the group, Iris, were all that was left at the "party."

About 12:15 A.M., two free drinks arrived at their table, followed by two young guys in tight jeans. Glenda doesn't remember much of what happened after that. There was more drinking and laughing, some dancing she thought . . . then a big argument, first inside then outside the bar. The police arrived. . . .

She awoke in her apartment. As she sat up on her bed, still in the clothes she had worn the night before, she saw that it was noon. Her ankle was swollen and very sore, and a glance into her dresser mirror revealed a bruise around her left eye. Had she fallen? Who brought her home? She felt terrible, and she was due at work in a few hours. She reached for the phone to call in sick.

INTRODUCTION

The use, misuse, and abuse of mind-altering substances undoubtedly predates our recorded history. It is perhaps part and parcel of human nature to wish to experience strange and unusual feelings or changes in mood and perceptions. Early humans used drugs as a vehicle to communicate with spirits. Even today, drugs are used for this purpose in some cultures.

For many Americans, drug taking is experimental or social, a temporary departure from a natural, nondrugged physical and mental state. For many others, it is a misguided attempt to solve personal problems such as loneliness, guilt, or low self-esteem. For a small but significant segment of the population, drug taking ceases to be a matter of conscious choice; these people have become chronic drug abusers. In most cultures, chronic alcohol or other drug abuse is regarded as destructive behavior, both to oneself and to the community.

Scope of the Problem

Those abusing alcohol and other drugs represent serious health threats to themselves, their families, and their communities. They are a threat to themselves because they put themselves and their families personally at risk for physical, mental, and financial ruin. The habitual drug user may develop a psychological and/or physical dependence on the drug and thus experience great difficulty in discontinuing use (abuse), even in the face of worsening health and emotional and financial deterioration. If the drug is an illegal one, its use constitutes criminal activity and carries the risks of arrest and incarceration.

Abusers of alcohol and other drugs represent a serious threat to the community because they have greater health care needs, suffer more injuries, and are less productive than those who do not. Community consequences range from loss of economic opportunity and productivity to the destruction of the community (see Table 12.1).

Those who abuse drugs also perpetrate more violent acts that result in economic loss, injury, and death. The violence associated with the abuse of alcohol and other drugs is depicted in Figure 12.1.[1]

The annual economic loss from alcohol and other drug use has been placed at $400 billion.[37] These costs include direct costs, such as those associated with treatment, mortality, and loss of productivity; and indirect costs, including the costs of law enforcement, courts, jails, and social work. The burden on the health care system, its providers, and third-party payers is also considerable. Clearly, the abuse of alcohol and other drugs is one of America's most expensive community health problems.

When the words *drug abuse* are mentioned, most people think of illicit drugs, such as heroin, LSD, cocaine, and other illegal substances. While the abuse of illicit drugs is certainly a major problem in America, it should be kept in perspective with other drug problems, such as alcohol consumption and smoking.

According to the 1993 survey on drug use, abuse of illicit drugs among young Americans in high school and college has continued to decline from the highest use year, 1979. Still, 27.1% of all high school seniors and 30.6% of college students took at least one illicit drug during the previous year.[2]

Marijuana is the Number 1 illicit drug used by these groups; 11.9% of high school seniors reported marijuana use within the past 30 days (see Table 12.2). This figure, while still too high, represents a significant decline in use from past years. A decline was also noted in the use of cocaine including crack cocaine. At its peak of popularity

Table 12.1

Consequences of Drug Use

Personal Consequences	Community Consequences
Absenteeism from school or work	Loss of productivity and revenue
Underachievement at school or work	Lower average SAT scores
Scholastic failure/interruption of education	Loss of economic opportunity
Loss of employment	Increase in public welfare load
Marital instability/family problems	Increase in number of broken homes
Risk of infectious diseases	Epidemics of sexually transmitted diseases
Risk of chronic or degenerative diseases	Unnecessary burden on health care system
Increased risk of accidents	Unnecessary deaths and economic losses
Financial problems	Defaults on mortgages, loans/bankruptcies
Criminal activity	Increased cost of insurance and security
Arrest and incarceration	Increased cost for police/courts/prisons
Risk of adulterated drugs	Increased burden on medical care system
Adverse drug reactions or "bad trips"	Greater need for emergency medical services
Drug-induced psychoses	Unnecessary drain on mental health services
Drug overdose	Unnecessary demand for medical services
Injury to fetus or newborn baby	Unnecessary use of expensive neonatal care
Loss of self-esteem	Increase in mental illness, underachievement
Suicide	Damaged and destroyed families
Death	

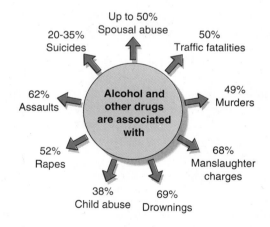

FIGURE 12.1

Violence associated with the use of alcohol and other drugs.

From: Prevention Plus II (1989). Rockville, Md.: Substance Abuse Prevention.

in 1985, 6.7% of high school seniors reported that they had used cocaine within the past 30 days; in 1992, only 1.3% were current users (Table 12.2).

While illicit drugs are still a serious problem, it appears that some progress has been made in the reduction of the abuse of these drugs. The question is, to which of the many approaches to reducing the drug problem may we ascribe the success: public education? school health programs? improved parental supervision and involvement? military interdiction? changes in police activity? changes in drug laws, such as asset seizure laws?

While the abuse of illicit drugs has declined, little reduction is evident in the rate of consumption of two legal drugs, alcohol and nicotine (tobacco). Alcohol remains our

Table 12.2
Percentage of High School Seniors Who Have Used Drugs— Class of 1992

	Ever Used	Past Month	Daily Use
Alcohol	87.5%	51.3%	3.4%
Cigarettes	61.8	27.8	17.2
Marijuana	32.6	11.9	1.9
Stimulants	13.9	2.8	0.2
Inhalants	16.6	2.3	0.1
Cocaine	6.1	1.3	0.1
Tranquilizers	6.0	1.0	*
Hallucinogens	9.2	2.1	0.1
Sedatives	6.1	1.2	0.1
Crack	2.6	0.6	0.1
PCP	2.4	0.6	0.1
Heroin	1.2	0.3	*

*Less than 0.05%

From: Johnston, L. D., P. M. O'Malley, and J. G. Bachman (1993). *National Survey Results on Drug Use from the "Monitoring the Future Study," 1975–1992.* Vol. I: "Secondary School Students" (NIH pub. no. 93-3597). Washington, D.C.: U.S. Government Printing Office.

most serious drug problem, and statistics cited in this chapter confirm this assertion. Nearly half a million people die each year from causes related to cigarette smoking.

Yet another drug problem is the overuse and misuse of therapeutic drugs. Millions of people misuse over-the-counter and prescription drugs each year, resulting in a waste of valuable resources and unnecessary medical expense. Sometimes the result of the misuse of prescription drugs can have deadly consequences.

Definitions

As we begin a discussion of alcohol and other drugs as a community health prob-lem, it is important to define some terms. A **drug** is a substance, other than food or vitamins, which upon entering the body in small amounts, alters one's physical, mental, or emotional state. **Psychoactive drugs** are drugs that affect the central nervous system.

In this chapter, the term **drug use** is a nonvaluative term referring to drug-taking behavior in general, regardless of whether the behavior is appropriate. **Drug misuse** refers primarily to the inappropriate use of legally purchased prescription or non-prescription drugs. Drug misuse occurs when one discontinues the use of a prescribed antibiotic before the entire prescribed dose is completed or when one takes four aspirin rather than two as specified on the label. **Drug abuse** can be defined in several ways depending upon the drug and the situation. Drug abuse occurs when one takes a prescription or nonprescription drug for a purpose other than that for which it is medically approved. For example, drug abuse occurs when one takes a prescription diet pill for its mood altering effects (stimulation). The abuse of legal drugs such as nicotine or alcohol is said to occur when one is aware that continued use is detrimental to one's health. Because illicit drugs have no approved medical uses, any illicit drug use is considered drug abuse. Likewise, the use of alcohol and nicotine by those under the legal age is considered drug abuse.

---

drug A substance other than food that when taken in small quantities, alters one's physical, mental, or emotional state.

psychoactive drugs Drugs that affect the central nervous system.

drug misuse Inappropriate use of prescription or nonprescription drugs.

drug abuse Use of a drug when it is detrimental to one's health or well-being.

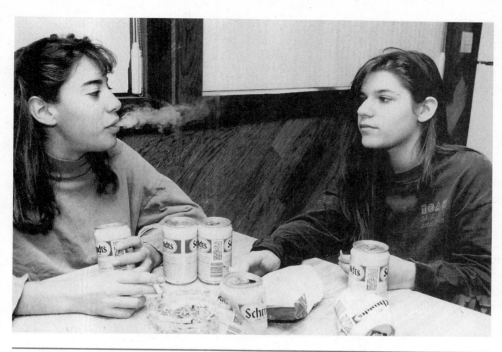

FIGURE 12.2

While abuse of illicit drugs has declined, little reduction is evident in the use of alcohol and nicotine.

Drug (chemical) dependence occurs when a user feels that a particular drug is necessary for normal functioning. Dependence may be **psychological,** in which case the user experiences a strong emotional or psychological desire to continue use of the drug, or **physical,** in which discontinuation of drug use results in clinical illness. Often, both psychological and physical dependence are present at the same time, making the discontinuation of drug use very difficult. Such is frequently the case with cigarette smoking.

drug (chemical) dependence A psychological and sometimes physical state characterized by a craving for a drug.

psychological dependence A psychological state characterized by an overwhelming desire to continue use of a drug.

physical dependence A physiological state in which discontinued drug use results in physical illness.

FACTORS THAT CONTRIBUTE TO SUBSTANCE ABUSE

The factors that contribute to the abuse of alcohol and other drugs can be either genetic (inherited) or environmental. Numerous studies have concluded that inherited traits can increase one's risk of developing dependence on alcohol, and it is logical to assume that susceptibility to other drugs might also be inherited. Environmental risk factors, such as one's home and family life, school and peer groups, and society and culture have also been identified.

Inherited Risk Factors

The vast majority of the data supporting the notion that the risk of drug dependence can be inherited comes from studies on alcoholism. Evidence for the heritability of risk for alcoholism is provided by numerous studies,[3, 4, 5] which have been reviewed by Tabakoff and Hoffman[6] in the *Seventh Special Report to the U.S. Congress on Alcohol and Health,* from the Secretary of Health and Human Services.[7] Studies of alcoholics' families have found that there are at least two types of inherited alcoholism[4], now referred to as Type I, or milieu limited, and Type II, or male limited alcoholism.[7] These observational studies of alcoholics' families are supported by research using genetic and biological markers in animal models. Some of these markers predispose an individual biochemically to increased susceptibility to developing alcohol-related problems while others may actually be protective in nature. For example, genes which code for enzymes that inhibit the normal metabolism of alcohol could cause one to respond positively to the effects of alcohol and thus drink more, or respond negatively to alcohol and thus drink less or not at all.[6] The heritability of susceptibility to other drugs is still under investigation.

Environmental Risk Factors

There are a great many environmental factors, both psychological and social, that influence the use and abuse of alcohol and other drugs. Included are personal factors, the influences of home and family life, school and peer groups, and the sociocultural environment.

Personal Factors

Personal factors include personality traits, such as impulsiveness, depressive mood, susceptibility to stress, or possibly, personality disturbances. Some of these factors have been reviewed by Needle[8] and by Naelge.[9] While models that involve personal factors provide frameworks for research and theorizing about the etiology of alcohol and drug abuse, they have their limitations. It is difficult to determine the degree to which these factors are inherited or are simply the product of the family environment. For example, one's choice to use alcohol or drugs in response to a stressful situation (and the outcome of that decision) could be the result of either inherited characteristics, learned behavior, or a combination of these factors.

Home and Family Life

The importance of home and family life on alcohol and drug abuse has been the subject of numerous studies, some of which have been reviewed by Meller[10] and Needle et al.[9] Research demonstrates that not all family-associated risk is genetic in origin. Family structure, family dynamics, and family problems can all contribute to drug experimentation by children and adolescents (see Figure 12.3). Major negative family events (death, divorce, parental drug use, or other family turmoil) have been associated with the initiation of alcohol and other drug use.[8]

The development of interpersonal skills, such as communication skills, independent living skills, and learning to get along with others, are nurtured in the home. The failure of parents to provide an environment conducive to the development of these skills can result in the loss of self-esteem and in-

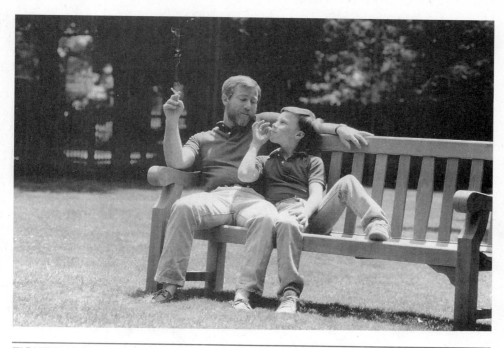

FIGURE 12.3

Influences of home and family life can affect one's decisions about alcohol, tobacco, and other drugs.

crease in delinquency, nonconformity and sociopathic behavior, all personal risk factors for alcohol and drug abuse.[7]

Finally, family attitudes toward alcohol and drug use influence adolescents' beliefs and expectations about drugs' effects. These expectations have been shown to be important factors in adolescents' choices to initiate and continue alcohol use.[7]

School and Peer Groups

Perceived and actual drug use by peers influences attitudes and choices by adolescents (see Figure 12.4). Some studies have shown that perceived support of drinking by peers is the single most important factor in an adolescent's choice to drink.[7] Peers can also influence expectations for a drug. Alcohol may be perceived as "a 'magic elixir' that can enhance social and physical plea-

sure, sexual performance and responsiveness, power and aggression and social competence."[7] It is interesting to note that these are precisely the mythical qualities about alcohol portrayed in advertisements for beer and other alcoholic beverages.

Sociocultural Environment

The notion of environmental risk includes the effects of sociocultural and physical settings on drug-taking behavior. The study of the effects of the physical and social environment upon the individual is termed *social ecology*.[11] Environmental risk for drug taking can stem from one's immediate neighborhood or from society at large. For example, living in the inner city—with its sordidness, physical decay, and threats to personal safety—could set into motion a variety of changes in values and behaviors, in-

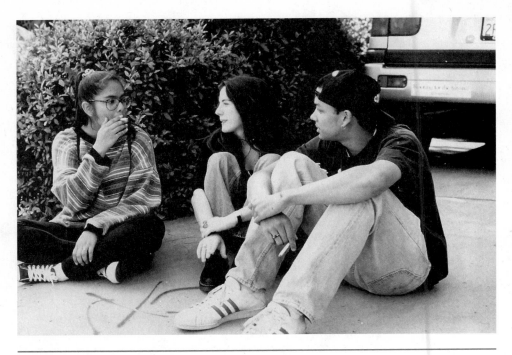

FIGURE 12.4

Peers can influence one's expectations of the effects of a drug.

cluding some related to alcohol or drug use. Likewise, federal, state, and local enforcement policies and educational efforts can influence individual choices about drug use.

TYPES OF DRUGS ABUSED AND RESULTING PROBLEMS

Almost any psychoactive drug available is subject to abuse by at least some segment of the population. Classification systems of drugs of abuse are many, but none of them are perfect. Problems of classification arise because all drugs have multiple effects and because the legal status of some drugs varies with formulation or with age of user.

In this chapter, our classification system includes legal drugs and illegal drugs. Legal (licit) drugs include alcohol, nicotine, nonprescription and prescription drugs. Illegal (illicit) drugs can be classified further on the basis of physiological effects as stimulants, depressants, narcotics, hallucinogens, marijuana, and other drugs.

Legal Drugs

Legal drugs include some that are closely regulated, like morphine; others that are lightly regulated, like alcohol; and still others that are not regulated at all, like caffeine.

Alcohol

Alcohol is the Number 1 problem drug in America by almost any standard of measurement—the number of those who abuse it, the number of injuries and deaths it causes, and its economic cost to society. Alcohol is consumed in a variety of forms including beer, wine, fortified wines and brandies, and distilled spirits.

Drinking by high school and college students continues to be very widespread, despite the fact that it is illegal for virtually all high school students and for most college students to purchase these beverages. Ninety percent of high school seniors report having tried alcohol at least once, and 32% report occasions of heavy drinking (consuming five or more drinks in a row at least once in the prior two-week period). Of college students, 41% report occasions of heavy drinking.[2]

Most of those who experiment with alcohol begin use in a social context and become light or moderate drinkers. Alcohol use is reinforcing in two ways: it lowers anxieties and produces a mild euphoria. For the majority, alcohol use does not become a significant problem, but for a significant minority it does. Some of these become **problem drinkers;** that is, they begin to experience social, legal, or financial problems because of their alcohol consumption. For still others—perhaps 10% of those who drink—use becomes intensified and dependence develops. Physical dependence on alcohol and the loss of control over one's drinking are two important characteristics of **alcoholism.** A revised definition of alcoholism has recently been published in the *Journal of the American Medical Association:*[12]

> **Alcoholism** is a primary, chronic disease with genetic, psychosocial, and environmental factors influencing its development and

manifestations. The disease is often progressive and fatal. It is characterized by impaired control over drinking, preoccupation with the drug alcohol, use of alcohol despite adverse consequences, and distortions in thinking, most notably denial. Each of these symptoms may be continuous or periodic.

The cost of alcohol-related injuries alone is estimated at $47 billion each year—that is, $188 for every man, woman, and child. "Every single hour our nation spends over $5 million for alcohol-related injuries."[37] More than 60% of the cost is due to lost employment or reduced productivity, and 13% of the cost is due to medical and treatment costs. Health care costs for alcoholics are about twice those for nonalcoholics.[7]

Alcohol and other drugs are contributing factors to a variety of unintentional injuries and injury deaths. Approximately 40% of all crashes with occupant deaths involve drivers who have **blood-alcohol concentrations (BACs)** of 0.10% or higher (see Figure 12.5), and 53% of drivers killed in single-vehicle crashes in 1989 had illegal BACs.[13] Alcohol-impaired drivers also kill nondrinking motor vehicle occupants. One study found that of the children aged 1–14 years who died in motor vehicle crashes, more than one-fourth died in *alcohol-related* motor vehicle crashes. (See Box 12.1.)

Alcohol has also been found to increase one's risk of involvement in other types of unintentional injuries, such as drowning, falls, fires, and burns. Associations between unintentional injuries and the abuse of other drugs is less well documented, but given a knowledge of the effects of such drugs, one can assume that they increase neither the user's alertness nor coordination.

Alcohol also contributes to intentional violence in the community. For example, 50%

---

problem drinker   One for whom alcohol consumption results in a medical, social, or other type of problem.

alcoholism   A disease characterized by impaired control over drinking, preoccupation with drinking, and continued use of alcohol despite adverse consequences.

---

blood-alcohol concentration (BAC)   The percentage of concentration of alcohol in the blood.

of spouse abuse, 49% of murders, 62% of assaults, 52% of rapes, 38% of child abuse cases, and 20%–35% of suicides are traceable to alcohol consumption (see Figure 12.1).

Nicotine

Nicotine is the psychoactive and addictive drug present in tobacco products, such as cigarettes, cigars, smokeless tobacco (chewing tobacco and snuff), and pipe tobacco. Tobacco use is legal for those 18 years of age and over in most states. Unfortunately, the most popular form of tobacco use, cigarette smoking, is the Number 1 modifiable cause of death in the United States. Nonetheless, some 28% of high school seniors reported having smoked cigarettes in the past month in 1992, and cigarettes remain the class of substance most frequently used on a daily basis by that group. Nearly one in five high school seniors smoked cigarettes daily in 1990.[2] This level has not dropped appreciably since 1980, despite adverse publicity and increasingly restrictive legislation (see Figure 12.6). The rates of cigarette smoking among high school seniors is about the same for males as it is for females (17%).[2] While it is true that some of these students are light smokers (less than half a pack a day) studies show that many light smokers become heavy smokers (more than half a pack a day) as they become older. The prevalence of cigarette smoking in people aged 20 and older is 29%.[14]

The health consequences of tobacco use are familiar to all, even smokers. They include increased risks for heart disease, lung cancer, chronic obstructive lung disease, stroke, emphysema, and other conditions.[15] Annually, smoking accounts for more than 400,000 deaths in the United States and 2.5 million deaths worldwide.[16] The economic costs of tobacco smoking were estimated to be $52 billion ($221 per person per year) in

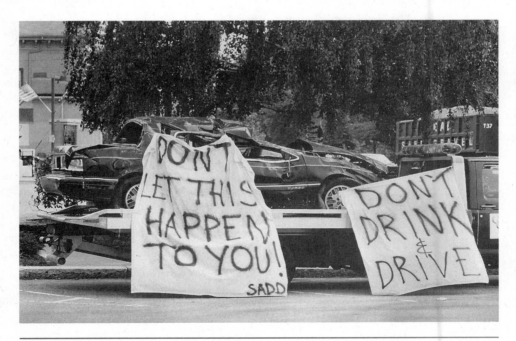

FIGURE 12.5

Forty percent of all crashes with occupant deaths involved drivers with BACs of greater than 0.10%.

BOX 12.1
Healthy People 2000—Objective

4.1   Reduce deaths caused by alcohol-related motor vehicle crashes to no more than 8.5 per 100,000 people. (Age-adjusted baseline: 9.8 per 100,000 in 1987)

Special Population Targets

	Alcohol-Related Motor Vehicle Crash Deaths (per 100,000)	1987 Baseline	2000 Target	Percent Decrease
4.1a	American Indian/Alaska Native men	52.2	44.8%	
4.1b	People aged 15–24	21.5	18	

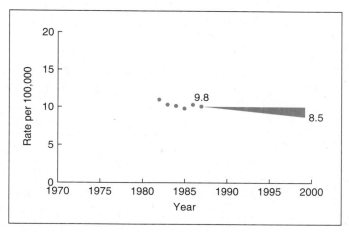

Baseline data source: Fatal Accident Reporting System, U.S. Dept. of Transportation.

Age-adjusted alcohol-related motor vehicle crash death rate.

For Further Thought

Approximately one-half of the fatal motor vehicle crashes are alcohol related. In addition, alcohol-related traffic crashes are the leading cause of spinal cord injuries for young Americans. With such negative statistics, why do you think that some states still do not have laws that make it illegal to drink and drive?

the United States in 1985.[7] Obviously, tobacco use and nicotine addiction continue to be a burden on society.

Recent research has demonstrated that one does not have to use tobacco products to be adversely affected. The 1986 Surgeon General's report on the effects of **environmental tobacco smoke (ETS)** indicated that adults and children who inhale the tobacco smoke of others are also at increased risk for cardiac and respiratory illnesses.[17, 18]

environmental tobacco smoke (ETS)   Tobacco smoke in the ambient air.

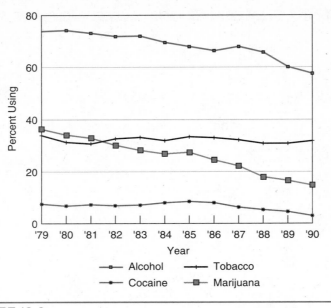

FIGURE 12.6

Drug use by high school seniors, past 30 days, 1979–1990.

From: Johnston, L.D. et al. (1991). "Drug Use Among American High School Seniors, College Students and

These findings resulted in new smoking regulations in many indoor environments. Then in December 1992, the Environmental Protection Agency (EPA) released its report, "Respiratory Health Effects of Passive Smoking: Lung Cancer and other Disorders."[19] Among their findings were that ETS is a human carcinogen, responsible for 3,000 lung cancer deaths annually among nonsmoking Americans. ETS exposure is causally associated with as many as 150,000–300,000 cases of lower respiratory infections (such as bronchitis and pneumonia) in infants and young children up to 18 months of age. The EPA study also found that ETS aggravates asthma in children and is a risk factor for new cases of asthma in children who do not have it.

The use of smokeless (chewing) tobacco also carries with it serious health risks. These include addiction, periodontal disease, and oral cancer.[19] Approximately 5% of 12- to 17-year-old males and 11% of 18- to 25-year-old males report using smokeless tobacco within the past 30 days.[20] The majority of users are white males, who reported a 30-day use rate of 7.6% for all age groups.

Over-the-Counter (OTC) Drugs

Over-the-counter (OTC) drugs are those drugs, with the exception of tobacco and alcohol, that can be purchased without a physician's prescription. Included in this category are internal analgesics such as aspirin, acetaminophen (Tylenol), and ibuprofin (Advil); cough and cold remedies (Robitussin, Contac); emetics; laxatives; mouthwashes; vitamins; and many others. More than 100,000

over-the-counter (OTC) drugs (nonprescription drugs) Drugs (except tobacco and alcohol) that can be legally purchased without a physician's prescription.

different OTC products are sold by pharmacies, supermarkets, convenience stores and in vending machines. These products are manufactured and sold to those who self-diagnose and self-medicate their own illnesses. While the Food and Drug Administration assures the safety and effectiveness of these products when used according to label directions, no person or agency supervises the actual purchase or use of these substances.

Naturally, some of these substances are misused and abused. Examples of misuse were given at the beginning of this chapter. A specific example of OTC drug abuse is the taking of laxatives or emetics to lose weight or to avoid gaining weight. Other OTC drugs that are often abused are appetite suppressants (Dexatrim), stimulants (NoDoz), and nasal sprays (Neo-Synephrine).

Most OTC drugs merely provide symptomatic relief and do not provide a cure. For example, cough and cold remedies relieve the discomfort that accompanies a cold but do not in anyway rid a person of the cold virus that is causing these symptoms. Therefore, a real danger of OTC drug misuse and abuse is that symptoms that should be brought to the attention of a physician remain unreported. Another danger is that those who abuse these drugs may become dependent, unable to live normally without them. Lastly, abuse of OTC drugs may establish a pattern of dependency that predisposes the abuser to developing dependent relationships with prescription drugs or illicit drugs.

Prescription Drugs

Because all prescription drugs have serious side effects for some people, they can be purchased only with a physician's (or dentist's) written instructions (prescription). More than 2,500 drugs are listed in each annual edition of the *Physician's Desk Reference*.[21] The written prescription connotes that the prescribed drugs are being taken by the patient under the prescribing physician's supervision. Each prescription includes the patient's name, the amount to be dispensed, and the dosage. Nonetheless, prescription drugs are also subject to misuse and abuse. Types of misuse include those cited above for the OTC drugs and also the giving of one person's prescription drug to another. Certain prescription drugs such as stimulants (amphetamines), depressants (Valium), and narcotics (morphine, codeine) have a higher potential for abuse than others. Because prescription drugs are usually stronger or more concentrated than OTC drugs, there is a greater risk of developing dependence or taking an overdose from these drugs. Those who develop dependence may try to obtain duplicate prescriptions from other physicians or steal the drugs from hospital dispensaries or pharmacies.

While the abuse of prescription drugs is a concern, levels of abuse are much lower for these drugs than for alcohol and tobacco. Only about 2% of 12- to 17-year-olds, 3% of 18- to 25-year-olds and 2% of the 26- to 34-year-olds report having abused a psychotherapeutic drug in the past 30 days.[20]

One serious consequence of the misuse of prescription drugs is the development of drug resistant strains of pathogens. A prime example is the tuberculosis bacillus. When patients fail to complete the entire antibiotic treatment, some of the bacteria survive and multiply, reinfecting the body with drug resistant organisms. Succeeding treatments are less effective. When this strain of the disease is transmitted to another, the antibiotic treatment fails. New drugs are sometimes used to treat these patients, but as drug misuse continues to occur, multidrug resistant tuberculosis (MDR-TB) develops. It is now clear than MDR-TB is the most serious aspect of the current increase in TB cases in the United States.[22]

Illicit (Illegal) Drugs

Illicit (illegal) drugs are those substances, that cannot be cultivated, manufactured, bought, sold, or used within the confines of the law (see Figure 12.7). They include marijuana (including hashish and hash oil), opium and heroin, cocaine, and a group of substances known as *dangerous drugs*. These include the hallucinogens, such as lysergic acid diethylamide (LSD); designer drugs, such as alpha methyl fentanyl (China white); phencyclidine (angel dust); methylenedioxymethamphetamine (MDMA); stimulants such as the amphetamines; depressants such as the barbiturates and benzodiazapines; and anabolic drugs, including steroids.[23]

Marijuana

Of all illicit drugs abused in the United States, marijuana is the most common. **Marijuana** and the related products, hashish and hash oil, are derived from the hemp plant, *Cannabis sativa*. The products are most commonly used by smoking but can also be ingested. While marijuana abuse has declined, it remains a concern for several reasons. First, it is illegal, and therefore brings the user into contact with those involved in illegal activities. Second, the act of smoking is detrimental to one's health. Third, marijuana smoking often occurs in conjunction with the drinking of alcohol or the use of other drugs. The effects of **polydrug use** (the use of more than one drug at a time) may be more serious than those of single-drug use. Lastly, as is true of all drugs, the adolescent who uses marijuana is delaying the accomplishment of

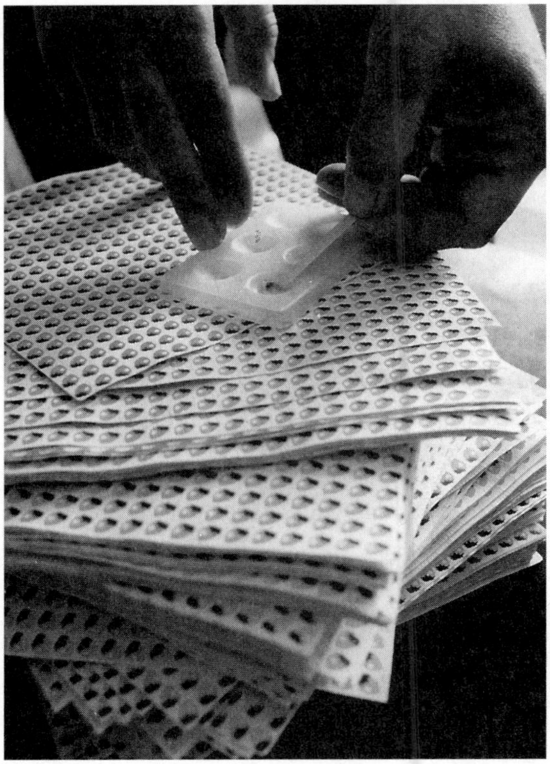

FIGURE 12.7

Illicit drugs, like LSD shown here, cannot be legally manufactured, bought, or sold.

developmental tasks such as attaining an adult self-identity, achieving independence, and developing the interpersonal skills necessary for successful independent living.

The percentage of college students who report having smoked marijuana in the past 30 days dropped from 34% in 1980 to 14.6% in 1992.[2] There are data to suggest that the perceived risk of regular marijuana use may have contributed to the decline in actual use. In 1980, only 44% of 19- to 22-year-olds studied reported believing that great risk was associated with regular marijuana use; in 1992, 69% felt that way.[2]

---

illicit (illegal) drugs Drugs that cannot be legally manufactured, distributed, or sold and that usually lack recognized medical value.

marijuana Dried plant parts of *Cannabis sativa*.

polydrug use Concurrent use of multiple drugs.

The acute health effects of marijuana use include reduced concentration, slowed reaction time, impaired short-term memory, and impaired judgment. Naturally, these effects can have serious consequences for someone operating a motor vehicle or other machinery. Marijuana use in combination with alcohol can be especially dangerous because the two drugs in combination may affect the brain differently.[24] The chronic effects of smoking marijuana include damage to the respiratory system by the smoke itself and for some, the development of **amotivational syndrome,** a chronic apathy toward maturation and the achievement of the developmental tasks listed above (e.g., developing skills for independent living, setting and achieving goals, and developing an adult self-identity). See Box 12.2.

Opium, Morphine, and Heroin

Opium and its derivatives, morphine and heroin, come from the oriental poppy plant, *Papaver somniferum.* These **narcotics** numb the senses and reduce pain. As such, they have a high potential for abuse. In 1990, between 500,000 and 1 million people used heroin in the United States.[20] However, it is acknowledged that this survey missed a great many addicts who may be homeless and living in shelters; thus, this estimate may be low.

Narcotics produce euphoria, analgesia, and drowsiness. They reduce anxiety and pain without affecting motor activity the way alcohol and barbiturates do. If use continues, the body makes physiological adjustments to the presence of the drug. This **tolerance** means that larger and larger doses

---

BOX 12.2
Healthy People 2000— Objective

4.6 Reduce the proportion of young people who have used alcohol, marijuana, and cocaine in the past month, as follows:

Substance/Age	1988 Baseline	2000 Target
Alcohol/aged 12–17	25.2%	12.6%
Alcohol/aged 18–20	57.9	29
Marijuana/aged 12–17	6.4	3.2
Marijuana/aged 18–25	15.5	7.8
Cocaine/aged 12–17	1.1	0.6
Cocaine/aged 18–25	4.5	2.3

Note: The targets of this objective are consistent with the goals established by the Office of National Drug Control Policy, Executive Office of the President.

Baseline data source: National Household Survey of Drug Abuse, ADAMHA.

For Further Thought

What benefits do you see for the United States if the above objective can be reached? Are there any disadvantages to trying to meet this objective? If yes, what are they?

---

are required to achieve the same euphoria and numbing as the initial dose. While tolerance develops rapidly to the euphoric effects, the depressing effects on respiration may continue to increase with dose level, increasing the risk of a fatal overdose. As the cost of the drug habit becomes higher, the abuser

---

amotivational syndrome A pattern of behavior characterized by apathy, loss of effectiveness, and a more passive, introverted personality.
narcotics Drugs similar to morphine that reduce pain and induce a stuporous state.

tolerance Physiological and enzymatic adjustments that occur in response to the chronic presence of drugs and which are reflected in the need for ever-increasing doses.

usually attempts to quit. This results in withdrawal illness, because the body has become physically dependent upon the drug.

Heroin addicts have a difficult time changing their life-style for several reasons. First there is the addiction itself, both physical and psychological. Often too, there are underlying psychosocial problems, such as poor self-image, lack of job skills, and absence of supporting family and friends. Addicts usually mistrust official programs set up to help them. They are usually in poor health mentally and physically. Since the duration of action of heroin is only four to five hours, the addict is usually too concerned with finding the next dose or recovering from the previous one to be productive in the community.

The community is affected by more than the loss of productivity, however. The addict must obtain money to purchase heroin, and the price of the habit can be very high—as much as $200 per day. The money is usually obtained illegally through burglaries, thefts, robberies, muggings, prostitution (male and female), and selling drugs (see Figure 12.8). If a prostitute can make $50 dollars a "trick," he or she needs to "turn" at least four tricks a day just to maintain the habit. The result is not only a deteriorating community but also epidemics of sexually transmitted diseases, such as gonorrhea, syphilis, chlamydia, herpes, and AIDS. Since most heroin addicts inject the drug, there are also epidemics of blood-borne diseases, such as AIDS and hepatitis. In this way, drug abuse increases the burden on community health resources. Addicts who turn to dealing drugs to support their habit do even more damage, because they increase the availability of the

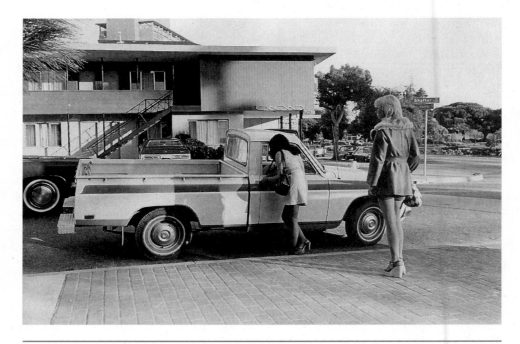

FIGURE 12.8

The community is affected by the increase in criminal activity associated with illicit drug use.

drug and may introduce it to first-time users. When caught, they use resources of the justice system.

Cocaine

Cocaine is the psychoactive ingredient in the leaves of the coca plant, *Erythoxolyn coca,* which grows in the Andes Mountains of South America. Cocaine is a **stimulant;** that is, it increases the activity of the central nervous system. For centuries, natives of the Andes Mountains chewed the leaves to improve stamina during work and long treks. In its more purified forms, as a salt (white powder) or dried paste (crack), cocaine is a powerful euphoriant/stimulant and very addictive.

Cocaine use among college students peaked in 1982, when 7.9% reported use within the past 30 days. In 1992, only 1.0% reported monthly use.[2] Still, estimates for 1991 indicate that as many as 2 million Americans have used cocaine or crack in the past 30 days.[20] Therefore, cocaine remains a serious drug problem in the United States.

Dangerous Drugs

Dangerous drugs are substances that have a high potential for abuse and have no accepted medical uses and no acceptable standards of safe use. Dangerous drugs include all the remaining illicit drugs, such as the hallucinogens and designer drugs and illegally acquired or manufactured prescription drugs, such as stimulants, depressants, and anabolic steroids. Also included as dangerous drugs are substances known as *inhalants.*

Hallucinogens

Hallucinogens are drugs that produce illusions, hallucinations, and other changes in one's perceptions of the environment. These effects are due to the phenomenon known as **synesthesia,** a mixing of the senses. Hallucinogens include both naturally derived drugs like mescaline, from the peyote cactus, and psilocybin and psilocin, from the Psilocybe mushroom; and synthetic drugs, such as LSD. While physical dependence has not been demonstrated with the hallucinogens, tolerance does occur. Though overdose deaths are rare, "bad trips" (unpleasant experiences) do occur. Since there are no legal sources for these drugs, the user is always at risk for taking fake, impure, or adulterated drugs.

Designer Drugs

Designer drugs is a term that describes psychoactive drugs prepared illegally by amateur chemists in secret laboratories. The drugs are designed to mimic popular psychoactive compounds such as amphetamines or narcotics, but their chemical structures are altered slightly to evade detection and law enforcement. Examples of designer drugs include designer narcotics like "china white" (alpha methyl fentanyl and other analogues of fentanyl), MPPP (1-methyl-4 phenyl-4 proprionoxypiperidine), and analogues of meperidine (Demerol); the dissociative anesthetics like angel dust (phencyclidine or PCP and its many analogues); and the psychedelic amphetamines such as MDMA (3, 4-methylenedioxy-methamphetamine). The Controlled Substances

---

cocaine The psychoactive ingredient in the leaves of the coca plant, *Erythoxolyn coca.*

stimulant A drug that increases the activity of the central nervous system.

dangerous drugs Any controlled substances other than cocaine, opiates (narcotics), and *cannabis* products (such as marijuana).

hallucinogens Drugs that produce profound distortions of the senses.

synesthesia Impairment of mind characterized by a sensation that senses are mixed.

designer drugs Drugs synthesized illegally that are similar to, but structurally different from, known controlled substances.

Analogue Act of 1986 was enacted to reduce the flow of these drugs into the market and make it easier to prosecute those involved in manufacturing and distributing designer drugs.

Stimulants

Stimulants are drugs that increase the activity level of the central nervous system. Examples include the **amphetamines,** such as amphetamine itself (bennies), dextroamphetamine (dexies); methamphetamine (meth, crystal, crank, go fast) and dextromethamphetamine (ice); and a new drug, methcathinone (cat). Amphetamine and dextroamphetamine are prescription drugs that were widely abused in the past. The increased regulatory efforts that reduced the availability of these drugs for abuse probably contributed to the rise in the cocaine trade in the 1980s. The decline in cocaine's popularity in the late 1980s was accompanied by a return to the abuse of amphetamines produced in clandestine laboratories. "Crank" or "crystal" (methamphetamine) abuse became epidemic in the Southwestern states in the late 1980s, while "ice" (dextromethamphetamine) became a problem in Hawaii at about the same time.

Presently, a new stimulant has appeared on the street. **Methcathinone ("cat")** is a methamphetamine-like analog of cathinone, a chemical found in the khat plant of east Africa, *Cathis edulis*. Methcathinone was first encountered in Michigan in 1991, and its use is now spreading to other areas of the United States.[25]

Depressants

The **barbiturates, benzodiazapines, methaqualone,** and other **depressants,**

slow down the nervous system. They are attractive to some people because, like alcohol, among the first effects of taking these drugs are the lowering of anxiety and the loss of inhibitions. These effects produce the feeling of a "high," even though these drugs depress the central nervous system. As one continues to use these drugs, tolerance develops and the user experiences the need for greater and greater doses in order to feel the same effects as the previous dose provided. Strong physical dependence develops, so that abstinence results in severe clinical illness; thus abusers of these substances must often rely on medical assistance during detoxification and recovery.

Anabolic Drugs

Anabolic drugs are protein-building drugs. Included are the anabolic/androgenic steroids (AS), testosterone, and human growth hormone (HGH). These drugs have legitimate medical uses, such as the rebuilding of muscles after starvation or disease and the treatment of dwarfism. But they are sometimes abused by athletes as a shortcut to increasing muscle mass, strength, and endurance. They are believed to improve performance and, in body building, where size equals performance, they do. Abuse of steroids is accompanied by numerous acute and chronic side effects including (for men): acne, gynecomastia (the development of breasts), baldness, reduced fertility, and reduction in testicular size. Side effects for women are masculinizing: development

---

amphetamines A group of synthetic drugs that act as stimulants.
methcathinone ("cat") An illicit, amphetamine-like, designer drug.

barbiturates Depressant drugs based on the structure of barbituric acid.
benzodiazapines Nonbarbiturate depressant drugs.
methaqualone An illicit depressant drug.
depressant A drug that slows down the central nervous system.
anabolic drugs Compounds, structurally similar to the male hormone testosterone, that increase protein synthesis and thus muscle building.

of a male physique, increased body hair, failure to ovulate (menstrual irregularities), and a deepening of the voice.[26] Long-term abuse of anabolic steroids can result in psychological dependence, making the discontinuation of use very difficult.

In the late 1980s, it became apparent that increasing numbers of boys and young men of high school and college age were taking anabolic steroids as a shortcut to muscle building or to maturity. Because of this trend, the Anabolic Steroids Control Act of 1990 was enacted; and in 1991, federal law-enforcement agencies initiated regulatory, enforcement, and demand reduction efforts.[23] As these regulatory and enforcement activities began to take effect, some steroid users began using veterinary steroids and "steroid alternatives" such as gamma hydroxybutyrate (GHB) and clenbuterol. Use of these drugs, which is illegal and dangerous, has resulted in serious health problems and several deaths.[27]

Inhalants

Inhalants are a collection of psychoactive, breathable chemicals. They include paint solvents, motor fuels, cleaners, glues, aerosol sprays, cosmetics, and other types of vapors (see Figure 12.9). Because of their easy availability and low cost, they are often the drug of choice for the young. The effects of most of the inhalants is depression. As with alcohol, the user may at first experience a reduction of anxieties and inhibitions, making the user feel high. Continued use may result in hallucinations and loss of consciousness. Many of these chemicals are extremely toxic to the kidneys, liver, and nervous system. The use of inhalants by youth results from boredom and perhaps peer pressure and represents a maladaptation to these conditions.

---

inhalants Breathable substances that produce mind-altering effects.

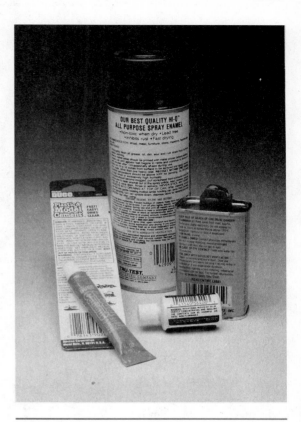

FIGURE 12.9

Many inhalants are extremely toxic to the kidneys, liver, and nervous system.

PREVENTION AND CONTROL OF DRUG ABUSE

The prevention and control of alcohol and other drug abuse require a knowledge of the causes of drug-taking behavior, sources of illicit drugs, drug laws, and treatment programs. It also requires community organization skills, persistence, and cooperation among a vast array of official and unofficial agencies.

From a theoretical standpoint, the activities of these agencies and organizations can be viewed as chronic disease prevention activities. This approach, involving three different levels of prevention, was discussed in Chapter 4.

Levels of Prevention

Drug abuse prevention activities can be viewed as primary, secondary, or tertiary, depending upon the point of intervention. *Primary prevention* programs are aimed at those who have never used drugs, and their goal is to prevent or forestall the initiation of drug use. Drug education programs that stress primary prevention of drug and alcohol use are most appropriate and successful for children at the elementary school age. In a broader sense, almost any activity that would reduce the likelihood of primary drug use could be considered primary prevention. For example, raising the price of alcohol, increasing cigarette taxes, arresting a neighborhood drug pusher, or destroying a cocaine crop in Bolivia could be considered primary prevention if it forestalled primary drug use in at least some individuals.

Secondary prevention programs are aimed at those who have begun alcohol or other drug use but who have not become chronic abusers and have not suffered significant physical or mental impairment from their drug or alcohol abuse. Alcohol and other drug abuse education programs that stress secondary prevention are often appropriate for people of high school or college age. They can be presented in educational, workplace, or community settings.

Tertiary prevention programs are designed to provide treatment for abuse and aftercare, including relapse prevention programs. As such, they are usually designed for adults. Tertiary programs for teenagers are far too uncommon. Tertiary prevention programs may receive clients who "turn themselves in" for treatment voluntarily, but more often than not, their clients are referred by the courts.

Official Agencies and Programs

Official agencies involved in drug abuse prevention, control, and treatment include a multitude of federal, state, and local agencies. At each of these levels of government, there are numerous offices and programs aimed at reducing either the supply of, or the demand for, drugs.

Federal Agencies and Programs

On September 5, 1989, then president George Bush presented the first National Drug Control Strategy to Congress.[28] This plan was formulated in response to the acknowledged and visible effects of widespread drug use in this country. Cited examples of these effects were the rising rates of violent crime, damage to the nation's health and economy, and strains on relationships with international allies. The plan included funding for both the "supply" variable and the "demand" variable but was weighted heavily in favor of programs to reduce supply. The federal budget still reflects this bias—in part, for good reason. There are simply some aspects of drug control that only the federal government can undertake. These include border control, interdiction in foreign countries and on the high seas, and measures against international money laundering. Other activities most easily supported by federal efforts include large-scale criminal investigations and long-term scientific research studies. Finally, some federal programs provide information, advice, and even training for state and local agencies and their personnel.

The federal budget request for fiscal 1993 was $12.7 billion more than a sevenfold increase over the 1981 budget (see

Figure 12.10).[29] The distribution of this budget is shown in Figure 12.11: 43% is earmarked for the criminal justice system; 14% for drug treatment; 13% for education, community action, and the workplace; 18% for border interdiction and security; and 12% for research, intelligence gathering, and international activities.

At least 12 cabinet-level departments and numerous other offices are involved in drug control at the federal level (see Table 12.3) and receive federal funds to reduce alcohol and other drug abuse problems. Those who received the most funds in 1992 were the Department of Justice at $4,425 million, the Department of Health and Human Services at $1,823 million, the Department of Defense at $1,158 million, and the Department of the Treasury at $950 million (Table 12.4).[29]

Department of Justice (DOJ)

By far, the largest budget for fighting the drug abuse problem is that of the Department of Justice (DOJ) (see Table 12.5). The DOJ addresses the supply side of the drug trade most directly by identifying, arresting, and prosecuting those who break drug laws. It tries to protect the welfare of society by incarcerating the most serious offenders, deterring others from becoming involved in drug trade, and providing a clear picture to all of the cost of drug trade and abuse. Regarding the latter, the DOJ indirectly contributes to reducing the demand for drugs.

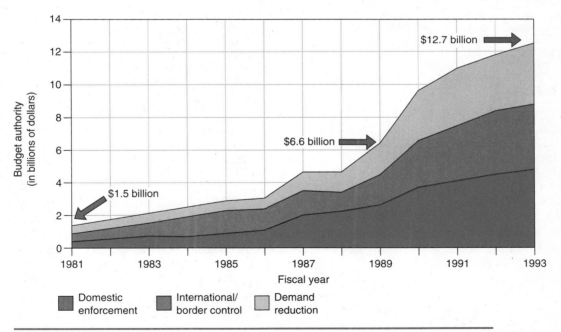

FIGURE 12.10

National drug control budget, 1981–1993.

From: Office of the National Drug Control Policy (1991). National Drug Control Policy (S/N 040-000-00550-1. Sup. Gov. Doc. G.P.O.) Washington, D.C.: The White House.

Table 12.3
National Drug Control Program Agencies and Accounts

ACTION

Agency for International Development

Department of Agriculture
  Agricultural Research Service
  U.S. Forest Service

Central Intelligence Agency

Department of Defense

Department of Education
  Educational Research and Improvement
  Elementary and Secondary Education
  Post-Secondary Education
  Special Education and Rehabilitation Services

Department of Health and Human Services
  Administration for Children and Families
  Alcohol, Drug Abuse, and Mental Health
    Administration
  Centers for Disease Control
  Food and Drug Administration
  Indian Health Service

Department of Housing and Urban Development

Department of the Interior
  Bureau of Indian Affairs
  Bureau of Land Management
  Fish and Wildlife Service
  National Park Service
  Office of Territorial and International Affairs

The Judiciary

Department of Justice
  Assets Forfeiture Fund
  U.S. Attorneys

  Bureau of Prisons
  Criminal Division
  Drug Enforcement Administration
  Federal Bureau of Investigation
  Immigration and Naturalization Service
  INTERPOL/U.S. National Central Bureau
  U.S. Marshals Service
  Office of Justice Programs
  Organized Crime Drug Enforcement Task Forces
  Support for Prisoners
  Tax Division

Department of Labor

Office of National Drug Control Policy

Small Business Administration

Department of State
  Bureau of International Narcotics Matters
  Bureau of Politico/Military Affairs
  Emergencies in the Diplomatic and Consular Service

Department of Transportation
  U.S. Coast Guard
  Federal Aviation Administration
  National Highway Traffic Safety Administration

Department of the Treasury
  Bureau of Alcohol, Tobacco, and Firearms
  U.S. Customs Service
  Federal Law Enforcement Training Center
  Financial Crimes Enforcement Network
  Internal Revenue Service
  U.S. Secret Service

U.S. Information Agency

Department of Veterans Affairs

From: Office of National Drug Control Policy (1992). *National Drug Control Strategy: A Nation Responds to Drug Use.* Washington, D.C.: Executive Office of the President, The White House, p. 146.

The DOJ's budget is extremely large, because in addition to its enforcement responsibilities, the department maintains prisons and prisoners, a responsibility that consumes one-third of its budget. The DOJ employs not only those who manage the penal system but also many marshals, attorneys, and judges. The DOJ also operates treatment, education, and rehabilitation programs in these prisons.

Within the DOJ are several important drug-fighting agencies. The lead agency in this respect is the Drug Enforcement Agency (DEA), with an annual budget of $748 million. The DEA "investigates and assists in the prosecution of drug traffickers and their accomplices in the United States and abroad, and seizes the drugs as well as the assets on which they depend."[28] The DEA employs 6,389 agents and support personnel.

Two other very important agencies in the DOJ are the Federal Bureau of Investigation (FBI) and the Immigration and Naturalization Service (INS). The FBI investigates multinational organized-crime

Table 12.4
National Drug Control Budget Authority (in millions)

Department	1991 Actual	1992 Estimate	1993 Request
Department of Justice	3,824.4	4,283.7	4,694.5
Department of the Treasury	977.6	1,069.0	1,105.2
Department of Transportation	749.6	706.3	724.1
Department of State	257.6	293.2	314.6
Department of Agriculture	16.1	16.1	16.1
Department of the Interior	35.7	45.2	42.7
Department of Health and Human Services	1,924.9	1,993.1	2,222.3
Department of Defense	1,042.5	1,274.6	1,223.4
Department of Housing and Urban Development	150.0	165.0	165.0
Department of Education	683.1	715.6	751.0
Department of Labor	67.6	73.2	72.6
Department of Veterans Affairs	473.1	544.2	590.6
ACTION	12.5	12.3	13.4
The Judiciary	294.1	347.7	429.9
Total	10,841.4	11,953.1	12,714.3

From: Office of National Drug Control Policy (1992). *National Drug Control Strategy: A Nation Responds to Drug Use.* Washington, D.C.: Executive Office of the President, The White House, p. 144–155.

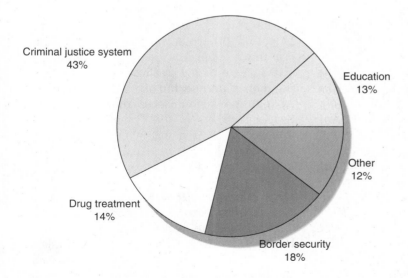

FIGURE 12.11

Distribution of national drug control budget, 1992.

Table 12.5
National Drug Control Budget Summary Department of Justice

Department	1991 Actual	1992 Estimate	1993 Request
Department of Justice			
Assets Forfeiture Fund	421.1	421.0	439.0
U.S. attorneys	161.6	188.7	215.9
Bureau of Prisons	1,027.5	1,293.5	1,454.4
Criminal Division	18.5	17.2	17.2
Drug Enforcement Administration	692.4	720.2	819.3
Federal Bureau of Investigation	180.3	231.4	243.7
Immigration and Naturalization Service	130.7	138.0	156.5
INTERPOL	1.3	1.8	1.9
U.S. Marshals Service	202.5	210.3	227.8
Office of Justice programs	535.7	543.5	530.2
Organized Crime Drug Enforcement task forces	334.5	363.4	399.1
Support of U.S. prisoners	135.1	153.4	187.9
Tax division	1.2	1.3	1.5
Total	10,841.4	11,953.1	12,714.3

From: Office of National Drug Control Policy (1992). *National Drug Control Strategy: A Nation Responds to Drug Use.* Washington, D.C.: Executive Office of the President, The White House, pp. 144–155.

networks that control the illegal drug market, and the INS works to deport alien drug traffickers currently detained in our federal prisons.

Another important agency in the DOJ is the Organized Crime Drug Enforcement Task Force, with a budget of $402 million. This task force works with state and local task forces, enabling authorities to apply enforcement pressure on illegal drug organizations along several levels and fronts at the same time.

The Department of the Treasury

The DOJ and its agencies work closely with the agencies of other cabinet-level departments to control the drug problem. Two such agencies are in the Department of the Treasury: the United States Customs Service and the Internal Revenue Service

(IRS). The United States Customs Service works with the DEA to target the transportation of drugs and to interdict drugs crossing our borders (see Figure 12.12). The IRS targets major traffickers by investigating money laundering operations and prosecuting tax evasion cases. Another agency in the Department of the Treasury is Alcohol, Tobacco, and Firearms, which is responsible for the regulation of our two most used and abused drugs, alcohol and tobacco.

Department of Health and Human Services (DHHS)

In 1991, the Department of Health and Human Services (DHHS) received nearly $1.5 billion for drug prevention education, treatment programs, and research. This figure increased to $1.8 billion in 1992 (Table 12.6).[29] The preponderance of these funds is

Table 12.6
National Drug Control Budget Summary, Department of Health and Human Services

Agency	1991 Actual	1992 Estimate	1993 Request
Administration for Children and Families	106.3	111.0	121.5
Alcohol, Drug Abuse, and Mental Health Administration	1,557.0	1,609.9	1,793.9
Centers for Disease Control	29.3	28.8	31.5
Food and Drug Administration	6.5	6.7	7.0
Health Care Financing Administration	190.5	210.5	231.5
Indian Health Service	35.3	35.2	37.0
	1,924.9	1,993.1	2,222.3

From: Office of National Drug Control Policy (1992). *National Drug Control Strategy: A Nation Responds to Drug Use.* Washington, D.C.: Executive Office of the President, The White House, pp. 144–155.

spent to reduce the *demand* for drugs. The approach of DHHS to the drug problem is broad, including research, treatment, and educational activities.

The misuse and abuse of tobacco, alcohol, and other drugs are addressed primarily as life-style problems—as *health promotion* issues, like physical fitness and nutrition. As such, DHHS recognizes that the problems of drug misuse and abuse are complex—involving environmental, social, and economic causes. Therefore, the solutions are also viewed as being complex. The typical approach involves the application of the three levels of prevention; primary, secondary, and tertiary (explained in Chapter 4 and referred to earlier in this chapter). It also recognizes the importance of incorporating the three primary prevention strategies of education, regulation, and automatic protection, which are discussed in greater detail in Chapter 17.

The DHHS has published health status, risk reduction, and service and protection objectives of the use of tobacco, alcohol, and other drugs in *Healthy People 2000.*[14] These objectives set the direction and standards for success of all our national drug control efforts.

The lead agency within DHHS is the Substance Abuse and Mental Health Services Administration (SAMHSA). Within SAMHSA there are three centers: The Center for Substance Abuse Prevention (CSAP); the Center for Substance Abuse Treatment (CSAT); and the Center for Mental Health Services (CMHS). In addition to SAMHSA, there are two other important agencies that deal with the problems of alcohol and other drugs: the National Institute of Drug Abuse and the Food and Drug Administration.

The National Institute of Drug Abuse (NIDA), is the largest institution devoted to drug abuse research in the world. At NIDA, research efforts are aimed at understanding the causes and consequences of drug abuse and at evaluating prevention and treatment programs. NIDA's budget approaches $400 million.[30]

Within NIDA are several important divisions and centers such as the Division of Clinical Research, the Division of Epidemiology and Prevention Research, the Di-

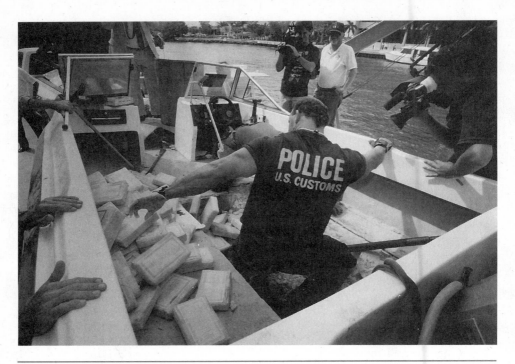

FIGURE 12.12

Customs agents assist in the arrest and prosecution of those involved in drug trafficking.

vision of Preclinical Research, the Division of Applied Research, the Medications Development Division, and the Addiction Research Center. These agencies conduct research and publish articles on the causes, prevention, and treatment of tobacco, alcohol, and drug abuse.

Another important agency in DHHS is the Food and Drug Administration (FDA). The FDA is the agency responsible for the regulation of all prescription and nonprescription drugs. The FDA dictates which drugs reach the market, and how they must be labeled, packaged, and sold. The FDA is more concerned with drug misuse than abuse.

Other Federal Agencies

Other agencies involved in drug abuse prevention and control are the Department of Transportation (DOT), the Department of State (DOS), the Department of Defense (DOD), the Department of Housing and Urban Development (HUD), and the Department of Education. Agencies in the DOT that assist with drug control efforts include the United States Coast Guard, the Federal Aviation Administration, and the National Highway Traffic Safety Administration. Of these agencies, the United States Coast Guard has the largest budget, at about $700 million.

Agencies in the DOS include the Bureau of International Narcotics Matters, the Agency for International Development (AID), and the United States Information Agency (USIA). The State Department also provides military assistance to foreign countries. Through various diplomatic efforts, including various "drug summits," DOS attempts to achieve a reduction in the production and shipment of illicit drugs into this country.

The Department of Education, under the direction of then secretary William J. Bennett, launched a program to support drug-free schools and communities. The effort was aimed at encouraging schools to adopt clear "no drug use" policies and to provide a message that both communities and schools do not condone or approve of alcohol or drug use by minors. A handbook entitled *What Works: Schools Without Drugs* was prepared and distributed to schools and communities.[31] Federal funds were made available to assist communities in adopting and implementing these policies.

State and Regional Agencies and Programs

While tremendous economic power can be brought to bear on the drug problem at the federal level, it is becoming increasingly clear that to achieve success, the drug war in America must be fought at the local level—in homes, neighborhoods, and schools. Inasmuch as state governments are able to support these efforts, they are helpful. State support usually comes in the form of expertise in law enforcement, education, and mental health, and sometimes funding initiatives. It is usually up to local citizens to put these state initiatives into action or begin initiatives of their own.

State Government

State agencies that address drug abuse problems include state departments of health, offices of education, departments of mental health, state police, and other agencies of the executive branch. The following is an example of a state initiative for drug abuse prevention and control. It is the Governor's Commission for a Drug-Free Indiana. Initiated in 1989 by Governor Evan Bayh, the commission has as its primary goal the coordination and expansion, at both the state and local levels, of all efforts to combat alcohol and other drug abuse in the state. At the state level, coordination is achieved through the Interagency Council on Drugs, an organization of all state agencies involved in alcohol and other drug programming. At the local level, the commission hopes to develop and expand similar coordinating councils and assist them in developing comprehensive plans. In this way, the Governor's Commission hopes to assure that funding actions for community-based programs are in concert with local coordinated efforts. Finally, to supplement other sources, a Drug-Free Communities Fund was established to give assistance to local grass-roots efforts.

Regional Coordinating Offices

In the Indiana system, local coordinating councils, which are communitywide consortiums representing all agencies involved with alcohol and other drug problems, are assisted by one of ten regional coordinating offices (RCOs). The RCO facilitates citizen involvement and assists communities in the development of a coordinated community-based comprehensive drug prevention and control strategy. In some cases, where turfism or personalities require it, the RCO must actually assist in the formation of the local coordinating council. Through the RCOs, the state can respond to local needs and efforts.

Local Programs and Agencies

Local Coordinating Councils

The local coordinating council (LCC) has as its goals educating the community about alcohol and other drug problems; assessing local needs; and initiating, coordinating, and implementing comprehensive local alcohol and other drug plans. The major thrusts of the LCC are: (1) prevention via education, (2) intervention and treatment, and (3) law enforcement. The local coordinating council should include a wide diversity of participating groups. Membership on the local coordinating council might include representatives from the following: local health department; housing authority; neighborhood associations; mental health association; city government; city and county schools; children and family services; parents; chamber of commerce; city police; county sheriff; religious leaders; prosecutor's office; judges; justice/law enforcement task force; high school students; local treatment facilities; and representatives from labor, management, and employee assistance programs.

It is the goal of the governor's initiative that, through better coordination of all the groups involved with the problems of alcohol and other drug abuse, significant progress in the reduction of the pervasiveness and seriousness of this problem can be achieved. Specifically, it is hoped that educational efforts will be communitywide, not just centered in schools, that city and county law enforcement will be able to work toward consistency in enforcement, and that local treatment and support group resources be coordinated for optimal effectiveness.

Unofficial Programs and Agencies

Community-Based Drug Education Programs

Community-based drug education can occur in a variety of settings such as child care facilities, public housing, religious institutions, businesses, and health care facilities. Information about the abuse of alcohol, tobacco, and other drugs can be disseminated through television and radio programs, movies, newspapers, and magazines.

Community-based drug education programs are most likely to be successful when they include six key features:[32]

1. A comprehensive strategy.
2. An indirect approach to drug abuse prevention.
3. The goal of empowering youth.
4. A participatory approach.
5. A culturally sensitive orientation.
6. Highly structured activities.

Community-based drug education programs that address broader issues (e.g., coping and learning skills) are most effective, as are those embedded in other existing community activities. Participation can be increased by planning drug education programs around sporting or cultural events. Culturally sensitive programs are crucial for reaching minorities in the community. Use of the appropriate language, reading level, and spokespersons can mean the success or failure of a program.

The importance of the media in communicating antidrug messages cannot be overestimated. One of the most successful antidrug programs was the 1989 *Partnership for a Drug-Free America* media campaign.[33] Television and print ads showed a fried egg in a frying pan with the message, "This is your brain on drugs." In areas of high media exposure, marijuana use declined 33% and cocaine use decreased 15% between 1988 and 1989. Whereas, in areas of little of no media exposure, marijuana and cocaine use declined 15% and 2% respectively. Although the media alone probably do not create lasting changes in behavior, media campaigns in combination with multiple strategies are very effective. The goal of media-based education is to educate the public about the harmful effects of alcohol and other drugs and about how to reduce risk factors and strengthen the community. The media are powerful partners in shaping community opinions, values, and norms (see Figure 12.13).

Individual initiatives can successfully influence the outcome of community coalitions in changing alcohol and drug policies. The question is sometimes where to start. Based on the results of the 1992 national policy panel of over 100 community leaders representing a diverse group of coalitions, the following recommendations to Congress have been proposed in regard to underage access to drinking:[34]

1. It should be illegal for individuals under age 21 to drive with any amount of alcohol in their bodies. Violation of the zero tolerance law would result in license suspension.

2. There should be a 5-cent per drink increase in current federal excise tax on all alcoholic beverages. Revenues would be used for school education and law enforcement.

3. All retail outlets should be held liable for providing alcohol to minors. Negligence in illegally selling or serving underage individuals would result in revocation or suspension of liquor licenses.

4. Media that promote alcohol through advertising should be required to provide equal time for counteradvertisement about the health risks of alcohol use. Warning labels should appear on all advertisements.

5. Local coalitions should systematically evaluate underage access to alcohol and find ways to discourage easy access.

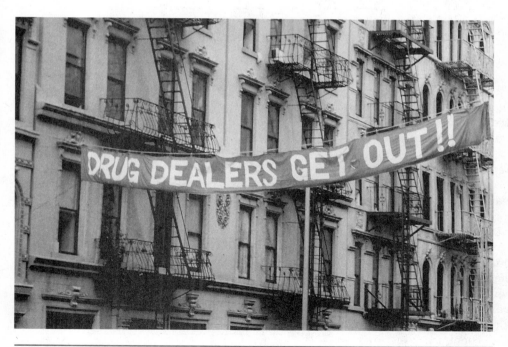

FIGURE 12.13

Community efforts to get rid of drug dealers can be successful.

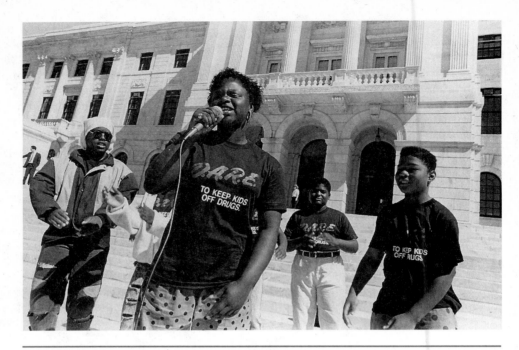

FIGURE 12.14

Drug Abuse Resistance Education (DARE) programs involve police in school drug education.

Project ASSIST is another community-based strategy for influencing public policy. The aim of *Project ASSIST* is to change tobacco-related policies to limit youth access and minimize the harm to society caused by tobacco.

School-Based Drug Education Programs

Most health educators believe that a strong, comprehensive school health education program (see Chapter 6)—one that occupies a permanent and prominent place in the school curriculum—is the best defense against all health problems, including drug abuse. However, many schools lack these strong programs and, in their absence, substitute drug education programs developed specifically for school use.

One such program is the Drug Abuse Resistance Education (DARE) program, which began in Los Angeles. In the DARE program, local police enter the classroom to teach grade school children about drugs (see Figure 12.14). While imparting some knowledge, the program's primary approach is to change attitudes and beliefs about drugs. It is also successful in improving children's images of the police themselves.

Another program that takes place in schools is *Here's Looking at You 2000*. This commercially produced health education program includes a drug education module. Books, transparencies, and videotapes are provided for each grade level.

Student assistance programs (SAPs) are school-based programs modeled after employee assistance programs in the work-

---

student assistance programs (SAPs) School-based drug education programs to assist students who have alcohol or other drug problems.

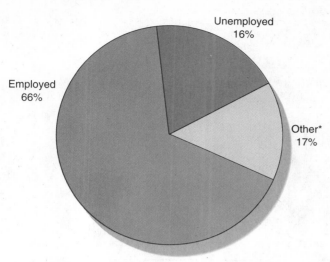

Unemployed
16%

Employed
66%

Other*
17%

* Homemakers, students, and retirees   Source: NIDA National Household Survey on Drug Abuse, 1991

FIGURE 12.15

Employment status of current adult drug users, 1991.
From: NIDA, National Household Survey on Drug Abuse, 1991.

place. They are aimed at identifying and intervening in cases of drug problems. **Peer counseling programs** are also present in some schools. In these programs, students "rap" about mutual problems and receive support and perhaps coping skills from peers who do not use drugs.

Workplace-Based Drug Education Programs

In recent years, attention has been focused on alcohol and other drug use in the workplace. It has become a broadly held viewpoint that drug abuse is not just a personal health problem and a law enforcement problem but also a behavior that affects the safety and productivity of others, especially

at work. Studies have shown that substance abusers: (1) are less productive, (2) miss more work days, (3) are more likely to injure themselves, and (4) file more workers' compensation claims than their non-substance-abusing counterparts.[35]

While a substantial part of the problem can be attributed to alcohol consumption, illicit drug use is also a serious problem in many workplaces. One study shows that two-thirds of all current users of illicit drugs are employed either full or part time (see Figure 12.15).[28] Statistics further suggest that nearly 10 million employed people are current drug users.[29]

Data such as these led then president Ronald Reagan, in September of 1986, to sign Executive Order Number 12564, proclaiming a Drug Free Federal Workplace.[36] The rationale for the order was cited in the document itself: the desire and need for the

---

peer counseling programs   School-based programs in which students discuss alcohol and other drug-related problems with peers.

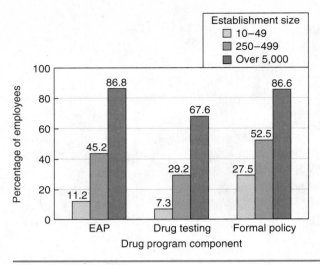

FIGURE 12.16

Establishments with antidrug programs, 1988.

From: Bur. of Labor Statistics, 1989.

well-being of employees, the loss of productivity caused by drug use, the illegal profits of organized crime, the illegality of the behavior itself, the undermining of public confidence, and the role of the federal government as the largest employer in the nation to set a standard for other employers to follow in these matters.

The Drug Free Federal Workplace order required federal employees to refrain from using illegal drugs, and it required agency heads to develop plans for achieving drug-free workplaces for employees in their agencies. The order further required the setting up of drug testing programs and procedures and employee assistance programs that would include provisions for rehabilitation.[36] Similar workplace substance abuse programs are now in place in companies in the private sector.[29]

A typical workplace substance abuse program has five facets.[34] The first is a formal written substance abuse policy that reflects the employer's commitment to a drug-free workplace. The second is an employee drug education and awareness program. Third is the supervisor training program. Fourth is the **employee assistance program (EAP),** to help those who need counseling and rehabilitation. The last component is a drug testing program. Large companies are more likely than small companies to have the major components of a drug-free workplace program (see Figure 12.16).

Voluntary Health Agencies

Drug prevention and control programs are carried out at the local level with the cooperation and effort of many members of the community. Some of these programs are of local origin while others have received national recognition and even endorsement.

---

employee assistance program (EAP) A workplace drug program designed to assist employees in recovering from their alcohol or other drug problems.

The people who actually deliver drug abuse prevention programs include teachers, community health educators, social workers, law enforcement officers, and volunteers.

The programs presented vary greatly in their message and approach. Some programs seek to educate or provide knowledge, others seek to change beliefs or attitudes about alcohol or other drug use, while still others seek to alter behavior by providing new behavior skills. Studies have shown that programs incorporating all these approaches are most successful.

A large number of voluntary health agencies have been founded to prevent or control the social and personal consequences of drug and alcohol abuse. Among these are such agencies as **Mothers Against Drunk Driving (MADD), Students Against Driving Drunk (SADD), Alcoholics Anonymous (AA), Narcotics Anonymous (NA),** the **American Cancer Society (ACS),** and many others. Each of these organizations is active locally, statewide and nationally.

An important function of community leaders is to encourage parents, school officials, law enforcement people, businesses, social groups, community health workers, and the media to work together in an effort to reduce the abuse of alcohol and other drugs. Every approach should be used, including seeking favorable legislation and judicial appointments, fairness in advertising, school and community education and treatment, and law enforcement. Only through citizen support and vigilance can there be a reduction in the threat that alcohol and other drugs pose to our community.

CHAPTER SUMMARY

The abuse of alcohol and other drugs is a major community health problem in the United States. Alcohol and other drug abuse affects not only in-

dividuals but also communities. The cost of this problem, in terms of lives and dollars, is a substantial drain on our society.

Investigations into the causes of drug experimentation and drug abuse indicate that both inherited and environmental factors contribute to the problem. While the abuse rates of many of the illicit drugs have leveled off or declined, those for alcohol and tobacco remain much too high. Chronic alcohol and tobacco use result in the loss of thousands of lives and millions of dollars in America each year. The misuse of prescription and nonprescription drugs is also widespread.

There are substantial federal, state, and local efforts to reduce the use, misuse, and abuse of drugs in the United States. Federal agencies involved include the Departments of Justice, Treasury, Health and Human Services, and many others. Efforts at the state level vary from state to state but usually include attempts to coordinate federal and local efforts.

SCENARIO: ANALYSIS AND RESPONSE

1. Would spending a Saturday night in the emergency room of a large community hospital change your view of drinking? How?

2. Why hadn't Glenda's friends mentioned their concern about her drinking? Are there any danger signs that you detect?

3. What risks did Glenda take to her personal health? To the health of others? How is Glenda's behavior a community concern?

4. What do you think happened that Glenda can't recall?

5. To what degree is alcohol or other drug impairment a problem in the medical or allied health professions?

6. Can you think of any alcohol impaired co-workers? Have you confronted them with your concern about this?

7. How much do you drink or use other drugs? Have you ever put another person in the community at risk through your drinking or other drug-taking behavior?

REVIEW QUESTIONS

1. What are some personal consequences resulting from the abuse of alcohol and other drugs?

2. What are some community consequences resulting from the abuse of alcohol and other drugs?

3. What are the recent trends in drug use by high school seniors?

4. What is our most serious drug problem?

5. Explain the difference among *drug use, misuse,* and *abuse.*

6. How are physical and psychological dependence different?

7. What are the two primary factors that contribute to substance abuse?

8. Name the four categories of environmental risk factors that contribute to substance abuse and give an example of each.

9. What are the two major types of abused drugs? Give examples of each.

10. Why is alcohol considered the Number 1 problem drug in America?

11. In what forms do Americans consume nicotine, and in what groups of people do we see the heaviest users?

12. What effect do over-the-counter drugs have on illness?

13. What information is included in a doctor's prescription?

14. What is the most commonly used illicit drug? Why is this drug a concern?

15. What is meant by *dangerous drugs*? Give some examples.

16. What are the side effects for both men and women that result from the use of anabolic drugs?

17. What are the two major approaches to attacking the drug problem in this country?

18. What role has the Department of Justice played in preventing and controlling drug abuse? The Department of the Treasury? The Department of Health and Human Services?

19. What role do state governments play in preventing and controlling drug abuse? Local governments?

20. List and describe some community-based and school-based drug education programs.

ACTIVITIES

1. Schedule an appointment with the vice president of Student Affairs or the dean of students on your campus to find out more about drug (including alcohol) problems. Find out what the greatest concerns are and how the administration is trying to deal with the issues.

2. Make an appointment with the health educator or another employee in your local health department to find out more about the existing alcohol and other drug problems in the community. Collect the same information as noted in question 1 above, except find it for the community, not the campus.

3. Find six articles that appeared in your local paper during the past two weeks that dealt with drugs. Find two that related to problems at the national or international level, two at the state level, and two at the local level. Summarize the articles and present your reaction to these in a written paper.

4. Conduct a survey of at least 100 students on your campus. Try to get a random sample of people. Interview these people and find out what they think are the major drug problems on your campus and how they might be solved. Feel free to include other questions on your survey. Summarize the results in a two-page paper.

REFERENCES

1. Office for Substance Abuse Prevention (1989). *Prevention Plus II* (DHHS pub. no. ADM-89-1649).

Washington, D.C.: U.S. Government Printing Office, p. 3.

2. Johnston, L. D., P. M. O'Malley, and J. G. Bachman (1993). National Survey Results on Drug Use from the monitoring the future study, 1975–1992. Volume I. Secondary School Students. NIH pub. no. 93-3597.

3. Cotton, N. S. (1979). "The Familial Incidence of Alcoholism: A Review." *J Stud Alcohol* 40: 89–116.

4. Cloninger, C. R., M. Bohman and S. Sigvardsson (1981). "Inheritance of Alcohol Abuse." *Arch Gen Psychiatry* 38: 861–868.

5. Schuckit, M. A., S. C. Risch, and E. O. Gold (1988). "Alcohol Consumption, ACTH Level, and Family History of Alcoholism." *Am J Psychiatry* 145(11): 1391–1395.

6. Tabakoff, B., and P. L. Hoffman (1988). "Genetics and Biological Markers of Risk for Alcoholism." *Public Health Report* 103(6): 690–698.

7. U.S. Dept. of Health and Human Services (1990). *Seventh Special Report to the U.S. Congress* (DHHS pub. no. ADM-90-1656). Washington, D.C.: U.S. Government Printing Office.

8. Needle, R., Y. Lavee, S. Su, et al. (1988). "Familial, Interpersonal, and Intrapersonal Correlates of Drug Use: A Longitudinal Comparison of Adolescents in Treatment, Drug-Using Adolescents Not in Treatment, and Non-Drug-Using Adolescents." *Int J Addict* 239(12): 1211–1240.

9. Naegle, M. A. (1988). "Theoretical Perspectives on the Etiology of Drug Abuse." *Holistic Nurs. Pract.* 2(4): 1–13.

10. Meller, W. H., R. Rinehart, R. J. Cadoret, and E. Troughton (1988). "Specific Familial Transmission in Substance Abuse." *Int'l. J. Addict.* 23(10): 1029–1039.

11. Dembo, R., W. R. Blount, J. Schmeidler, and W. Burgos (1986). "Perceived Environmental Drug Use Risk and the Correlates of Early Drug Use or Nonuse Among Inner-City Youths: The Motivated Actor." *Int'l. J. Addict.* 21(9 and 10): 977–1000.

12. Morse, R. M., and D. K. Flavin (1992). "The Definition of Alcoholism." *JAMA* 268(8): 1012–1014.

13. Baker, S. P., B. O'Neill, M. J. Ginsburg, and G. Li (1992). *The Injury Fact Book,* 2nd ed. New York: Oxford Univ. Press.

14. U.S. Dept. of Health and Human Services (1991). *Healthy People 2000: National Health Promotion and Disease Prevention Objectives.* (DHHS pub. no. PHS-91-510212). Washington, D.C.: U.S. Government Printing Office.

15. U.S. Dept. of Health and Human Services (1989). *Reducing the Health Consequences of Smoking: 25 Years of Progress. A Report of the Surgeon General.* Office on Smoking and Health. Public Health Service, Centers for Disease Control. (DHHS pub. no. CDC-89-

8411). Washington, D.C.: U.S. Government Printing Office.

16. American Cancer Society (1992). *Cancer Facts and Figures—1992.* Atlanta: Author, 30 pp.

17. U.S. Dept. of Health and Human Services (1986). *The Health Consequence of Involuntary Smoking. A Report of the Surgeon General.* Public Health Service, Centers for Disease Control (DHHS pub. no. CDC-87-8398). Washington, D.C.: U.S. Government Printing Office.

18. Byrd, J. C., R. S. Shapiro, and D. L. Schiedermayer (1989). "Passive Smoking: A Review of Medical and Legal Issues." *Am. J. Publ. Health* 79(2): 209–215.

19. Environmental Protection Agency (1991). *Respiratory Health Effects of Passive Smoking: Lung Cancer and Other Disorders* (EPA/600/6-90/006F). Washington, D.C.: Indoor Air Quality Clearinghouse.

20. National Institute of Drug Abuse (1991). *National Household Survey on Drug Abuse Population Estimates 1991.* (DHHS pub. no. ADM-92-1887). Washington, D.C.: U.S. Government Printing Office.

21. No author. *Physician's Desk Reference,* 44th ed. (1991). Oradell, N.J.: Medical Economics Company.

22. Centers for Disease Control (1992). "National Action Plan to Combat Multidrug-Resistant Tuberculosis; Meeting the Challenge of Multidrug Resistant Tuberculosis: Summary of a Conference; Management of Persons Exposed to Multidrug-Resistant Tuberculosis." *MMWR* 41 (RR-11): 1–71.

23. Drug Enforcement Agency, National Narcotics Intelligence Consumers Committee (NNICC) (1992). *The NNICC Report 1991: The Supply of Illicit Drugs to the United States.* Washington, D.C.: Author.

24. Lucas, S., J. Mendelson, J. Henry, L. Amass, and A. Budson (1988). *Ethanol Effects on Marijuana-Induced Intoxication and Electroencephalographic Activity. Problems of Drug Dependence* (Research Monograph Series 90). Rockville, Md.: National Institute of Drug Abuse, p. 62.

25. Drug Enforcement Agency, Dept. of Justice (1993). "Schedules of Controlled Substances: Placement of Methcathinone into Schedule I." *Federal Register* 58(198) (Oct. 15, 1993): 53404–53406

26. Friedl, K., D. Pearson, C. Maresh, W. Kraemer, and D. Catlin (1989). "What the Coach, Athlete and Parent Need to Know About Anabolic Drugs: A Fact Sheet." *NSCA Journal* 11(6): 10–13.

27. Mishra, R. (1992). *Steroids and Sports: A Losing Proposition* (DHHS pub. no. FDA-92-1187). Reprinted from *FDA Consumer Magazine,* Sept. 1991.

28. Office of National Drug Control Policy (1991). *National Drug Control Strategy.* Washington, D.C.: The White House, 180 pp.

29. Office of National Drug Control Policy (1992). *National Drug Control Strategy: A Nation Responds to Drug Use.* Washington, D.C.: The White House, 215 pp.

30. National Institute of Drug Abuse (1991). "History of NIDA." *NIDA Notes* 5(5): 1–40.

31. U.S. Dept. of Education (1987). *What Works: Schools Without Drugs.* Washington, D.C.: Author, 78 pp.

32. Brown, M. E. (1993). "Successful Components of Community and School Prevention Programs." *National Prevention Evaluation Report: Research Collection* 1 (1): 4–5.

33. Black, G. S. (1989). *Changing Attitudes Toward Drug Use: The First Year Effort of the Media-Advertising Partnership for a Drug-Free America, Inc.* Rochester, N.Y.: Gordon S. Black.

34. Join Together (1993). *Who Is Really Fighting the War on Drugs?: A National Study of Community-based Anti-Drug and Alcohol Activities in America.* Boston, Mass.: Author.

35. U.S. Dept. of Labor (1991). *What works: Workplaces Without Alcohol or Other Drugs* (pub. no. 282-148/54629). Washington, D.C.: U.S. Government Printing Office.

36. Drug-Free Federal Workplace (1986). (Executive Order 12564 of Sept. 15, 1986). *Federal Register* 51(180), Sept. 17, 1986. Presidential Documents 32893.

37. Center for Substance Abuse Prevention, Substance and Mental Health Services Administration (1993). *Prevention Works: A Discussion Paper on Preventing Alcohol, Tobacco and Other Drug Problems.* PHS DHHS pub. no. (SMA)93-2046.

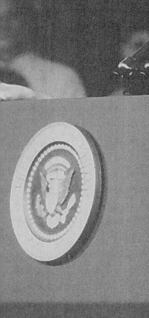

UNIT III

HEALTH CARE
DELIVERY

HOPKINS

Chapter 13

HEALTH CARE SYSTEM: STRUCTURE

Chapter Outline

Chapter Objectives

After studying this chapter, you will be able to:

1. Define the term *health care system*.
2. Trace the history of health care delivery in the United States from the mid-nineteenth century to the present.
3. Discuss and explain the concept of the spectrum of health care delivery.
4. Distinguish between the different kinds of health care, including: preventive, primary, secondary, tertiary, restorative, and continuing care.
5. List and characterize the various groups of health care providers.
6. Explain the differences among allopathic, osteopathic, and nonallopathic providers.
7. Explain why there is a need for health care providers.
8. Prepare a list of the different types of facilities in which health care is delivered.
9. Explain the differences among private, public, and voluntary hospitals.

Marcus had had a busy summer. Not only was he working 45 hours a week in order to earn enough money to return to college in the fall, but he was a member of two different softball teams and played in the golf league sponsored by his summer employer. He really enjoyed sports. In fact, one of his softball teams was a traveling team that played a 60-game schedule, traveling as far as 100 miles away to play in some tournaments.

Marcus was an aggressive softball player who enjoyed good competition and was always willing to slide hard into second base to break up a double play. In fact, it was his excessive sliding into the different bases that led to his medical problem. Toward the end of the season, Marcus had realized that the scab on his leg really never got a chance to heal over the summer because of his sliding, and now it was getting tender and a redness appeared around it. So he decided to go see his physician. After a quick look and a little probing, Dr. Schudel said "Marcus, you have a basic infection. Are you allergic to any antibiotics?" When Marcus said no, Dr. Schudel wrote a prescription and sent him on his way.

Two weeks passed. Marcus had taken all his medication, but his leg didn't look any better. He called Dr. Schudel for another appointment. At the second appointment, Dr. Schudel took another look at the leg and prescribed a second medication. Another two weeks passed and still no change. So at his third visit, Dr. Schudel ordered a number of tests and prescribed several different medications. Marcus's condition still persisted. When Marcus returned for his fourth visit, Dr. Schudel stated, "I'm not sure what the problem is. I'd like to refer you to a specialist. I think you should see Dr. McCallum, the dermatologist."

INTRODUCTION

Health care in the United States is delivered by a variety of **providers** in a variety of settings. Although reference is often made to the American health care delivery system, many people feel that the delivery of health care in the United States is *not* systematically organized. A close examination reveals that, at best, health care in the United States is delivered by providers who are linked by informal cooperation. The providers:

operate independently and autonomously, each being responsible for only a small portion of what might be called the "total care" of the patient. As a result, patients may receive excellent care for particular health problems, but gaps in meeting their overall health care needs can occur because of inadequate coordination among the kaleidoscope of health care providers. The system gives high priority to acute care and pays little heed to the other ends of the spectrum, preventive care and continuing care.[1]

Ubell[2] presents an interesting critique of the process of health care delivery in the United States.

Like the Holy Roman Empire, which was neither Holy nor Roman nor an Empire, the

---

providers Those individuals educated and trained to provide health care.

Health-Care System often spoken of refers not to Health nor to Care nor is it a System. Ninety-five percent of the medical effort in the United States goes to disease not health, provides medical treatment not care, and it is in no way a System; rather it is a vast haphazard conglomeration of medical entrepreneurs, be they doctors, pharmacies, pharmaceutical manufacturers, hospitals or insurance companies.

In a true system, a newborn would enter into a health care system in which his or her records and health information were centrally located and available throughout his/her lifetime. All providers would communicate with each other and all procedures at every age would be recorded. Whether or not health care delivery in the United States should be called a "system," there is a process in place in which health care workers, located in a variety of facilities, provide services to deal with disease and injury for the purpose of promoting, maintaining, and restoring health to the citizens (see Figure 13.1). In this chapter, we will outline the history of health care delivery in the United States, examine the spectrum of health care delivery, and describe the various types of health care providers and the facilities in which health care is delivered.

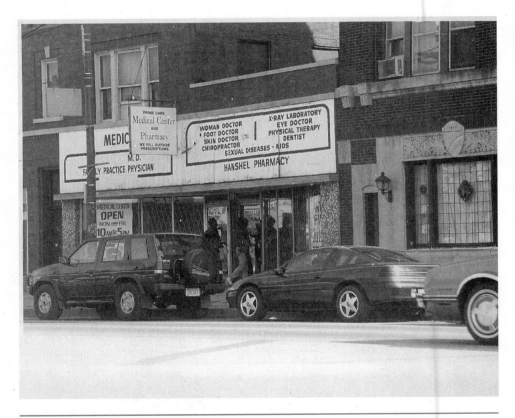

FIGURE 13.1
Do we really have a health care system?

A BRIEF HISTORY OF HEALTH CARE DELIVERY IN THE UNITED STATES

For as long as humankind has been concerned with disease, injury, and health, there has always been a category of health care in which people have tried to help or treat themselves. This category of care is referred to as self-care or self-treatment. For example, in most American homes, there are usually provisions to deal with minor emergencies, nursing care, and the relief of minor pains or ailments. This type of care continues today and includes actions taken with the goal of preventing problems before they occur. The following discussion of the history of health care in the United States does not include self-care, since it is assumed that most people would engage in some type of self-care prior to seeking professional help. Instead, we will review the development of professional care provided by those who have been formally educated in some aspect of health care.

Before 1850, health care occurred primarily in a physician-patient relationship, with most of the treatment taking place in the patient's home. This is not to say that physicians did not see patients in their offices; but it was more frequent for the physician to visit the patient at his or her home.

In the mid- to late-nineteenth century, formal health care gradually moved from the patient's home to the physician's office and into the hospital. The primary reason for this change was the building and staffing of many new hospitals. It was felt that patients could receive better care in a setting designed for patient care, staffed with trained people, and equipped with the latest medical supplies and instruments. In addition, physicians could treat more patients in a central location because of the reduced travel time.

It was also during the latter portion of the nineteenth century that the scientific method began to play a more important role in health care. Medical procedures backed by scientific findings began to replace "rational hunches," "good ideas," and "home remedies" as the standards for medical care. With the acceptance of the germ theory of disease and the identification of infectious disease agents, there was real hope for the control of communicable diseases, which were the leading health problems of that period.

Other significant milestones in public health occurred during this period. Milk was pasteurized for the first time, bacteriology was studied in botany classes, septic tanks were developed for sewage treatment, and the American Public Health Association was founded.[3] (For other historical milestones, the reader is referred to Chapter 1.)

At the beginning of the twentieth century, great strides in health care took place. New medical procedures such as X-ray therapy, specialized surgical procedures, and chemotherapy were developed, group medical practices were begun; and new medical equipment and instruments such as the electrocardiograph to measure heart function were invented. The training of doctors and nurses improved and became more specialized. Although communicable diseases were still the leading causes of deaths, mortality rates began to decline. By 1929, the United States was spending about 3.9% of its gross domestic product (GDP) on health care.

By 1940, communicable diseases were no longer the leading causes of death and Americans had become increasingly concerned about the noncommunicable, chronic diseases. It was also a time when the country was facing another war. Huge technical strides were made in the 1940s and 1950s as medical developments that occurred during World War II found applications in civilian medicine. However, adequate health facilities to treat long-term diseases were lacking in many areas of the country. The **Hospital Survey and Construction Act of 1946,** better known as the **Hill-Burton Act** (after the authors of the legislation), provided substantial funds for hospital construction. The infusion of federal funds helped to remedy the serious hospital shortage caused by the lack of construction during the Depression and World War II. Hill-Burton was primarily a federal-state partnership. State agencies were given grants to determine the need for hospitals and then were provided with seed money to begin construction of the facilities.[1] However, the major portion of construction dollars came from state and local sources.[4] Through the years, the Hill-Burton Act has been amended several times to help meet the health care needs in the United States. As such, funds have been made available for additional construction, modernization, and replacement of other health care facilities and for comprehensive health planning.

With improved procedures, equipment, and facilities, the cost of health care began to rise. As the cost of health care rose, it became too expensive for some people. Concerns were expressed about who should receive health care and who should pay for it. The debate over whether health care is a basic right or a privilege in America began in earnest. By the end of the 1950s, there remained an overall shortage of quality health care in America. There was also a maldistribution of health care services—metropolitan

areas being better served than the less-developed rural areas.

In the 1960s, there was an increased interest in health insurance, and it became common practice for workers and their bargaining agents to negotiate for better health benefits (see Figure 13.2). Undoubtedly, some employers preferred to increase benefits rather than to raise wages. Few could foresee then the explosion in health care costs Americans are experiencing now. Thus, the **third-party payment system** for health care became solidified as the standard method of payment for health care costs in the United States. The third-party payment system gets its name from the fact that the insurer—either government or a private insurance company (third party)—pays the health care bills instead of the patient (first party) or the provider (second party).[5] (A detailed explanation of the third-party payment system is presented in Chapter 14.) It should be noted that government and private insurers pay the bills with tax dollars and collected premiums, respectively—not with their own funds.

With the growth of the third-party system of paying for health care, the cost of health care rose even more rapidly than before, because patients enjoyed increased access to care without out-of-pocket expenses. However, those without insurance found it increasingly difficult to afford care. When the Democrats regained the White House in the 1960s, they led a federal policy change to increase citizen access to health care, which culminated in 1965 with the authorization of Medicare and Medicaid by Titles XVIII and XIX, respectively, of the Social Security Act. These programs, which were enacted to help provide care for the elderly,

---

Hospital Survey and Construction Act of 1946 (Hill-Burton Act) Federal legislation that provided substantial funds for hospital construction.

third-party payment system A health insurance term indicating that bills will be paid by the insurer and not the patient or the health care provider.

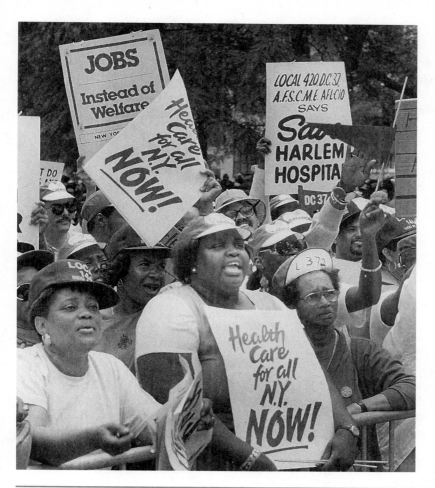

FIGURE 13.2

New York State health care workers rallying for health care benefits.

the disabled, and the poor, are also discussed at length in Chapter 14. Also in the 1960s, the federal government increased funding for medical research and technology to support transplants and life extension.

By the late 1960s and early 1970s, it had become apparent that the Hill-Burton Act had stimulated not only the growth of health care facilities but also demand for health care services. With this growth came a continuing rise in health care costs and a need for better planning in health care delivery.

Among the early attempts at planning were the 1964 amendments to the Hill-Burton Act. The amendments called for comprehensive planning on a regional level. Their purpose was to make more efficient use of federal funds by preventing the duplication of facilities. However, they depended on good faith efforts and could not be enforced. It soon became evident that more-powerful legislation was needed to control costs and to coordinate and control rapid growth in health care facilities. Another attempt was made to encourage better planning two years later. The Comprehensive Health Planning and Public Service Amendments of 1966 authorized funds for state and areawide Comprehensive Health Planning Agencies. These too failed because they had no "teeth." Then, in 1974, Public Law 93-641 was passed. This law, known as the National Health Planning and Resources Development Act of 1974, combined several pieces of previous legislation to put teeth into comprehensive planning efforts. There were high hopes and expectations that these pieces of legislation would provide reason and order to the development and modification of health care services.[6] This legislation led to the formation of Health Systems Agencies throughout the entire country. Their purpose was to cut costs by preventing the building of "unnecessary" facilities or the purchase of unnecessary equipment. While some money may have been saved, the Health Systems Agencies were viewed by some as yet another unnecessary government bureaucracy, and when President Reagan took office in 1980, he, along with Congress, eliminated this program.

The 1980s brought many changes to the health care industry. Probably the most notable was the deregulation of health care delivery. In 1981, with Ronald Reagan in the White House, it was announced that the administration would let the competitive market, not governmental regulation, shape health care delivery.[7] Open competition is a philosophy of allowing consumers to regulate delivery by making choices about where and from whom they receive their care. In theory, those who provide good care will get more patients and in turn be able to offer the care at a lower price.

There are some economists, however, who do not believe that the health care system behaves like a normal market. For example, it is not likely that a sick patient will shop for a cheaper physician. Physicians do not advertise their prices. Also, it is the physician who tells the patient which hospital to go to and when to check in and out, because of the admitting privileges that physicians have. In addition, providers tend to offer more and more services to entice the market to "shop with us," which in effect drives up health care spending. For these reasons, the competitive market approach is of questionable value in lowering health care costs.

The 1980s also saw a proliferation of new medical technology (MRI, ultrasound, etc.). With this new technology have come new health care issues such as medical ethics (e.g., prolonging life and ending life) and more elaborate health insurance programs (e.g., policies that cover specific diseases such as cancer and AIDS, home care, and rehabilitation).

Health care costs continue to rise in the 1990s. The total health care bill for the United States in 1992 was $817 billion, 14% of the gross national product (GNP).[8] Health care is the one segment of the United States economy that continues to grow faster than the cost of inflation (see Table 13.1 and Figure 13.3). Ever-newer technology, ever-

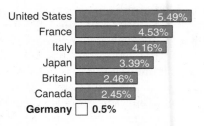

FIGURE 13.3

Real growth in health care costs in seven countries, 1987–1990.

From: Muncie, Ind., Star. (July 19, 1992):6B.

Table 13.1
Consumer Price Index and Average Annual Percentage of Change for All Items and Selected Items: United States, Selected Years 1950–1992

(Data are based on reporting by samples of providers and other retail outlets)

Year	All Items	Medical Care	Food	Apparel and Upkeep	Housing	Energy	Personal Care
			Consumer Price Index				
1950	24.1	15.1	25.4	40.3	—	—	26.2
1955	26.8	18.2	27.8	42.9	—	—	29.9
1960	29.6	22.3	30.0	45.7	—	22.4	34.6
1965	31.5	25.2	32.2	47.8	—	22.9	36.6
1970	38.8	34.0	39.2	59.2	36.4	25.5	43.5
1975	53.8	47.5	59.8	72.5	50.7	42.1	57.9
1980	82.4	74.9	86.8	90.9	81.1	86.0	81.9
1985	107.6	113.5	105.6	105.0	107.7	101.6	108.3
1990	130.7	162.8	132.4	124.1	128.5	102.1	130.4
1991	136.2	177.0	136.3	128.7	133.6	102.5	134.9
1992	140.3	190.1	137.9	131.9	137.5	103.0	138.3
			Average Annual Percent Change				
1950–1992	4.3	6.2	4.1	2.9	6.2*	4.9†	4.0
1950–1955	2.1	3.8	1.8	1.3	—	—	2.7
1955–1960	2.0	4.1	1.5	1.3	—	—	3.0
1960–1965	1.3	2.5	1.4	0.9	—	0.4	1.1
1965–1970	4.3	6.2	4.0	4.4	—	2.2	3.5
1970–1975	6.8	6.9	8.8	4.1	6.9	10.5	5.9
1975–1980	8.9	9.5	7.7	4.6	9.9	15.4	7.2
1980–1985	5.5	8.7	4.0	2.9	5.8	3.4	5.7
1985–1990	4.0	7.5	4.6	3.4	3.6	0.1	3.8
1990–1991	4.2	8.7	2.9	3.7	4.0	0.4	3.5
1991–1992	3.0	7.4	1.2	2.5	2.9	0.5	2.5

*Data are for 1970–1992.

†Data are for 1960–1992.

Date from: Bureau of Labor Statistics, U.S. Dept. of Labor: Consumer Price Index. Various releases.

Source: U.S. Dept. of Health and Human Services (1993). *Health United States 1992 and Healthy People 2000 Review* (DHHS pub. no. PHS-93-1232) Hyattsville, MD.: U.S. Government Printing Office, p. 164.

Note: 1982–1984 = 100.

increasing demand for the best care; growing medical liability; new diagnostic procedures; more people living longer; and newly identified diseases such as Legionnaires disease, Lyme disease, and AIDS, put great demands on the system.

THE SPECTRUM OF HEALTH CARE DELIVERY

Because health care in the United States is delivered by a variety of practitioners in a variety of settings, reference is sometimes made to the **spectrum of health care delivery** (see Figure 13.4). The spectrum of health care delivery refers to the array of types of care—from preventive care to continuing, or long-term, health care. This spectrum comprises six levels of care: preventive, primary, secondary, tertiary, restorative, and continuing.[1]

You may remember that we used the terms *primary, secondary,* and *tertiary* given earlier, in Chapter 4, as they related to levels of prevention. These terms have a similar meaning here, but now they are applied to health care delivery rather than prevention.

Preventive Care

Preventive care refers to the care provided to healthy individuals to keep them healthy. The primary component of preventive care is education. If people are going to behave in a way that will promote their health and the health of their community, they first must know how to do so. Health education not only provides such informa-

tion but also attempts to empower and motivate people to put this information to use by discontinuing unhealthy behaviors and adopting healthy ones. This type of care takes place in a variety of settings such as schools, well-clinics, fitness programs, family planning clinics, and physicians' and dentists' offices. Those who provide this level of care include school nurses, nurse practitioners, nutritionists, physicians, health educators, and dental hygienists, to name but a few.

Primary Care

Primary care is "front-line" or "first-contact" care. It is "person-centered (rather than disease- or organ system–centered), and comprehensive in scope, rather than being limited to illness episodes or by the organ system or disease process involved."[9] Primary health care includes routine medical care to treat common illnesses or to detect health problems in their early stages. Primary care includes such things as semiannual dental checkups, annual physical exams, health screenings for hypertension (high blood pressure) and breast or testicular cancer, and sore throat cultures. Primary health care usually is provided in practitioners' offices, clinics, and other outpatient facilities. This is the type of care that is the most difficult for the poor and uninsured to obtain (see Box 13.1).

The World Health Organization has stated that

> Primary health care rests on the following eight elements:
>
> • education concerning prevailing health problems and the methods of preventing and controlling them.

---

preventive care   Care given to healthy people to keep them healthy.

primary care   Regular and routine front-line health care.

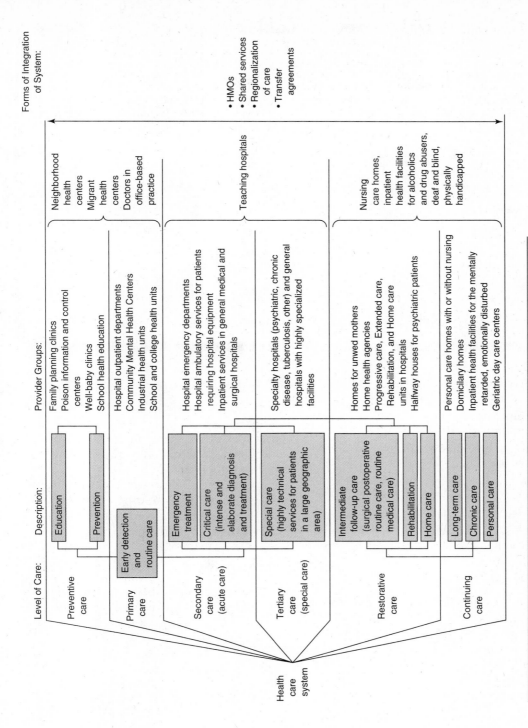

FIGURE 13.4

Spectrum of health care delivery.

From: Cambridge Research Institute (1976). Trends Affecting the U.S. Health Care System (DHEW pub. no. HRA 75-14503). Washington, D.C.: U.S. Government Printing Office, p. 262.

BOX 13.1
Healthy People 2000—Objective

21.3 Increase to at least 95% the proportion of people who have a specific source of ongoing primary care for coordination of their preventive and episodic health care. (Baseline: Less than 82% in 1986, as 18% reported having no physician, clinic, or hospital as a regular source of care)

Special Population Targets

Percentage with Source of Care	1986 Baseline	2000 Target	Percent Increase
21.3a Hispanics	70%	95%	
21.3b Blacks	80	95	
21.3c Low-income people	80	95	

Baseline data source: The Robert Wood Johnson Foundation, 1986.

For Further Thought

Why is it important that the United States reach the objective noted above by the year 2000?

- Promotion of food supply and proper nutrition.
- An adequate supply of safe water and basic sanitation.
- Maternal and child health care, including family planning.
- Immunization against the major infectious diseases.
- Prevention and control of locally endemic diseases.
- Appropriate treatment of common diseases and injuries.
- Provision of essential drugs.[10]

In the United States, the supplies of food and clean water are taken for granted. But other elements, such as maternal and child health services, immunizations, and routine dental and medical care, are not available to large segments of our population—primarily for economic reasons.

Secondary Care

Secondary (acute) care is care that involves intense and elaborate diagnosis and treatment. Secondary care includes emergency care and often is provided to patients who are not ambulatory. This type of care usually takes place in hospital emergency rooms, free-standing emergency centers, trauma centers, outpatient clinics, and other departments of hospitals.

Tertiary Care

Tertiary (special) care is advanced care that often requires highly technical services for patients. This care is not usually

---

secondary (acute) care That which includes intense and elaborate diagnosis and treatment.
tertiary (special) care Advanced care that often requires highly technical services for patients.

performed in smaller hospitals; however, it is provided in specialty hospitals or on specialized floors of general hospitals. Such facilities are equipped and staffed to provide advanced care for people with illnesses such as AIDS, cancer, and heart disease.

Restorative Care

Restorative care is the health care provided to patients after surgery or other successful treatment, during remission in cases of an oncogenic (cancerous) disease, or when the progression of an incurable disease has been arrested (see Figure 13.5). This level of care includes follow-up to secondary and tertiary care, rehabilitative care, therapy, and home care. Typical settings for this type of care include both inpatient and outpatient rehabilitation units, nursing homes, halfway houses, and private homes.

Because of the high cost of inpatient health care and changes in health insurance guidelines, care in personal residences—**home health care**—is becoming more and more common. Home health care involves providing health care via health personnel and medical equipment to individuals and families in their places of residence, for the purpose of promoting, maintaining, or restoring health or to maximize the level of independence while minimizing the effects of disability and illness, including terminal disease.[5] Such care includes prehospital care and testing, such as being prepared for surgery; posthospital treatment; and hospice care.

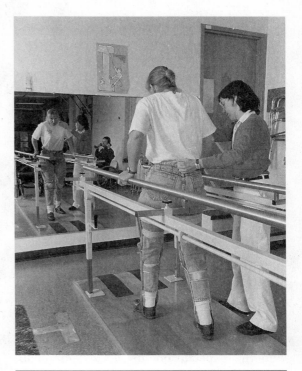

FIGURE 13.5

Restorative care can follow either secondary or tertiary care.

Continuing Care

The final level in the health care delivery spectrum is **continuing care.** Continuing care includes long-term care, care for chronic problems, and personal care. Continuing care is provided in nursing homes, facilities for the mentally and emotionally disturbed, adult and senior day care centers, and in the home. Continuing care is often provided on a 24-hour basis and is often required by patients for even basic life functions.

---

restorative care Care provided after an successful treatment or when the progress of a incurable disease has been arrested.

home health care Care that is provided in the patient's residence for the purpose of promoting, maintaining, or restoring health.

---

continuing care Long-term care for chronic health problems.

TYPES OF HEALTH CARE PROVIDERS

To offer comprehensive health care that includes services at each of the six levels just mentioned, a great number of health care workers are needed. Between 1990 and 1991, the number of civilians employed in the health service industry grew by 4% to 9.8 million, compared with a 0.9% decrease in total civilian employment (see Table 13.2). More than 8% (9.8 million) of all employed civilians in the United States work in the health care industry.

Despite this recent increase in numbers of health care workers, the demand for health care workers is expected to continue to grow. The primary reasons for this growth are the aging U.S. population (by the year 2030 it is estimated that one in five people will be 65 years old or older) and the expectation for more demand for long-term health care.[11] Because of the continuing geographic maldistribution of health care workers, the need will be greater in some settings than in others. The settings of greatest need will continue to be the rural and inner-city areas.[13] (See Box 13.2.)

Approximately half (49%) of all the health care workers are employed in hospitals, 17% in nursing homes, and 12% in physicians' offices.[12] The remaining 20% practice in a variety of settings, including official and unofficial health agencies, home health care, and other private practices. These proportions of health care workers by setting have changed in recent years, with fewer persons working in hospitals and more employed in nursing homes and ambulatory care settings such as surgical and emergency centers.[12] This trend is also expected to continue in the future.

BOX 13.2
Healthy People 2000— Objective

21.8 Increase the proportion of all degrees in the health professions and allied and associated health profession fields awarded to members of underrepresented racial and ethnic minority groups as follows:

Degrees Awarded to:	1985–1986 Baseline	2000 Target
Blacks	5%	8%
Hispanics	3	6.4
American Indians/ Alaska Natives	0.3	0.6

Note: Underrepresented minorities are those groups consistently below parity in most health profession schools—blacks, Hispanics, American Indians, and Alaska Natives.

Baseline data source: Bureau of Health Professions (HRSA).

For Further Thought

Minority and disadvantaged Americans lag behind the general U.S. population on virtually all health status indicators. Furthermore, among the poor, minorities, and the uninsured, access to medical care has been deteriorating. What impact do you think meeting the above objective will have on the community health problem? Please defend your response.

There are well over 200 different careers in the health care industry.[13] To help simplify the discussion of the different types of health care workers, they have been categorized into five different groups: independent providers, limited care providers, nurses, allied health care professionals, and public health professionals.

Table 13.2

Persons Employed in Health Service Sites: United States, Selected Years 1970–1991

(Data are based on household interviews of a sample of the civilian noninstitutionalized population.)

Site	1970*	1975	1980	1983	1984	1985	1986	1987	1988	1989	1990	1991
	Number of Persons in Thousands											
All employed civilians	76,805	85,846	99,303	100,834	105,005	107,150	109,597	112,440	114,968	117,342	117,914	116,877
All health service sites	4,246	5,945	7,339	7,874	7,934	7,910	8,129	8,478	8,781	9,110	9,447	9,817
Offices of physicians	477	618	777	888	896	894	896	950	985	1,039	1,098	1,128
Offices of dentists	222	331	415	441	468	480	497	552	521	560	580	574
Offices of chiropractors†	19	30	40	54	61	59	66	72	77	97	90	105
Hospitals	2,690	3,441	4,036	4,348	4,288	4,269	4,368	4,444	4,520	4,568	4,690	4,839
Nursing and personal care facilities	509	891	1,199	1,342	1,362	1,309	1,339	1,337	1,467	1,521	1,543	1,626
Other health service sites	330	634	872	801	859	899	963	1,123	1,211	1,325	1,446	1,545
	Percent of Employed Civilians											
All health service sites	5.5	6.9	7.4	7.8	7.6	7.4	7.4	7.5	7.6	7.8	8.0	8.4
	Percent Distribution											
All health service sites	100.0	100.0	100.0	100.0	100.0	100.0	100.0	100.0	100.0	100.0	100.0	100.0
Offices of physicians	11.2	10.4	10.6	11.3	11.3	11.3	11.0	11.2	11.2	11.4	11.6	11.5
Offices of dentists	5.2	5.6	5.7	5.6	5.9	6.1	6.1	6.5	5.9	6.1	6.1	5.8
Offices of chiropractors†	0.4	0.5	0.5	0.7	0.8	0.7	0.8	0.8	0.9	1.1	1.0	1.1
Hospitals	63.4	57.9	55.0	55.2	54.0	54.0	53.7	52.4	51.5	50.1	49.6	49.3
Nursing and personal care facilities	12.0	15.0	16.3	17.0	17.2	16.5	16.5	15.8	16.7	16.7	16.3	16.6
Other health service sites	7.8	10.7	11.9	10.2	10.8	11.4	11.8	13.2	13.8	14.5	15.3	15.7

*April 1, derived from decennial census; all other data years are annual averages from the *Current Population Survey.*

†Data for 1980 are from the American Chiropractic Assn.; data for all other years are from the U.S. Bur. of Labor Statistics.

Data from: U.S. Bur. of the Census: 1970 Census of Population, occupation by industry. Subject Reports. Final Report PC(2)-7C. Washington. U.S. Government Printing Office. Oct. 1972; U.S. Bur. of Labor Statistics: *Labor Force Statistics Derived from the Current Population Survey: A Databook,* vol. I. Washington. U.S. Government Printing Office, Sept. 1982; *Employment and Earnings,* Jan 1983–1992. vol. 30, no. 1, vol. 31, no. 1, vol. 32, no. 1, vol. 33, no. 1, vol. 34, no. 1, vol. 35, no. 1, vol. 36, no. 1, vol. 37, no. 1, vol. 38, no. 1, and vol. 39, no. 1. Washington, D.C.: U.S. Government Printing Office, Jan. 1983–92; American Chiropractic Assn.: Unpublished data.

Source: U.S. Dept. of Health and Human Services (1993). *Health United States 1992 and Healthy People 2000 Review* (DHHS pub. no. PHS-93-1232) Hyattsville, Md.: U.S. Government Printing Office, p. 140.

Notes: Totals exclude persons in health-related occupations who are working in nonhealth industries, as classified by the U.S. Bur. of the Census, such as pharmacists employed in drugstores, school nurses, and nurses working in private households. Totals include federal, state, and county health workers. In 1970–1982, employed persons were classified according to the system used in the 1980 Census of Population. Beginning in 1983, persons were classified according to the industry groups used in the 1970 Census of Population.

Independent Providers

Independent providers are those health care workers that have the specialized education and legal authority to treat any health problem or disease that an individual has. This group of workers can be further divided into allopathic, osteopathic, and nonallopathic providers.

Allopathic and Osteopathic Providers

Allopathic providers are those who use a system of medical practice in which specific remedies for illnesses, often in the form of drugs or medication, are used to produce effects different from those of diseases.[14] The practitioners who fall into this category are those who are referred to as Doctors of Medicine (MDs). The usual method of practice for MDs includes the taking of a health history, a physical examination, perhaps with special attention to the area of the complaint, and the provision of specific treatment, such as antibiotics for a bacterial infection or a tetanus injection and sutures for a laceration.

Another group of physicians that provide services similar to those of MDs are **osteopathic providers**—Doctors of Osteopathic Medicine (DOs). At one time, MDs and DOs would not have been grouped together, because of differences in their formal education, methods, and philosophy of care. While the educational requirements and methods of treatment used by MDs have remained essentially consistent over the years, those of DOs have not. The practice of osteopathy began in the later half of the nineteenth century. At that time, the education and training of osteopaths was aimed at a thorough understanding of the musculoskeletal system, because, according to osteopathic theory, all health problems, including diseases, could be cured by manipulating this system. During that time, DOs were often referred to as "bone doctors" and were often called upon to set fractured bones.[14] During the twentieth century, osteopathic medicine changed. It is now based on a philosophy of health care that emphasizes the interrelationships of the body's systems in the prevention, diagnosis, and treatment of illness, disease, and injury. The distinctive feature of osteopathic medicine is the recognition of the reciprocal interrelationship between the structure and function of the body.[15] The actual work of DOs and MDs is very similar today. Both types of physicians use all available scientific modalities, including drugs and surgery, in providing care to their patients. Few if any patients today would be able to tell the difference between the care given by a DO and an MD.

The educational requirements for MD and DO degrees are very similar. Both educational programs generally accept students into their classes after they have completed a bachelor's degree. Medical school education takes four years to complete. The first two years include course work in the sciences, while the final two years emphasize clinical experiences and rotations through the specialty areas of medicine. Upon completion of the degree (MD or DO), the students are then eligible to sit for the licensing examination in the state or territory in which they wish to practice. If they pass the exam, they are then entitled to practice medicine. At this

---

independent providers Health care professionals with the education and legal authority to treat any health problem.

allopathic providers Independent providers whose remedies for illnesses produce effects different from those of the disease.

osteopathic providers Independent providers whose remedies emphasize the interrelationships of the body's systems in prevention, diagnosis, and treatment.

point in time, some begin their practice while others join the staff of a hospital as **interns.** This internship provides the new physicians with an opportunity to gain valuable working experience and helps them decide if they want to pursue an area of specialization. If they decide to specialize in a particular field of medicine, they can apply for acceptance into a residency program. Those accepted are given the title of **resident** and the opportunity to develop the knowledge and skills necessary for the specialty. After completing the residency, which may last two to five years, they are eligible to sit for another examination to become "board certified" in the specialty. A list of such medical care specialties and subspecialties is presented in Table 13.3.

In July 1988, there were 126 accredited medical schools and 15 accredited schools of osteopathy in the United States. While the total number of applicants for openings in these schools has declined in recent years, the proportion of applications from minorities and women has increased.[12,16]

Nonallopathic Providers

Nonallopathic providers are identified by their nontraditional means of providing health care. Included in this group of providers are chiropractors, acupuncturists (those who use acupuncture as a therapy, see Figure 13.6), naturopaths (those who use natural therapies), homeopaths (those who use drugs in small doses for therapy), and naparapaths (those who use therapeutics to alter connective tissue, the root of many diseases).

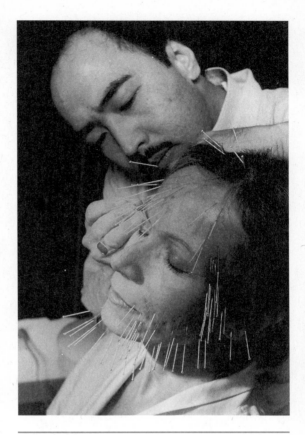

FIGURE 13.6

Many people still seek out nontraditional means of health care, such as acupuncture.

The best known and most often used nonallopathic providers in the United States are **chiropractors.** The underlying premise of the care provided by chiropractors is that all health problems are caused by misalignments of the vertebrae in the spinal column. The chiropractic approach to the treatment is (1) the identification of the misalignment through X-rays and (2) the realignment of the bones

---

intern A physician who, after passing a licensing examination, joins the staff of a hospital for practical experience.

resident A physician who is training in a specialty.

nonallopathic providers Independent providers who provide nontraditional forms of health care.

---

chiropractor A nonallopathic, independent, health care provider who treats health problems by adjusting the spinal column.

through a series of treatments called "adjustments." Chiropractors do not use more traditional therapeutic techniques such as medications, immunizations, surgery, or laboratory analyses of human tissue.

Chiropractors are educated in four-year chiropractic colleges. As with allopathic programs, students usually enter chiropractic programs after earning a bachelor's degree. Over the years, the educational standards for chiropractors have improved, but many people still question their ability to help the ill and injured. However, it should be noted that the American Public Health Association recognizes chiropractors as a professional group, and many insurance companies and Medicare and Medicaid provide reimbursement for chiropractic care.

Limited-Care Providers

Much health care is provided by **limited-care providers,** who have advanced training in a health care specialty. Their specialty allows them to provide care for a specific part of the body. This group of providers includes but is not limited to dentists (teeth), optometrists (eyes), podiatrists (feet), and psychologists (mind).

Nurses

We have categorized nurses into a group of their own because of their unique degree programs, the long-standing tradition of nursing as a profession, and their overall importance in the health care industry. It has been estimated that there are between 3 and 4 million individuals who work in the nursing profession (see Figure 13.7). These include registered nurses, licensed practical/vocational nurses, and ancillary nursing

personnel such as nurses aids.[16] Nurses outnumber physicians, dentists, and every other single group of health care workers in the United States (see Table 13.4).[11]

Training and Education of Nurses

Nurses can be divided into two subcategories based on their level of education and type of preparation. The first are those who are prepared as licensed practical/vocational nurses. Once they complete their one to two years of education in a vocational, hospital, or associate degree program and complete a licensure examination, these nurses are referred to as **licensed practical nurses (LPNs)** and **licensed vocational nurses (LVNs).** They then are able to work under the supervision of physicians or registered nurses. They usually perform routine duties and provide nontechnical bedside nursing care. The present trend is to phase out LPN/LVN training programs.

The second group of nurses includes those who have successfully completed an associate or baccalaureate degree and a state licensing (registration) examination. They are referred to as **registered nurses (RNs).** Associate degree–prepared RNs are referred to as **technical nurses.** Technical nurses provide care consisting of technical skills, including the treatments prescribed by physicians, giving medication, monitoring patient progress, and starting intravenous lines.

The third group of nurses includes the baccalaureate prepared nurses who hold the

---

limited-care providers Health care providers who provide care for a specific part of the body.

licensed practical nurse (LPN)/licensed vocational nurse (LVN) Those prepared in one- to two-year programs to provide nontechnical bedside nursing care under the supervision of others.

registered nurse (RN) An associate- or baccalaureate degree–prepared nurse who has passed the state licensing examination.

technical nurse An associate degree–prepared registered nurse.

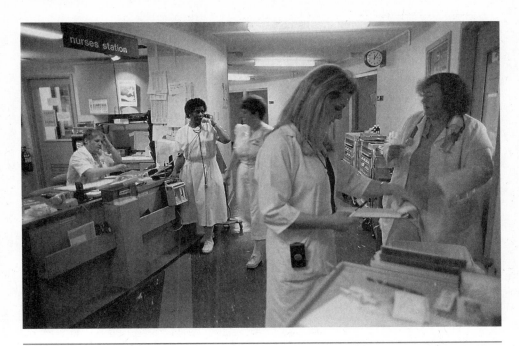

FIGURE 13.7

There is still a critical need for more nurses.

degree of Bachelor of Science in Nursing (BSN). These nurses also must pass a state licensing examination to become registered nurses (RNs). RNs holding BSN degrees are referred to as **professional nurses** and are considered to have been more thoroughly prepared for additional activities involving independent judgment. The total number of licensed RNs in the United States in 1990 exceeded 2 million. Eighty percent of these were employed either full or part time in the nursing profession.

Specialized and Advanced Training in Nursing

With advances in technology and the development of new areas of medical specialization, there is a growing need for spe-

cialty-prepared nurses. Such preparation can be received either through formal academic degree-granting programs that prepare nurses (BSN) for advanced clinical, administrative, or teaching positions, or through continuing education programs that provide specialized skills and techniques.[14] Of the advanced formal academic degrees, the master's degree programs are aimed primarily at clinical specialties. In 1990, approximately 5% of RNs held master's degrees; that percentage is expected to reach 10% by the twenty-first century. The relatively few nurses who hold doctorate degrees in nursing are highly sought after as university faculty. Nurses with doctorates teach and otherwise prepare other nurses or hold administrative (leadership) positions in health care institutions. See Table 13.4 for information on RNs holding advanced degrees.

---

professional nurse (BSN)   A registered nurse holding a bachelor of science degree in nursing.

Table 13.3
Listing of Medical Specialties and Subspecialties

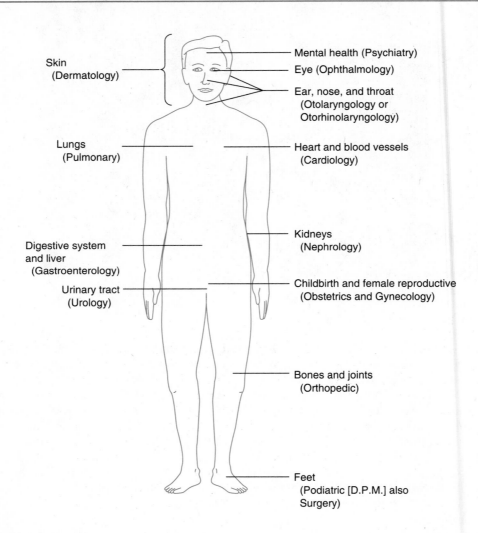

Skin
(Dermatology)

Mental health (Psychiatry)

Eye (Ophthalmology)

Ear, nose, and throat
(Otolaryngology or
Otorhinolaryngology)

Lungs
(Pulmonary)

Heart and blood vessels
(Cardiology)

Digestive system
and liver
(Gastroenterology)

Kidneys
(Nephrology)

Urinary tract
(Urology)

Childbirth and female reproductive
(Obstetrics and Gynecology)

Bones and joints
(Orthopedic)

Feet
(Podiatric [D.P.M.] also
Surgery)

Allergy and immunology (immune systems)

   Diagnostic laboratory immunology

Anesthesiology (administer drugs for pain during surgery)

   Critical care medicine

Cardiology (heart and circulatory system)

Colon and rectal surgery

Dermatology (skin)

   Dermatologic immunology/diagnostic and
   laboratory immunology

Dermatopathology

Emergency medicine

Family practice (general family health)

Table 13.3 (continued)

Geriatric medicine

Internal medicine
  Cardiovascular medicine
  Clinical cardiac electrophysiology
  Critical care medicine
  Diagnostic laboratory immunology
  Endocrinology (endocrine glands)
  Gastroenterology (digestive organs)
  Geriatric medicine
  Hematology (blood, spleen, and lymph glands)
  Infectious disease
  Medical oncology (cancer)
  Nephrology (kidney)
  Pulmonary disease (lungs)
  Rheumatology (joints, muscle, bones, and tendons)

Neurological surgery (central, peripheral, and autonomic nervous system)

Nuclear medicine (use radioactive substances to diagnose, research, and treat disease)

Obstetrics and gynecology (female reproductive system, the fetus, and the newborn)
  Critical care
  Gynecologic oncology
  Maternal-fetal medicine
  Reproductive endocrinology

Ophthalmology (eye)

Orthopedic surgery (musculoskeletal problems)

Otolaryngology (ear and throat)

Otorhinolaryngology (ear, nose, and throat)

Pathology
  Blood banking/ transfusion medicine
  Cytopathology (tumors)
  Dermatopatholgy
  Forensic pathology (cause of death)
  Hematology
  Immunopathology
  Medical microbiology
  Neuropathology
  Pediatric Pathology
  Radioisotopic pathology

Pediatrics (children)
  Adolescent medicine (adolescents and young adults)
  Diagnostic laboratory immunology
  Neonatal—prenatal medicine (problems of the fetus and newborns)
  Pediatric cardiology
  Pediatric critical care workers
  Pediatric emergency medicine
  Pediatric endocrinology
  Pediatric gastroenterology
  Pediatric hematology-oncology
  Pediatric infectious disease
  Pediatric nephrology
  Pediatric rheumatology
  Pediatric sports medicine

Physical medicine and rehabilitation
  Sports medicine

Plastic and reconstructive surgery
  Cosmetic surgery
  Hand surgery

Preventive medicine
  Public health and general preventive medicine
  Aerospace medicine
  Occupational medicine

Psychiatry and neurology
  Neurology
  Psychiatry

Radiology (radiation to diagnose and treat disease)
  Radiation oncology
  Diagnostic radiology
  Diagnostic radiology with special competence on nuclear radiology

Surgery
  General vascular surgery
  Hand surgery
  Pediatric surgery
  Surgical critical care
  Thoracic surgery (chest area)

Urology (genitals and urinary tract)

Table 13.4
Active Health Personnel and Number per 100,000 Population, According to Occupation and Geographic Region: United States, 1970, 1980, and 1990

(Data are compiled by the Bur. of Health Professions)

Year and Occupation	Number of Active Health Personnel	United States	Geographic Region			
			Northeast	Midwest	South	West
			Number per 100,000 population[1]			
1970						
Physicians	—	—	—	—	—	—
Federal[2]	—	—	—	—	—	—
Nonfederal	290,862	142.7	185.0	127.5	114.8	158.2
Doctors of medicine[2,3]	279,212	137.0	178.7	118.2	111.5	154.8
Doctors of osteopathy	11,650	5.7	6.3	9.3	3.3	3.4
Dentists[4]	95,700	47.0	58.9	46.3	35.3	54.9
Optometrists	18,400	9.0	9.7	10.3	6.6	10.5
Pharmacists	112,570	55.4	60.1	57.5	50.6	52.9
Podiatrists	7,110	3.5	6.0	3.6	1.6	3.0
Registered nurses	750,000	368.9	491.2	367.5	281.8	355.9
Veterinarians	25,900	12.7	8.3	16.1	11.8	15.0
1980						
Physicians	427,122	189.8	—	—	—	—
Federal[2]	17,642	7.8	—	—	—	—
Doctors of medicine[2,3]	16,585	7.4	—	—	—	—
Doctors of osteopathy	1,057	0.5	—	—	—	—
Nonfederal	409,480	182.0	224.5	165.2	157.0	200.0
Doctors of medicine[2,3]	393,407	174.9	216.1	153.3	152.8	195.8
Doctors of osteopathy	16,073	7.1	8.4	11.9	4.2	4.2
Dentists[4]	121,240	53.5	66.2	52.7	42.6	59.2
Optometrists	22,330	9.8	9.9	10.9	7.7	11.6
Pharmacists	142,780	62.5	66.5	67.8	62.1	51.8
Podiatrists	8,880	4.0	6.3	3.9	2.5	4.1
Registered nurses	1,272,900	560.0	736.0	583.6	443.4	533.7
Associate and diploma	908,300	399.9	536.0	429.2	316.5	351.1
Baccalaureate	297,300	130.9	161.0	127.8	103.8	148.1
Master's and doctorate	67,300	29.6	39.0	26.7	23.0	34.6
Veterinarians	36,000	16.3	10.8	19.9	16.0	18.5

(continued)

Allied Health Care Professionals

Allied health describes a large group of health-related professions that fulfill necessary roles in the health care delivery system. These professionals assist, facilitate, and complement the work of physicians and other health care specialists.[17] These health care workers provide a variety of services that are essential to the care of the patient. **Allied health care professionals** include: dieticians; occupational, physical, and

---

allied health care professionals Health care workers who provide services that assist, facilitate, and complement the work of physicians and other health care specialists.

Table 13.4 (continued)

Year and Occupation	Number of Active Health Personnel	United States	Geographic Region			
			Northeast	Midwest	South	West
			Number per 100,000 population[1]			
1990						
Physicians	567,611	230.2	—	—	—	—
Federal[2]	20,784	8.4	—	—	—	—
Doctors of medicine[2,3]	19,166	7.7	—	—	—	—
Doctors of osteopathy	1,618	0.7	—	—	—	—
Nonfederal	546,827	221.8	285.5	203.9	195.5	223.3
Doctors of medicine[2,3]	520,451	211.1	271.6	186.8	188.6	216.9
Doctors of osteopathy	26,376	10.7	13.9	17.1	6.9	6.3
Dentists[4]	145,500	58.4	70.9	58.0	48.5	62.7
Optometrists	26,000	10.4	—	—	—	—
Pharmacists	161,900	64.4	—	—	—	—
Podiatrists	12,000	4.8	—	—	—	—
Registered nurses	1,715,600	690.0	859.1	738.7	583.7	622.3
Associate and diploma	1,077,800	433.4	536.7	464.4	379.5	367.4
Baccalaureate	517,800	208.2	256.6	223.4	166.1	208.8
Master's and doctorate	120,000	48.3	65.7	51.0	38.0	45.9
Veterinarians	51,000	20.4	—	—	—	—

[1]Ratios for physicians and dentists are based on civilian population; ratios for all other health occupations are based on resident population.

[2]Starting in 1989 data for doctors of medicine are as of Jan. 1; in earlier years these data are as of Dec. 31.

[3]Excludes physicians not classified according to activity status from the number of active health personnel.

[4]Excludes dentists in military service.

Sources: Division of Health Professions Analysis, Bur. of Health Professions: *Supply and Characteristics of Selected Health Personnel.* (DHHS pub. no. HRA-81-20). Health Resources Administration. Hyattsville, Md., June 1981 and *Eighth Report to the President and Congress on the Status of Health Personnel in the United States.* Health Resources and Services Administration. (DHHS pub. no. HRS-P-OD-92-1). Rockville, Md., 1991; American Medical Association: *Physician Characteristics and Distribution in the U.S.* 1981 edition; 1992 edition. Chicago, 1981; 1992; unpublished data; American Osteopathic Association: 1980–81 *Yearbook and Directory of Osteopathic Physicians.* Chicago, 1980. American Association of Colleges of Osteopathic Medicine: *Annual Statistical Report* 1990. Rockville, Md., 1990; unpublished data.

From: U.S. Dept. of Health and Human Services (1993). *Health United States 1992 and Healthy People 2000 Review* (DHHS pub. no. PHS-93-1232). Hyattsville, Md.: U.S. Government Printing Office, p. 145.

respiratory therapists; radiographers (X-ray technicians); medical technologists (clinical laboratory workers); medical record keepers; paramedics and emergency medical technicians; nuclear medicine technicians; speech pathologists and audiologists; and medical secretaries. The educational backgrounds of allied health workers range from vocational training to master's degrees. Most of these professionals also must pass a state or national licensing examination before they can practice.

The demand for allied health care workers in all of the areas noted above is expected to continue well into the twenty-first century. The primary reasons for this are the growth of the entire health care industry and the impending arrival of the baby boomers as senior citizens.

Public Health Professionals

A discussion about health care providers would be incomplete without the

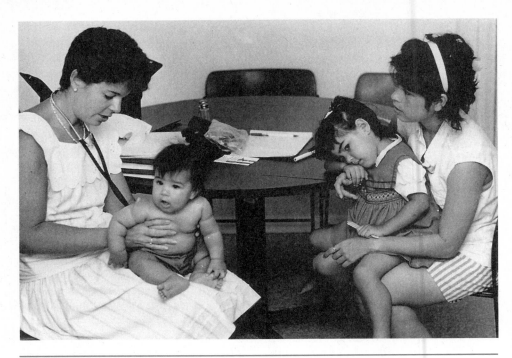

FIGURE 13.8

Public health workers make up a key component of the health care system.

mention of a group of health workers who provide unique health care services to the community—**public health professionals.** Public health professionals support the delivery of health care by such hands-on providers as public health physicians, dentists, nurses, and nutritionists, who work in public health clinics sponsored by federal, state, local, and voluntary health agencies (see Figure 13.8). Examples of public health professionals are environmental health workers, public health administrators, epidemiologists, health educators, and biostatisticians. Public health professionals often make possible such care as is practiced in immunization clinics; nutritional programs for women, infants; and children (WIC)

dental health clinics; and sexually transmitted disease clinics. The school nurse is also considered a public health professional. These services are usually financed by tax dollars and, while available to most taxpayers, serve primarily the economically disadvantaged.

HEALTH CARE FACILITIES

Health care facilities are the physical settings in which health care is actually administered. They include practitioners' private offices, public and private clinics, hospitals, rehabilitation centers, and continuing care facilities.

---

public health professional   A health care worker who works in a public health organization.

Practitioner Offices

The setting for much of the preventive and primary care provided in America is the offices of health care practitioners. Practitioner offices are privately owned buildings such as physicians' and dentists' offices, where care is provided by the practitioner and his or her staff. Because it is very expensive to set up a private practice, it is increasingly common to see more than one practitioner sharing both office and staff. These practices are often referred to as *group practices* to distinguish them from *solo (single practitioner) practices*.

Clinics

When two or more physicians practice as a group, the facility in which they provide medical services is called a *clinic*. Some clinics are small, with just a few providers, while others are very large with many providers, such as the Mayo Clinic in Rochester, Minnesota, or the Cleveland Clinic in Cleveland, Ohio. Some clinics provide care only for individuals with special health needs such as treatment of cancer or diabetes or assistance in family planning; others accept patients with a wide range of problems. A misconception held by many is that clinics are not much different from hospitals. A big difference is that clinics do not have inpatient beds, and hospitals do. Some clinics do have an administrative relationship with inpatient facilities so that if a person needs to be admitted to a hospital, it is a relatively simple process; other clinics may be free-standing, independent of all other facilities.

Clinics funded by tax dollars are public health clinics. Most of these are located in large urban areas or in rural areas that are underserved by the private sector.

Hospitals

Like clinics, hospitals vary in size, mission, and organizational structure. The major purpose of hospitals is to provide secondary (acute) and tertiary (special) care. It was once thought that most needs for emergency care should be directed toward hospitals, but the advent of the "emergicenters" and ("docs in the box") facilities and the overcrowding of many hospital emergency rooms has changed that thinking. These facilities, which offer both emergency and primary care, often can provide quicker service with less paperwork, particularly for those with cash or credit cards.

However, a majority of patients with life-threatening conditions are still taken to hospital emergency rooms, where top-of-the-line, advanced life support equipment and emergency physicians are on staff. Although emergency rooms are expensive for hospitals to maintain, they obviously perform a needed service. In addition, from a client standpoint, emergency rooms provide hospitals with patients, because many emergency patients remain for tertiary care.

Hospitals can be categorized in several different ways; one way is by hospital ownership (see Figure 13.9). A **private or proprietary hospital** is one that is owned as a business for the purpose of making a profit. A second type is the publicly owned **government hospital.** These hospitals are tax-supported and are usually found in larger cities. Public hospitals are often teaching hospitals—hospitals that have, as a part of their mission, the responsibility to prepare new health care providers. Examples of hospitals operated by the federal government include Walter Reed Army

---

private (proprietary) hospitals   For-profit hospitals.
government hospital   One that is partially or fully funded by tax dollars.

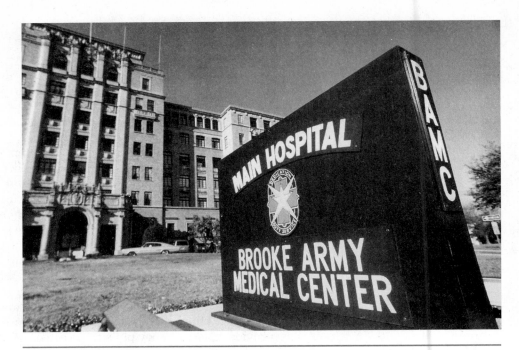

FIGURE 13.9

Hospitals are often categorized by ownership.

Hospital, Bethesda Naval Hospital, and the many hospitals run by the Veterans Administration and Indian Health Service. There are also hospitals that are owned or partially financed by states and local governments. Examples include university hospitals, state mental hospitals, and local city and county hospitals. **Voluntary (independent) hospitals** make up the third category of hospitals. These are nonprofit hospitals administered by religious, fraternal, and other charitable community organizations. Examples of this latter group are the Southern Baptist hospital, the many Shriners' hospitals, and many community hospitals.

A second means of categorizing hospitals is by the services offered. **Full-service hospitals** are those that offer care at all or most of the six levels of care discussed earlier in the chapter. These are the most expensive hospitals to run and are usually found in metropolitan areas. **Limited-service hospitals** offer the specific services needed by the population served, such as emergency, maternity, general surgery, and so on, but they lack much of the sophisticated technology available at full-service hospitals. This type of hospital is more common in rural areas. Many limited-service hospitals were

voluntary (independent) hospital   Nonprofit hospital administered by charitable community organizations.

full-service hospitals   Hospitals that offer services in all or most of the six levels of care defined by the spectrum of health care.

limited-service hospitals   Hospitals that offer only the specific services needed by the population served.

once full-service hospitals but have become limited service because of the low volume of patients, a shortage of health care personnel, and financial distress.[17]

Rehabilitation Centers

Rehabilitation centers are health care facilities in which patients work with health care providers to restore functions lost because of injury, disease, or surgery. These centers are sometimes part of a clinic or hospital but may also be stand-alone facilities. Rehabilitation centers may operate on both an ambulatory and an inpatient basis. Those providers who would commonly work in a rehabilitation center would include physical, occupational, and respiratory therapists as well as exercise physiologists.

Continuing Care Facilities

Not too many years ago, when the topic of continuing care was mentioned, most people thought of nursing homes and state hospitals for the mentally ill and emotionally disabled. Today, however, the term *continuing care* includes not only long-term care, but also *chronic, respite, hospice,* and personal home health care. These are facilities that provide both intermediate (limited service to patients) and skilled nursing services (time-intensive skilled care). The traditional facilities known for providing continuing care are nursing homes and inpatient mental facilities, but newer additions to this group are halfway houses, group homes, and special day care facilities for young, old, and other people with health problems that require special care. Recent growth in new continuing care came about as a result of

the current trend to discharge patients from hospitals earlier in their recovery to reduce health care costs. Some of these individuals no longer in need of tertiary care are still unable to care for themselves completely but can be discharged to continuing care facilities prior to returning home.

CHAPTER SUMMARY

The concept of a health care system has been and continues to be questioned in the United States. Is it really a system or is treatment provided in an informal cooperative manner? Health care in the United States has evolved from the modest services of the independent country doctor who often visited the sick in their homes to a highly complex $800 billion plus industry. Today there are medical specialists of all types and health care facilities for almost every type of illness and health problem. Whether we classify the health care delivery in the United States as a system or not, health care services are available in a broad spectrum. That spectrum includes six levels of care: preventive, primary, secondary, tertiary, restorative, and continuing.

Types of health care providers include the independent providers: allopathic, osteopathic, and nonallopathic; limited care providers; nurses; allied health care professionals; and public health professionals. These providers perform services in a variety of settings including practitioners' offices, clinics, hospitals, rehabilitation centers, and continuing care facilities.

SCENARIO: ANALYSIS AND RESPONSE

1. Have you ever experienced a situation similar to the one described in the scenario? If so, briefly describe it.

2. If we truly had a "health care system" in this country, how would this scenario be different?

3. If you were Marcus, how would you have handled this situation?

---

rehabilitation center A facility in which restorative care is provided following injury, disease, or surgery.

REVIEW QUESTIONS

1. Why have some questioned whether or not the United States really has a health care system?

2. Describe some of the major changes that have taken place in health care delivery over the years?

3. What is meant by *third-party payment?*

4. Why has the cost of health care in the United States continued to grow faster than the cost of inflation?

5. What is meant by a *spectrum of health care?*

6. What are the six different levels of care noted in the spectrum of care?

7. Is there a demand for health care workers in the United States today? If so, why?

8. In what type of facility are most health care workers employed?

9. What is the difference between independent and limited-care providers?

10. What are the differences between allopathic and nonallopathic health care providers?

11. What kind of education do limited-care providers have?

12. What is the difference between LPNs/LVNs and RNs? Between technical and professional nurses?

13. What role do public health professionals play in health care delivery?

14. What is meant by a *continuing care facility?* Give two examples.

ACTIVITIES

1. Using Figure 13.4 from this chapter, identify two different health care facilities in your community for each of the levels of care. Briefly describe each facility and determine whether each one is private, public, or voluntary.

2. Make an appointment to interview three health care workers in your community who have different kinds of jobs. Ask them what they like and dislike about their jobs, what kind of education they needed, whether they are happy with their work, and whether they would recommend that others seek this line of work. Summarize your findings in a written paper.

3. Obtain a copy of a local newspaper and look through the want ads for health care worker jobs. In a one-page paper, briefly describe what you have found and summarize the status of health care position openings in your community.

4. Create a list of all the health care providers from whom your family has sought help in the past five years. Group the individuals into the five provider groups outlined in the chapter. When appropriate, identify the providers' specialties and whether they were allopathic, osteopathic, or nonallopathic providers.

5. Make an appointment to interview an administrator in the local (city or county) health department. In the interview, find out what kind of people, by profession, work in the department. Also find out what type(s) of health care services and clinics are offered by the department. Summarize your findings in a paper.

REFERENCES

1. Cambridge Research Inst. (1976). *Trends Affecting the U.S. Health Care System.* (DHEW pub. no. HRA 75-75-14503). Washington, D.C.: U.S. Government Printing Office, p. 261.

2. Ubell, E. (July 21, 1974). "'Health" (Letter to the Editor). *The New York Times Book Reviews,* p. 19.

3. American Public Health Assn. (1975). "The Note of Official Local Health Agencies." *American Journal of Public Health* 65(2): 189–196.

4. U.S. Dept. of Health, Education, and Welfare; Health Resources Admin. (Sept. 1974). *Fact Sheet: The Hill-Burton Program.* Washington, D.C.: U.S. Government Printing Office.

5. Lokkeberg, A. R. (1988). "The Health Care System." In E. T. Anderson and J. M. McFarlane, eds. *Community as Client: Application of the Nursing Process.* Philadelphia: J.B. Lippincott, pp. 3–14.

6. Koff, S. Z. (1987). *Health Systems Agencies: A Comprehensive Examination of Planning and Process.* New York: Human Services Press.

7. Stockman, D. A. (1981). "Premises for a Medical Marketplace: A Neoconservative's Vision of How to Transform the Health System." *Health Affairs* 1(1): 5–18.

8. No Author (July 1987). "Health Care Dollars." *Consumer Reports,* pp. 435–448.

9. Hibbard, H., and P. A. Nutting (1991). "Research in Primary Health Care: A National Priority." In M. L. Grady, ed. *AHCPR Conference Proceedings—Primary Care Research: Theory and Methods.* Rockville, Md.: Agency for Health Care Policy and Research.

10. World Health Organization (1990). *Facts About WHO.* Geneva, Switz.: Author, p. 6.

11. Rice, D. P. (1990). "The Medical Care System: Past Trends and Future Projections. In P. R. Lee and C. L. Estes, eds. *The Nation's Health,* (3rd. ed.), pp. 72–93. Boston: Jones and Bartlett.

12. U.S. Dept. of Health and Human Services (1993). *Health United States 1992 and Healthy People 2000 Review.* (DHHS pub. no. PHS-93-1232). Hyattsville, Md.: U.S. Government Printing Office.

13. National Health Council, Inc. (1985). *200 Ways to Put Your Talent to Work in the Health Field.* New York: Author.

14. Payne, W. A., and D. B. Hahn (1992). *Understanding Your Health,* 3rd ed. St. Louis, Mo.: Mosby-YearBook.

15. University of Osteopathic Medicine and Health Sciences (UOMHS) (1992). *1992–1994 Catalog.* Des Moines, Ia.: Author.

16. U.S. Dept. of Health and Human Services (1990). *Seventh Report to the President and Congress on the Status of Health Personnel in the U.S.* (DHHS pub. no. HRS-P-0D-90-1). Washington, D.C.: U.S. Government Printing Office.

17. Gupta, G. C. (1991). Student Attrition: A Challenge for Allied Health Education Programs. *Journal of the American Medical Association.* 266(7): 963–967.

Chapter 14

HEALTH CARE SYSTEM: FUNCTION

Chapter Outline

Chapter Objectives

After studying this chapter you will be able to:

1. Explain what is meant by a fee-for-service system of payment.
2. Briefly describe the purpose and concept of insurance.
3. Define the term *insurance policy.*
4. Explain the insurance policy terms: *deductible, coinsurance, copayment, fixed indemnity, exclusion,* and *preexisting condition.*
5. Explain what is meant when a company or business is said to be self-insured.
6. List the different types of medical care usually covered in a health insurance policy.
7. Briefly describe Medicare, Medicaid, and medigap insurance.
8. Explain the difference between catastrophic and long-term care health insurance.
9. List four problems of the present health care system.
10. Explain how health maintenance organizations differ from our traditional fee-for-service system of payment.
11. Briefly describe the four different types of HMOs.
12. Define the terms *PPO* and *EPO* and explain how these organizations function.
13. Explain the concept behind ambulatory care centers.
14. Identify the strengths and weaknesses of national health indid2path: Cannot open: No such file or directorying the Oregon Health Plan.

Greg, a young father, is awakened in the middle of the night by his 8-year-old son, Zack, who has all the typical signs and symptoms of influenza. Greg does not want to disturb his family physician at this time of night, but he does want Zack to receive appropriate medical care. Therefore, he decides to take Zack to the hospital emergency room for treatment. After examining the boy, Dr. Rainey, the attending physician, declares that Zack has the flu. Dr. Rainey then instructs Greg that Zack should drink plenty of clear fluids, take a nonaspirin analgesic for his fever, and get plenty of rest. Dr. Rainey concludes by indicating that the illness should pass in a couple of days. As Greg and Zack leave the hospital, they stop at the business desk to pay the bill. The billing clerk informs Greg that there is no charge. "You have zero deductible health insurance." The bill was for $223.00.

INTRODUCTION

In Chapter 13, we described the structure of the health care delivery system in the United States, including such concepts as the spectrum of care and levels of care. We also surveyed the various types and levels of health care providers and the types of facilities in which health care is provided. In this chapter, we will build on that information by explaining how people obtain health care services, how these services are paid for, and by whom. We will also discuss two serious shortcomings of our traditional health care delivery system—access and cost—and examine some current and potential solutions to these shortcomings.

GAINING ACCESS TO AND PAYING FOR HEALTH CARE IN THE UNITED STATES

Access to Health Care

The services offered by health care providers in the United States are perhaps the best offered anywhere in the world. Unfortunately, the services are not accessible to all Americans. Access to health care services has been and continues to be a major health policy issue in the United States (see Figure 14.1). Although the majority of people (approximately 86%) in the United States do have access to health care, millions, especially the poor and the working poor, do not. Interestingly enough, the poor do not lack emergency or urgent care because no one needing such care and willing to go to a hospital will be turned away. However, they usually do not have access to primary care, such as checkups, screenings for chronic illnesses, and prenatal care (see Figure 14.2). Without adequate primary care, many patients eventually find themselves in need of more-costly and often less-effective medical treatment. The primary factors that limit access to this type of care are total lack of health insurance, inadequate insurance, and poverty. Those who are unable to receive primary medical care because they cannot afford it are referred to as "medically indigent."[1] The medically indigent in America include people and families with income above the poverty level but who are unable to afford health care or health in-

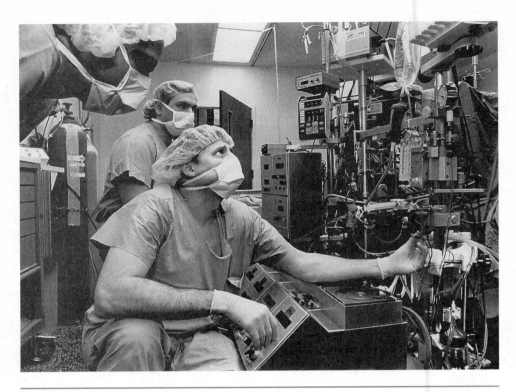

FIGURE 14.1

We have the finest health care in the world, but at what cost?

surance. In many cases, these people may be working full time at low-paying jobs that provide no health care benefits. This group of people has also been referred to as the "working poor." The poorest of the poor may not be the medically indigent because of public health insurance for the poor, Medicaid (see Box 14.1).

Paying for Health Care

Health care in America has not only been labeled the best, but also the most expensive (see Table 14.1). Health care is the single largest expenditure in the country, surpassing defense, education, and housing. America spends more per capita annually on health care (approximately $2,900) than any other nation. The next closest country,

---

BOX 14.1
Healthy People 2000— Objective

21.4 Improve financing and delivery of clinical preventive services so that virtually no American has a financial barrier to receiving, at a minimum, the screening, counseling, and immunization services recommended by the U.S. Preventive Services Task Force. (Baseline data not available.)

For Further Thought

In your opinion, what kinds of things will have to happen by the year 2000 for the above objective to be met? Do you think this objective will be met? Why or why not?

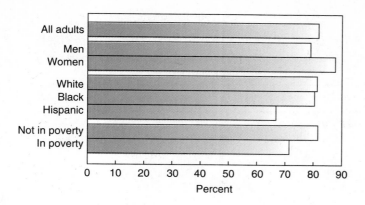

Characteristics	1991
All adults	80
Men	74
Women	86
White	81
Black	79
Hispanic	64
Not in poverty	82
In poverty	72

Note: Related tables in *Health, United States, 1992,* are 78–81.

From: U.S. Dept. of Health and Human Services, National Center for Health Statistics (1993). *Healthy People 2000 Review 1992* (DHHS pub. no. PHS 93-1232-1). Washington, D.C.: U.S. Government Printing Office.

FIGURE 14.2

Adults with a usual source of medical care, according to selected characteristics related to year 2000 objectives, United States, 1991.

Canada, spends almost $1,000 less per capita.[2] Under the U.S. system, the actual cost of the service is usually not known until after the service has been provided, unless the patient is bold enough to inquire ahead of time—most are not.

Payments for the 1991 U.S. health care bill of $660 billion came from four sources (see Figure 14.3). The first is the patients themselves. These, *direct* or *out-of-pocket payments,* represent approximately one-fifth of all payments. The remaining portion of health care payments, four-fifths, comes almost entirely from *indirect,* or *third-party, payments.* The first source of third-party

payments is private insurance companies. These payments are made from premiums paid to the insurance company by the patients and/or their employers. The second source of third-party payments is public or governmental insurance programs (i.e., Medicare, Medicaid, Veterans Administration, Indian Health Service, or military). These government programs are funded by a combination of taxes and premiums from those insured (in the case of PART B Medicare coverage). And lastly, a small percentage of health care bills are paid by private philanthropy—personal donations to help cover costs.

Table 14.1

Total Health Expenditures as a Percent of Gross Domestic Product and Per Capita Expenditures in Dollars: Selected Countries and Years, 1960–1991

(Data compiled by the Organization for Economic Cooperation and Development)

Country	1960	1965	1970	1975	1980	1985	1988	1989	1990	1991*
	Health Expenditures as a Percent of Gross Domestic Product									
Australia	4.9%	5.1%	5.7%	7.5%	7.3%	7.7%	7.7%	7.8%	8.2%	8.6%
Austria	4.4	4.7	5.4	7.3	7.9	8.1	8.4	8.4	8.3	8.4
Belgium	3.4	3.9	4.1	5.9	6.6	7.4	7.7	7.6	7.6	7.9
Canada	5.5	6.0	7.1	7.2	7.4	8.5	8.8	9.0	9.5	10.0
Denmark	3.6	4.8	6.1	6.5	6.8	6.3	6.5	6.5	6.3	6.5
Finland	3.9	4.9	5.7	6.3	6.5	7.2	7.2	7.2	7.8	8.9
France	4.2	5.2	5.8	7.0	7.6	8.5	8.6	8.7	8.8	9.1
Germany	4.8	5.1	5.9	8.1	8.4	8.7	8.8	8.3	8.3	8.5
Greece	2.9	3.1	4.0	4.1	4.3	4.9	5.0	5.4	5.4	5.2
Iceland	3.5	4.2	5.2	6.2	6.4	7.1	8.6	8.6	8.3	8.4
Ireland	4.0	4.4	5.6	8.0	9.2	8.2	7.3	6.9	7.0	7.3
Italy	3.6	4.3	5.2	6.1	6.9	7.0	7.6	7.6	8.1	8.3
Japan	3.0	4.5	4.6	5.6	6.6	6.5	6.6	6.6	6.5	6.6
Luxembourg	—	—	4.1	5.6	6.8	6.8	7.2	6.9	7.2	7.2
Netherlands	3.9	4.4	6.0	7.6	8.0	8.0	8.2	8.1	8.2	8.3
New Zealand	4.3	—	5.2	6.7	7.2	6.5	7.1	7.2	7.3	7.6
Norway	3.3	3.9	5.0	6.7	6.6	6.4	7.7	7.4	7.4	7.6
Portugal	—	—	3.1	6.4	5.9	7.0	7.1	7.2	6.7	6.8
Spain	1.5	2.5	3.7	4.8	5.6	5.7	6.0	6.3	6.6	6.7
Sweden	4.7	5.6	7.2	7.9	9.4	8.8	8.6	8.6	8.6	8.6
Switzerland	3.3	3.8	5.2	7.0	7.3	7.6	7.8	7.5	7.8	7.9
Turkey	—	—	—	3.5	4.0	2.8	3.8	3.9	4.0	4.0
United Kingdom	3.9	4.1	4.5	5.5	5.8	6.0	6.1	6.1	6.2	6.6
United States	5.3	5.9	7.4	8.4	9.2	10.5	11.1	11.5	12.2	13.2
	Per Capita Health Expenditures†									
Australia	$99	$127	$207	$438	$663	$998	$1,171	$1,225	$1,310	$1,407
Austria	69	94	163	369	683	984	1,191	1,298	1,383	1,448
Belgium	55	84	128	303	571	879	1,081	1,153	1,242	1,377
Canada	109	154	253	435	743	1,244	1,558	1,666	1,811	1,915
Denmark	70	125	212	340	582	807	972	1,013	1,051	1,151
Finland	57	95	164	305	517	855	1,044	1,147	1,291	1,426
France	75	124	203	386	698	1,083	1,295	1,415	1,528	1,650

Table 14.1 (continued)

Country	1960	1965	1970	1975	1980	1985	1988	1989	1990	1991*
Germany	98	135	216	458	811	1,175	1,409	1,412	1,522	1,659
Greece	16	27	58	102	184	282	334	384	400	404
Iceland	53	88	137	290	581	889	1,331	1,373	1,379	1,447
Ireland	38	53	97	231	449	572	620	651	748	845
Italy	51	83	153	280	571	814	1,058	1,150	1,296	1,408
Japan	27	64	127	256	517	792	992	1,092	1,175	1,267
Luxembourg	—	—	154	326	632	930	1,219	1,267	1,392	1,494
Netherlands	74	106	207	410	696	931	1,101	1,176	1,286	1,360
New Zealand	94	—	180	364	562	747	900	954	995	1,047
Norway	49	77	134	306	549	846	1,112	1,128	1,193	1,305
Portugal	—	—	46	157	238	398	493	548	554	624
Spain	14	38	82	187	325	452	598	682	774	848
Sweden	94	151	271	470	855	1,150	1,303	1,390	1,455	1,443
Switzerland	96	141	268	512	839	1,224	1,435	1,498	1,640	1,713
Turkey	—	—	—	36	64	66	110	118	133	142
United Kingdom	79	102	147	273	458	685	858	912	985	1,043
United States	143	204	346	592	1,063	1,711	2,146	2,351	2,600	2,868

*Preliminary figures.

†Per capita health expenditures for each country have been adjusted to U.S. dollars using gross domestic product purchasing power parities for each year.

Note: Some numbers in this table have been revised and differ from previous editions of *Health,* United States.

Sources: Schieber, G. J., J. P. Poullier, L. G. Greenwald, "U.S. health expenditure performance: An international comparison and data update." *Health Care Financing Review* 13(4). HCFA pub. no. 03331. Health Care Financing Administration. Washington, D.C. U.S. Government Printing Office, Sept. 1992; Office of National Health Statistics, Office of the Actuary. "National health expenditures, 1991." *Health Care Financing Review.* 14(2) HCFA pub. no. 03335. Health Care Financing Administration. Washington, D.C. U.S. Government Printing Office, Winter 1992; Unpublished data.

From: U.S. Dept. of Health and Human Services (1993). *Health United States 1992 and Healthy People 2000 Review* (DHHS pub. no. PHS-93-1232) Hyattsville, Md.: U.S. Government Printing Office, p. 161.

The most traditional system of health care financing is known as a **fee-for-service system.** Under this system, people select a provider, receive care (service), and pay the bill (a fee). Those who seek health care are obligated to pay their fee at the time the service is rendered. The fee-for-service system still predominates in the United States for most kinds of medical services from routine preventive examinations to the most advanced hospital care.

fee-for-service A method of paying for health care in which after the service is rendered, a fee is paid.

In the past, some physicians provided care when needed and worried about payment later. Others often accepted "in kind" payment, such as farm produce or other products or services as payment in full for a medical service rendered. Today, in order for patients to receive care, they are often required to demonstrate the ability to pay (to assume financial responsibility for the fee) before the service is rendered. A physician's receptionist may ask, "How do you plan to settle your bill?" In other cases, providers have signs placed around the

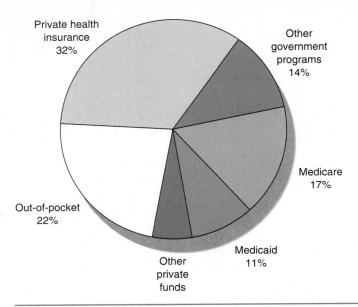

FIGURE 14.3
Who paid the health care bill in 1991?

waiting room that state, "Payment is expected when service is rendered, unless other arrangements have been made prior to the appointment."

Third-Party Payment

The process for receiving a third-party payment usually begins when a health care provider or his or her staff requests information about the insured's health insurance plan. They normally request the name of the insuring company (Blue Cross/Blue Shield, for example), the policy number, and a personal identification number (PIN). This information is usually provided to the insured on a wallet-sized card by the insurer. The provider may then ask the patient to sign an insurance claim form (see Figure 14.4) in two places. The first signature indicates that the service has been provided and authorizes the provider to submit patient information with the claim for payment. The second signature instructs the

insurance company to make the payment directly to the provider. Upon receiving and reviewing the completed and signed form, the insurance company then issues payments to the provider for services based upon the provisions of the insurance policy. Depending upon the level of reimbursement for the claim, the provider will either consider the bill paid in full or will request payment from the patient in the amount of the difference between the provider's full fee and the portion paid by the insurance company.

HEALTH INSURANCE

The concept of health insurance is not a new one in this country. Group health and life insurance are considered American inventions of the early twentieth century. Montgomery Ward and Company in 1911 sold health insurance policies based upon

ATTENDING DENTIST'S STATEMENT

CHECK ONE:

☐ DENTIST'S PRE-TREATMENT ESTIMATE

☐ DENTIST'S STATEMENT OF ACTUAL SERVICES

Send Completed Claim Forms To:

1. PATIENT NAME
2. RELATIONSHIP TO EMPLOYEE — SELF | SPOUSE | CHILD | OTHER
3. SEX — M | F
4. PATIENT BIRTHDATE — MO | DAY | YEAR
5. IF FULL TIME STUDENT — SCHOOL — CITY

6. EMPLOYEE/SUBSCRIBER NAME — FIRST — MIDDLE — LAST
7. BC/BS ID NO.
9. ACCOUNT NO — BENEFIT CODE

8. EMPLOYEE/SUBSCRIBER MAILING ADDRESS

CITY STATE ZIP

10. EMPLOYER (COMPANY) NAME AND ADDRESS

11. GROUP NUMBER
12. LOCATION (LOCAL)
13. ARE OTHER FAMILY MEMBERS EMPLOYED? — EMPLOYEE NAME — SOC. SEC. NO
14. NAME AND ADDRESS OF EMPLOYER IN ITEM 13

15. IS PATIENT COVERED BY ANOTHER DENTAL PLAN? — DENTAL PLAN NAME — UNION LOCAL — GROUP NO. — NAME AND ADDRESS OF CARRIER

I HAVE REVIEWED THE FOLLOWING TREATMENT PLAN. I HEREBY AUTHORIZE ANY INSURANCE COMPANY, ORGANIZATION, EMPLOYER OR PROVIDER OF SERVICE TO RELEASE TO ASSOCIATED INSURANCE COMPANIES, INC. PRIOR TO OR AFTER PAYMENT ANY AND ALL INFORMATION RELATED TO THIS CLAIM.

SIGNED (PATIENT OR PARENT IF MINOR) — DATE

I HEREBY AUTHORIZE PAYMENT DIRECTLY TO THE BELOW-NAMED DENTIST OF THE GROUP INSURANCE BENEFITS OTHERWISE PAYABLE TO ME. A PERSON WHO KNOWINGLY AND WITH INTENT TO DEFRAUD AN INSURER, FILES A STATEMENT OF CLAIM CONTAINING ANY FALSE, INCOMPLETE, OR MISLEADING INFORMATION COMMITS A FELONY.

SIGNED (INSURED PERSON) — DATE

16. DENTIST NAME

17. MAILING ADDRESS

CITY STATE ZIP

18. DENTIST SOC. SEC. OR T.I.N.
19. DENTIST PROVIDER NO.
20. DENTIST PHONE NO.

21. FIRST VISIT DATE CURRENT SERIES
22. PLACE OF TREATMENT — OFFICE | HOSP | ECF | OTHER
23. RADIOGRAPHS OR MODELS ENCLOSED? — NO | YES | HOW MANY?

	NO	YES	
24. IS TREATMENT RESULT OF OCCUPATIONAL ILLNESS OR INJURY?			IF YES, ENTER BRIEF DESCRIPTION AND DATES
25. IS TREATMENT RESULT OF AUTO ACCIDENT?			
26. OTHER ACCIDENT?			
27 ARE ANY SERVICES COVERED BY ANOTHER PLAN?			
28 IF PROSTHESIS, IS THIS INITIAL PLACEMENT?			(IF NO, REASON FOR REPLACEMENT) — 29 DATE OF PRIOR PLACEMENT
30. IS TREATMENT FOR ORTHODONTICS?			IF SERVICES ALREADY COMMENCED, ENTER — DATE APPLIANCES PLACED — MOS. TREATMENT REMAINING

IDENTIFY MISSING TEETH WITH "X"

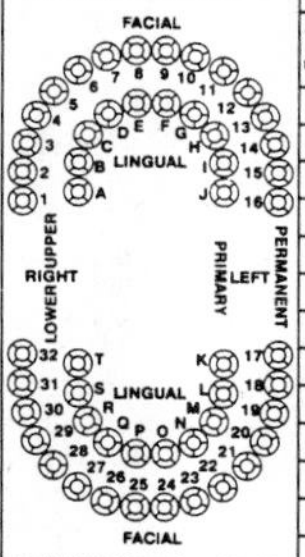
FACIAL
1 2 3 4 5 6 7 8 9 10 11 12 13 14 15 16
A B C D E F G H I J
LINGUAL
UPPER
LOWER
RIGHT
LEFT
PRIMARY
PERMANENT
T S R Q P O N M L K
LINGUAL
32 31 30 29 28 27 26 25 24 23 22 21 20 19 18 17
FACIAL

32. REMARKS FOR UNUSUAL SERVICES

31. EXAMINATION AND TREATMENT PLAN - LIST IN ORDER FROM TOOTH NO. 1 THROUGH TOOTH NO. 32 - USE CHARTING SYSTEM SHOWN

TOOTH # OR LETTER	SURFACE	DESCRIPTION OF SERVICE (INCLUDING X-RAYS, PROPHYLAXIS, MATERIALS USED, ETC.) LINE NO.	DATE SERVICE PERFORMED MO DAY YEAR	PROCEDURE NUMBER	FEE	FOR ADMINISTRATIVE USE ONLY

I HEREBY CERTIFY THAT THE PROCEDURES AS INDICATED BY DATE HAVE BEEN COMPLETED.

SIGNED (DENTIST) — DATE

TOTAL FEE CHARGED	
MAX. ALLOWABLE	
DEDUCTIBLE	
CARRIER %	
CARRIER PAYS	
PATIENT PAYS	

FORM APPROVED BY THE COUNCIL ON DENTAL CARE PROGRAMS OF THE ADA 1975 ADS (75)

21J-016 R8(6-91)

FIGURE 14.4

Insurance claim form.

the principles still used today in the business. Now, more than 800 companies sell health and life insurance policies.[3]

Because of the expense of health care, those without health insurance find it difficult to pay for the care. If people do not have insurance, they are more likely to not have a usual source of primary medical care.[4] It was estimated in 1993 that at any particular point in time there are approximately 37 million Americans without health insurance; this amounts to almost 14% of the population and is up from 13% in 1984. Those most likely to be without coverage included younger persons, males, nonwhites, those with low incomes, persons 18 years of age and older who are unemployed or who had less than 12 years of education, residents of the South and West regions of the country, and residents of central cities in metropolitan statistical areas. However, it should be pointed out that 13.9% of the employed are still not covered, because their employers do not provide such benefits.[5,6]

Health insurance, like all other types of insurance, is a risk- and cost-spreading process. That is, the cost of one person's injury or illness is shared by all in the group. Each person in the group has a different chance (or risk) of having a problem and thus needing health care. Some members of the group, for example those who are obese or those who suffer from congenital health problems, will probably need more care while others in the group will need less. The concept of insurance has everyone in the group, no matter what their individual risk, helping to pay for the collective risk of the group. The risk of costly ill health is spread in a reasonably equitable fashion among all persons purchasing insurance, and everyone is protected from having to pay an insurmountable bill for a catastrophic injury or illness.

There are some exceptions to the "equitable fashion." If someone in the group knowingly engages in a behavior that increases his or her risk, such as smoking cigarettes or driving in a reckless manner, that person may have to pay more for the increased risk. Likewise, if someone enters the group with a **preexisting condition,** a medical condition that carries a higher-than-average risk, such as a long history of heart disease, that person may have to pay more (see Figure 14.5). In short, the greater the risk, the more the individual or group has to pay for insurance.

The Health Insurance Policy

A policy is a written agreement between a private insurance company (or the government) and an individual or group of individuals to pay for certain health care costs in return for regular, periodic payments (a set amount of money) called *premiums*. The insurance company benefits in that it anticipates collecting more money in premiums than it has to pay out for services; hence, it anticipates a profit. The insured benefits by not being faced with medical bills he or she cannot pay, because the insurance company can and will pay them. The added benefit for those insured as a group is that group premiums are less expensive than premiums for individuals.

The expectations of both insurers and insurees are not always met. An insurer occasionally has to pay out more than it collects in premiums. Alternatively, the insured often purchases insurance that is never used.

Although the language of health insurance policies can be confusing, everyone

---

preexisting condition A medical condition that exists prior to the insured being covered by an insurance policy.

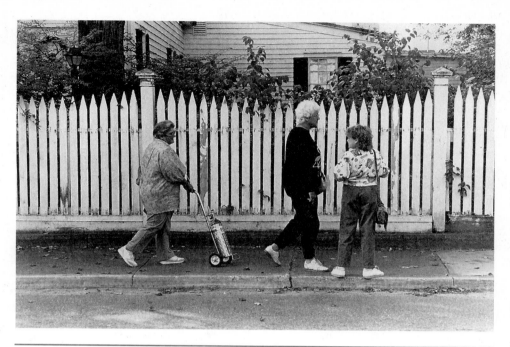

FIGURE 14.5

Preexisting conditions are often excluded from policies.

needs to understand several key terms. One of the most important is **deductible.** The deductible is the amount of expenses (money) that the beneficiary (insured) must incur (pay) before the insurance company begins to pay for covered services. A common deductible level is $200 per individual policy holder, or a maximum of $500 per family. This means that a family must pay the first $500 of medical costs before the insurance company begins paying. The higher the deductible of a policy, the lower the premiums.

Another key term, **coinsurance,** refers to the portion or percentage of insurance company's approved amounts for covered services that the beneficiary is responsible for paying. The coinsurance clause may be invoked after the deductible limits have been met and the insurance company begins to pay. Coinsurance, also known as **copayment,** is paid by both the insured and insurer. For example, a policy that states the coinsurance is 20/80 requires the insured to pay 20% of the remainder of the bill after the deductible is paid while the insurer pays 80%. The greater the proportion of coinsurance paid by the insured, the lower the premiums.

A third key term, **fixed indemnity,** refers to the maximum amount an insurer will pay for a certain service. For example, a

---

deductible The amount of expense that the beneficiary must incur before the insurance company begins to pay for covered services.

coinsurance The portion of the insurance company's approved amounts for covered services that a beneficiary is responsible for paying.

---

fixed indemnity The máximum amount an insurer will pay for a certain service.

policy may state that the maximum amount of money paid for AIDS treatment is $15,000. Depending upon the language of a policy, the fixed indemnity benefit may or may not be subject to the provisions of the deductible or coinsurance clause. Costs above the fixed indemnity amount are the responsibility of the insured.

Another key term related to health insurance is **exclusion.** When an exclusion is written into a policy, it means that a specified health condition is excluded from coverage. That is, the policy does not pay for service to treat the condition. Cancer treatment is often an excluded health condition. However, one can purchase special cancer insurance policies to help pay for such care. A special type of exclusion often written into policies is an exclusion for preexisting health conditions. For example, a policy could have a clause about an exclusion for a preexisting heart condition. This would mean that if a person with heart disease took out a policy with this clause in it, he or she would not be covered by the policy for service to treat the heart condition.

Self-Insured Organizations

With the high cost of health care today, some of the institutions that provide health insurance for their employees are deciding to cut their costs by becoming self-insured. Most organizations that do this hire an insurance company to manage the program for them. Basically a **self-insured organization** is one that pays the health care costs of its employees with the premiums

---

exclusion A health condition written into the health insurance policy indicating that which is not covered by the policy.

self-insured organization One that pays the health care costs of its employees with the premiums collected from the employees and the contributions made by the employer.

collected from the employees and the contributions made by the employer. In doing so, the organization gets to set most of the parameters of the policy: deductibles, coinsurance, fixed indemnities, and exclusions. If the organization wants to exclude some services and include others, it can. For example, if the organization has an older work force, it may wish to delete obstetrics from the policy but include a number of preventive health services. If at the end of a year the amount paid for the plan by both the employer and employees is less than expenditures for health services, the premiums and contributions must be increased the following year. If there is a surplus of money at the end of a year, the premiums and contributions the following year could be reduced or a refund could be made to the contributors.

For self-insurance to work, there must be a sizable group of employees over which to spread the risk. Larger organizations usually find it more useful than smaller ones.

The Cost of Health Insurance

The cost of health care in the past two decades has skyrocketed and, with it, the cost of health insurance. In 1992, it cost U.S. businesses an average of $5,000 per employee to provide health insurance; and it was estimated that it would increase at about 15% annually, so that if it goes unchecked, it could reach $16,800 annually per employee in the year 2012. The automobile industry has estimated that workers' health insurance adds somewhere between $700–800 to the cost of every new car.[7] The actual cost of a policy is determined by two major factors—the risk of those in the group and the type of coverage provided. An increase in either risk or coverage will result in an increase in the cost of the policy.

Table 14.2
Types of Health Insurance Coverage

dental—Dental procedures.

disability—Income when insured is unable to work because of a health problem.

hospitalization—Inpatient hospital expenses including room, patient care, supplies, and medications.

major medical—Large medical expenses usually not covered by regular medical or dental coverage.

optical—Nonsurgical procedures to improve vision.

regular medical—Nonsurgical service provided by health care providers. Often has set amounts (fixed indemnity for certain procedures).

surgical—Surgeons' fees (for inpatient or outpatient surgery).

Types of Health Care Coverage

As has been noted in the previous discussions, there are a number of different types of services that health insurance policies cover. The more common types of coverage include hospitalization, surgical, regular medical, major medical, dental, and disability. Table 14.2 presents a short overview of each of these.

HEALTH INSURANCE PROVIDED BY THE GOVERNMENT

Although there are many in the United States who would like to see all health insurance provided by the government—a national health insurance—at the present time, government health insurance plans are only available to select groups in the United States. The only government health insurance plans that exist today are Medicare and Medicaid, Veterans Administration benefits (see Figure 14.6), Indian

Health Service, and health care benefits for the uniformed services. Our discussion here will be limited to Medicare and Medicaid. These programs were created in 1965 by amendments to the Social Security Act and implemented for the first time in 1966.

Medicare

Medicare is a federal health insurance program for people 65 years of age or older, people of any age with permanent kidney failure, and certain disabled people under 65. It

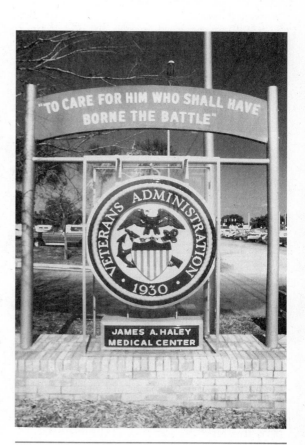

FIGURE 14.6

Insurance provided for veterans is one of four major insurance plans paid for by the U.S. government.

is administered by the Health Care Financing Administration (HCFA) of the U.S. Department of Health and Human Services (USDHHS). The Social Security Administration, also part of USDHHS, provides information about the program and handles enrollment.[8] Medicare has two parts; hospital insurance (Part A) and medical insurance (Part B). Medicare is considered a contributory program, in that employers and employees are required to contribute a percentage of each employee's wages/salaries via Social Security (FICA) tax to the Medicare fund. In 1992, both employer and employees paid a Medicare tax of 1.45% on the first $130,200 of covered wages. If people were self-employed, their Medicare tax was 2.9%.[9]

The Medicare hospital insurance (Part A) portion is mandatory and is provided for those eligible without further cost. While it has deductible and coinsurance provisions, it pays for an inpatient semiprivate hospital room, inpatient care in a skilled nursing facility, inpatient care in a psychiatric hospital, home health care, and hospice care.[8] It also covers some follow-up care equipment, and supplies. Those enrolled in Part A are automatically enrolled in Part B unless they state they do not want it. Part B is financed 75% by the federal government and 25% by premiums of those wanting it. In 1993 the premium was $36.60 per month.[8] This portion of Medicare covers physicians' fees and selected other health care services. Part B also has a deductible ($100 per year) and coinsurance (80/20). Both portions of Medicare are subject to yearly changes in coverages and administrative procedures. Finally, it should be noted that when health care providers take assignment (willing to accept Medicare patients) on a Medicare claim, they agree to accept the Medicare-approved amount as payment in full. These providers are paid directly by the Medicare carrier, except for the deductible and coinsurance amounts.[8]

Medicare, like private health insurance programs, is affected by the high costs of health care and, therefore, the government is always looking for ways of cutting the costs of the programs. One procedure added in 1983 that has helped to control the costs is the **prospective pricing system (PPS).** In the PPS, hospitals are paid predetermined amounts of money per procedure for service provided to Medicare patients. The predetermined amounts are based upon over 470 **diagnosis-related groups (DRGs)** rather than the actual cost of the care rendered. Each hospital stay by a Medicare patient is assigned a DRG. "The correct DRG for each patient is decided by considering the patient's major or principal diagnosis; any complications or other problems that might arise; any surgery performed during the hospital stay; and other factors."[10] The amount of money assigned to each DRG is not the same for each hospital. The figure is based on a formula that takes into account the type of service, the type of hospital, and the location of the hospital. Using this prospective pricing system, hospitals are encouraged to provide services at or below the DRG rate. If the hospital delivers the service below the DRG rate, the hospital can retain the difference. If it is delivered above the DRG rate, the hospital incurs the extra expenses. "However, when a Medicare patient's condition requires an unusually long hospital stay or exceptionally costly care, Medicare makes additional payment to the hospital."[10] Because of DRGs, some have felt that hospitals are quicker to discharge Medicare patients to

---

prospective pricing system One in which providers are paid predetermined amounts of money per procedure for services provided.

diagnosis-related groups (DRGs) A procedure used to classify the health problems of all Medicare patients when they are admitted to a hospital.

keep their expenses down. This phenomenon has resulted in an increase in the need for skilled nursing care in homes, in adult day care facilities, and in nursing homes.

Medicaid

A second type of government health insurance is Medicaid, a health insurance program for the poor. Eligibility for enrollment in Medicaid is determined by each state. Many Medicaid recipients are also enrolled in other types of public assistance programs (welfare). Unlike Medicare, there is no age requirement for Medicaid, eligibility requirements are strictly financial. Also, unlike Medicare, Medicaid is a noncontributory program jointly administered through federal and state governments. Both programs cover nursing home care but under different conditions.

In theory, both Medicare and Medicaid programs seem to be sound programs that help provide health care to two segments of the society who would otherwise find it difficult or impossible to obtain health insurance. In practice, there are two recurrent problems with these programs. One problem is that some physicians and hospitals do not accept Medicare and Medicaid patients because of the tedious and time-consuming paperwork, lengthy delays in reimbursement, and insufficient reimbursement. As a result, it is difficult if not impossible for many of those eligible for Medicare and Medicaid to receive health care. The second problem occurs when physicians and hospitals file Medicare and Medicaid paperwork for care or services not rendered or rendered incompletely. This is known as *Medicare/Medicaid fraud.*

A third drawback to these public insurance programs is the lack of coverage for catastrophic illness and long-term care, two situations that could quickly deplete the lifetime savings of an individual or family.

People who wish to be protected in these situations must purchase their own catastrophic and long-term care insurance. Former president Reagan proposed that catastrophic illness insurance be included with Medicare; and, in fact, Congress approved it in 1988 for implementation in 1990, but it was repealed in 1989 because the elderly objected to the increased cost.

SUPPLEMENTAL HEALTH INSURANCE

Medigap

As noted earlier, both portions of Medicare have deductibles and coinsurance stipulations. To help cover these out-of-pocket costs, some people purchase supplemental policies from private insurance companies. These policies have come to be known as **medigap** policies. Recent changes in federal law have mandated national standardization of medigap policies. Under these standards, insurance companies can offer no more than ten standardized plans (see Box 14.2) that have been developed by the National Association of Insurance Commissioners. Each of these ten plans is required to have a core set of benefits. The plans vary from simple (core benefits only) to more-complex plans with additional benefits. The plans are identified by the letters A–J. By law, the letters and benefits of the individual plans cannot be changed by the insurance companies. However, they may add names or titles to the letter designations. While companies are not required to offer all the plans, they must make Plan A available if they sell any of the other nine plans in a state.[8]

---

medigap Private health insurance to supplement Medicare benefits.

BOX 14.2
Ten Standard Medicare Supplement (Medigap) Benefit Plans

	Plan									
	A	B	C	D	E	F	G	H	I	J
Core Benefits										
Part A hospital (days 61–90)	X	X	X	X	X	X	X	X	X	X
Lifetime reserve days (91–150)	X	X	X	X	X	X	X	X	X	X
365 life hospitalization days—100%	X	X	X	X	X	X	X	X	X	X
Parts A and B, blood	X	X	X	X	X	X	X	X	X	X
Part B coinsurance—20%	X	X	X	X	X	X	X	X	X	X
Additional Benefits										
Skilled nursing facility coinsurance (days 21–100)			X	X	X	X	X	X	X	X
Part A deductible		X	X	X	X	X	X	X	X	X
Part B deductible			X			X				X
Part B excess charges						100%	80%		100%	100%
Foreign travel emergency			X	X	X	X	X	X	X	X
At-home recovery				X			X		X	X
Prescription drugs								1	1	2
Preventive medical care					X					X

Core Benefits

Core Benefits pay the patient's share of Medicare's approved amount for physician services (generally 20%) after $100 annual deductible, the patient's cost of a long hospital stay ($169/day for days 60–90, $338/day for days 91–150, approved costs not paid by Medicare after day 150 to a total of 365 days lifetime), and charges for the first three pints of blood not covered by Medicare.

Drug Benefits

Two prescription drug benefits are offered:

1. A "basic" benefit with $250 annual deductible, 50% coinsurance, and a $1,250 maximum annual benefit (Plans H and I above).
2. An "extended" benefit (Plan J above) containing a $250 annual deductible, 50% coinsurance, and a $3,000 maximum annual benefit.

From: U.S. Dept. of Health and Human Services (1993). *1993 Guide to Health Insurance for People with Medicare* (pub. no. HCFA-02110). Washington, D.C.: U.S. Government Printing Office, p. 14.

Other Supplemental Insurance

Medigap is a supplemental insurance program specifically designed for those on Medicare. However, a number of supplemental insurance policies exist for people regardless of their age. Included are specific-disease insurance, hospital indemnity insurance, and long-term care insurance. Specific-disease insurance, not available in some states, provides benefits for only a single disease (such as cancer) or a group of specific diseases. Most policies are written as fixed-indemnity policies. Hospital indemnity coverage is insurance that pays a fixed amount for each day a person is hospital-

ized, up to a designated number of days. Long-term care insurance, which covers nursing home and skilled nursing care, is of great concern to many people.[8] For that rea-

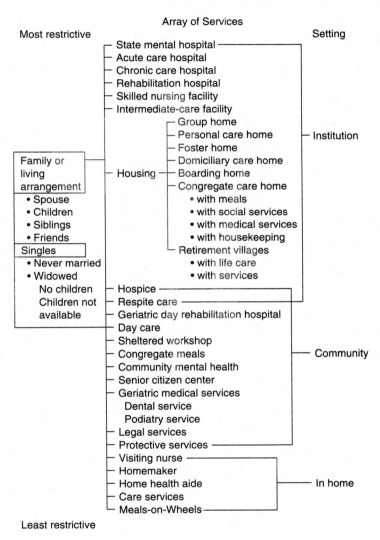

FIGURE 14.7

Inventory of recommended available services appropriate to a long-term care support system.

From: Manson, S. M., and D. G. Callaway (1990). "Health and Aging Among American Indians: Issues and Challenges for the Geriatric Sciences." In M.S. Harper (ed.), Minority Aging: Essential Curricular Content for Selected Health and Allied Health Professions *(DHHS pub. no. HRS-P-DV90-4). Washington, D.C.: U.S. Government Printing Office, p. 99. Manson and Callaway adapted this from Brody, S. J., and C. Mascrocchi. "Data for Long-Term Care by Health Systems Agencies."* American Journal of Public Health 70(2):1197.

son, a separate subsection on the topic is presented below.

Long-Term Care Insurance

Because it can cost from $2,200 to $4,000 or more per month to stay in a nursing home, the cost of long-term care (see Figure 14.7) has many people worried about their financial future. Much of the cost of long-term care is paid directly by the patient until those funds are exhausted; only then does Medicaid payment begin. A 1990 study showed that 48.5% of all nursing home costs were paid by Medicaid, 48.3% were paid by patients and their families, and only the remaining 3.2% was paid for by Medicare or private insurance.[11] The national average cost for one year of nursing home care ranges from $25,000 to $40,000 or more, depending on the services provided and the geographic location of the home. It was projected that a person reaching 65 years of age in 1990 would have to put $27,600 per year into savings to pay for future nursing home use.[12, 13]

Health care provided in the patient's home is also expensive. The estimated cost of three *unskilled* home health aide visits per week for one year would amount to more than $5,000. Three visits by a *skilled* aide could cost as much as $10,000 per year. The majority of Americans are impoverished within the first year of making long-term health care payments. Those caring for a spouse find that they quickly exhaust both their spouse's resources and their own. Suggestions for careful purchasing of long-term care insurance have been provided by Weissert[14] and appear in Table 14.3.

Table 14.3
Suggestions for Buying a Long-Term Care Policy

1. A reasonable *annual premium for people age 65* ranges from $700 to $1,400. Since this type of insurance is to protect the estates of the elderly, Weissert feels that their children should pay the premiums. "Not everyone will agree with that, of course," he acknowledges.

2. Select a policy with the *maximum number of benefit years* you can find. Some policies only cover three or four years.

3. Policies that require *a prior hospitalization* adversely affect the chances of a payout. People with chronic conditions who have not been hospitalized will be at a disadvantage. Likewise, some home care policies require the patient to have been in a nursing home first.

4. Choose a policy with as long a *grace period* as possible between hospital discharge and nursing home admission. A longer time allows a comprehensive search for the right nursing home.

5. The best policies offer *four levels of nursing care,* some of which will not be appropriate for the patient. Consumers should seek out policies that cover intermediate and custodial care, not just skilled care. Your coverage should not require a skilled stay first.

6. Look for policies that will cover *Alzheimer's disease,* even if they exclude other kinds of mental illness.

7. It might be best to choose a policy with a *higher premium and fewer deductible days,* because some patients will experience several short stays and may have to meet the deductible each time.

8. Look for policies that will *waive the premium* if the patient is confined to a nursing home for longer than three to six months.

From: Weissert, W. G. (1991). "Choose Long-Term Care Insurance with Caution." *Findings,* 6(2). A publication of the School of Public Health, Univ. of Michigan, Ann Arbor.

ALTERNATIVES TO THE CURRENT SYSTEM

Although most people in the United States are content with the way they are now receiving health care, this system is not without its problems. It is expensive, limits access to health care for certain groups, does not insure against financial bankruptcy, is burdened with paperwork and red tape, and is subject to fraud. These shortcomings are not new: the United States has struggled with some of them for years.

Recent surveys of Americans indicate that there is widespread dissatisfaction with the way the United States finances and controls the cost of health care.[15] This is especially true when Americans see the shortcomings of the U.S. system being effectively handled in other countries. Many other industrialized nations have health care systems that assure access to all, produce health status indicators that are equal to or exceed those of the United States, and, accomplish all this at a lower cost[15] (see Box 14.3 for comparative data).

The debate seems to be not *whether* the U.S. system of health care should be changed, but rather *how* it should be changed. There is no shortage of ideas. In fact, an entire issue of the *Journal of the American Medical Association* (May 15, 1991) was devoted to explanations of different plans. Several additional alternatives surfaced in the 1992 presidential election. Proposed solutions range from minor adjustments to our present system to a total revamping of the entire health care delivery system. In the information that follows on the next several pages, several alternative approaches to the present system are discussed. Some of these have already been put into practice while others have merely been proposed.

Existing Alternatives

Several alternatives to the traditional health care delivery system are already in use today. These include health maintenance organizations, preferred provider organizations, exclusive provider organizations, and ambulatory care centers.

Health Maintenance Organizations

The **health maintenance organization (HMO)** is an alternative to the fee-for-service system of health care. With an HMO, the insurance coverage and the delivery of medical care are combined into a single organization. The organization then hires doctors (on straight salaries) or contracts with a specific group of doctors to provide care and either builds its own hospital or contracts for the services of a hospital within the community.[16] No fee is exchanged when service is provided. Instead, subscribers (or their employers) make regular payments in advance on a fixed contract fee to the HMO. For example, if a husband and wife with three children choose to enroll in an HMO, their monthly fixed contract fee might be $250. In return, the "HMO is contractually obligated to provide this family with a comprehensive range of outpatient and inpatient services without imposing significant additional fees."[17]

How do HMOs make a profit? An HMO's focus of care is different from that of a traditional fee-for-service provider. In an HMO, ill and injured patients become a "cost." An HMO does not make money on the ill but on keeping people healthy. The less the providers of an HMO see a patient, the lower the costs and the more profitable the organization. Therefore, most HMOs emphasize

---

health maintenance organizations (HMOs) Groups that supply prepaid comprehensive health care with an emphasis on prevention.

Comparing International Health Care Systems

How the U.S. Health Care System Compares to Other Industrialized Countries

	United States	Canada	France	Germany	Japan	United Kingdom
Health spending per capita 1970	$346	$274	$192	$199	$126	$144
Health spending per capita 1990	2,566	1,795	1,379	1,287	1,113	909
Health spending as percent of GDP	12.4%	9.0%	8.9%	8.1%	6.5%	6.1%
Number of doctors per 100,000 population	234	215	250	281	157	137
Life expectancy, men	71.5	73.0	72.3	71.8	75.5	72.4
Life expectancy, women	78.3	80.2	81.6	78.4	82.3	78.1

Three Basic Models

Health care systems in developed countries fall into three basic models:

1. A national health service model with universal coverage and general tax-financed government ownership of the facilities and doctors as public employees. Examples: United Kingdom, Spain, Italy, Greece, and Portugal.
2. A social insurance model providing universal coverage under social security, financed by contributions paid by employers and employees. In Canada, contributions are made to a government entity. In France and Germany, contributions are going to nonprofit funds with national negotiation on fees. Japan also has a compulsory system that relies heavily on employer-based coverage.
3. A private insurance model with employer-based or individual purchase of private health insurance and private ownership and control of inputs to the health sector. The United States and South Africa are the only examples of this system.

From: The Muncie (Ind.) Star, Sept. 26, 1993.

health promotion activities and primary and secondary care. Critics of HMOs often express the concern that people will not receive all the care they need because the care cuts into the profits. There are no data to support this concern.

There are four main organizational models of HMOs. They include (1) staff, (2) group, (3) network, and (4) individual practice models.[18] (See Figure 14.8.)

Staff Model

In **staff model HMOs,** salaried physicians provide services only to HMO members, those who join the HMO and pay monthly premiums. The physicians, whose offices and examining rooms are housed in

---

staff model HMO A health maintenance organization that hires its own staff of physicians.

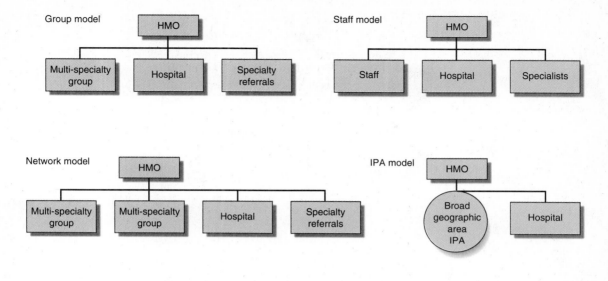

FIGURE 14.8

HMO model types.

---

the building paid for by the HMO, work only for the HMO. They do not have their own private practices.

Group Model

In a **group model HMO,** a physicians' group practice contracts with an HMO to provide care for the members of the HMO. With this model, the group practice sees not only the HMO members but also other patients who are not enrolled HMO members.

Network Model

In the **network model,** two or more group practices contract with an HMO to provide service to the members. The groups involved in the network model also see patients other than those belonging to the HMO.

---

group model HMO An HMO that contracts with a physicians' group practice to provide care for a specific number of HMO enrollees.

network model HMO An HMO that contracts with several physicians' group practices to provide care for a specified number of enrollees.

Independent Practice Association Model

In the **independent practice association model (IPA),** individual physicians contract with an HMO to provide care for members. The physicians "are paid a capitated sum per enrollee or a discounted fee for services."[17] These physicians also have their own private practices.

While the number of HMOs has grown steadily since 1970 (see Table 14.4), it is difficult to predict whether their popularity will increase or decrease in the future (see Figure 14.9). Some of the bigger and better known HMOs today include Kaiser Permanente (also the oldest), The Health Group of Puget Sound, and Cigna. One team of researchers[19] predict an HMO boom. They state that the future trends for HMOs will be largely driven by the relative competitive strengths of the different types of HMOs in

---

independent practice association (IPA) model HMO An HMO in which individual physicians contract with the HMO to provide care for a certain number of enrollees.

Table 14.4

Health Maintenance Organizations and Enrollment, According to Model Type, Geographic Region, and Federal Program: United States, Selected Years 1976–1992

(Data are based on a census of health maintenance organizations)

Plans and Enrollment	1976	1980	1984	1985[1]	1986	1987	1989	1990	1991	1992
Plans					*Number*					
All plans	174	235	304	478	623	647	604	572	553	555
Model type[2]:										
Individual practice association[3]	41	97	125	244	384	409	385	360	346	340
Group[4]	122	138	179	234	239	238	219	212	168	166
Mixed	—	—	—	—	—	—	—	—	39	49
Geographic region:										
Northeast	29	55	67	81	105	114	118	115	116	111
Midwest	52	72	106	157	202	203	183	160	157	165
South	23	45	66	141	188	194	172	176	163	161
West	70	63	65	99	128	136	131	121	117	118
Enrollment[5]					*Number of Persons in Thousands*					
Total	5,987	9,078	15,101	21,005	25,725	29,232	31,883	33,028	34,004	36,076
Model type[2]:										
Individual practice association[3]	390	1,694	2,929	6,379	9,932	12,014	13,542	13,741	13,619	14,665
Group[4]	5,562	7,384	12,172	14,625	15,793	17,217	18,342	19,287	17,063	16,543
Mixed	—	—	—	—	—	—	—	—	3,322	4,868
Federal program[6]:										
Medicaid[7]	—	265	349	561	802	811	1,043	1,187	1,446	1,728
Medicare	—	391	671	1,064	1,490	1,674	1,761	1,842	2,029	2,161

(continued)

meeting the needs of the local consumer and employers. Each of the four models mentioned earlier has strengths and weaknesses, so it is unlikely that any one of them will dominate the future market.

Preferred Provider Organizations

The **preferred provider organizations (PPO)** is another alternative form of health care delivery. While maintaining some fee-for-service characteristics, the PPO differs from the traditional system in

---

preferred provider organization (PPO) An organization that buys fixed-rate health services from providers and sells them to consumers.

that the fee has been fixed through a negotiation process between a health care provider (e.g., physicians, dentists, hospitals, etc.) and the PPO. It works in the following manner: A PPO approaches a provider, such as a group dental practice, and contracts with the dentists to provide dental services to all those covered by the PPO's insurance plan at a fixed (discount) rate. To the extent that the PPO succeeds in obtaining favorable prices, it can offer lower premiums and hence can attract more patients to enroll in its insurance plan.[16] Advantages for the providers are that they are assured: (1) a certain volume of patients and (2) that the patients will pay promptly (via the

Table 14.4 (continued)

Plans and Enrollment	1976	1980	1984	1985[1] 1992	1986	1987	1989	1990	1991
				Number Enrolled per 1,000 Population					
Geographic region:									
Northeast	19.9	31.4	57.8	79.4	100.5	117.0	137.7	145.6	153.7	161.1
Midwest	15.2	28.1	61.6	96.8	116.4	130.5	129.2	126.2	126.5	128.3
South	4.3	8.3	20.4	37.5	54.4	64.2	70.5	70.5	71.4	78.1
West	96.9	121.8	148.0	172.5	190.4	205.6	225.5	232.1	237.7	247.0

[1]Increases partly due to changes in reporting methods.

[2]Eleven HMOs with 35,000 enrollment did not report model type in 1976.

[3]An HMO operating under an individual practice association model contracts with an association of physicians from various settings (a mixture of solo and group practices) to provide health services.

[4]Group includes staff, group, and network model types.

[5]Open-ended enrollment in HMO plans, amounting to 1.2 million on Jan. 1, 1991, is not included in this table.

[6]Federal program enrollment in HMOs refers to enrollment by Medicaid or Medicare beneficiaries, where the Medicaid or Medicare program contracts directly with the HMO to pay the appropriate annual premium.

[7]Data for 1989 and later include enrollment in managed care health insuring organizations.

Notes: Data as of June 30 in 1976–1984, Dec. 31 in 1985–1987, and Jan. 1 in 1989–1992. Medicaid enrollment in 1989–1990 is as of June 30. HMOs in Guam are not included.

Sources: Office of Health Maintenance Organizations: *Summary of the National HMO census of prepaid plans—June 1976 and National HMO Census 1980.* Public Health Service. Washington, D.C.: U.S. Government Printing Office. (DHHS pub. no. PHS 80-50159). InterStudy: *National HMO Census: Annual Report on the Growth of HMO's in the U.S., 1984–1985 Editions;* The InterStudy Edge, 1989, 1990, vol. 2; Competitive Edge, vols. 1 and 2, issues 1, 1991 and 1992; 1986 Dec. Update of Medicare Enrollment in HMOs. 1988 Jan. Update of Medicare Enrollment in HMOs. Excelsior, Minn. (Copyrights 1983, 1984, 1985, 1986, 1987, 1988, 1989: Used with the permission of InterStudy); U.S. Bur. of the Census: *Current Population Reports.* Series P-25, Nos. 998 and 1058. Washington, D.C. U.S. Government Printing Office, Dec. 1986 and Mar. 1990. U.S. Dept. of Commerce: Press release CB 91-100. Mar. 11, 1991. Health Care Financing Administration: Unpublished data; Centers for Disease Control and Prevention, National Center for Health Statistics: Data computed by the Division of Analysis.

From: U.S. Dept. of Health and Human Services (1993). *Health United States 1992 and Healthy People 2000 Review* (DHHS pub. no.

PPO). Providers and patients see the PPO as a compromise between traditional practice and an HMO.[17]

The one major objection to both HMOs and PPOs is that the patients cannot freely select their provider. They are restricted to those with whom the company has contracted. Some employers have solved this problem by allowing employees to visit the provider of their choice. In this case, however, the employer pays only the amount for care that it would have paid if the employee had gone to the preferred provider. The difference between the actual provider's fee and what the company pays must then be paid by the patient.[18, 19]

Exclusive Provider Organization

Exclusive Provider Organizations (EPOs) are much like PPOs except that they have stronger financial incentives for enrolled consumers to use the exclusive (only) provider. For example, the employees of a company that enrolled in an EPO may have only a single choice for a hospital if they want the insurance company to pay the bill. If the employees were to go to another hospital, they would be responsible for the *whole* bill. Typically, the number of providers (physicians, dentists, hospitals,

---

exclusive provider organization (EPO) Like a PPO but with fewer providers and greater discounts.

etc.) is much smaller in an EPO, which strengthens the ability of the organization to receive a greater discount since the providers are guaranteed a larger share of patients. Because of such arrangements, a business or corporation is able to create a more stringent utilization and monitoring program with an EPO.

Ambulatory Care Centers

Other alternatives to the traditional means of offering health care in the United States are the relatively new emergicenters and surgicenters. These free-standing, fee-

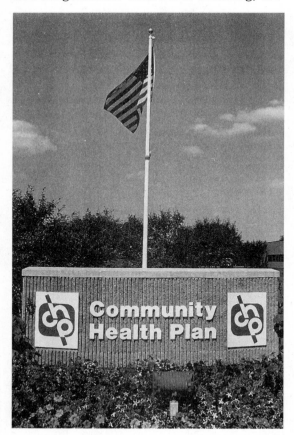

FIGURE 14.11

HMOs are an alternative to the fee-for-service system of health care.

for-service facilities provide acute care to walk-in (ambulatory) patients without the hotel-like services traditionally available in hospitals (see Figure 14.10). These alternative sites for acute care have been successful because they are efficient and cost-effective. These facilities (often not much larger than a fast-food restaurant) have sometimes been referred to as "Docs in Box"! Their smaller size, fewer employees, and less technical equipment allows these centers to offer care at a lower price. These facilities do not perform major surgery, such as heart transplants, and most have a transfer arrangement with a full-service hospital nearby for patients who need extended care.

The establishment of a new ambulatory care facility in a community is not always received with enthusiasm. In previously underserved communities, fast-growing communities, or communities with many temporary residents, such as resort communities, they have been well received. However, in stable or shrinking communities where there is an adequate number of health providers, the arrival of a new free-standing acute-care facility is sometimes viewed as unfriendly competition.

Innovative Programs

New Programs in Hospitals

In order to keep their share of the market, some hospitals are creating services not traditionally offered through hospitals. Two such services are sick-child day care and minorcare centers. Sick-child day care has come about because of the increase in numbers of single-parent and dual-career families. Both types of families have problems when children are sick and cannot attend school or go to their normal day care center. Where can a sick child receive better health care than in a hospital? Thus, hospitals are accepting these children on a daily basis to

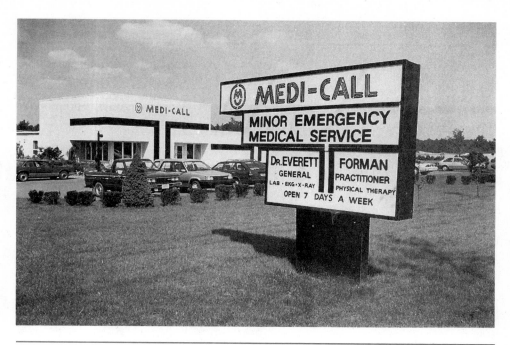

FIGURE 14.10

Ambulatory Care Centers provide medical services efficiently without the overhead of a hospital clinic.

provide a needed service, fill their empty beds, and keep their health care workers working. For the same reasons, hospitals are creating minorcare centers. The centers, located in hospitals, are now providing services that have traditionally been offered in physicians' offices and in the new emergicenters, such as treating sore throats, flu, and childhood diseases. They advertise drop-in visits, no appointments necessary, and they offer their services at a somewhat lower cost than emergency rooms.

National Health Insurance

National health insurance or *national health care* suggests a system in which the federal government assumes the responsibility for the health care costs of the entire population. Obviously, the costs would be paid for with tax dollars. Presently among all the developed countries of the world, there are only two that do not provide such a plan for their citizens: South Africa and the United States. When one considers the level of satisfaction with health care in other countries and the better access to these services in these countries, one must ask why the United States has not adopted such a program. It is not because the United States has not considered such a plan. President Harry Truman presented a proposal to Congress on two different occasions, only to have it defeated.[20] Other attempts at national health care legislation were made during the Kennedy and Nixon administrations, but they also failed.

The 1992 presidential campaign again brought attention to America's problems with health care delivery. Bill Clinton, then overnor of Arkansas, based his election campaign strategy on being a new kind of Democrat—one who could take on the nation's domestic ills. He saw health care as one of those ills, because the present system failed to cover all and the spiraling costs threatened to bankrupt the government and cripple American industry.

Shortly after being elected president, Mr. Clinton appointed the first lady, Hillary Rodham Clinton, to head a committee to develop a plan to overcome the shortcomings of the present health care system. The first lady and the committee spent a great deal of time during the spring and summer of 1993 gathering information to identify approaches and clarify alternatives. By fall 1993, a plan had been completed. The president then presented it to a joint session of Congress in front of a national television audience (see Figure 14.11). The detailed plan, referred to informally as the President's Health Security Plan and formally as the American Health Security Act of 1993, was over 1,500 pages in length.

The plan rested on six major points.[6] The first was security. Security will be provided by the plan's call for universal coverage; a guaranteed national benefits package; protection from catastrophic costs; coverage regardless of one's employment status, medical condition, or age; and support for long-term care.

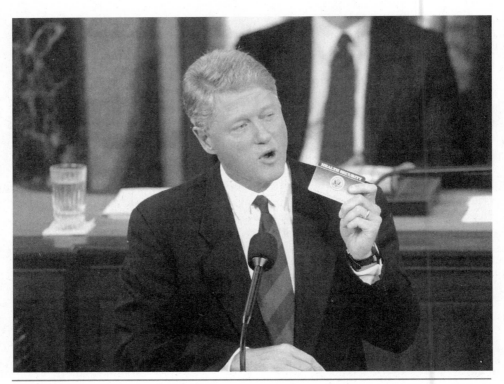

FIGURE 14.11

President Bill Clinton presents his health care reform proposal, the American Health Security Act of 1993, to a joint session of Congress and to the American people.

The second major point was to control cost. The plan is designed to bring health care cost growth in line with growth in the gross domestic product (GDP) by 1997. It is to accomplish this goal by increasing competition in health care, reducing administrative costs, and imposing budget discipline. Most of the cost controls are based on the ideas of managed care and managed competition. "Managed care is a comprehensive approach to health care delivery that encompasses planning, education, monitoring, coordinating and controlling quality, access, and cost considering the interests of patients, providers and payers."[21] When implemented, this means of controlling health care costs uses such techniques as limiting services to those deemed "medically necessary," utilization reviews, and case management.[22]

Managed competition, an approach that has not been tried anywhere in the world, emphasizes using incentives to motivate consumers (patients), insurers (payers), and providers to be more cost conscious. It tries to penetrate the health care system with efficiency, flexibility, and innovation of competitive markets, without the undesirable outcomes of the present system.[23] Managed competition is an approach that creates competition based on costs, quality, and access. With this approach, purchasers of health care are usually health purchasing cooperatives or alliances representing all people in a given geographic area. The regulator (possibly the government) determines such elements as the basic benefits package, accountability for providing access and quality of care to all eligible, and the monitoring of costs.[22]

In order for managed competition to reduce overall health care costs, the type of health care people receive and the manner in which it is delivered would have to differ significantly from the way it is received and delivered now. With managed competition, consumers would probably have less choice, more limited access to many providers, fewer services, and slower access to new technology. Furthermore, the number of payers (insurers) could drop dramatically, and providers would be paid at lower rates and would face more extensive guidelines when making clinical decisions.[23]

The third major point of the American Health Security Act was enhancing quality. The plan improves the quality of health care by creating standards and guidelines for practitioners, reorienting quality assurance to measure outcomes rather than regulate process, increasing the national commitment to medical research, and promoting more and better preventive and primary care. This point was also to be enhanced by the ideas of managed care and competition.

The fourth point of the plan was expanding access to care to areas that have been traditionally underserved: rural communities and urban neighborhoods. To meet this concern, incentives are to be provided to encourage providers to locate in these areas and to encourage communities to develop new programs such as school-based and school-linked clinics.

Reducing bureaucracy was the fifth point of the plan. The plan is to streamline the system for both the consumer and providers. Included in this point are things like having only one standard insurance claim form and reducing the billing and regulating requirements.

The final major point of the plan was to reduce fraud and abuse. The plan cracks down on health care providers and institutions that impose excessive charges or engage in fraudulent practices by setting tougher accountability standards and imposing stiffer criminal and civil monetary penalties.

President Clinton's health care plan was much discussed in Congress in 1994 but failed to come to a vote before Congress adjourned. Because of the complexity of both health care delivery and the proposed act itself, it is anticipated that discussion will continue for some time. There are some who predict that the entire plan will not be decided before the end of President Clinton's first term of office.

Even prior to the passage of a new health care act, students can learn much about national health insurance by the plans of other countries. Characteristics of such plans for other countries are presented in Figure 14.12. Because of cultural similarities and the geographic proximity to Canada, we describe the Canadian system in more detail below.

Canadian Health Care System

Canada has provided its legal residents with universal health insurance coverage since 1972 through a program that is jointly financed by their federal government and the ten provincial and two territorial governments. The program is designed by the individual provincial and territorial authorities according to federal standards. Each provincial and territorial authority must ensure that: all residents have access to care regardless of cost; necessary hospital and physician services are available; residents have continuous coverage as they travel from one province to another; and that the provincial programs are run as nonprofit organizations.[24]

The Canadian federal government's financial support to this program is based on block grants to the provinces and territories. The government provides grants based on an equal per capita figure. The figures are adjusted annually to take into account the GNP. These grants cover about 30%–40% of the total cost of health care. Since the beginning of the use of block grants, the percentage of the total cost paid for by the federal government has continued to decrease. About 25% of the total comes from private sources, and the remaining portion must be financed by the provinces. Provinces can tax the people via sales or payroll taxes, or they can charge premiums; but they cannot impose user fees or extra billing without loss of federal support.[24]

The Canadian health care system is not a socialized system of health care. It is a system whereby the government is the third-party payer. Canadian residents get to select their physicians, who are independent physicians working for themselves—not the government. It is a fee-for-service program. Providers must accept the provincial plan reimbursement as payment in full if the province is to receive maximum federal support. In addition, there are no maximum limits on the amount of care provided as long as it is deemed medically necessary. And finally, Canada prohibits private health insurance except for items not covered under the provincial plan.[15]

Compared to the American health care system, the Canadian system has four major strengths (see Figure 14.13). The first is that "no Canadian is without health insurance. There is equity across income groups. The poor are treated as well as the rich."[25] The second is that the administrative costs of the Canadian system are under control. It has been estimated if the United States implemented the Canadian system, we would save about $30 billion, or 0.5% of the GNP, on administrative cost reductions alone.[26] (A number of people in the United States who are presently not being treated could be treated with the savings.) Third, overall, the Canadian system is less expensive to run. In 1991, the per capita expenditure on health care in Canada was $1,915 compared to $2,868 in the United States. These health care costs amount to 10% of the Canadian GNP versus 13.2% in the United States. Those figures have continued to rise, with

Spain
Virtually everyone covered by public plan. Six percent deducted from paychecks to finance health care and unemployment programs, with matching funds from employers. Despite complaints about waiting for surgery and checkups, public system rated higher than private care.

Britain
Government pushing free-market reforms on National Health Service, which provides care for all. Financed 80% from general revenues and partly from payroll deductions. Local health authorities allowed to contract with hospitals and other facilities. Doctors free to contract with hospitals to care for their patients. Elective surgery often requires long wait. Private care available.

Denmark
Government-run and financed by general taxation, with optional private insurance for expenses not covered. Some competition being introduced, such as patients allowed to chose among hospitals and doctors. Some discussion of allowing supermarkets to sell painkillers in competition with pharmacies.

Israel
Choice of four funds costing $150 to $200 a month per family. Medicines heavily subsidized. Dentistry not covered. Largest fund is $1 billion in debt. Government preparing changes under which citizens would pay government and it would reimburse clinics. About 7% of the population not covered by insurance, particularly recent immigrants.

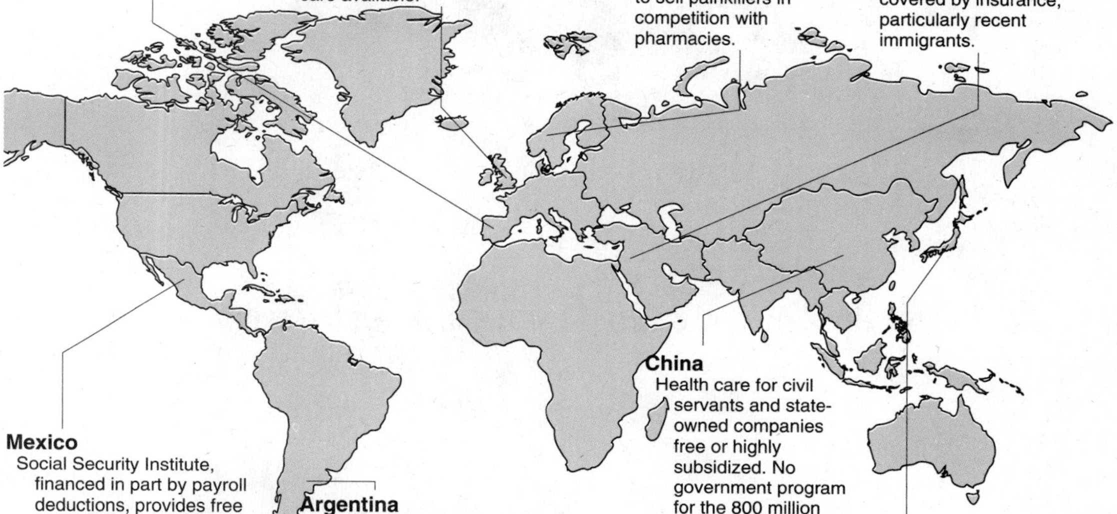

Mexico
Social Security Institute, financed in part by payroll deductions, provides free medical and hospital care, ambulances, and medicines to all employed people. No provision for unemployed. Complaints about quality of care are common. Those who can afford it use private doctors and hospitals.

Argentina
Two public systems, one government, the other run by trade unions. Government system includes hospitals run by municipalities and largely financed by proceeds from government gambling operations. As of March 1, 1993, Argentina ended a union monopoly on providing health care for members, giving workers a choice.

China
Health care for civil servants and state-owned companies free or highly subsidized. No government program for the 800 million peasants, who pay themselves or buy insurance. Several experiments under way, modeled after insurance programs in South Korea, Hong Kong, and United States.

Japan
Cheap, equal medical care and insurance for everyone. Average payroll tax of 8.2%, with some paying only 3%, depending on insurance plan.

Public Money

Seventeen OECD countries put more money into health care than the United States, where 57.6% of expenditures come from insurance and other private sources. Public-sector share of health spending:

United States	42.4%	Greece	76.0	Norway	95.7
Australia	69.5	Iceland	86.9	Portugal	61.7
Austria	66.5	Ireland	73.8	Spain	78.4
Belgium	82.5	Italy	75.9	Sweden	89.5
Canada	74.1	Japan	71.9	Switzerland	68.1
Finland	78.8	Luxembourg	91.4	Turkey	35.6
France	74.2	Netherlands	72.6	United Kingdom	84.5
Denmark	82.8	New Zealand	81.7	OECD	74.5
Germany	73.2				

FIGURE 14.12

Health care around the world: A look at a variety of health care systems.

From: "Health Care Around the World," Muncie (Ind.) Star, Feb. 14, 1993.

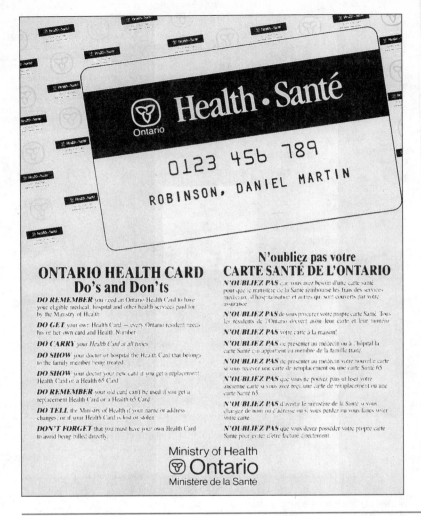

FIGURE 14.13
The United States health care system has often been compared to the Canadian universal health care system.

today's figures being slightly over 10% of the Canadian GNP and now over 14% in the United States.[2]

The fourth strength of the Canadian system is the emphasis it places on prevention and primary care. The U.S. health care system has a wealth of high-technology equipment and specialized physicians but falls short in the areas of prevention and primary care. Roughly 40% of children aged 1 to 4 lack basic immunizations for childhood infectious diseases. One result of this failure to provide adequate disease prevention measures was the measles epidemic of

1984, when 18,000 cases of measles were reported in the United States. About 20% of white mothers and 40% of black mothers do not receive prenatal care in the first trimester of pregnancy.[27] (Refer to Chapter 8.)

The Canadian system is not without its disadvantages.[28] The major complaint with the system has been the rationing of certain types of care requiring high-technology equipment and specialized physicians. The Canadian system does not limit care for life-threatening conditions but does have a tight supply for things such as cardiac bypass surgery, lens implants, and the use of magnetic resonance imaging (MRI). This tight supply has created waiting lists for certain types of care in some provinces. Those critical of the Canadian system argue that the availability of innovative technologies conflicts with the quality-of-care concerns.[15] Those Canadians who can afford it have gotten around this limitation by coming to the United States to get needed care.

Even with the many benefits of the Canadian system, the likelihood of a Canadian-type system in the United States is very small. The political and economic barriers are too great. Politically, there are too many people who benefit from not having such a program. Economically it has been estimated the implementation of a Canadian-type system in the United States would require $250 billion in new taxes.[29] In addition, because of the size of the country, it would be difficult for the national government to be sensitive to regional and local differences and needs. As has been the case with Medicare, it is difficult to provide consistent and equitable administration of the program when the national government delegates authority to state or local agents.[1]

The Oregon Health Plan

Because of the slow pace at which the federal government is approaching health care reform, several states including Florida, Hawaii, Minnesota, Oregon, and Vermont, have passed major health care reform packages aimed at providing increased access to health insurance and basic health services to all or most of their residents. Of all of these reform movements, the one that attracted the most publicity was the one in the state of Oregon.

While the Canadian plan addresses access first and cost second, the Oregon plan addresses the problem of cost primarily, with the expected result of greater access. In short, the state of Oregon has revised its Medicaid coverage. Oregon, like all other states, has a finite number of dollars to spend on health care and a significant number of people who lack access because of no health insurance. Unlike other states, Oregon has attempted to come to grips with the question of whether to spend $250,000 dollars to try to save a prematurely born infant with little hope of a normal life or to spend the same amount to provide maternal and child health services for 400 families.

In 1989, three state laws were passed in Oregon to put in place a plan that would allow every Oregonian to be covered by third-party health insurance. More specifically, the plan reforms Medicaid, creates incentives for employers to provide health insurance for their employees, and creates a high-risk insurance pool coordinated by state government. The cornerstone of the plan is the idea that benefit packages should be built on a list of health care services priorities. The entire list comprises 709 line items. Each line consists of a health condition and its associated treatment. The list was created and prioritized by a state commission after 18 months of statewide hearings and community meetings featuring public input and expert testimony and a random-sample survey. The list is subdivided into 17 categories (priorities). Category 1

Categories of Services Used in the Prioritization Process and Examples of Condition-Treatment (CT) Pairs

Category	Description
"Essential" services	
1. Acute fatal	Treatment prevents death with full recovery. Example: appendectomy for appendicitis.
2. Maternity care	Maternity and most newborn care. Example: obstetrical care for pregnancy.
3. Acute fatal	Treatment prevents death without full recovery. Example: Medical therapy for acute bacterial meningitis.
4. Preventive care for children	Example: Immunizations.
5. Chronic fatal	Treatment improves life span and quality of life. Example: Medical therapy for asthma.
6. Reproductive services	Excludes maternity/infertility services. Example: Contraceptive management.
7. Comfort care	Palliative therapy for conditions in which death is imminent. Example: Hospice care.
8. Preventive dental care	Adults and children. Example: Cleaning and fluoride applications.
9. Proven effective preventive care for adults	Example: Mammograms.
"Very important" services	
10. Acute nonfatal	Treatment causes return to previous health state. Example: Medical therapy for vaginitis.
11. Chronic nonfatal	One-time treatment improves quality of life. Example: Hip replacement.
12. Acute nonfatal	Treatment without return to previous health state. Example: Arthroscopic repair of internal knee derangement.
13. Chronic nonfatal	Repetitive treatment improves quality of life. Example: Medical therapy for chronic sinusitis.
Services that are "valuable to certain individuals"	
14. Acute nonfatal	Treatment expedites recovery of self-limiting conditions. Example: Medical therapy for diaper rash.
15. Infertility services	Example: In-vitro fertilization.
16. Less effective preventive care for adults	Example: Screening of nonpregnant adults for diabetes.
17. Fatal or nonfatal	Treatment causes minimal or no improvement in quality of life. Example: Medical therapy for viral warts.

Source: Oregon waiver application, Aug. 1991.

From: Congress of the United States, Office of Technology Assessment (May 1992). *Summary: Evaluation of the Oregon Medicaid Proposal* (pub. no. OTA-H-532). Washington, D.C.: U.S. Government Printing Office, p. 6.

has the highest priority. Categories 1–9 are considered essential components, 10–13 very important, and 14–17 valuable to individuals but not certain to improve the health status of the population. It should be noted that the categories are not absolutely discrete. Some items conceptually belong in one category but have special characteristics that led the commission to place them in another (see Box 14.4).

With the list in place, the state legislature then had to determine how many of the 709 services it could fund with the finite dollars available. They determined that there were enough state dollars available to fund items 1–587. Items 588–709, or 121 services, would not be funded by state money. By funding through line 587, the state of Oregon was able to fund 98% of categories 1–9, 82% of categories 10–13, and 7% of categories 14–17.

Those who oppose this process do so primarily because they say it rations health care: A person who needs a health service below item 587 on the list will not get it without being able to pay for it himself or herself. Thus, the plan rations care, as even the plan's developers will agree. However, the plan's proponents say that the previous system rationed care based on ability to pay; at least now it is rationed through a policy developed with input from those who are to pay for and receive the care—the citizens of the state.

The final step in the approval process for the Oregon plan had to come in the form of a waiver from the federal Health Care Financing Administration. Since Medicaid is a jointly funded federal-state program, approval has to be given by HCFA to those states who in changing their program take away services once offered to Medicaid recipients. Obviously, some of the 121 services and procedures that are no longer to be offered are cur-

rently available to those on Medicaid. Thus the need for the waiver.

The waiver was not easily obtained. The state of Oregon applied for the waiver in August 1991. The primary complaint from those in Washington, D.C., was that those most affected by the process, the poor women and children on Medicaid, were underrepresented at the public hearings, and that the wealthy consumers and health care providers were overrepresented. Therefore, the prioritized list really did not represent the true wish of the people. A second concern of those in Washington was that the cutoff point on the list in 1992 was Number 587, but in future years, it might be 560, 500, or 450 because of the possibility of fewer dollars to pay for the plan. At what point will the cutoff point stop descending down the list?

The waiver was finally approved in spring 1993. Only time will tell if the plan will provide the benefits its creators proposed. Many hope that it will, but even if it does not, at least the process created many new ideas and much debate. Best of all, the process showed that there are alternatives to the present system and that legislators can create a useful policy if they put their minds to it.

CHAPTER SUMMARY

In this chapter, we have provided an overview of how health care is financed in America. We have also discussed access to the health care system in the United States and some of the barriers to access: no health insurance, inadequate insurance, and poverty. We explained the concept of insurance and discussed private health insurance, including such pertinent terms as *deductible, coinsurance, fixed indemnity, exclusion,* and *preexisting condition.* We also described and explained health insurance plans like Medicare, Medicaid, and medigap programs as well as other supplemental insurance programs including long-term care insurance.

We presented alternatives to our traditional method of health care delivery, including some currently available programs such as HMOs, PPOs, and EPOs. We described alternatives to full-service hospitals and outlined the yet-to-be-implemented American Health Security Act of 1993. Lastly, we discussed the Canadian health care program and the new Oregon health care plan.

SCENARIO: ANALYSIS AND RESPONSE

1. Reread the scenario. In your opinion, did the father make the right decision in taking his son to the emergency room? Why or why not?

2. What other actions could the father have taken? What would you have done?

3. What impact do you think a zero deductible health insurance policy has on the health care system? What do you see as the advantages and disadvantages of such a policy? Explain your answer.

4. Do you think all people in the United States should have zero deductible health insurance? Why or why not?

5. If we had national health insurance, how would this scenario differ?

6. Under the Oregon Plan, as you understand it, how would this scenario differ?

REVIEW QUESTIONS

1. What is meant by *fee-for-service?* What are the alternatives to it?

2. Upon what basic concept is insurance based?

3. What is meant by the following insurance policy provisions:
   a. $200 deductible.
   b. 20/80 coinsurance.
   c. $4,500 fixed indemnity for a basic surgical procedure.
   d. An exclusion of the preexisting condition of lung cancer.

4. What is the difference between Medicare and Medicaid? What relationship does medigap insurance have to Medicare and Medicaid?

5. In what ways is the American health care system better than the Canadian system? In what ways is the Canadian system better than that of the United States?

6. Distinguish between the four different models of HMOs: staff, group, network, and IPA.

7. Briefly explain the differences among HMOs, PPOs, and EPOs.

8. Why might a company want to enter into an agreement with a preferred provider organization?

9. What are the advantages of ambulatory care centers?

10. Why was the Oregon health care plan considered so innovative?

ACTIVITIES

1. Obtain a copy of the student health insurance policy available at your school. After reading the policy, summarize in writing what you have read. In your summary, provide the premium costs and list specifics about the deductible, coinsurance, fixed indemnity, and any exclusions.

2. Contact the office in your community that handles the Medicaid insurance program. Find out who is qualified for coverage in your state and the process one must go through to get registered for such coverage.

3. Visit an HMO in your area and find the answers to the following: (a) What type of HMO is it? (b) How does one enroll? (c) What does it cost? (d) What services are provided? and (e) Why should someone get his or her health care from an HMO instead of the more traditional private-practice physician?

4. Write a two-page position paper on one of the following topics:

   The United States federal government should provide national health insurance.

   The United States federal government should not provide national health insurance.

   Health care is a right.

   Health care is a privilege.

REFERENCES

1. Butler, P. A. (1988). *Too Poor to Be Sick: Access to Medical Care for the Uninsured.* Washington, D.C.: American Public Health Association.

2. U.S. Dept. of Health and Human Services (1993). *Health United States 1992 and Healthy People 2000 Review* (DHHS pub. no. PHS-93-1232). Washington, D.C.: U.S. Government Printing Office.

3. No author (1992). "Health Insurance Relationship Allows Employees to Share Risks, Benefits." *Campus Update* 13(3):3. Muncie, Ind.: Ball State Univ.

4. Cornelius, L., K. Beauregard, and J. Cohen (1992). "Usual Sources of Medical Care and Their Characteristics, Government Handling of Health Insurance Would Worsen Crisis." *Campus Update* 12(22). Muncie, Ind.: Ball State Univ.

5. Ries, P. (1991). "Characteristics of Persons With and Without Health Care Coverage: United States, 1989." *Advance Data from Vital and Health Statistics,* no. 201. Hyattsville, Md.: National Center for Health Statistics, Centers for Disease Control.

6. The White House Domestic Policy Council (1993). *The President's Health Security Plan: The Clinton Blueprint.* New York: Times Books.

7. No author (Sept. 1992). "The crisis in health insurance: Part II." *Consumer Reports,* pp. 608–617.

8. U.S. Dept. of Health and Human Services (1993). *1993 Guide To Health Insurance for People with Medicare.* (pub. no. HCFA-02110). Washington, D.C.: U.S. Government Printing Office.

9. U.S. Dept. of Health and Human Services (1992). *Social Security Administration: Personal Earnings and Benefits Estimate Statement.* Washington, D.C.: U.S. Government Printing Office.

10. U.S. Dept. of Health and Human Services (1989). *Your Hospital Stay Under Medicare's Prospective Payment System* (pub. no. HCFA 02163). Washington, D.C.: U.S. Government Printing Office, p.2.

11. Office of National Cost Estimates (1990). "National Health Expenditures, 1988." *Health Care Financing Review* 11(4): 1–41.

12. The State Teachers Retirement System of Ohio (1992). *Long-Term Care Insurance Through the ORS-LTC Plan.* Columbus: Author.

13. Kemper, P., B. C. Spillman, and C. M. Murtaugh (1991). "A Lifetime Perspective on Proposals for Financing Nursing Home Care." *Inquiry* 28 (Winter): 333–344.

14. Weissert, W. G. (Spring/Summer 1991). "Choose Long-Term Care Insurance with Caution." *Findings* 6(2): 18. Ann Arbor: School of Public Health, Univ. of Michigan.

15. U.S. General Accounting Office (1991). *Canadian Health Insurance: Lessons for the United States* (pub. no. GAO/HRD-91-90). Washington, D.C.: Author.

16. Phelps, C. E. (1992). *Health Economics.* New York: HarperCollins.

17. Brown, L. D. (1985). "The Managerial Imperative and Organizational Innovation." In E. Ginzberg, ed. *The U.S. Health Care System: A Look to the 1990s,* pp. 28–47. Totowa, N.J.: Rowman & Allanheld.

18. U.S. Dept. of Health and Human Services (1991). "What Future Do HMOs Face?" *Research Activities: Agency for Health Care Policy and Research,* no. 145 (pub. no. AHCPR 91-0048). Rockville, M.D.: Agency for Health Care Policy and Research.

19. Christianson, J. B., S. M. Sanchez, D. R. Wholey, and B. A. Shadle (1991). "The HMO Industry: Evolution in Population Demographics and Market Structures." *Medical Care Review* 48(1): 3–46.

20. Ginzberg, E. (1990). *The Medical Triangle: Physicians, Politicians, and the Public.* Cambridge, Mass.: Howard Univ. Press.

21. American Managed Care and Review Assocns., as printed in the American Public Health Assn. (Sept. 1993). "Definitions of Health Care Terminology." *Section Letter—Alcohol, Tobacco, and Other Drugs.* Washington, D.C.: Author.

22. American Public Health Assn. (Sept. 1993). "Definitions of Health Care Terminology." *Section letter—Alcohol, Tobacco, and Other Drugs.* Washington, D.C.: Author.

23. Congress of the United States, Congressional Budget Office (May 1993). *Managed Competition and its Potential to Reduce Health Spending.* Washington, D.C.: U.S. Government Printing Office.

24. Fuchs, B. C., and J. Skolovsky (1990). *CRS Report for Congress: The Canadian Health Care System.* Washington, D.C.: Congressional Research Service, Library of Congress.

25. Holahan, J., M. Moon, W. P. Welch, and S. Zuckerman (1991). "An American Approach to Health System Reform." *Journal of the American Medical Association* 265(19): 2537–2540.

26. Evans, R. G., J. Lomas, M. L. Barer, et al. (1989). "Controlling Health Expenditures—the Canadian Reality." *New England Journal of Medicine* 320: 571–577.

27. Enthoven, A. C. (1992). "A Cure for Health Costs." *World Monitor* 5(4): 34–39.

28. Rachlis, M., and C. Kusher (1989). *Second Opinion: What's Wrong with Canada's Health Care System and How to Fix It.* Toronto: HarperCollins.

29. The Pepper Commission—U.S. Bipartisan Commission on Comprehensive Health Care (Sept. 1990). *A Call for Action: Final Report.* Washington, D.C.: U.S. Government Printing Office.

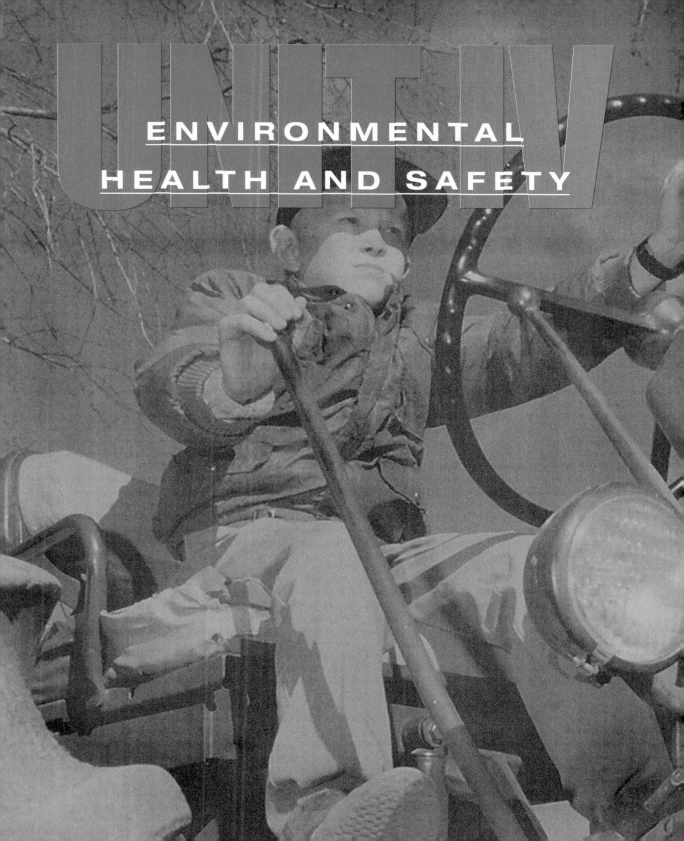

UNIT IV

ENVIRONMENTAL HEALTH AND SAFETY

Chapter 15

ENVIRONMENTAL CONCERNS:
WASTES AND POLLUTION

Chapter Outline

SCENARIO

INTRODUCTION

THE ENVIRONMENTAL SYSTEM
Life Support Systems
Human Activities
Residues and Wastes
Environmental Hazards

WASTES AND POLLUTION

SOLID WASTE
Sources of Solid Waste
Solid Waste Management

HAZARDOUS WASTE
Hazardous Waste Defined
Hazardous Waste Management
Hazardous Waste Cleanup

AIR POLLUTION
Contaminants of Outdoor Air
The Pollutant Standard Index
Special Concerns with Outdoor Air
Protection of Outdoor Air Through
Regulation
Indoor Air

WATER AND ITS POLLUTION
Sources of Water
Treatment of Water for Domestic
Use
Sources of Water Pollution
Types of Water Pollutants
Water-Related Issues
Strategies to Insure Safe Water

RADIATION
Sources of Radiation

The Danger of Radiation
Policy Related to Nuclear Waste
Disposal

NOISE POLLUTION
What Is Noise and How Is It
Measured?
Approaches to Noise Abatement

CHAPTER SUMMARY

REVIEW QUESTIONS

SCENARIO: ANALYSIS AND
RESPONSE

ACTIVITIES

REFERENCES

Chapter Objectives

After studying this chapter you will be able to:

1. List the four major components of Purdom's environmental system and explain the contribution of each.
2. Identify four major reasons why we are facing more environmental problems today than ever before.
3. Name the primary sources of solid waste.
4. List and briefly explain the four methods of dealing with solid waste.
5. Define *hazardous waste*.
6. Explain the difference between sanitary and secured landfills.
7. Identify six ways to deal with hazardous wastes.
8. Explain what is meant by the term *Superfund*.
9. Explain the Pollutant Standard Index (PSI).
10. Briefly describe acid rain, ozone layer, global warming, and photochemical smog.
11. Identify the major indoor air pollutants.
12. Explain the difference in point source and nonpoint source pollution.
13. Identify the three categories of water pollution.
14. Briefly describe waste water treatment.
15. List means of conserving water.
16. Name the primary sources of radiation.
17. Explain how nuclear wastes are handled in the United States.
18. Identify the two basic characteristics of sound.
19. Identify steps to deal with noise pollution.

Tom and Mary recently accepted jobs as teachers in the Blackford School Corporation. When they moved to the Blackford community, they purchased a modest home on five acres of land outside the city. They had only been living in their new home two months when they noticed that their water was beginning to taste "different." The source of their water was a well on their own property. A testing of the water by the local health department sanitarian revealed that their water was contaminated with lead and perhaps other chemicals. The sanitarian recommended that Tom and Mary drink bottled water until the well water could be tested further. After some investigation, county officials determined that Mary and Tom's 15-year-old home had been built close to a former landfill that had been closed about 20 years earlier. Tom and Mary were now faced with an expensive, unforeseen, and long-term problem, not to mention the devaluation of their property.

INTRODUCTION

As human beings, we are a part of the environment in which we live. Our lives and health are affected by the quality of our environment, and the way we live our lives influences the quality of the environment. This chapter explains in detail and illustrates with examples the ways in which human interactions with the environment have direct consequences for the quality of life. While this chapter seeks to describe and define wastes and pollution, Chapter 16 examines the specific health consequences of these environmental hazards.

THE ENVIRONMENTAL SYSTEM

In order to fully understand the environmental concerns that threaten the health of a community, one must understand how humans interact with their environment. The study of these interactions is referred to as **ecology.** One scientist, P. W. Purdom, has provided a useful model of these interactions, which he calls the **environmental system**[1] (see Figure 15.1). Purdom's system has four major components: life support systems, human activities, residues and wastes, and environmental hazards. The interaction of these four components creates either a healthy or an unhealthy environment, which in turn impacts the health of individuals and the greater community (see Figure 15.2).

Life Support Systems

Life support systems include those elements in the environment that provide the basis for life. These include energy, geophysical systems, the biological system, those items that humans have built, and the social interactions of people.

Energy, an essential element of the life support system, exists in two forms: nutri-

---

ecology Interrelationship of organisms and their environments.

life support systems Those elements in the environment that provide the basis for life.

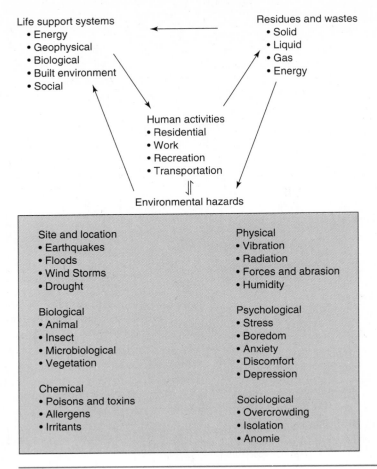

Life support systems
• Energy
• Geophysical
• Biological
• Built environment
• Social

Residues and wastes
• Solid
• Liquid
• Gas
• Energy

Human activities
• Residential
• Work
• Recreation
• Transportation

Environmental hazards

Site and location
• Earthquakes
• Floods
• Wind Storms
• Drought

Biological
• Animal
• Insect
• Microbiological
• Vegetation

Chemical
• Poisons and toxins
• Allergens
• Irritants

Physical
• Vibration
• Radiation
• Forces and abrasion
• Humidity

Psychological
• Stress
• Boredom
• Anxiety
• Discomfort
• Depression

Sociological
• Overcrowding
• Isolation
• Anomie

FIGURE 15.1

The environmental system.

From: Purdom, P.W. (1980). "Environment and Health." In P.W. Purdom, ed. Environmental Health, *2nd ed. San Diego: Academic Press, p. 8.*

tive and nonnutritive. **Nutritive energy** is food, for which the need is obvious. While the majority of Americans enjoy adequate nutrition, some do not. Whether or not there is enough nutritive energy to support the world's population is arguable, but there is no doubt that it is maldistributed. **Nonnutritive energy** includes energy sources that provide our shelter, fiber, heat, and transportation; these include oil, electricity, gas, solar power, etc. This type of energy is needed to carry out much of our daily work.

The **geophysical system** comprises the earth itself, its water, and its atmosphere. The importance of an optimally balanced at-

---

nonnutritive energy Energy sources that provide shelter, fiber, heat, and transportation.

geophysical system Comprises the earth, its water, and its atmosphere.

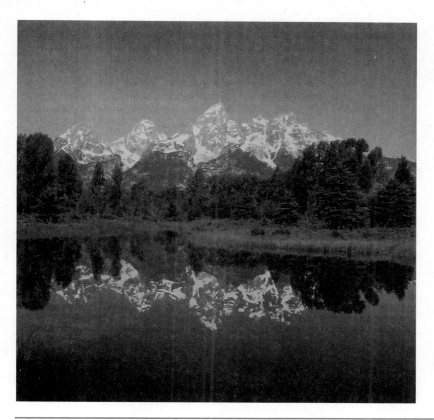

FIGURE 15.2

A healthy environment supports a healthy community.

mosphere with regard to oxygen and nitrogen cannot be overemphasized. Atmospheric changes could alter the earth's temperature, reduce nutritive energy production (by plants), and threaten the planet's ability to sustain life. Inadequate quantities of clean water could also limit life.

The **biological system** contributes to life support as well. Here, the key element is diversity, because a diverse **biosphere** is more stable than one with fewer species. The nutritive and nonnutritive energy re-

quirements of one type of living organism are often the residues and wastes of other organisms. For example, the carbon dioxide expelled by human beings via exhalation is required by plants for photosynthesis, a nutrient-building process that provides oxygen to the atmosphere.

The **built environment** (versus the natural environment) is also important in supporting life. Examples of the built environment include human dwellings, industrial plants and factories, water and sewage

biological system All living organisms and their interactions.

biosphere Sum total of all life forms on earth.

built environment Portion of the environment built by human beings.

systems, communication networks, and transportation systems.

Social interaction between members of the human community also sustains life. Few humans could survive without the support of others. All people have shortcomings and something to offer in exchange (e.g., goods, services, psychological support, etc.) with others. It is through the social support system that civilization has advanced to its present complexity.

Human Activities

Human activities include the building of homes and other shelters, manufacturing clothing, acquiring food, traveling and relocating, recreating, washing and cleaning. These activities and the environmental elements reciprocally impact each other. For example, the weather dictates the work schedules of some people and the recreation activities of many. In turn, one of the most important human activities and one that impacts heavily on the rest of the environment is the extraction, conversion, and expenditure of energy—particularly fossil fuels such as oil and coal but also nuclear fuels such as uranium. In this regard, humans are unlike any other part of their environment, and it is these activities that threaten the balance of the environmental system.

Residues and Wastes

As people participate in their daily activities, they continually produce **residues and wastes.** These products occur as solids, liquids, gases, and energy. A typical day for a person in the United States might gener-

ate the following list of residue and waste products:

1. Human body wastes: urine and feces.
2. Excess materials and foods: trash and garbage.
3. Vegetation wastes: grass clippings and tree branches.
4. Construction and manufacturing wastes: scrap wood and metal, contaminated water, solvents, and excess heat and noise.
5. Transportation wastes: carbon monoxide, nitrous oxides, hydrocarbons, other gaseous pollutants, and used motor oil.
6. Energy production wastes: mining wastes, electrical power (combustion of coal), nuclear power (radioactive) wastes, and weapons production (radioactive) wastes.

As noted in Figure 15.1, the residues and wastes created by human activity can affect life support systems positively, by creating products needed to sustain life, or negatively, by creating environmental hazards that threaten life. If one assumes that living things are optimally adapted to an environment that has been stable for thousands of years, it seems logical to suspect that substantial changes to the earth's environment resulting from human activities are more likely to have an overall negative effect than a positive one on life.

Environmental Hazards

The fourth component of the environmental system is environmental hazards. **Environmental hazards** result from natural phenomena as well as human activities. Environmental hazards impact the life

---

human activities Includes all actions performed by human beings.
residues and wastes Unwanted by-products of human activities.

environmental hazards Conditions that threaten the well-being of the environment.

support systems, and hence, human well-being. The attention given to the environment in recent years has been focused on controlling environmental hazards.

Purdom classifies environmental hazards into six groups: site and location, biological, chemical, physical, psychological, and sociological.[1] Site and location hazards, or natural hazards,[2] include such events as avalanches, droughts, earthquakes, floods, hurricanes, lightning, tornados, volcanos, and the like. Site and location hazards usually impact only those in the immediate area and often are unpredictable. Sometimes, however, these events are cyclical or repetitive, allowing communities to prepare in advance. In these cases, their impact on health is directly related to the preparation of the communities. For example, the annual flooding of a river is expected and planned for in some communities. Likewise, Hawaiians are less surprised than visitors when the Mt. Kilauea volcano erupts.

Biological hazards are threats to society that result from disease-producing agents. Examples include malaria, plague, and AIDS. Biological hazards and their resulting epidemics were the topic of Chapter 4 and will not be discussed here.

Chemicals are nonbiological substances that can adversely affect the environment, and hence, human health. Whether chemicals are considered chemical hazards depends upon their toxicity, concentration, and the duration of human exposure.[1] Chemical hazards occur in three physical states: gases, liquids, and solids. They can enter the body several ways: absorption, ingestion, and inhalation.

Physical hazards are extremes in conditions of the physical environment. They include things such as natural and industrial radiation, extremes in air temperature and humidity, unsafe design or usage of tools and equipment, and mechanical noise and vibration.

Psychological hazards affect people's outlook on life. Psychological hazards are just as real and damaging to health as physical hazards. Boredom, stress, fear, and depression represent psychological hazards that consume significant health care dollars of communities. A workplace can be most unproductive if the workers are highly stressed, bored, or depressed. The fear of losing a job and other economic factors can also weigh heavily on members of a community. Entire communities may have problems if their young people are bored and frustrated.

The final classification of environmental hazards is that of sociological hazards. Sociological hazards occur when societies interact in destructive ways or fail to interact in productive ways. Overcrowding and war are sociological hazards (see Figure 15.3). Some would say Adolph Hitler, the German dictator, was a sociological hazard before and during World War II; others might nominate Saddam Hussein, the leader of Iraq, or late drug kingpin Pablo Escobar.

The four components of the environmental system—life support systems, human activities, residues and wastes, and environmental hazards—are interrelated. No single component can be changed without affecting the other three components, thus, in dealing with environmental issues, the environmental system must be dealt with as a whole.

During the American presidential campaign of 1992, Americans were asked to consider various environmental issues at local, national, and international levels:

1. The inability to locate and open new landfills in the face of a growing waste disposal problem. (Citizen concern has been referred to as the NIMBY syndrome, "Not in my back yard!")

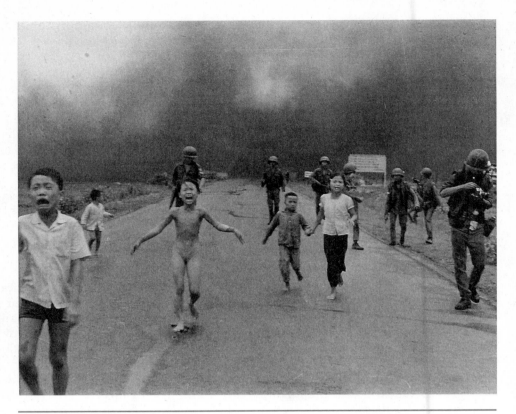

FIGURE 15.3
War is one of the most feared sociological hazards.

2. The need to convert communities from a cheaper short-term solution of solid-wastes disposal in landfills to more expensive long-term solutions of source reduction, recycling, composting, and incineration.

3. The limiting of harvesting of trees to save the spotted owl population in the northwestern United States.

4. The implementation of high-tech solutions to environmental problems which would put a great strain on outdated U.S. factories and an uneducated work force but could create new jobs and a stronger economy in the future.

5. The implementation of worldwide carbon dioxide emission controls was a topic for debate at the United Nations Conference on Environment and Development (better known as Earth Summit '92 in Rio de Janeiro, Brazil) to curb global warming. (The United States argued that such control would negatively impact industry and the economy.)

Lasting solutions to environmental problems will become evident only when special-interest groups both understand and work toward decisions that take into account the balance of the entire environmental system. While it is unrealistic to believe humans can have a pollution-free environment, pollution cannot be allowed to occur unchecked. As the dominant species on this planet, our very survival depends upon our recognition of the deleterious effects our activities have on the other components of the environmental system and our taking responsibility for minimizing these effects.

WASTES AND POLLUTION

If the environmental system is to stay in balance, the frequency and severity of environmental hazards must be reduced. Unfortunately, in recent years, this has not been the case. One example is society's inability to control the generation and proper disposal of residues and wastes. While it may be within society's technical capabilities to solve this problem, this has yet to occur. One reason may be the difficulty of changing attitudes and altering behaviors. Attitudes that prevent implementation of solutions are summed up in the following statements: "I don't need to worry about the water, I have city water not a well," "Why should I worry about acid rain? I don't burn coal," "Car pools are too inconvenient," "The solution to pollution is dilution," and "One soft drink can won't destroy the environment; besides, littering creates jobs for others."

Several factors have contributed to an increasing number of environmental hazards: (1) urbanization, (2) industrialization, (3) population growth, and (4) the production and use of disposable products and containers. **Urbanization,** the process in which people come together to live in cities, often results in people living in overcrowded conditions without ade-

quate space for the disposal of wastes; urbanization has made waste management more difficult. Concomitant industrialization, resulting in the generation of new types of wastes, has complicated the waste disposal problem; one example is nuclear waste.

Overall population growth has also contributed to the overall waste disposal problem, as has the reliance on disposable containers. Not only are there more people than there were 30 years ago, but the amount of refuse generated by each person in the 1990s is much greater than it was in the 1960s, when reusable containers and products began to fall into disfavor and to be replaced by more convenient but less environmentally sound throwaway containers (see Table 15.1).

SOLID WASTE

Household trash, grass clippings, tree trimmings, manure, excess stone generated from mining, and steel scraps from automobile

---

urbanization The process by which people come together to live in cities.

Table 15.1
Reusable Versus Throwaway Consumer Goods

Reusable Goods	Throwaway Goods
Milk bottles	Cardboard cartons and plastic jugs
Returnable soft drink bottles	Aluminum cans and plastic bottles
Cloth diapers	Disposable diapers
Garbage cans	Trash bags
Lunch boxes	Paper bags
Cloth napkins	Paper napkins
Refillable pens	Disposable pens
Handkerchiefs	Facial tissues
Cloth towels or rags	Paper towels
Ceramic or plastic dishes	Paper plates

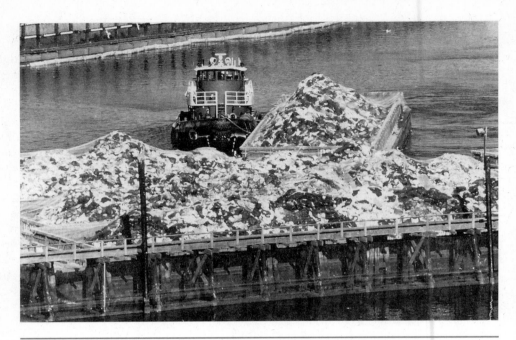

FIGURE 15.4

Solid waste is becoming such a problem in some areas that it is shipped elsewhere.

plants are all examples of **solid waste.** Solid waste is a part of modern life, just as it was in antiquity.

Archaeologists and anthropologists have gleaned much about previous cultures and societies from the bits of solid waste that they left behind. Today we are generating solid wastes in record quantities. In the last 30 years, the daily solid waste production per person in the United States jumped from just over 2.5 pounds to almost 4 pounds.

Today, we are generating waste faster than we can dispose of it in an environmentally sound way (see Figure 15.4). Take for example the 1987 Islip, New York,

solid waste Solid refuse from households, agriculture, and businesses.

garbage problem. In March of that year, 3,186 tons of refuse was turned away from the Islip landfill because of insufficient space. The refuse was then loaded onto a barge to be transported to another state for disposal. The barge traveled to six states and then to three other countries trying to unload the unwanted trash, only to be turned down by each. After sailing for five months and over 6,000 miles, the barge returned to New York, where its overripe cargo was burned in a Brooklyn incinerator. A similar incident occurred during the summer of 1992, when a trainload of garbage left New York City for a landfill in Illinois. The garbage could not be disposed of in Illinois because the contract had expired between the haulers and those who were supposed to unload it. The trash train tried to unload at other landfills in Missouri, Kansas, and Illinois, but was turned away by court orders. It returned to New York 26 days later, where the garbage was unloaded and buried in a landfill on Staten Island. In both of these examples, the cost of labor and transportation was extensive.

Sources of Solid Waste

Most solid waste can be traced to four major sources: agriculture, mining, industry, and municipalities (domestic sources). By far, agriculture generates the greatest volume of solid waste. Examples of agricultural wastes include crop residues, manures, and other vegetation trimmings. Most solid waste generated by farming will decompose, enriching the soil, or it can be fed to animals or otherwise used as energy. Farms have long been known for recycling their own nonhuman solid waste.

Unlike agricultural waste, mining waste does not decompose in any reasonable period of time, nor can it be reused in any other manner. As the extraction of the earth's natural resources intensifies, mining wastes will constitute even greater problems.

The solid waste resulting from industrial production is quite varied, each industry producing a different type of waste. Examples include paper, wood chips, and highly complex chemicals. Certain industrial waste products are especially hazardous because of their toxicity, corrosiveness, or flammability.

The last source of solid waste is household or municipal waste. According to Environmental Protection Agency (EPA) statistics, only about 5% of all solid waste each year is generated by individual households, businesses, and institutions located within municipalities. This waste is known as **municipal waste.** Agricultural and mining wastes make up about 91% of the total solid wastes while industry contributes about 4%.[3] (See Figure 15.5.) While it makes up only 5% of the total volume, municipal solid waste receives considerable attention because it is visible, malodorous, and considered a threat to human health if not disposed of properly.

The heterogeneous makeup of municipal solid waste precludes efficient disposal. There are seven major categories: paper, yard waste, rubber, textiles and wood, metal, glass, plastic, and food wastes (see Figure 15.6). Thirty to forty years ago, food wastes were the primary component in municipal solid waste, but garbage disposals in homes and the preprocessing of foods have reduced that greatly. Today, paper and paper products make up 39% of the total. Much of it is packaging.[4]

Solid Waste Management

Though the preponderance of solid waste is created by agriculture and mining, the following discussion of solid waste management is aimed primarily at municipal and industrial wastes, which create greater problems in the environmental system.

In 1976, Congress passed the first comprehensive law to address the collection and disposal of wastes. This law, known as the

---

Environmental Protection Agency (EPA) The federal agency primarily responsible for setting, maintaining, and enforcing environmental standards.

municipal waste Waste generated by individual households, businesses, and institutions located within municipalities.

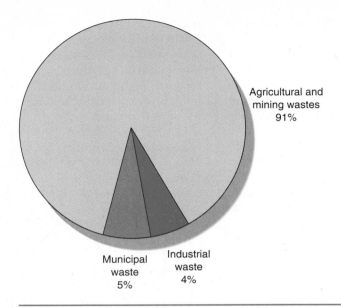

FIGURE 15.5

Sources of solid waste.

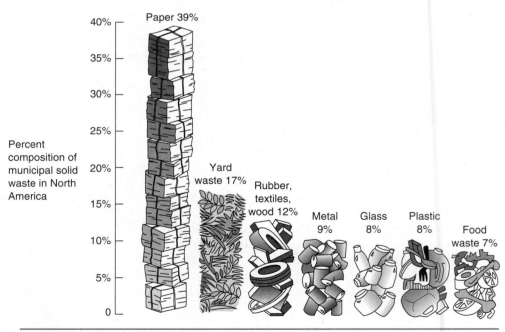

FIGURE 15.6

Types and percentages of municipal solid waste.

From: Enger, E. D., and B. F. Smith (1991). Environmental Science: A Study of Interrelationships, *4th ed. Dubuque, Ia.: Wm. C. Brown, p. 431.*

Resource Conservation and Recovery Act of 1976 (RCRA, pronounced Rick-Rah) and its 1984 amendments, provide for "cradle-to-grave" regulation of solid and hazardous wastes. However, many environmentalists feel that even these laws do not adequately protect the environment. While RCRA was due to be reauthorized in 1988 with certain amendments, this did not occur because of "congressional gridlock." Environmentalists want more restrictions to protect our natural resources while economists feel such restrictions will not allow the economy to grow. As of this writing, the future of RCRA remains uncertain.

Collection

The handling of municipal solid waste can be divided into two steps: collection and disposal. Approximately 80% of the money spent on waste management is spent on the collection process. Faced with ever-increasing amounts of waste, greater efficiency is needed in collecting the wastes so that more money can be spent on environmentally sound disposal. Traditionally, municipal wastes have been collected at the curb or alley by crews of three people and a large truck. However, experience has shown that crew size, truck size, and special-feature trucks, like those that can be operated by a single person or those with different storage compartments for separating the trash, can improve efficiency and reduce cost (see Figure 15.7). Moreover, the collecting and transporting of trash through pipelines hydraulically and/or pneumatically (the method used at Disney World) can make collection even more efficient.

Disposal

Currently, most municipalities dispose of their wastes in **sanitary landfills,** sites judged suitable for inground disposal of

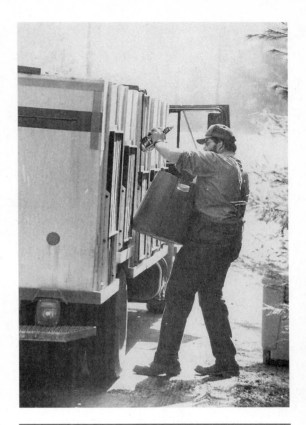

FIGURE 15.7

Household waste picked up at the curbside with a segregated container, recycling truck.

solid waste. However, many of these municipal landfills are filling up, and the availability of land suitable for new landfill sites near cities is quickly disappearing. Disposal of municipal solid waste on unsuitable land can result in the contamination of groundwater (water found in the ground), which may be the community's only source of drinking water. To meet the need for better management of solid waste, the EPA is suggesting that each community adopt an **integrated waste management approach.**

---

integrated waste management approach An approach to disposing of solid waste that includes sanitary landfills, incineration, recycling, and source reduction.

This approach combines the following four methods in a way best suited to local needs and capabilities: (1) sanitary landfills, (2) incineration, (3) recycling, and (4) source reduction.[4]

Sanitary Landfills

Prior to the mid-1970s, much of the solid waste in the United States was simply placed in a hole in the ground with little thought given to the underlying soil type, location, and depth of groundwater and little concern for neighbors. This process, known as dumping, was cheap and convenient. These open **dumps** were unsanitary because they supported large populations of rodents, flies, and vermin. Such dumps were found to produce **leachates,** liquids created when water mixes with wastes and removes soluble constituents from them by percolation; these liquids then find their way into the groundwater. Dumps also reduced the value of adjacent property because of their obnoxious odors, their unsightliness, and their generally unsanitary conditions.[3]

The passage of RCRA in 1976 provided legislation that phased out open dumps and required that the disposal of solid waste be done in sanitary landfills. Sanitary landfills differ from open dumps in several ways. First, they are located at sites that can geographically and geologically support them. Landfill sites selected should have natural clay soil or be clay-lined. They must not be located over sand or gravel deposits that would allow leachates to reach ground water. Second, in sanitary landfills, all refuse is spread and compacted in thin layers by bulldozers. Once the compacted layers are about eight to ten feet thick, they are cov-

ered with about six inches of soil, compacted again, and readied for another layer of refuse. At the end of each day, unlike an open dump, refuse is again covered with a layer of soil. This process continues until the landfill is full, at which time a final layer of soil about two feet thick is placed on the top. When this process is strictly followed, sanitary landfills provide little refuge for rodents and insects, and there is no reason why the area cannot be used for recreation. In fact, there is a ski slope in Michigan that was created by using this process.

Sanitary landfills are still not without problems. The production of leachates and contamination of groundwater can still occur if the clay seal breaks or if the landfill is located improperly. Some local governments have enacted legislation that requires sanitary landfills to be lined or double-lined with plastic liners. Another concern is the possibility of explosions and fires caused by the accumulation of dangerous amounts of methane gas created by the anaerobic decomposition of refuse.[3] However, it should be noted that some communities have systems in place to harness the methane gas and use it as an energy source.

Today, about 73% of all municipal waste goes into landfills. However, the number of existing landfills in the United States has declined from approximately 20,000 in 1978 to fewer than 6,000 in 1991.[5] At this rate, only one of every six landfills that was operating in 1979 will still be open in the year 2000. This means that: (1) it will be more costly to use existing landfills in the future because of supply and demand, (2) new sites for landfills will be needed, and (3) alternative means of waste disposal must be developed.

The decline in the number of sanitary landfills is the direct result of the difficulty of finding new locations that are suitable for

---

dumps   Open pits in which solid waste is placed.
leachates   Liquids created when water mixes with wastes and removes soluble constituents from them by percolation.

landfill use. There are those, however, who seek other environmentally sound approaches to the solid waste problem, such as incineration, recycling, and source reduction (reducing the production of solid waste).

Incineration

Incineration, or the burning of wastes, is the second major method of refuse disposal. The passage of the Clean Air Act of 1970 severely restricted the rights of individuals and municipalities to burn refuse because most could not comply with the strict emission standards. Today, only about 14% of all municipal waste is incinerated. Most of the nearly 200 municipal incinerators are **waste-to-energy (WTE) plants.** That is, they are able to convert some of the heat generated from the incineration process into steam and electricity to operate municipally owned equipment or to be sold to a utility. Some high-tech waste-to-energy plants also include the separation of waste prior to incineration so that glass and metals can be recycled.

Incineration greatly reduces the weight and volume of solid waste. Generally, volume is reduced by as much as 90% and weight is reduced by as much as 80%. While incineration might seem to be the ultimate solution to the solid waste disposal problem, it is not without serious drawbacks. First of all, large commercial incinerators are expensive. Start-up costs can approach a quarter of a billion dollars. Some environmentalists feel that there are too many unanswered questions about incinerators to invest that type of money. One of their questions is about air quality. While most modern incinerators use filters to reduce harmful emissions, they do not eliminate them entirely. A second environmental concern has to do with the remaining ash. The ash may be toxic, particularly when plastics have been incinerated, which occurs with increasing frequency. A third concern is that at least 10% of the volume (20% of the weight) of the original wastes remains to be dealt with. Most of this ash enters landfills, but because of its toxicity, it poses a threat to local groundwater. Also, it now appears that future restrictions on items placed in landfills may prohibit the disposal of the ash.

Finally, since incinerators require large amounts of wastes to operate efficiently, there is concern that the existence of community incinerators might impede the development of recycling and source reduction programs. However, it would seem logical in these times that incineration and waste reduction could coexist.

Recycling (Resource Recovery)

Recycling is the collection and reprocessing of a resource so that it can be reused for the same or another purpose. This process yields three major benefits. First, it conserves resources. If we recycle paper, we do not need to cut down as many trees to generate new paper. Second, recycling conserves energy. It takes less energy to recycle an aluminum soft drink can than it does to create a new one. Third, recycling conserves sanitary landfill space that can be used for the disposal of nonrecyclable waste.[3]

Though recycling makes perfectly good sense, Americans recycle only a small percentage of what could be recycled (see Figure 15.8). Overall, only 13% of all municipal solid waste is being managed through recycling. In contrast, Japan recycles ap-

---

waste-to-energy (WTE) plants Incinerators that are able to convert some heat generated from the burning of trash into steam and electricity.

recycling The collection and reprocessing of a resource after use so it can be reused for the same or another purpose.

proximately 45% of its municipal solid waste.[4] In an effort to encourage recycling, the EPA has set a goal of recycling 25% of municipal solid wastes by the mid-1990s, and several municipalities in the United States have set even higher standards for themselves (see Box 15.1).

The primary reasons why Americans have been slow to embrace recycling are: (1) the absence of reliable markets for the recycled materials, (2) the lack of incentives for people to recycle, and (3) the inconvenience of recycling. Nadakavukaren[3] has reviewed the following five reasons for low market demand:

1. Virgin materials are generally cost-competitive with, or cheaper than, recycled materials and are usually perceived by manufacturers as superior in quality.
2. The composition of virgin materials is usually more homogeneous than that of recycled materials, making them more suitable for new-product creation.
3. Manufacturing processes that use virgin materials are well established while

processes to use recycled materials are not.
4. Some products that are potential candidates for recycling are composed of a mixture of synthetic and natural materials that cannot be easily separated for recycling.
5. Artificial economic barriers (e.g., tax depletion allowances, differential freight rates, and government subsidies to producers of virgin materials) favor the use of virgin materials.

The second reason for the low volume of recycling in the United States is the lack of incentives for people to recycle. While it could be argued that incentives should not be necessary, most people do not change their behavior until they realize their health or prosperity is in danger. Recycling generally requires a behavioral change.

Probably the greatest recycling efforts in the United States took place during World War II, when resources were scarce. It was a patriotic thing to do and people believed it was important. The end of the war was followed by great industrial growth and prosperity, and recycling faded quickly. Over the next 20 years, America became a "throwaway society." It was not until the late 1960s that the concerns about the environment caused people to think once again about recycling. Now in the 1990s, without much national leadership, some communities are providing incentives—both punitive and economic—to recycle. Examples include laws that mandate the recycling of certain materials and centers that will purchase used materials, like aluminum and paper, from the average citizen. In areas of the country where these incentives do not exist, fewer people recycle.

When most people think of recycling, they think of paper, glass, aluminum, and plastic. But one solid waste that can easily be recycled and currently consumes almost

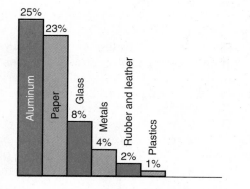

FIGURE 15.8

Percent of waste being recycled, by type of waste.

From: Enger, E. D., and B. F. Smith (1991). Environmental Science: A Study of Interrelationships, *4th ed. Dubuque, Ia.: Wm. C. Brown, p. 438.*

BOX 15.1
One Corporation's Response to Environmental Responsibility

When Americans think about those symbols around us that are truly "American," thoughts of baseball and apple pie come to mind. When we are asked to think about corporations that are truly American, the McDonald's Corporation—the hamburger people—come to mind. In each of their restaurants, they provide information for the customers about the nutritional value of their foods and other interesting bits of information about the company. In recent years, McDonald's has presented information about their support of recycling. They have stated that they are the largest user of recycled paper in their business. Specifically, they use recycled paper for trayliners, brown carryout bags, Happy Meal bags, corrugated shipping containers, wash-room tissue, office stationery, and towels. In addition, they are redesigning dozens of other packaging items they use in order to reduce the amount of material in them.

The corporation estimated that by recycling corrugated cardboard shipping containers nationwide, they could reduce the amount of waste McDonald's restaurants formerly sent to landfills by 30%–40%.

It is efforts like that of the McDonald's Corporation that will help us reach our future recycling goals.

Note: For more information on the recycling program of McDonald's Corporation write: McDonald's Environmental Affairs, McDonald's Corp., Oak Brook, IL 60521.

20% of the solid waste going into landfills is yard waste—grass clippings, leaves, and shrub and tree trimmings. Yard waste can be recycled by composting. **Composting** utilizes the natural aerobic biodegradation process of microorganisms to convert organic plant and animal matter to compost, which can then be used as a mulch or fertilizer. Composting can be done by individuals collecting household yard wastes for their own compost piles or on a communitywide basis. In communitywide composting programs, communities collect and transport the wastes to a central composting area, where they are shredded, processed, and made available to citizens either free or for a nominal fee. Because yard wastes take up so much space in a municipal landfill, a number of municipalities and even some states have banned them from landfills.

For recycling to be successful, it must be made more convenient. Many believe that recycling is less convenient than disposing of wastes in the traditional manner, and in some cases, they are right. For example, it is not convenient for families to transport their trash to a central location for recycling, which is the only option in some communities. On the other hand, separating paper, glass, aluminum, and plastic for pickup at the curbside is not too inconvenient for most. Similarly, the disposal of hazardous substances like paint thinner or oil-based paint can be made convenient. Monthly pickups of these hazardous substances, as opposed to annual pickups, will result in better compliance from households and less disposal of toxins in unsecured municipal landfills.

---

composting The natural, aerobic biodegradation of organic plant and animal matter to compost.

Another way to entice people to recycle is to artificially add value to items to be recycled. This approach is exemplified by "**bottle bills,**" laws that require consumers to pay refundable deposits (usually 5–10 cents) on beer and soft drink containers. Currently, bottle bill laws exist in ten states (see Table 15.2). Bottle bills benefit the environment by reducing litter and encouraging recycling of glass, plastic, and aluminum. In states with bottle bills, 90% of all such containers are returned for recycling, as opposed to only 54% for the nation as a whole.[3]

Bottle bills are not without problems. Many consumers dislike paying the refundable deposits; others dislike the inconvenience of storing the empty containers and having to return them to a store. Retail merchants also dislike handling the dirty containers and providing storage space for them. Even with these disadvantages, bottle bills still seem to make good sense.

Source Reduction

The ultimate means of dealing with solid waste is to limit its creation in the first place; this approach is referred to as **source reduction.** One way to reduce solid waste is to select products made from materials that can be reused, such as cloth diapers. Another approach is to reduce the packaging of groceries and carry out foods such as hamburgers and pizzas. (A cardboard round and a paper bag constitute less packing than an entire corrugated cardboard box.) Lightweight containers like aluminum soft drink cans create less to recycle than heavier ones. A third approach is to sell products in concentrated form so they can be pack-

---

bottle bills Laws that require consumers to pay refundable deposits on beverage containers.

source reduction Reduction or elimination of materials that produce an accumulation of solid waste.

Table 15.2
States with Bottle Bills

Effective Date	States
1972	Oregon
1973	Vermont
1978	Maine
1979	Iowa, Michigan
1980	Connecticut
1983	Delaware, Massachusetts, New York
1987	California

aged in smaller containers. Examples are frozen orange juice and laundry detergent. With regard to packaging, it has been estimated that about 9% of grocery bills can be attributed to costs associated with packaging of the products.

Solid waste management has come a long way in the past 20 years. Today, most people know what is and what is not environmentally sound management; and the necessary technology to insure appropriate disposal of waste is available. One question still remains: When will protecting the environment become a high enough priority for most Americans to act and demand wise waste management? (See Box 15.2.)

HAZARDOUS WASTE

Like solid waste, **hazardous waste,** waste that is dangerous to human health or the environment, has become the subject of intensified concern in recent years. Improperly handled hazardous waste can result in an immediate threat to human health or to the environment. Until 1976

---

hazardous waste Waste that is dangerous to human health or the environment.

BOX 15.2
Tips for Reducing Solid Waste

Reduce

1. Reduce the amount of unnecessary packaging.
2. Adopt practices that reduce waste toxicity.

Reuse

3. Consider reusable products.
4. Maintain and repair durable products.
5. Reuse bags, containers, and other items.
6. Borrow, rent, or share items used infrequently.
7. Sell or donate goods instead of throwing them out.

Recycle

8. Choose recyclable products and containers and recycle them.
9. Select products made from recycled materials.
10. Compost yard trimmings and some food scraps.

Respond

11. Educate others on source reduction and recycling practices. Make your preferences known to manufacturers, merchants, and community leaders.
12. Be creative—find new ways to reduce waste quantity and toxicity.

From: U.S. Environmental Protection Agency (1992). *The Consumer's Handbook for Reducing Solid Waste.* Washington, D.C.: U.S. Government Printing Office, p. 7.

Americans are faced with the dual problem of (1) appropriately disposing of new hazardous waste while (2) working to correct the errors of mishandling of hazardous waste in the past. There are untold numbers of hazardous waste sites that are "polluted" from past actions, legal and illegal, that must be cleaned up. Meanwhile, the production of hazardous wastes continues at a record pace. The United States alone produces almost 300 million metric tons of hazardous industrial waste annually. That is more than 1 ton of waste for every person living in the country. This figure does not include any wastes that are discarded improperly or illegally.

Hazardous Waste Defined

The accepted definition for hazardous waste in the United States can be found in the Resource Conservation and Recovery Act of 1976. This act states that

> the term "hazardous waste" means a solid waste, or combination of solid wastes, which, because of its quantity, concentration, or physical, chemical, or infectious characteristics may (1) cause or significantly contribute to an increase in mortality or an increase in serious irreversible, or incapacitating reversible, illness; or (2) pose a substantial present or potential hazard to human health or the environment when improperly treated, stored, transported, or disposed of, or otherwise managed.

It is the responsibility of the EPA to implement the legislation created by the RCRA. In doing so, the agency has identified hazardous waste by two means: listing and testing. Listing involves compiling a list of hazardous materials. It is the most common means of defining hazardous waste in European countries and is also used by some states in their statutes.[4] Testing, the second

and the passage of RCRA, hazardous waste could be disposed of in the same way that other solid wastes were; that is, by placing it in a dump or landfill. In addition, a great deal of hazardous waste was illegally buried or discarded into waterways. Today,

method of identifying hazardous wastes, is conducted by the EPA to determine if a new and unknown substance is hazardous. Following these tests, the substance may be added to the list. There are four characteristics, any one of which can make a waste hazardous. They are ignitability (ability to catch fire), corrosiveness (the ability to weaken and destroy), reactivity (explosiveness), and toxicity (poisonousness). There are now more than 400 substances that are considered hazardous wastes in the United States. The EPA list includes neither radioactive wastes, which are controlled by the Nuclear Regulatory Commission, nor biomedical wastes, which are regulated by the individual states.

Hazardous Waste Management

There are several approaches to managing hazardous waste (see Figure 15.9). During the 1980s, about 89% of the hazardous waste in the United States was placed in the earth via land disposal (67%) or discharged into sewers, rivers, or streams (22%). The remaining 11% was either distilled for recovery of solvents (4%), burned in industrial boilers (4%), chemically treated (1%), land treated (for biodegradable waste) (1%), incinerated (1%), or processed for recovery of metals (<1%).[6] While there is now legislation in place that regulates the disposal of all hazardous wastes, illegal dumping still occurs.

Secured Landfill

The least expensive, and perhaps least environmentally sound means of disposing of hazardous waste is placing it in a **secured landfill** (see Figure 15.10). Such a

---

secured landfill   A double-lined landfill located above flood plain and away from a fault zone, equipped with monitoring pipes for seepage, used primarily for hazardous waste.

landfill differs from a sanitary landfill in its location, design, and its ability to be monitored. Some of the requirements for secured landfills are that they must be: located above the 100-year flood plain and away from fault zones; double-lined with clay or a synthetic material; and equipped with pipes that enable them to be monitored for any seepage. The owner must provide for area wells for the monitoring of groundwater, as well as monitor the surrounding **surface water** (water on the earth's surface).

There are several drawbacks of the use of secured landfills for the discarding of hazardous waste. Some authorities feel that even the best built secured landfill will eventually leak because the clay liners will crack or the synthetic liners will break. Because of this concern, the legislation governing secured landfills continues to mount. There are now specific standards that stipulate which hazardous wastes can and cannot be placed in secured landfills without further processing (some wastes must undergo prior treatment before being placed in the landfill). Many authorities desire this means of disposal to be phased out.

Deep Well Injection

Another means of disposing of hazardous waste is deep well injection, a form of disposal developed by petroleum refineries. Deep well injection consists of pumping the hazardous waste, by way of lined wells, far below drinking water aquifers into layers of permeable rock that are surrounded by impermeable rock. About 25% of all hazardous waste in the United States is disposed of by deep well injection. The major objection to deep well injection is that, like the secured landfill, there may be seepage of hazardous waste out of the well and into the water supply.

---

surface water   Water found on the earth's surface.

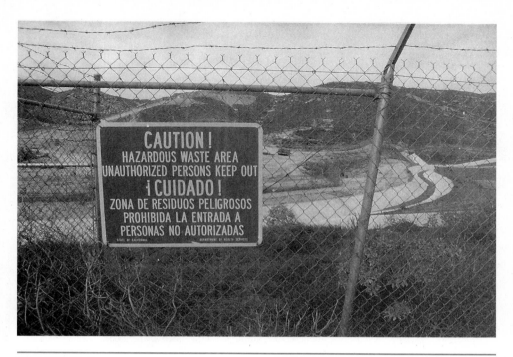

FIGURE 15.9

The management of hazardous wastes is becoming big business.

Incineration of Hazardous Waste

Appropriately controlled incineration is one of the most efficient means of managing hazardous waste; however, it is also one of the most expensive. Nadakavukaren[3] identified four major benefits of this means of disposal: (1) conversion of toxic compounds to harmless ones, (2) reduction in the volume of waste, (3) destruction instead of isolation of waste, and (4) possible energy recovery during combustion.

This method of disposal consists of burning the wastes at very high temperatures. It requires the appropriate mixture of air and an adequate supply of fuel to ensure complete combustion. Gaseous by-products are recombusted to minimize the release of hydrocarbons and other harmful gases. Airborne products of combustion are subject to special filtration (scrubbers and electro-static precipitators) to eliminate air pollution. In 1993, the EPA began looking closely at hazardous waste incinerators to make sure they were operating safely.

Hazardous Waste Recycling

The best solution to hazardous waste disposal is recycling in a system in which a hazardous waste created by one process becomes the raw material for another. Unfortunately, finding someone who can use your hazardous waste is not easy. In Europe, **waste exchanges** have been created to help parties carry out mutually agreeable exchanges. These waste exchanges are managed by "intermediaries"

---

waste exchanges Managed exchanges in which a contract is written between those who want to dispose of hazardous wastes and those who can use them as raw materials.

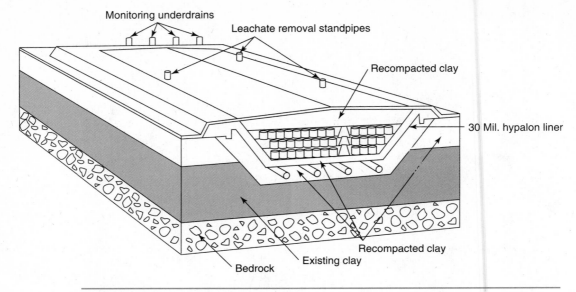

FIGURE 15.10

Diagram of a secured landfill.

From: Nadakavukaren, A. (1990). Man and Environment: A Health Perspective, *3rd ed. Prospect Heights, Ill.: Waveland Press, p. 489.*

who help to establish contacts between those who want to dispose of hazardous wastes and those who can use them as raw materials.[7]

Neutralization of Hazardous Waste

Small amounts of certain types of hazardous waste can be neutralized by physical, chemical, or biological processes. Examples include extracting toxic metals from waste, adding a base to an excessively acidic waste, and promoting the growth of microbes that feed on hazardous waste—a method that has been used successfully with oil spills.

Source Reduction

Source reduction represents the best solution to the problem of hazardous waste. Increased public concern and the high cost of disposal have led hazardous waste producers to invest in technological research to reduce the amount of waste produced. Unfortunately, this approach is limited because there are still few incentives for source reduction. Some state and federal laws support research into source reduction technology; but, for most wastes, the cost of disposal is, in the short run, less expensive than investing money for an eventual reduction at the source. Environmental experts say this is a shortsighted solution.

Hazardous Waste Cleanup

Managing present and future hazardous wastes is one issue; dealing with the inappropriate past disposal of hazardous wastes is another. Much of the past disposal, while inappropriate, was not illegal because not until 1976 was hazardous waste defined in the United States. Prior to this date, our best knowledge for disposal of hazardous waste was to bury it. It should be noted here that the problem of hazardous waste cleanup is not limited to the United States but extends throughout most of the industrialized world. The following discussion, however, is limited to efforts to clean up hazardous waste in the United States.

The primary participant in the cleanup of hazardous waste in America has been the federal government. In 1980, Congress passed the **Comprehensive Environmental Response, Compensation, and Liability Act (CERCLA)** in response to the public's demand to clean up leaking dump sites. This law, which has become known as **Superfund,** was created primarily to cleanup abandoned hazardous waste sites. The law also supports the advancement of scientific and technological means of managing hazardous wastes. With regard to cleanup, CERCLA:

1. Created a national priority list (NPL) of sites to be cleaned up.
2. Stated that the government would make responsible parties pay for those cleanups whenever possible.
3. Provided up to $1.6 billion to support the identification and cleanup of the sites from 1980 to 1985, hence, the name *Superfund.*

The EPA was responsible for creating the NPL in cooperation with the individual states. Sites were placed on the list in order of priority based upon the threat to public health or the environment. Once on the NPL, sites were eligible for Superfund dollars. These dollars could be used for removing and destroying wastes and for the temporary or permanent relocation of residents impacted by the wastes, but not for compensation to victims for related health problems. At the time the bill expired, in September 1985, only 13 sites had been cleaned up and most believe that those 13 cleanups were done improperly.

In 1986, the fund was reauthorized with the **Superfund Amendments Reauthorization Act (SARA).** Because of Congress's dissatisfaction with the way cleanups were handled under CERCLA, specific directions about how they should be conducted were given to the EPA with SARA. This time, Congress designated specific sites to be cleaned up and required that such cleanup efforts were to permanently reduce the amount of hazardous waste, not just move it from one site to another (see Figure 15.11). SARA also increased Superfund allocations to $9 billion to be spent by 1991. While this seems like a lot of money, it has not gone very far in hazardous waste cleanup. It has been estimated that hazardous waste cleanup can cost as much as $1 million per acre.[8]

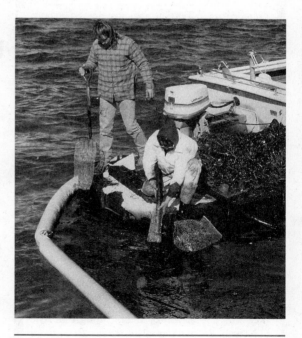

FIGURE 15.11

Workers cleaning up a kerosene spill on the Hudson River.

Table 15.3
Different Government Agency Projected Estimates of Hazardous Waste Cleanup Sites and Costs

	Estimated	
Agency	Sites	Costs
Environmental Protection Agency (EPA)	2,500	$30 billion
Government Accounts Office (GAO)	4,000	40 billion
U.S. Office of Technology Assessment (OTA)	10,000	100 billion

The Superfund bill was up for reauthorization again in 1991. The major issues of concern for the second reauthorization were how to pay for cleanup of the nearly 1,300

sites still on the NPL and what new sites should be added to the priority list. It was obvious in 1991 that the number of sites to be cleaned up had been underestimated. It is still unclear how many sites and what the final total cleanup costs will be (see Table 15.3). At the time of this writing, the Superfund legislation still had not been reauthorized as it was supposed to have been in 1991. As with other environmental legislation, political posturing between environmentalists, economists, and industrialists has slowed the process (see Box 15.3).

AIR POLLUTION

Until a few hundred years ago, air pollution could be attributed entirely to natural causes: dust and sand storms, forest fires, volcanic eruptions, and the gases escaping from deep within the earth or given off by decaying organic matter. These forms of air pollution still exist today, and at times cause serious threats to the environment and health. However, in addition to these natural pollutants, there are now additional waste products created by a modern industrialized civilization. These products of modern society threaten the quality of the air breathed not only in this country but around the world. Since there is little that can be done about natural air pollutants,

---

BOX 15.3
Healthy People 2000— Objective

11.14 Eliminate significant health risks from National Priority List hazardous waste sites, as measured by performance of cleanup at these sites sufficient to eliminate immediate and significant health threats as specified in health assessments completed at all sites. (Baseline: 1,082 sites were on the list in March of 1990; of these, health assessments have been conducted for approximately 1,000)

Baseline data sources: *Federal Register* March 14, 1990 EPA National Priorities List Update (final rule); 55 FR 55 (50):9688; Agency for Toxic Substances and Disease Registry.

For Further Thought

Do you feel it is the responsibility of the party who created a hazardous waste site to pay for the cleanup, even though at the time the site was created it was not illegal to dispose of the waste in such a manner? Why or why not?

the discussion in this section will concentrate on the concerns associated with those created by human beings.

Contaminants of Outdoor Air

Air pollution is the contamination of the air by substances in amounts great enough to interfere with comfort, safety, and health of living organisms. These contaminants, or substances, occur as gases, liquids, or solids. The most prevalent sources of air pollution in the United States are: (1) transportation, including privately owned motor vehicles; (2) electric power plants fueled by oil and coal; and (3) industry, primarily mills and refineries. In addition to these major sources, there are many smaller sources such as wood and coal burning stoves, fireplaces, and other incinerators.

The six most pervasive air pollutants in the United States have been labeled by the federal government as the **criteria pollutants.** These are: carbon monoxide, lead, nitrogen dioxide, ozone, particulate matter, and sulfur dioxide (see Table 15.4). The EPA has established national standards for allowable concentration levels of each of these six pollutants and nine others in the ambient (outdoor) air and closely monitors their levels. These standards are known as the **National Ambient Air Quality Standards (NAAQSs).**

The widespread concern about the possible ill effects of these criteria pollutants has led to efforts to reduce their concentrations in ambient air (see Figure 15.12). Between 1975 and 1989, the United States

reduced the ambient air concentrations of lead by 93%, carbon monoxide by 47%, ozone by 14%, particulate matter by 20%, nitrogen oxides by 17%, and sulfur dioxide by 46%[5] (see Box 15.4).

---

air pollution Contamination of the air that interferes with the comfort, safety, and health of living organisms.
criteria pollutants The six most pervasive air pollutants in the United States.
National Ambient Air Quality Standards (NAAQSs) Standards created by the EPA for allowable concentration levels of outdoor air pollutants.

BOX 15.4
Healthy People 2000— Objective

11.5 Reduce human exposure to criteria air pollutants, as measured by an increase to at least 85% in the proportion of people who live in counties that have not exceeded any Environmental Protection Agency standard for air quality in the previous 12 months. (Baseline: 49.7% in 1988)

Proportion Living in Counties That Did Not Exceed Criteria Air Pollutant Standards in 1988

Pollutant	Percentage
Ozone	53.6%
Carbon monoxide	87.8
Nitrogen dioxide	96.6
Sulfur dioxide	99.3
Particulates	89.4
Lead	99.3
Total (any of above pollutants)	49.7

Note: An individual living in a county that exceeds an air quality standard may not actually be exposed to unhealthy air. Of all criteria air pollutants, ozone is the most likely to have fairly uniform concentrations throughout an area. Exposure is to criteria air pollutants in ambient air. Due to weather fluctuations, multi-year averages may be the most appropriate way to monitor progress toward this objective.

Baseline data source: Office of Air and Radiation, EPA.

For Further Thought

Have you or any members of your family done anything during the past year to help reduce air pollution?

Table 15.4
Criteria Pollutants

Pollutants (Designation)	Form(s)	Major Sources (in order of percentage of contribution)
Carbon monoxide (CO)	Gas	Transportation, industrial processes, other, solid waste, stationary fuel combustion.
Lead (Pb)	Metal or aerosol	Transportation, industrial processes, stationary fuel combustion, solid waste.
Nitrogen dioxide (NO_2)	Gas	Stationary fuel combustion, transportation, industrial processes, solid waste, other.
Ozone (O_3)	Gas	Transportation, industrial processes, solid waste, other, stationary fuel combustion.
Particulate matter (total suspended particles—TSP)	Solid or liquid	Industrial processes, stationary fuel combustion, transportation, solid waste, other.
Sulfur dioxide (SO_2)	Gas	Stationary fuel combustion, industrial processes, transportation, other.

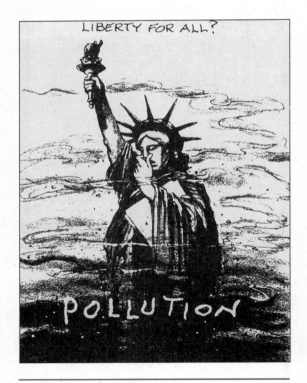

FIGURE 15.12

People are now more concerned with air pollution than they were ten years ago.

The Pollutant Standard Index

The deleterious effects of air pollution are many, including reduced visibility, weakened or ruined fabrics, and defaced buildings and monuments. Other effects are damaged paint on automobiles and injured or killed vegetation and aquatic life. Given these observations, there is naturally a concern about the effects of air pollution on human health.

Sensitivities to air pollutants vary with each individual. Variations are attributed to such chronic diseases as heart disease, lung diseases, and allergies. Other factors may be age, skin color, and history of exposure to the pollutants. For those most susceptible individuals, it is important to be able to measure the quality of ambient air. Therefore, the EPA developed a **Pollutant Standard Index (PSI).** It is a scale that relates pollutant concentrations to health effects. Thus, with a single numeric figure, air-quality professionals can provide the

Pollutant Standard Index (PSI) A scale developed by the EPA that relates the air pollutant concentrations to health effects.

Table 15.5

Comparison of Pollutant Standard Index (PSI) Values with Pollutant Concentrations and Health Effects*

Index Value	Air quality Level	Pollutant Levels					Health Effect Descriptor	General Health Effects	Cautionary Statements
		TSP (24-Hour) µg/m³	SO₂ (24-Hour) µg/m³	CO (8-Hour) µg/m³	O₃ (1-Hour) µg/m³	NO₂ (1-Hour) µg/m³			
500	Significant harm	1,000	2,620	57.5	1,200	3,750		Premature death of ill and elderly. Healthy people will experience adverse symptoms that affect their normal activity.	All persons should remain indoors, keeping windows and doors closed. All persons should minimize physical exertion and avoid traffic.
400	Emergency	875	2,100	46.0	1,000	3,000	Hazardous	Premature onset of certain diseases in addition to significant aggravation of symptoms and decreased exercise tolerance in healthy persons.	Elderly and persons with existing diseases should stay indoors and avoid physical exertion. General population should avoid outdoor activity.
300	Warning	825	1,600	34.0	800	2,260	Very unhealthful	Significant aggravation of symptoms and decreased exercise tolerance in persons with heart or lung disease, with widespread symptoms in the healthy population.	Elderly and persons with existing heart or lung disease should stay indoors and reduce physical activity.
200	Alert	375	800	17.0	400	1,130	Unhealthful	Mild aggravation of symptoms in susceptible persons, with irritation symptoms in the healthy population.	Persons with existing heart or respiratory ailments should reduce physical exertion and outdoor activity.
100	NAAQS	260	365	10.0	160	†			
50	50% of NAAQS	75‡	80‡	5.0	80	†	Moderate		
0		0	0	0	0	†	Good		

*From: Council on Environmental Quality, 1977.

†400 µg/m³ was used instead of the O₃ alert level of 200 µg/m³.

‡Annual primary NAAQS.

From: Purdom, P. W. (1980). "Air Resources Management." In P. W. Purdom, ed., *Environmental Health*, 2nd ed. (pp. 276–277). San Diego: Academic Press, p. 277.

Table 15.6
Air Quality Trends in Major Urban Areas, 1982–1991
Number of PSI Days Greater than 100 at Trend Sites

PMSA	1982	1983	1984	1985	1986	1987	1988	1989	1990	1991
					Year					
Atlanta	5	23	8	9	17	19	15	3	16	5
Boston	5	16	7	3	2	5	12	2	1	3
Chicago	3	16	8	6	4	10	18	2	3	8
Dallas	12	18	11	15	5	8	3	3	5	0
Denver	52	67	61	38	45	36	18	11	7	7
Detroit	19	18	7	2	6	9	17	12	3	7
Houston	49	70	48	47	44	54	48	32	48	39
Kansas City	0	4	12	4	8	6	3	2	2	1
Los Angeles	195	184	208	196	210	187	226	212	164	156
New York	69	62	110	60	53	40	41	10	12	16
Philadelphia	44	56	31	25	21	36	34	19	11	24
Pittsburgh	13	33	15	5	6	14	26	11	11	3
San Francisco	2	4	2	5	4	1	1	0	1	0
Seattle	19	19	4	26	18	13	8	4	2	0
Washington	25	53	30	15	11	23	34	7	5	16
Total	512	643	562	456	454	461	504	330	291	285

Notes: PMSA=Primary Metropolitan Statistical Area. PSI=Pollutant Standards Index. The PSI index integrates information from many pollutants across an entire monitoring network into a single number which represents the worst daily air quality experienced in the urban area. Only carbon monoxide and ozone monitoring sites with adequate historical data are included in the PSI trend analysis above, except for Pittsburgh, where sulfur dioxide contributed a significant number of days in the PSI high range.

From: U.S. Environmental Protection Agency, Office of Air Quality Planning and Standards (Oct. 1992). *National Air Quality and Emissions Trends Report 1991* (pub. no. 450-R-92-001). Research Triangle Park, N.C.: Author.

public with an indication of the air quality. The higher the PSI, the poorer the air quality. The PSI and the major pollutant are often reported daily over television in conjunction with the weather report. Table 15.5 presents the PSI with pollutant concentration levels and the health effects on humans while Table 15.6 presents a comparison of air-quality trends in major urban areas from 1982 to 1991.

Special Concerns with Outdoor Air

The pollution of the outdoor air has resulted in a number of specific problems for the United States and the world. They include acid rain, destruction of the ozone layer, global warming, and photochemical smog.

Acid Rain

Acid deposition, often referred to as **acid rain** (also acid snow, acid dew, acid drizzle, acid fog, and acid sleet), includes both the wet and dry acidic deposits, which occur both within and downwind of areas

---

acid rain Both wet and dry acidic deposits, which occur both within and downwind of areas that produce emissions containing sulfur dioxide and oxides of nitrogen.

that produce emissions that contain sulfur dioxide (SO_2) and oxides of nitrogen (NO_2 and NO_3). These emissions, which result from the burning of fossil fuels—oil, coal, and natural gas—react in the atmosphere to form acidic compounds called *sulfates* and *nitrates*. These sulfates and nitrates combine with water vapor to form sulfuric and nitric acids, which fall to the earth as acid rain (see Box 15.5).

The primary problems associated with acid rain are the acidification of surface water, resulting in the death of certain species of water life, damage to vegetation primarily at higher elevations, the erosion of monuments and buildings, and reduced visibility (see Figure 15.13). Some researchers also feel that acidic air pollutants can contribute to respiratory problems in humans.

In North America, a significant proportion of the sulfur nitrogen emissions are produced in the Midwest. The resulting acid rain falls in Ohio, West Virginia, Pennsylvania, New York, New Jersey, Maryland, the New England states, and Ontario, Canada.

The realization that acid rain in Canada can be traced to emission of sulfur and nitrogen by American industry is the source of much dismay to the Canadians. While it is true that the United States is the recipient of some acid rain from Canada, it has been estimated that almost half of the acid rain that falls in Canada is created by emissions from the United States. The two countries have discussed the problem on many occasions, but no formal agreement has ever been reached. However, the United States is working to reduce the problem.

BOX 15.5
The pH Scale

The pH scale is used to measure the alkalinity or acidity of a solution. On this 14-point scale, 7 is considered neutral; while values below that represent acids, and values above that represent bases. A normal rain that is not subject to SO_2 and NO_x is naturally slightly acidic (average pH 5.6). Thus, any rain with a pH of less than 5.6 would be considered acid rain.

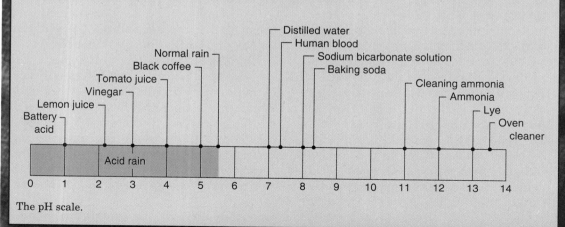

The pH scale.

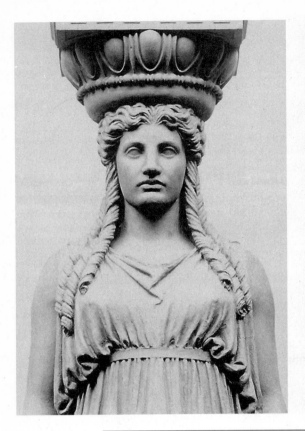 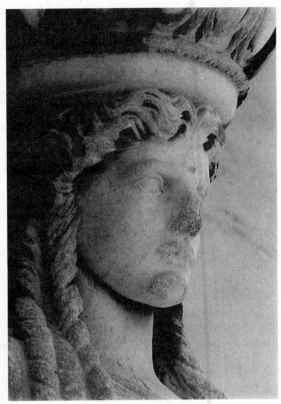

FIGURE 15.13

Acid rain defaces our art and our architecture and is hazardous to the environment.

As will be noted later in this chapter, the 1990 amendments to the U.S. Clean Air Act called for the reduction of sulfur dioxide emissions. In 1992, the EPA released regulations to implement the amendments. Under the regulations, the first round of reductions will affect the 110 largest electricity-producing power plants in the East and Midwest. They are to collectively reduce their emissions by 3.5 million tons by 1995. In the second phase, which begins in 2000, 6.5 million tons of additional reductions will be required of those large plants, together with 800 other utility plants around the country.

Destruction of the Ozone Layer

Although ground level ozone gas (O_3) is considered a criteria pollutant (see Figure 15.14), it provides a great benefit to the earth as it occurs in the stratosphere. This stratospheric **ozone layer** filters out much of the sun's harmful ultraviolet radiation. Without this protective filter, ultraviolet radiation would reach the earth's surface at dangerously high levels, causing increased rates of skin cancers and eye problems. Further, there would be an increase in the rate of mutations (genetic changes) and per-

ozone layer   Ozone gas (O_3) found in the stratosphere.

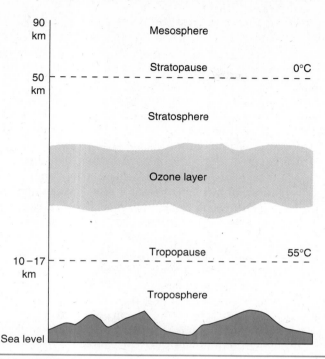

FIGURE 15.14

Regions of the atmosphere.

From: Nadakavukaren, A. (1990). Man and Environment: A Health Perspective, *3rd ed. Prospect Heights, Ill.: Waveland Press, p. 302.*

haps the disruption of the oceanic food chain.

The ozone layer is being depleted faster than originally believed. In fact, scientific evidence suggests that the rate of ozone depletion over the last decade is more than twice what was previously projected. Thinning of the ozone layer has been found over the polar regions and in the northern mid-latitudes.[5] Presently a hole exists in the ozone layer in the southern hemisphere, and it is anticipated that one will appear shortly in the northern hemisphere. Because of this thinning, it is anticipated that the ultraviolet radiation that reaches earth will increase 5%–20% over the next 40 years.

The primary cause of the depletion of the ozone layer is the presence in the atmos-

phere of **chlorofluorocarbons (CFCs).** CFCs are solely a product of the chemical industry. They do not occur naturally in the environment. CFCs are used for a wide range of purposes including propellants in aerosol cans, in the freon of air conditioners and refrigerators, and for blowing plastic foams. The problem with CFCs lies with the chlorine atom, which reacts with ozone (O_3) to form oxygen (O_2) and chlorine oxide (ClO). Because CFCs are implicated in both ozone depletion and global warming, considerable attention has been placed on controlling their production and release.[4] In September

chlorofluorocarbons (CFCs) A family of chemical agents used in industry for such items as propellants, refrigeration, solvent cleaning, and insulation.

1987, in Montreal, Canada, diplomats from 31 countries agreed to freeze the consumption of CFCs at 1986 levels by 1990 and reduce production by 50% by the year 2000. The United States went one step further with the amendments to the U.S. Clean Air Act of 1990 by banning CFC production in this country by the year 1996.

Global Warming

Global warming is the gradual increase in the earth's surface temperature. Whether or not global warming is occurring at present is a matter of debate. Records show that the average global temperature was 58.2°F (14.6°C) in 1880, but was 59.4°F (15.2°C) in 1980.[9] Some scientists do not regard this increase in the global temperature over the past 100 years as significant. Other scientists point to the fact that the yearly average is constantly rising. If global warming is occurring and if it continues to occur, a number of serious complications can be expected. A few degrees increase in the earth's surface temperature would cause major changes in water resources, sea level, agriculture, forests, biological diversity, air quality, human health, urban infrastructure, and the demand of electricity for cooling.[10]

One of the conditions that seems to be contributing to global warming is the increase in levels of **greenhouse gases,** namely carbon dioxide, CFCs, methane, and nitrous oxide, which are transparent to visible light but absorb infrared radiation. These gases permit the passage of sunlight to the earth's surface. However, when some of this energy is reradiated as infrared radiation (heat), it is absorbed by the gases causing the air temperature to rise. This process is known as the **greenhouse effect** because it is analogous to the process by which a greenhouse captures heat from sunlight (see Figure 15.15).

Carbon dioxide is the most important of the greenhouse gases because it is the most abundant since it is a normal by-product of plant and animal respiration. Today, however, excessive quantities of carbon dioxide are being released into the atmosphere by the combustion of fossil fuels. Two solutions to the problem of excessive levels of carbon dioxide in the atmosphere are to reduce excessive emissions and to remove carbon dioxide from the atmosphere. Emissions could be cut through greater use of alternative energy sources, such as nuclear or solar power, or by getting people to be more fuel efficient. Removal of carbon dioxide from the atmosphere occurs when plants use it during photosynthesis. If the amount of vegetation can be increased, more carbon dioxide would be depleted from the atmosphere. However, destruction of vegetation via the clearing of rainforests in tropical regions of the world and the logging of forests worldwide have worked against this solution.

Photochemical Smog

Photochemical smog is a secondary air pollutant created when primary pollutants including nitrogen oxides, hydrocarbons, and other secondary pollutants like ozone and peroxyacyl nitrates (PAN) react with oxygen and sunlight. The resulting photochemical smog can be seen in the air as a brownish haze. It is detrimental to human health and to the well-being of other living things.

---

global warming The gradual increase in the earth's surface temperature.

greenhouse gases Atmosphere gases, principally carbon dioxide, CFCs, methane, and nitrous oxide, that are transparent to visible light but absorb infrared radiation.

greenhouse effect The trapping of heat in the atmosphere by greenhouse gases.

photochemical smog A secondary air pollutant created when primary and other secondary pollutants react with oxygen and sunlight.

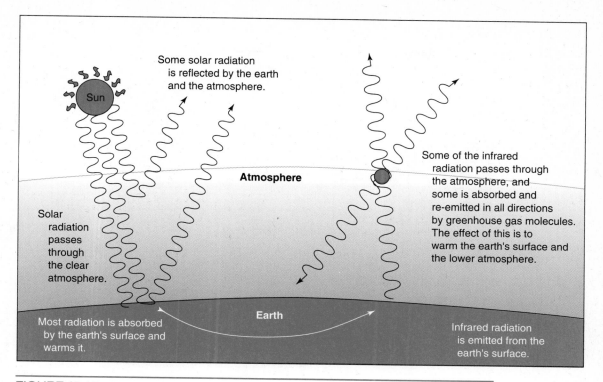

FIGURE 15.15

The greenhouse effect.

From: U.S. Department of State (1992). National Action Plan for Global Climate Change (USDS pub. no. 10026). Washington, D.C.: U.S. Government Printing Office, p. 6.

The effects of photochemical smog can be amplified by physical geography. For example, the cities of Denver, Los Angeles, Phoenix, and Salt Lake City are surrounded by mountains that restrict lateral air movement. This trapped air mass may also be subject to another phenomenon referred to as a **thermal inversion.** Normally, the air surrounding the earth's surface is heated by the sun and rises to mix with the cooler air above it. However, in cases of thermal inversion, a layer of warm air settles above the cooler air at the surface, preventing cooler air from rising. When the cool air is trapped,

it accumulates pollutants. If the thermal inversion continues, the pollutants can reach dangerously high levels[4] (see Figure 15.16).

Just as with other types of pollution, the best way to reduce photochemical smog is to reduce (or eliminate) emissions from the internal combustion engines of motor vehicles. Such a reduction can be achieved through more carpooling, better use of mass transit systems, and the development of electric and solar energy sources for motor vehicles.

Protection of Outdoor Air Through Regulation

So far, we have discussed several specific air pollution problems, their origins,

---

thermal inversion When warm air traps cooler air at the surface of the earth.

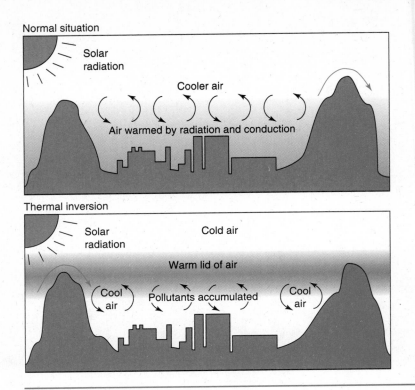

FIGURE 15.16

A thermal inversion.

and possible solutions. In this section, we review legislative efforts to protect the air. Air quality legislation is not new in the United States; the first emission control ordinance was adopted in Pittsburgh in 1815.[11] There have been many other local ordinances since that time. However, a national air-quality policy was not enacted until the second half of the twentieth century.

Steady deterioration of air quality in the 1950s and 1960s led to the signing of the first **Clean Air Act (CAA) (P.L. 88-206)** by president Lyndon Johnson on December 17, 1963. The CAA provided the federal government with authority to address interstate air pollution problems. The CAA was amended several times in the late 60s, but much of the regulation was based upon voluntary compliance.[3]

Public concern about air quality and other environmental issues continued to grow in the late 1960s and early 1970s. The concern became so great that the largest organized demonstration in U.S. history was held on April 22, 1970, to express dissatisfaction with the state of the environment and the policies to protect it. This demonstration marked the first national observance of **Earth Day.** On the first Earth Day, thousands of primary and secondary schools and colleges and universi-

Earth Day Annual public observance for concerns about the environment.

ties took part, along with millions of other citizens, to express their desire to work toward national environmental goals. The United States Congress adjourned for the day, New York's Fifth Avenue was closed, and hundreds of ecology fairs were held nationwide. Some experts have indicated that the first Earth Day gave birth to the modern environmental movement. The public outcry to preserve the environment helped convince Congress and then president Richard Nixon to establish the Environmental Protection Agency (EPA) and again amend the CAA in 1970. These two steps radically changed the course of pollution control.[12]

The 1970 amendments to the CAA provided the first comprehensive approach to dealing with air pollution nationwide. Three significant components of these amendments were the development of the National Ambient Air Quality Standards (NAAQSs) (see Table 15.5), tougher emission standards for automobiles, and **State Implementation Plans (SIPs).** The SIPs required each state to submit to the EPA its plan for achieving and maintaining air-quality standards.

The CAA was amended again in 1977. The 1977 CAA amendments empowered the EPA to regulate air quality. Specifically, the EPA was authorized to levy fines against those who violated the standards. The 1977 revisions were the last major revision to the CAA until president George Bush signed new amendments in November 1990. Key provisions of the 1990 amendments are: (1) mandates to reduce urban smog, sulfur dioxide, and nitrogen oxides; (2) tighter controls on auto emissions, including a guarantee that auto emission controls will last 100,000 miles; (3) power plants that are more efficient, and (4) a total ban on the production of CFCs by the year 1996.[4]

Indoor Air

As the outdoor air has become cleaner, the importance of indoor air in determining exposures to many inhaled pollutants has become increasingly evident. It is now clear that protection of public health requires satisfactory outdoor *and* indoor air quality. Moreover, the public also expects a degree of indoor air quality to assure comfort.[12]

It was once believed that the comfortable confines of the indoors were protected from the ills of air pollution. However, it is now known that indoor air pollution can be a greater threat to human health than outdoor air pollution. Unlike outdoor air pollutants, which are regulated and can be dispersed by the wind, indoor air pollutants can be trapped and concentrated to dangerous levels. This buildup of undesirable gases and particles with air inside a building has been termed **indoor air pollution.**[13] Poor indoor air quality combined with the fact that Americans spend 80%–90% of their time indoors[10] presents a potentially significant health concern.

Indoor Air Pollutants

Indoor air pollution can arise from a number of sources (see Figure 15.17). The presence of pollutants in a building does not necessarily mean people will be exposed to them. If there are excessive levels of gases in a building, chances are good that they will be inhaled by those in the building. However, the presence of other pollutants such as asbestos materials found in some buildings may not result in exposure except in situations where the material is disturbed or inadequately maintained.[14] At other times, a substance becomes a pollutant only when it is used improperly, such as when gasoline is used as a cleaning agent. The ma-

indoor air pollution The buildup of undesirable gases and particles in the air inside a building.

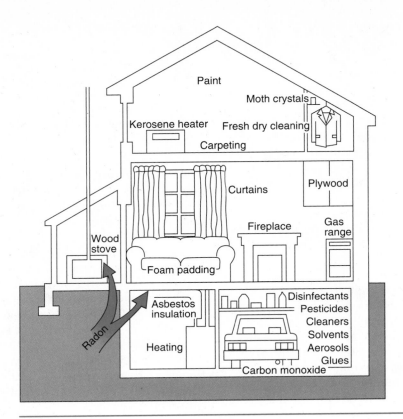

FIGURE 15.17

Air pollution sources in the home.

From: U.S. Environmental Protection Agency, 1991.

jor indoor pollutants and their sources are described in the paragraphs that follow.

Asbestos is a naturally occurring mineral fiber that was commonly used as an insulation and fireproofing material. It was often used in older buildings to insulate pipes, walls, and ceilings; as a component of floor and ceiling tiles; and sprayed in structures for fireproofing. It is relatively harmless if intact and left alone, but the loose fibers can cause serious health problems. **Aeroallergens** are biological organisms that float in the air. These organisms include fungal spores (e.g., mold, mildew), bacteria, viruses, pollens, arthropods, and protozoa. They can enter the human body by either being inhaled or being deposited on the skin surface. **Combustion by-products** include gases (e.g., CO, NO_2, and SO_2) and particulates (e.g., ash and soot). The major sources of these items are fireplaces, wood stoves, kerosene heaters, gas ranges and engines, candles and incense, second-hand tobacco smoke, and improperly main-

---

aeroallergens Biological organisms that float in the air and involve an immune response in humans.

combustion by-products Gases and particulates generated by controlled or uncontrolled burning.

tained gas furnaces. Prolonged exposure to these substances can cause serious illness and possibly death. **Formaldehyde (CH₂O),** a pungent water-soluble gas, is one of the most ubiquitous organic vapors indoors. It is a widely used chemical that can be found in hundreds of products. Some people associate it with science and medicine because of its use in preserving biological materials. However, many more Americans have been exposed to it when it evaporates from laminated wood products, such as plywood and particle board, in which it is a component of the glue binding these products together. Formaldehyde can also be found in products like grocery bags, wallpaper, carpet, insulation, wall paneling, and wallboard.[14]

Radon is a naturally occurring radioactive gas that cannot be seen, smelled, or tasted. Radon seeps into homes from surrounding soil, rocks, and water through openings (cracks, drains, wells, etc.) in the foundation and floor. The only way to determine if a building has elevated levels of radon is to test for it. The test is inexpensive and easy to conduct. The test can be administered by homeowners for themselves. Smokers and children are most sensitive to radon exposure.[15]

Environmental tobacco smoke (ETS), also known as **secondhand smoke,** includes both **mainstream smoke** (the smoke inhaled and exhaled by the smoker) and **sidestream** smoke (the smoke that comes off the end of a burning tobacco product. The inhalation of ETS by nonsmokers is referred to as **passive smoking.** There are

hundreds of toxic agents and more than forty **carcinogens** (cancer-causing agents) in secondhand smoke. A few of these harmful agents are carbon monoxide, nitrogen dioxide, carbon dioxide, hydrogen cyanide, formaldehyde, nicotine, and suspended particles.[16] According to Enger and Smith,[4] tobacco smoke may be the most important air pollution source in the United States in terms of human health. Approximately 420,000 people die from smoking-related causes each year. Of that number, 3,000 die due to secondhand smoke. It has been postulated that "banning smoking probably would save more lives than any other pollution control measure."[4] (See Box 15.6.)

Volatile organic compounds (VOCs) are compounds that exist as vapors over the normal range of air pressures and temperatures. In any one building, one might find hundreds of different VOCs. Sources of VOCs include construction materials (e.g., insulation, paint), structural components (e.g., vinyl tile, sheetrock), furnishings (e.g., drapes, upholstery fabric), cleansers and solvents (e.g., liquid detergent, chlorine bleach), personal care products (e.g., deodorant, eyeliner pencil), insecticides/pesticides, electrical equipment (e.g., computers, VCRs), and combustion of wood and kerosene.[14]

Protection of Indoor Air

Even though indoor air pollution may be more harmful to human health than outdoor air pollution, measures to monitor and correct indoor air pollution have been limited. Currently, there are two major ways that indoor air can be protected. They include formulating policy through legislation and/or modifying individuals' behavior.

---

formaldehyde (CH₂O) A water-soluble gas used in aqueous solutions in hundreds of consumer products.
radon A naturally occurring radioactive gas.
sidestream tobacco smoke The smoke that comes off the end of burning tobacco products.
passive smoking The inhalation of environmental tobacco smoke by nonsmokers.

---

volatile organic compounds (VOCs) Compounds that exist as vapors over the normal range of air pressures and temperatures.

BOX 15.6
Healthy People 2000—Objectives

3.12 Enact in 50 states comprehensive laws on clean indoor air that prohibit or strictly limit smoking in the workplace and enclosed public places (including health care facilities, schools, and public transportation). (Baseline: 42 states and the District of Columbia had laws restricting smoking in public places; 31 states restricted smoking in public workplaces; but only 13 states had comprehensive laws regulating smoking in private as well as public worksites and at least four public places, including restaurants, as of 1988)

Baseline data source: Office on Smoking and Health, CDC.

11.6 Increase to at least 40% the proportion of homes in which homeowners/occupants have tested for radon concentrations and that have either been found to pose minimal risk or have been modified to reduce risk to health. (Baseline: Less than 5% of homes had been tested in 1989)

Special Population Targets

Testing and Modification As Necessary	Baseline	2000 Target
11.6a Homes with smokers and former smokers	—	50%
11.6b Homes with children	—	50

Baseline data sources: Office of Radiation Programs, EPA; Center for Environmental Health and Injury Control, CDC.

For Further Thought

The two objectives above identify two of the primary concerns of indoor air quality. If you were given the opportunity to see that one of these two objectives was met by the year 2000, which one would you select? Why?

Policy

Policy regarding the quality of indoor air can be categorized into two major groups: **common law** (legal principles and rules based on past legal decisions; judge-made law) and **statutory law** (law passed by state or federal legislatures or another governing body).[17] For the most part, most laws dealing with indoor air quality—both common and statutory—focus primarily on public buildings or workplaces. The concept of the "sick building syndrome" emanates from common law. **Sick building syndrome** refers to the fact that the air quality in a building produces signs and symptoms of ill health in the building occupants. This phenomenon was first brought to the attention of public health authorities in the mid-1970s.[18] Armed with a knowledge of health effects of passive smoking, asbestos, radon, formaldehyde, and other substances, and with their lawyers and testifying environmental scientists, the public began suing architects, builders, contractors, building product manufacturers, realtors, building owners, building sellers, employers, and utility companies for their complicity in indoor air pollution. This type of action will obviously result in changes in building design and construction[19] (see Box 15.7).

---

sick building syndrome A term to describe a situation in which the air quality in a building produces signs and symptoms of ill health in the building's occupants.

BOX 15.7

Sick Building Syndrome Checklist

More employers and employees request health hazard evaluations on indoor air pollution than on any other problem. Indoor air pollution appears to be especially persistent in buildings constructed between 1972 and 1987, particularly those with locked windows.

Below is a checklist of questions that you can ask in identifying the likelihood that your building is contributing to respiratory health problems. Building managers should be able to assist you in answering these questions.

1. How much air does your building's ventilation system process?

   Your building's HVAC (heating/air conditioning) should process 20 cubic feet per minute (cfm) per person. HVACs in many sick buildings process only one-fourth that much air.

2. Where are your building's air intakes located?

   If your building's air intakes are located next to an alley where diesel trucks idle or next to a factory or other source of poor air, you're in trouble.

3. What kind of chemicals are used in cleaning your building?

   Many cleaning compounds are hazardous. You can identify contents by reading the container labels. You can call the Occu-

pational Safety and Health Administration, the Environmental Protection Agency or a chemistry department of a local school for guidance on potential health risks.

4. What kind of carpeting exists in your building? What ingredients were used in manufacturing the carpets?

   Many carpets are manufactured and treated with synthetic substances. Some of these belong to a set of chemicals known as volatile organic compounds, or VOCs, which may be emitted as vapors from the carpet and are suspected of causing upper respiratory tract irritation. Toluene, xylenes, and 4-phenylcyclohexene are all examples of such substances which may be used in carpet manufacture.

5. Are people allowed to smoke in your building?

   Second-hand tobacco smoke is associated with many respiratory problems. Even if you have a "smoke-free" office, people who smoke elsewhere on your floor or within the same building may be causing significant health problems for you.

Source: Prepared by the Healthy Office Research Program, National Safe Workplace Institute (1992). *Basic Information on Workplace Safety and Health in the United States.* Chicago: Author, p. 78.

Statutory law connected with indoor air quality is limited. The U.S. government has not yet established a framework for the development of indoor air policies as it has for outdoor air. It has, however, pursued voluntary industry standards. For example, there are safety codes for kerosene space heaters, an "action guideline" for radon, and smoking restrictions for commercial airlines. There has been federal guidance on the handling of asbestos in schools and a prohibi-

tion on new uses of asbestos. In the absence of a federal indoor clean air act, some states and municipalities have developed their own. Most of these acts are aimed at restricting smoking in public places.[20]

Individual Behavior

In the absence of any comprehensive policy, individual behavior becomes a factor in improving indoor air quality. One such behavior is the proper ventilation of buildings with high levels of VOCs. "Tight" buildings and those with climate control need frequent exchanges of air to assure an adequate level of indoor air quality.

In addition to assuring adequate ventilation, choices can be made to reduce or eliminate sources of indoor air pollution and improve air quality. These may include:

1. Selecting safer household products, such as a "pump" dispenser instead of a spray dispenser.
2. Venting dryers outdoors instead of indoors.
3. Avoiding products containing formaldehyde.
4. If loose asbestos fibers are found, having them professionally removed.
5. Limiting or prohibiting indoor smoking.
6. Maintaining heating, air conditioning, and ventilation systems in good working condition.
7. Periodically testing the building for radon.[13]

WATER AND ITS POLLUTION

Water is one of the basic elements of life in any ecosystem because it directly supports the first links in the food chain. While we can survive without food for several weeks, we would die within a few days without water (see Figure 15.18). Water makes up two-thirds of our bodies and covers three-fourths of the earth's surface. Water has been called the *universal solvent* because of its ability to break apart or dissolve many compounds and prevent them from recombining. As a solvent, water is essential to the processes of digestion, absorption, and excretion, but it is also vulnerable to contamination and pollution. Beyond its use to support life, wa-

ter is used to generate electric power, as a cooling agent for industry, and as a source of fun, relaxation, and recreation.[21, 22]

Most people take the supply of usable water for granted. Few steps have been taken to safeguard the quality and quantity of water for the future. As such, much of the water for human consumption has become polluted.

Sources of Water

The endless movement of water from the earth's surface to the atmosphere and back to the earth's surface is called the **hydrologic cycle** (see Figure 15.19). In this cycle, water evaporates from surface water, soil, and vegetation. The warm air containing the water vapor moves across the earth's surface until it cools. When it cools, water droplets are formed and fall to the earth as precipitation (rain, sleet, snow, hail). Some of the precipitation evaporates but most sinks into the soil or flows downhill into streams and rivers. The water that runs downhill (runoff) eventually becomes **surface water.** The water that sinks into the soil is referred to as *subsurface* or **groundwater.** Groundwater that is not absorbed by the roots of vegetation moves slowly downward until it reaches the underground reservoirs referred to as **aquifers.**[4, 21, 22, 23] Aquifers are found in the porous layers of underground rock.[17]

The majority (over 97%) of the world's water supply is in the oceans. The rest is found in ice sheets and glaciers (1.9%), groundwater (0.5%), nonocean surface water (0.02%), soil (0.01%) and in the atmosphere (0.0001%).[4] "The United States Geological

---

hydrologic cycle   The endless movement of water from the earth's surface to the atmosphere and back to the earth's surface.

aquifers   Underground water reservoirs.

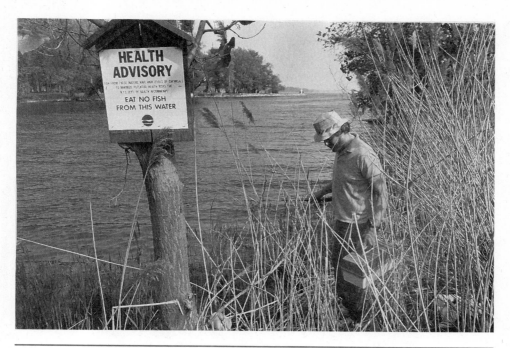

FIGURE 15.18

Clean water is one of the community's most precious resources.

Survey estimates the total amount of water on earth at 326,000,000 cubic miles, which is equal to 1,440,000,000,000,000,000 tons."[3] Even though this seems like an inexhaustible supply, over 97% of this water is salt water, thus it is not ready to be used by humans. While it is possible to remove salt from water by **desalinization,** it is a very expensive process.

The largest store of fresh water is in solid form as the ice sheets and glaciers at the North and South Poles. Its turnover to liquid or gaseous forms is too slow to be usable. Thus, almost all of the available fresh water of the world (96.5%) is found beneath the surface of the soil in the form of groundwater.[3]

It should now be clear why the contamination of our groundwater through the improper disposal of solid and hazardous waste is such a serious problem. "When one considers the amount of water too heavily polluted for use, or those sources too expensive or troublesome to utilize, we are left with only 0.003% of the world's water supply."[22] To put this fact in perspective, for every 55 gallons of water on earth, only one pint is available for human use.[22]

Surface and groundwater have very different characteristics. Surface water supports plant and animal life, including microorganisms, with the oxygen and nutrients that are contained in it. Conversely, groundwater is low in oxygen and contains few microorganisms. The microorganisms are filtered out as the water passes through the soil to the aquifers. The subsurface

---

desalinization The process used to remove salt from salt water.

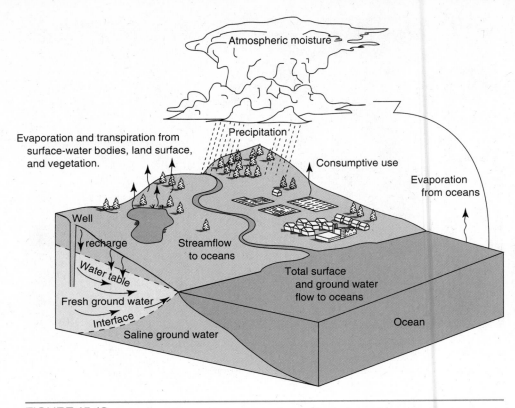

Atmospheric moisture

Precipitation

Evaporation and transpiration from surface-water bodies, land surface, and vegetation.

Consumptive use

Evaporation from oceans

Well

recharge

Water table

Streamflow to oceans

Fresh ground water

Total surface and ground water flow to oceans

Interface

Ocean

Saline ground water

FIGURE 15.19

The hydrological cycle.

From: Council of Environmental Quality (1989). Environmental Trends. *Washington, D.C.: CEQ, p. 21.*

water is, however, higher in minerals such as iron, chloride, and salts, because of its travel through the soil and rocks.[22] Each of these sets of characteristics is taken into account when preparing the water for human use.

Treatment of Water for Domestic Use

Domestic water use in the United States includes water for drinking, cooking, washing dishes and laundry, bathing, flushing toilets, and outdoor use such as watering lawns and gardens and washing cars. Most people are surprised to learn how much water we use in our homes. Estimates of water use per person per day in the United States range from 380 to 1,130 liters (100 to 300 gallons).[4,24] That amounts to over 100 billion liters of water used each day in the United States for domestic purposes.

While many rural residents in the United States obtain their water from untreated private wells (groundwater), urban residents obtain their water from municipal water treatment plants. About two-thirds of the municipalities use surface water, while one-third use groundwater.

The responsibility of municipal water treatment plants is to provide water that is chemically and bacteriologically safe for human consumption.[25] It is also desirable that the water be aesthetically pleasing in regard to taste, odor, color, and clarity. Above all, the municipal water supply must be reliable. Reliability with regard to both quantity and quality have always been regarded as "nonnegotiable" in planning a treatment facility.[24]

Virtually all surface water is polluted and needs to be treated before it can safely be consumed. The steps in surface water treatment vary from plant to plant, but the following four steps are almost always included:

1. *Coagulation and flocculation*—Alum (aluminum sulfate) is added to the water to cause suspended solids to attract one another and form larger particles (flakes).
2. *Sedimentation*—The water is permitted to stand so that the large particles (flakes) will settle out.
3. *Filtration*—The water is passed through filters (often sand filters) in order to remove any solids remaining after sedimentation.
4. *Disinfection*—Chlorine is added to the water to oxidize (kill) viruses, bacteria, algae, and fungi.

In many communities, chlorine is added in a pretreatment step before coagulation and flocculation, as well as during disinfection, which is sometimes referred to as *posttreatment*. In many communities, disinfection is accompanied by fluoridation, which helps prevent dental decay.

The treated water, now safe to drink, is pumped to community water storage tanks, many of which are familiar on the skylines of American towns. The water must then enter the distribution system through which it reaches homes. The integrity of this distribution system is not always reliable. There can be breaks in the pipes,

sometimes in the vicinity of sewer lines that also may be leaking. Therefore, a residual level of chlorine to kill bacteria must remain in the water until it reaches the tap. This is insurance against contamination during distribution.

Municipal water treatment plants are technologically complex, and it is important that well-trained and qualified personnel be entrusted with their operation. These facilities, which are either privately or municipally owned, are expensive to operate, especially since less than 2% of the water is used for drinking and cooking. The remaining 98% is used to flush toilets; take showers; do laundry; wash dishes, floors, or cars; and water the lawn or garden. There is no reason why water used for these purposes needs to be pure enough to drink.[4]

Sources of Water Pollution

Water pollution includes any physical or chemical change in water that can harm living organisms or make it unfit for other uses.[17] The sources of water pollution (see Figure 15.20) fall into two categories—point sources and nonpoint sources.[3] **Point source pollution** refers to a single identifiable source that discharges pollutants into the water, such as a pipe, ditch, or culvert. Examples of such might include release of pollutants from a factory or sewage plant.

Nonpoint source pollution includes all pollution that occurs through the runoff, seepage, or falling of pollutants into the wa-

---

water pollution Any physical or chemical change in water that can harm living organisms or make it unfit for other uses.

point source pollution A single identifiable source that discharges pollutants into the water.

nonpoint source pollution All pollution that occurs through the runoff, seepage, or falling of pollutants into the water.

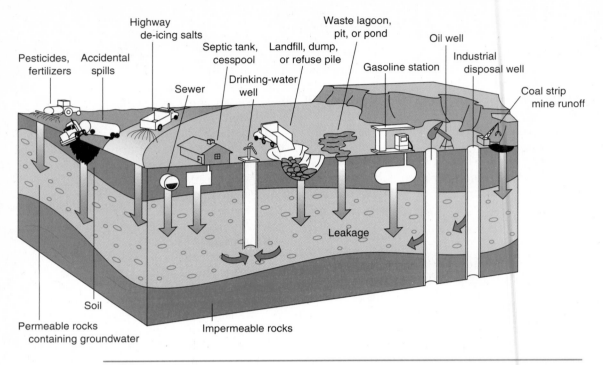

Pesticides, fertilizers · Accidental spills · Highway de-icing salts · Sewer · Septic tank, cesspool · Drinking-water well · Landfill, dump, or refuse pile · Waste lagoon, pit, or pond · Gasoline station · Oil well · Industrial disposal well · Coal strip mine runoff

Leakage

Soil

Permeable rocks containing groundwater

Impermeable rocks

FIGURE 15.20
Sources of groundwater contamination.
From: Environmental Protection Agency.

ter. Examples include the runoff of chemicals from farm fields, seepage of leachates from landfills, and acid rain. Of these two sources of pollution, nonpoint is the greater problem, because it is often difficult to track the actual source of pollution.

Types of Water Pollutants

As one might guess, the types and numbers of water pollutants are almost endless. For the ease of discussion, we have categorized pollutants into three different categories: biological, toxic, and miscellaneous.[3,22]

Biological Pollutants

Two major types of biological pollutants exist. The first includes pathogens such as parasites, bacteria, viruses, and other undesirable living microorganisms. Pathogens enter the water mainly through human and other animal wastes. This can occur when wastes are disposed of improperly, such as the flushing of wastes by boaters and runoff from farm fields. The second category of biological pollutants is the overgrowth of aquatic plants. This type of imbalance is usually caused by chemical pollution that favors plant growth. Such growth removes most of the dissolved oxygen and endangers other living organisms.

Toxic Pollutants

Toxic pollutants can be placed into three groups. One group includes inorganic chemicals. While these occur naturally, they become important as pollutants after they have been mined, processed, refined, and concentrated. Lead is an example of an inorganic, toxic pollutant.

A second group includes radioactive pollutants that can enter the water when not handled properly. Such cases have been reported at military bases and nuclear power plants.

A third group of toxic chemicals are synthetic organic chemicals (SOCs). These are chemicals that have been created by humans for a variety of purposes. They include industrial solvents such as trichloroethylene (TCE), pesticides such as dichlorodiphenyltrichloroethane (DDT), and the insulating chemicals used in transformers and electrical capacitors, such as the polychlorinated biphenyls (PCBs). There are also inks, plastics, tapes, paints, glues, waxes, and polishes. Lastly, there is dioxin (TCDD) a substance that is a by-product of the manufacture of certain herbicides when PCBs are burned.

Miscellaneous Pollutants

In recent years, there have been an increasing number of oil spills. Most of these occur at sea, but others, such as the Exxon *Valdez*, that polluted Alaska's Prince William Sound on March 24, 1989, result in a considerable loss of aquatic and terrestrial life.

Another type of miscellaneous pollution occurs when the water temperature is altered. **Thermal pollution** (heated water) can occur when factories discharge water that has been used as a cooling agent without proper cooling procedures for the water prior to returning it to the source.

Water-Related Issues

There are two major issues related to water. They are water quantity and water quality.[5]

Water Quantity

The United States, as a whole, is not running out of water. The hydrological cycle provides enough fresh water to meet the needs of all; and after the summer of 1993, many living along the Mississippi River would say too much! Yet there are times when unusually long, dry periods can reduce the amount of water available for use in some areas. The severity of these droughts depends primarily upon their length. Their overall effects on the community can be altered by: (1) the amount of water available from storage, (2) the amount of water consumed during the drought, and (3) the amount of new water created during the drought. When a water shortage appears imminent, communities with municipal water supplies often take steps to conserve water. These steps may range from voluntary compliance during the early drought (see Figure 15.21) to strict enforcement of water conservation policies (e.g., watering lawns and gardens only on alternate days or not at all). If the drought becomes severe, the washing of cars may be prohibited and the frequent flushing of toilets may be discour-

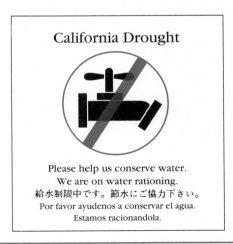

California Drought

Please help us conserve water.
We are on water rationing.
給水制限中です。節水にご協力下さい。
Por favor ayudenos a conservar el agua.
Estamos racionandola.

FIGURE 15.21

A citizen reminder to conserve water.

aged. Sometimes, the courtesy of serving water in restaurants is discontinued unless it is specifically requested by the customers.

In recent years, droughts have plagued much of the Southwest and Great Plains in the United States. Figure 15.22 shows the drought-severity index map for September 1991.

Water Quality

Water quality in the United States has been the target of increasingly careful scrutiny in recent years. Because of limited data, it is difficult, and perhaps meaning-less, to provide an assessment of the overall quality of water in the United States. The data that are available indicate that water quality has improved in some areas but has declined in others.[5]

Stewart[22] attributes the deterioration of water quality in the United States to four causes:

1. Population growth—an increase in the number of people generating waste.
2. Widespread and ever increasing chemical manufacture and usage, particularly synthetic organic chemicals (SOCs).

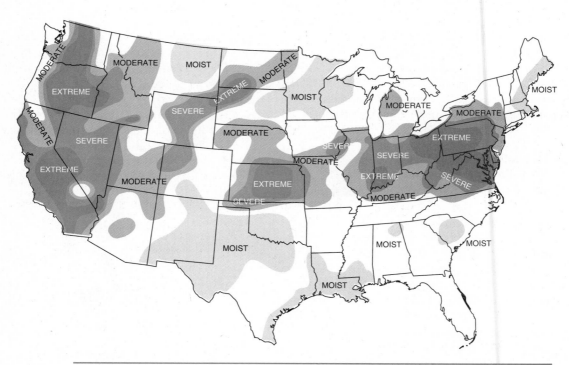

FIGURE 15.22

Drought-severity index map, 1991.

Note: The Palmer drought-severity index depicts prolonged abnormal dryness or wetness over months or years. The index responds slowly, changes little from week to week, and reflects long-term moisture runoff, recharge, and deep percolation, as well as evapotranspiration.

From: U.S. Department of Commerce NOAA/U.S. Department of Agriculture Joint Agricultural Weather Facility, Sept. 1991.

3. Gross mismanagement and irresponsible disposal of hazardous wastes.
4. Reckless land use practices that result in runoff of pollutants into waterways.

As the public's knowledge of the endangerment of water quality in the United States grows, so will the number of strategies and the public will to protect it.

Strategies to Insure Safe Water

Insuring safe water has been a concern for many years. Probably the best known epidemiological study of all time was done by John Snow in London, England, from 1849–1854 (see Chapter 3). This study confirmed that consumption of contaminated water from a city well caused cholera. John Snow interrupted the epidemic by removing the pump handle. This action made it impossible for the residents to obtain water from this well and thus eliminated any new cases of cholera. Strategies used to insure safe water in America today include public policy, proper treatment of water, and water conservation.

Policy

The earliest federal legislation dealing with water quality dates to 1914, but this legislation required only voluntary compliance and was ineffective. It was not until 1972 that a tough, comprehensive federal water-quality law was passed by Congress. The passage of the **Federal Water Pollution Control Act Amendments** (P.L. 92-500) in 1972 and additional amendments in 1977 radically changed the approach the U.S. government took to protecting its water resources. This act, now known as the **Clean Water Act (CWA),** contained provisions aimed at (1) ensuring water quality in such a way as to make all rivers swim-mable and fishable and (2) reducing the discharge of pollutants in U.S. waters to zero.

As with most other federal environmental legislation, the implementation of the CWA was given to the EPA, which in turn developed regulations to meet the goals of the act. A few of the more significant regulations include: limitation on industrial discharges of wastes, requirements for pollutant discharge permits, municipal sewage treatment plant discharge standards, and other water-quality standards.

The goals of the CWA have remained constant over the years, although there have been several amendments. Some amendments raised standards; others were necessary to keep up with new technology. The most recent reauthorization of the act by Congress occurred in 1987.

Another piece of legislation that has helped to ensure safe water is the 1974 **Safe Drinking Water Act (SDWA).** This is the only piece of federal legislation that deals with drinking water in a comprehensive manner. The act instructed the EPA to set maximum contaminant levels (MCLs) for specific pollutants in drinking water. There are hundreds of different pollutants, and by 1986, the EPA had set levels for only 23 of them. Congress was not pleased with this slow pace, so when they reauthorized the act in 1986, they strengthened it considerably and required the EPA to follow a strict timetable for setting MCLs for other pollutants.[3]

Waste Water Treatment

Waste water is the substance that remains after water has been used or consumed by humans. Such water, also sometimes referred to as *liquid waste* or *sewage,* consists of about 99.9% water and

---

waste water The substance that remains after water has been used or consumed by humans.

0.02%–0.04% solids. Included in the solids are human feces, soap, paper, garbage grindings (food parts), and a variety of other items that are put in to waste water systems from homes, schools, commercial buildings, hotels/motels, hospitals, industrial plants, and others connected to the system.[11]

The primary purpose of waste water treatment is to improve the quality of waste water to the point that it might be released into a body of water without seriously disrupting the aquatic environment, causing health problems in humans in the form of waterborne disease, or causing nuisance conditions. This is accomplished in two ways. One is by killing the pathogen organisms that enter the waste water as part of human wastes. The second is by converting organic wastes to inorganic wastes so that they will not unduly enrich the waters receiving the treated waste water.[3,11]

There are three stages of waste water treatment: primary, secondary, and tertiary (see Figure 15.23). Most municipalities and many large companies have waste water treatment plants, which incorporate these levels.

Primary Treatment

Primary treatment of waste water is a physical/mechanical process that results in the separation of liquids and solids. As water enters the treatment plant, large objects—which may include sticks, dead animals, rags, and so on—are removed from the water by screens. The waste water then passes through a large grinder, called a **comminutor,** to reduce the remaining particles to a uniform size so that they will not damage the equipment. The waste water then passes through a grit chamber, where sand, gravel, and other inorganic material

settles out. The waste water is then placed in a holding tank or settling pond or lagoon. In the settling tank, heavier solid particles settle to the bottom, forming a layer referred to as **sludge.** Sludge is a gooey solid mixture that includes bacteria, viruses, organic matter, toxic metals, synthetic organic chemicals, and solid chemicals.[17] Above the sludge remains water and all the dissolved substances, including many bacteria and chemicals. On top of the water layer is a layer of oils and fats. The layers of sludge and fat are removed, and the aquatic portion enters the secondary stage of treatment.

Secondary Treatment

While primary treatment involves the physical separation of liquids and solids, the secondary level is biological. In this stage, in the presence of adequate oxygen, aerobic bacteria break down the organic materials into inorganic carbon dioxide, water, and minerals. This is accomplished either through trickling filters (sprinkling systems over rocks) or an activated sludge process (agitation of waste water in a tank). After going through this secondary level of treatment, the water can be discharged into a waterway. It is estimated that about 90% of organic materials have been removed by this stage. However, the waste water still may contain some viruses, metals, dissolved minerals, and other chemicals. It was not until July 1988 (via the Clean Water Act of 1987) that this level of treatment was required of sewage treatment plants by the EPA.

This secondary level also produces sludge, but in much smaller quantities. In some treatment plants, sludge is put into a sludge digester. Under anaerobic condi-

---

comminutor A large grinder; part of a waste water system.

sludge A gooey mixture of solid waste.

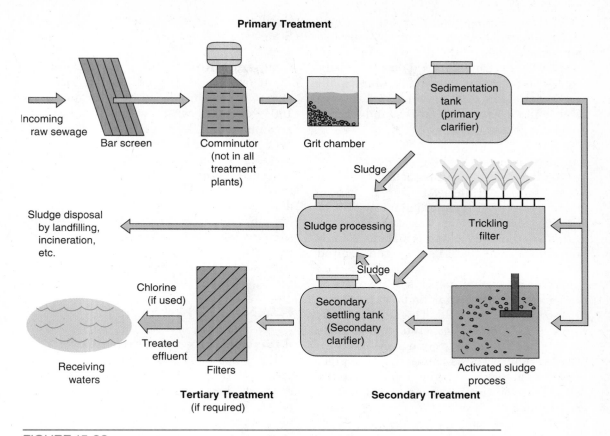

FIGURE 15.23

Schematic representation of the municipal waste water treatment process.

From: Nadakavukaren, A. (1990). Man and Environment: A Health Perspective, *3rd ed. Prospect Heights, Ill.: Waveland Press, p. 428.*

tions, the sludge produces methane gas, which can be sold. Most sludge is carried to landfills or lagoons, but some has been composted and used as fertilizer.[3, 4, 11]

Tertiary Treatment (Advanced Sewage Treatment)

The third level of treatment usually involves sand and charcoal filters, which can remove 90% of the remaining dissolved pollutants left behind after the first two treatment levels. The finished water is 99% pure and sometimes clearer than the river into which it is returned. Most treatment facilities in the United States do not have capabilities to perform tertiary treatment of waste water. There are two reasons for this. First is that it is not required by law, and second, the equipment to perform this treatment is very expensive.

Finally, whether or not waste water is discharged after secondary or tertiary treatment, it is recommended that the waste water be disinfected. The least expensive way of disinfecting is to chlorinate. About half of the waste water treatment plants in the

United States disinfect discharged water with chlorine. There are some who object to this because they feel that it has adverse effects on the environment and does not disinfect the water completely. Some municipalities do not disinfect at all while others have used a more expensive ultrasound energy process to do so.[3, 4]

Septic Systems

Septic systems are the means by which those who live in unsewered areas dispose of sewage. Presently, approximately 25% of all Americans live in unsewered areas.[3] Stated another way, there are about 20 million septic tanks in use in the United States.[4]

A septic system consists of two major components: a septic tank and a buried sand filter or absorption field. The **septic tank,** which is a watertight concrete or fiberglass tank, is buried in the ground some distance from the house and is connected by a pipe. The system works in the following way. Sewage leaves the home via the toilets or drains and goes through the pipe to the septic tank. In the tank, the sewage is partially decomposed by bacteria under anaerobic conditions. The sludge settles in the bottom while the liquid portions of the waste run out perforated pipes to the **absorption field.** The tanks have to be cleaned out (pumped out) periodically to remove the sludge. Sewage disposal by septic tanks is perfectly safe if the system is: (1) properly located in appropriate soil, (2) carefully constructed, and (3) properly maintained. Septic systems can contaminate groundwater if any of these conditions are not met.[3] It has been estimated that approximately one-

third of the present systems in the United States are operating improperly.[4]

Conservation

It has been estimated that the average person in the United States generates about 100 gallons of waste water a day.[3] That amount could be dramatically reduced if each of us took a few simple steps to conserve the water we use. Examples of domestic conservation include not letting the water run while brushing teeth, washing dishes, or washing a car. Also, shorter showers and water-saving shower heads conserve water. Box 15.8 gives you an opportunity to examine how you and your community might conserve water.

RADIATION

Radiation is the energy released when an atom is split. This process, called *fission,* produces radiation which travels through space in the form of waves or particles. If properly controlled, this energy can provide many benefits, as is the case when it is used in medicine and in the creation of nuclear power. The energy can also be destructive to both property and life, as in the case of the atomic bombs at the end of World War II and with the accidental release of radiation in 1986 at the nuclear power plant in Chernobyl, USSR.

Sources of Radiation

Although none of us expects to be exposed to extreme doses of radiation, such as those from a nuclear bomb or serious nuclear accident, each of us is exposed to low levels of radiation daily. This radiation

---

septic tank   A watertight concrete or fiberglass tank that holds sewage; one of two main parts of a septic system.

absorption field   The element of a septic system in which the liquid portion of waste is distributed.

---

radiation   Energy released when an atom is split during the process of fission.

BOX 15.8
More Efficient Water Use

What Individuals Can Do

More efficient water use begins with individuals in the home and workplace. Taking these and other steps and encouraging others to do so make good economic as well as environmental sense.

In the home

Install a toilet dam or plastic bottle in your toilet tank.

Install a water-efficient showerhead (2.5 gallons or less per minute).

When you buy a new toilet, purchase a low flow model (1.6 gallons or less per flush).

Outdoors

Water in the morning or evening to minimize evaporation.

Install a drip-irrigation watering system for valuable plants.

Use drought-tolerant plants and grasses for landscaping, and reduce grass-covered areas.

At work or school

Adopt the same water-saving habits that are effective at home.

Ask about installing water-efficient equipment and reducing outdoor water use.

Encourage employers to explore the use of recycled "gray-water" or reclaimed waste water.

What Communities Can Do

A water supplier or waste water system operator (public or private) has cost-effective options to process and deliver water more efficiently. A community can do the same and can foster ways to use water wisely.

Not all of these steps are expensive. The best choices vary by region and by community; start by asking if these are appropriate where you live and work.

A water supplier or waste water processor can:

Identify who uses water, and reduce unaccounted-for water use.

Find and repair leaking pipes.

Consider a new pricing scheme which encourages conservation.

Reduce excess pressure in water lines.

Explore the reuse of treated waste water for uses other than drinking water.

Charge hookup fees which encourage more efficient water use in new buildings.

Build water efficiency into future demand projections, facility planning, and drought planning.

A community can:

Adopt plumbing and building codes that require water-efficient equipment and practices.

Adopt a water-efficient landscaping ordinance to reduce the water used for golf courses and commercial landscapes.

Refit older buildings with water-efficient equipment, starting with public buildings.

Reduce municipal water use for landscaping and other uses.

Conduct a public education campaign.

Require developers to build in water efficiency measures.

From: Environmental Protection Agency (1990). *Preventing Pollution Through Efficient Water Use* (pub. no. OPPE [pm-222]) Washington, D.C.: Author.

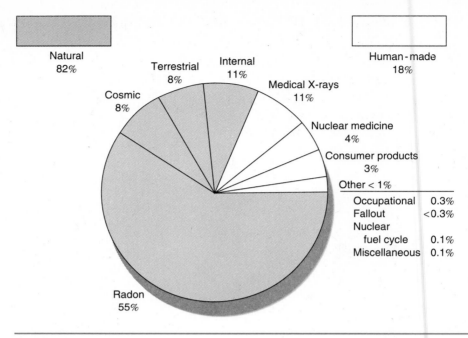

FIGURE 15.24

The percentage contribution of various radiation sources to the total average effective dose equivalent in the United States population.

From: National Council on Radiation Protection and Measurements, Report no. 93.

comes from one of three sources: naturally occurring, naturally occurring but enhanced by human behavior, or human-made radiation.[3] (See Figure 15.24.)

Naturally Occurring Radiation

Naturally occurring radiation comes from three sources. That which comes to the earth from outer space and the sun is referred to as **cosmic radiation.** Cosmic radiation is slightly more intense at higher elevations. The second source of naturally occurring radiation is the earth itself. **Terrestrial radiation** comes from radioac-

tive minerals that are within the earth: soil and rocks. Therefore people who live near these substances (which include traces of uranium), or who live or work in buildings made of brick and stone that could contain radioactive materials, would have greater exposure. Radon gas is the biggest contributor to terrestrial radiation. The third source of naturally occurring radiation is **internal radiation**—that is, internal to the human body. Exposure to such radiation occurs as a result of ingesting food and inhaling air.

Individual behavior plays a definite role in the amount of exposure one has to cos-

---

cosmic radiation Radiation that comes from outer space and the sun.

terrestrial radiation Radiation that comes from radioactive minerals within the earth.

internal radiation Radiation in the human body that occurs as a result of ingesting food and inhaling air.

mic, terrestrial, and internal radiation. For example, those who work outside, especially at higher elevations, increase their exposure to cosmic radiation. Included are individuals who choose to sunbathe and those who spend a lot of time at higher elevations, such as pilots and those who work in the mountains. Similarly, miners and bricklayers are at greater risk for terrestrial exposure. Those who drink from a contaminated well may be at greater risk of exposure to internal radiation.

Human-Made Radiation

Sources of human-made radiation include the radiation used in medical and dental procedures, such as X-rays, nuclear medicine diagnoses, and radiation therapy. Another source of human-made radiation is nuclear power plants (there are over 400 plants in the world, approximately 25% of them in the United States). Other sources include certain consumer products (such as smoke detectors), X-rays for security checks, tobacco, television and computer screens, and nuclear weapons.

The idea of using radiation for the benefit of our species brings with it a most controversial question. Do the benefits derived from the use of radiation outweigh the risks?[26] Most would agree that the use of radiation for medical purposes is justified. But there is less agreement about the cost/benefit question in the case of nuclear power plants. Yet there is a continually growing demand for energy in this country. The United States accounts for a little more than 25% of the total global energy consumption, a figure that is expected to grow at about 1% annually.[27] America's access to oil is not unlimited, and much of our coal contains sulphur, which contributes to acid deposition. While politicians, industrial leaders, and environmentalists continue to struggle with this question, all

Americans should become informed enough to have an opinion.

The Danger of Radiation

Since radiation is energy, it can damage living tissue. This damage can occur at the molecular, cellular, tissue, organ, or organism level. At the molecular level, biochemical changes can cause mutation or cell death. At the tissue level, there can be burns; if damage is severe enough, the organism can die.

"Human exposure to radiation is usually measured in **rems (roentgen equivalent man),** a measure of the biological damage to tissue."[4] The larger the dose of radiation, the greater the damage. However, the rate at which the dose is received, called **dose rate,** is also important. A single large dose of radiation produces more injury than many smaller doses over a period of time, because cells and tissues can repair themselves between doses.

The normal amount of radiation exposure for an American averages approximately 360 millirems (or 360/1,000 rems) a year or 1 millirem per day,[3] but this figure varies depending upon one's place of residence and one's occupation. The effects of large doses (1,000 + rems) can be easily quantified because of the high incidence of death. The effects of smaller doses (10–1,000 rems) are more difficult to measure, but they have been shown to cause miscarriages, cancer, and birth defects.[4] Table 15.7 shows the range of effects depending on the dose.

---

rems (roentgen equivalent man) A measure of the biological damage of radiation to human tissue.
dose rate The rate at which a dose of radiation is received.

Table 15.7
Radiation Effects

Source	Dose	Biological Effect
Nuclear bomb blast or exposure in a nuclear facility	100,000 rems/incident	Immediate death
X-rays for cancer patients	10,000 rems/incident	Coma, death within 1–2 days
	1,000 rems/incident	Nausea, lining of intestine damaged, death in 1–2 weeks
	100 rems/incident	Increased probability of leukemia
	10 rems/incident	Early embryos may show abnormalities
Upper limit for occupationally exposed people	5 rems/year	Effects difficult to demonstrate
X-ray of the intestine	1 rem/procedure	Effects difficult to demonstrate
Upper limit for release from nuclear installations (except nuclear power plants)	0.5 rem/year	Effects difficult to demonstrate
Natural background radiation	0.1–0.2 rem/year	Effects difficult to demonstrate
Upper limit for release by nuclear power plants	0.005 rem/year	Effects difficult to demonstrate

From: Enger, E. D., and B. F. Smith (1992). *Environmental Science: A Study of Interrelationships,* 4th ed. Dubuque, Ia.: Wm. C. Brown, p. 207.

Policy Related to Nuclear Waste Disposal

By the early 1980s, the public had become increasingly concerned with the problem of wastes from nuclear power plants. There was increasing pressure and criticism of the nuclear power industry. In 1982, Congress enacted the Nuclear Waste Policy Act (NWPA), which outlined the procedures for the disposal of the wastes. Specifically, the act designated the U.S. Department of Energy to oversee the development of a disposal site capable of safely receiving high-level nuclear wastes (from power plants) and to ensure that low-level wastes (from medicine, universities, and research labs) were also handled properly.

At the present time in the United States, there is no public waste facility capable of handling high-level wastes. American nuclear power plants and the U.S. military are storing their wastes above ground until such a facility is available. The NWPA made provisions to have a facility by 1998. The facility is planned for Yucca Mountain, Nevada, but protests over the facility have slowed its development. There is some doubt that it will ever be constructed. The more optimistic believe that the protests will keep it from completion until after the year 2000.

There are, however, three facilities in the United States (these are located in Beatty, Nevada, Barnwell, South Carolina, and Hanford, Washington) that are licensed to handle low-level wastes. These three landfills accept clothes, rugs, and other materials that have been contaminated. The space in these three facilities is becoming limited, and additional sites will probably be needed.

Americans may need to look for alternatives to burying nuclear wastes. For example, several European countries, including France and the United Kingdom, have reprocessing plants. In such facilities, spent nuclear fuel is reprocessed into new fuel rods, and the remaining wastes are solidified into glasslike material and either stored or buried. The reprocessing alternative is more expensive than manufacturing new fuel rods from ore, but it is a good alternative to waste storage.

NOISE POLLUTION

Of all environmental pollution, the type that receives the least attention in this country is **noise pollution:** excessive noise. Noise is something people have all grown up with, and as such, few people believe that much harm can come to the environment or our health because of it (see Figure 15.25). However, noise pollution can contribute to hearing loss, stress, and emotional problems, interrupting concentration and causing unintentional injuries.

What Is Noise and How Is It Measured?

Sound is the by-product of the conversion of energy. No process using energy is completely efficient; some energy always escapes either as heat, light, or sound waves. Sound is heard when energy from vibrations, traveling through air, liquid, or solid media as pressure waves, are received by the ear.[11] Unwanted sound is referred to as **noise.**[1,4,11] However, what constitutes unwanted sound is a matter of subjective judgment. What is a reasonable amount of sound to teenagers often is *noise* to their parents. In this regard noise is measured by an annoyance factor. Yet there are ways to scientifically measure and quantify noise (sound).

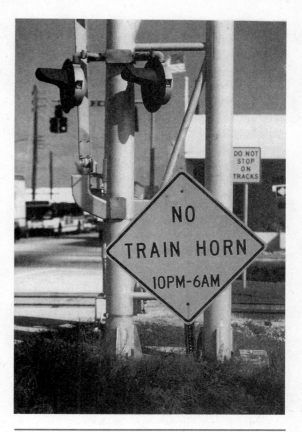

FIGURE 15.25

Noise is often the forgotten pollutant.

Sound-level meters, used to measure sound, take into account two basic characteristics of sound: frequency and amplitude. **Frequency** describes the rate of vibrations created by the transmission of energy. The more rapid the vibrations, the higher frequency of sound waves created. Frequency is measured in one of three ways: **cycles per second (cps), hertz (HZ),** or **vibra-**

---

noise pollution   Excessive sound.
noise   Unwanted sound.

---

sound-level meter   Instrument used to measure sound.
frequency   The rate of vibrations created by the transmission of energy.
cycles per second (cps), vibrations per second (vps), or **hertz**   Measures of sound frequency.

tions per section (vps). These are equivalent measures and express the number of sound waves passing by a certain point per second. People can hear sounds ranging from 20–20,000 Hz. Hearing acuity varies among individuals, but most people hear best when sound is in the 1,000–3,000 Hz range.

Amplitude refers to the sound volume; that is, its loudness or intensity. Amplitude is "measured and expressed as decibels—'deci' for one-tenth and 'bel' for Alexander Graham Bell."[11] The abbreviation for **decibels** is **dB.** The decibel scale, which is logarithmic in nature, ranges from zero dB, the faintest perceptible sound,[11] to 194 dB, which is regarded as the theoretic maximum for pure tones.[3] Thus, a sound measured at 10 dB is 10 times louder than zero dB, and 20 dB is 100 times louder than zero dB.

Though both frequency and amplitude are important characteristics of sound, it is the combination of the two that make sound "hearable." Sounds at the very low and very high ends of the audible frequency range are much fainter to our ears than those in the middle frequencies.

> for example, an extremely low-pitched [frequency] sound must have an amplitude [decibel reading] many times greater than a sound of medium pitch in order for both to be heard equally loud. For this reason, decibel values are sometimes weighted to take into account the frequency response of the human ear.[3]

Three standardized weightings—A, B, and C—are used. Currently, federal regulations require the use of the A network when measuring sound in environmental and occupational settings. Thus, the preferred notation using this network is dBA instead of dB. Most sound-level meters are calculated using dBA. Table 15.8 lists some commonly encountered sounds and their dBA levels.

Approaches to Noise Abatement

Since serious hearing problems can arise from noise pollution, communities need to take the necessary steps to control unwanted sound. To date, the most common means of dealing with noise pollution have been policy (legislation), educational programs, and environment changes.

Table 15.8
Intensity of Sounds

Sources of Sounds	Decibel Levels
Jet aircraft at takeoff	130–145
Air-raid siren	140
Hydraulic press	130
Jet airplane (160 meters overhead)	120
Rock concert	110–120
Subway train	90–100
Garbage truck	100
Gasoline lawnmower	95
City traffic	90
Food blender	90–95
Alarm clock	80
Garbage disposal	80
Freeway traffic	70
Dishwasher	65
Window air conditioner	60
Normal conversation	60
Light auto traffic	50
Living room	40
Library	30
Soft whisper	30
Barely audible	10
Hearing begins	0

---

amplitude The loudness or intensity of sound measured in decibels.

decibels (dB) A measure of sound amplitude.

Policy

The development of a federal policy for noise control has lagged behind that for other environmental problems—probably because by its very nature, noise is a local problem. As with most other public health issues, city governments were the first to recognize the need for limiting noise. The first noise ordinance was adopted September 30, 1850, in Boston, Massachusetts. Even today, the most effective noise policies are those developed at the local level, where they address specific noise issues.

It was not until 1972 that the Congress passed the **Noise Control Act (NCA) (P.L. 92-574).** This act was aimed at regulating noise emissions from new consumer products and did little to help communities deal with their problems. In 1978, Congress amended the NCA to include the Quiet Communities Act. This set of amendments authorized the EPA to assist local and state governments in developing noise reduction programs that would meet their specific needs. Through the amendments, federal dollars were provided to help the local governments put their programs into action.

Policy regarding noise pollution can be summed up by stating that most people see noise as a nuisance and not as a health problem. Until noise pollution becomes recognized as detrimental to health, it will continue to be overlooked and underfunded.

Educational Programs

Another approach to noise control is through education. The goal in this approach is to alter the behavior of those generating the noise, thereby reducing noise at the source. So far, little measurable progress has been achieved through noise education programs, and no model noise education program has been widely accepted. One that has been proposed by Purdom (1980) recommends the following activities:

workshops for both the public and private sectors; noise pollution reminders from the media; school curricula for noise pollution; and environmental graphics such as bumper stickers, posters, buttons and billboards to remind people of the need to control noise.

Environmental Changes

Once people are compelled to act, either by means of law or education, noise abatement can be achieved through environmental modification. This modification can be made at the source of the noise, to the path it travels, or to the exposed parties.[1] An example of reducing noise at its source is the common practice of placing a computer printer in a padded compartment. An example of altering the path on which noise travels can be seen in the large dirt mound placed at the beginning of the airport runway to absorb the jet engine sound from surrounding areas. Ways to protect against damaging effects of noise pollution include wearing ear protection in the form of earplugs or headsets, as is often practiced in manufacturing facilities.

CHAPTER SUMMARY

This chapter began with a discussion of the four components that make up our environmental system—life support systems, residues and wastes, human activities, and environmental hazards—and the importance of their interaction and synergistic existence. The remaining portions of the chapter provided overviews of the major wastes and pollution that the country deals with on a daily basis. Specifically, solid wastes, hazardous wastes, air pollution, water pollution, radiation and noise pollution were discussed. A common theme in each discussion was that, while most of these problems have been with us for years, it has only been recently (since the first Earth Day in April 1970) that public concern has forced the government to become active in dealing with these associated issues. For the most part, the solutions to correct each of these problems currently exist; however, the population as a whole has not placed a high enough priority on conserving the environment to preserve it.

REVIEW QUESTIONS

1. Name the four components of Purdom's environmental system. What is the contribution of each?

2. Why are there more environmental problems today than ever before?

3. What are the primary sources of solid waste? Why are municipal wastes such a problem?

4. What piece of federal legislation deals with "cradle-to-grave" regulation of solid and hazardous waste?

5. Define the following terms: *sanitary landfill, incineration, recycling,* and *source reduction.* Provide one advantage and one disadvantage for each process.

6. What is a bottle bill?

7. Define the term *hazardous waste* and give several examples.

8. How is a secured landfill different from a sanitary one?

9. The Superfund was part of what legislation? What is the Superfund used for?

10. What is the Number 1 source of air pollution?

11. In what forms can air pollutants be found?

12. What are the six criteria air pollutants?

13. What is the Pollutant Standard Index?

14. Outline the process and conditions that result in acid rain.

15. Why is the ozone layer thinning?

16. How does the greenhouse effect result in global warming?

17. What relationship is there between photochemical smog and thermal inversion?

18. Why was the Clean Air Act so important to the United States?

19. Name the six major indoor air pollutants.

20. Why is there so much concern about radon?

21. What is meant by *sick building syndrome?*

22. What makes water so important to life?

23. What is the difference between point source and nonpoint source pollution?

24. What are the two primary water-related issues?

25. How do the federal Water Pollution Control Act amendments and additional amendments help to protect the water supply?

26. Name and briefly describe the steps in waste water treatment.

27. What is a septic system?

28. What is radiation?

29. What types of human behavior increase exposure to radiation?

30. What type of radiation is most dangerous to humans? Why?

31. What is the most important part of the Nuclear Waste Policy Act?

32. What is noise?

33. Explain what is meant by *frequency* and *amplitude.*

34. What are decibels? What do they measure?

35. At what level of government does one find most of the noise ordinances?

SCENARIO: ANALYSIS AND RESPONSE

As you know from reading this chapter, the problem Mary and Tom face is not so uncommon. The National Priority List (NPL) associated with the Superfund legislation has over 1,300 known hazardous waste sites that still need to be cleaned up.

Knowing what you now know about polluted water, what could Mary and Tom have done before purchasing their house to try to insure against such a problem? If you were confronted with the problem that Mary and Tom now face, how would you handle it? Would you continue to live in the home, or would you move? If you planned to sell the house, would you tell the realtor or prospective buyers about the problem? Is it fair that Mary and Tom are faced with this problem? Name five things you could do to help prevent such a problem in the future.

ACTIVITIES

1. In order for all of us to be better stewards of our environment, we need to be aware of how our community handles various important environmental issues. Find the answers to the following questions about your community and state:

   How does your community dispose of solid waste?

   How far do you live from a secured landfill? What is the closest community to it?

   Where does your community get its water? If you personally get your water from a well, when was the last time the water was evaluated?

   Where is the closest nuclear power plant to your home? What are you supposed to do in case of an accident?

   Does your state/community have a clean indoor air act? If it does, briefly describe it.

   Does your community have a noise ordinance? If so, briefly describe it.

   What is the most recent piece of legislation your community has enacted to protect the environment? Do you agree with it? Why or why not?

2. Write a one-page paper describing either your support for or opposition to nuclear power plants.

3. In a one-page paper, identify what you feel to be the Number 1 waste or pollution problem faced by the United States, and then detail your rationale for feeling this way.

4. For two weeks, watch a television weather program that mentions the Pollutant Standard Index. During that two-week period, chart the PSI in a graph form and identify the major pollutant for each day.

5. During the next week, create a list of at least ten things you could have done to conserve the water you use.

REFERENCES

1. Purdom, P. W. (1980). Environment and Health. In P. W. Purdom, ed. *Environmental Health,* 2nd ed. San Diego: Academic Press, pp. 1–33.

2. White, G. F., ed. (1974). *Natural Hazards.* London: Oxford Univ. Press.

3. Nadakavukaren, A. (1990). *Man and Environment: A Health Perspective,* 3rd ed. Prospect Heights, Ill.: Waveland Press.

4. Enger, E. D., and B. F. Smith (1992). *Environmental Science: A Study of Interrelationships,* 4th ed. Dubuque, Ia.: Wm. C. Brown.

5. Curtis, D., and B. W. Walsh, eds. (1992). *Environmental Quality: The Twenty-Second Annual Report of the Council on Environmental Quality Together with the President's Message to Congress.* Washington, D.C.: U.S. Government Printing Office.

6. U.S. Congressional Budget Office (1985). *Hazardous Waste Management: Recent Changes and Policy Alternatives.* Washington, D.C.: U.S. Government Printing Office.

7. Hertzberg, R., and D. Kies (1983). "A Primer on Waste Exchanges." *Resource Recycling* 1(6).

8. Abelson, P. H. (1989). "Editorial: Cleaning Hazardous Waste Sites." *Science* 246(4934): 1.

9. Flavin, C. (1988). The Heat Is On. *World-Watch,* Nov.–Dec.: 10–20.

10. Piver, W. T. (1991). "Global Atmospheric Changes. *Environmental Health Perspectives* 96 (Dec.): 131–137.

11. Benarde, M. A. (1989). *Our Precarious Habitat: Fifteen Years Later.* New York: John Wiley & Sons.

12. Samet, J. M., and J. D. Spengler, eds. (1991). *Indoor Air Pollution: A Health Perspective.* Baltimore: The Johns Hopkins Univ. Press., p. 23.

13. Lioy, P. J. (1989). *INFO Sheet: Indoor Air Pollution.* Piscataway, N.J.: Environmental and Occupational Health Sciences Institute.

14. Spengler, J. D. (1991). Sources and Concentration of Indoor Air Pollution. In J. M. Samet and J. D.

Spengler, eds. *Indoor Air Pollution: A Health Perspective* (pp. 33–67). Baltimore: The Johns Hopkins Univ. Press.

15. American Medical Association (1990). *Radon: The Health Threat with a Simple Solution: A Physician's Guide.* Chicago: Author.

16. National Institute for Occupational Safety and Health (1991). *Environmental Tobacco Smoke in the Workplace: Lung Cancer and Other Health Effects* (DHHS [NIOSH] pub. no. 91-108). Cincinnati: Author.

17. Miller, G. T. (1990). *Living in the Environment,* 6th ed. Belmont, Calif.: Wadsworth.

18. Kreiss, K. (1990). "The Sick Building Syndrome: Where Is the Epidemiological Basis?" *American Journal of Public Health* 80(10): 1172–1173.

19. Kirsch, L. S. (1991). "Legal Aspects of Indoor Air Pollution." In J. M. Samet and J. D. Spengler, eds. *Indoor Air Pollution: A Health Perspective* (pp. 379–397). Baltimore: The Johns Hopkins Univ. Press.

20. Spengler, J. D. and J. M. Samet (1991). "A Perspective on Indoor and Outdoor Air Pollution." In J.

M. Samet and J. D. Spengler, eds. *Indoor Air Pollution: A Health Perspective* (pp. 1–29). Baltimore: The Johns Hopkins Univ. Press.

21. Null, G. (1990). *Clearer, Cleaner, Safer, Greener: A Blueprint for Detoxifying Your Environment.* New York: Villard Books.

22. Stewart, J. C. (1990). *Drinking Water Hazards: How to Know if There Are Toxic Chemicals in Your Water and What to Do if There Are.* Hiram, Oh.: Envirographics.

23. Piver, W. T. (1989). "Preface." *Environmental Health Perspectives* 83(Nov.): 3–4.

24. Lamb, J. C. (1985). *Water Quality and Its Control.* New York: John Wiley & Sons.

25. Hammer, M. J. (1975) *Water and Waste-Water Technology.* New York: John Wiley & Sons.

26. Shapiro, J. (1990). *Radiation Protection: A Guide for Scientists and Physicians,* 3rd ed. Cambridge, Mass.: Harvard Univ. Press.

27. Dreyfus, D. A., and A. B. Ashby (1990). "Fueling Our Global Future." *Environment* 32(4): 17–20, 36–41.

Chapter 16

THE IMPACT OF ENVIRONMENT ON HUMAN HEALTH

Chapter Outline

Chapter Objectives

After studying this chapter you will be able to:

1. Define *environmental health.*
2. Explain the relationship among environmental sanitation, sanitary engineers, and sanitarians.
3. Explain the meaning of *water-borne, food-borne,* and *vector-borne diseases.*
4. Define *vectors.*
5. Explain the relationship between vectors and human health.
6. Define *pest, pesticides, target organism, hard pesticides,* and *soft pesticides.*
7. Identify the major categories of pesticides.
8. Define *environmental tobacco smoke, mainstream smoke, sidestream smoke,* and *passive smoking.*
9. Describe the legislation in place to deal with environmental tobacco smoke.
10. Explain why exposure to lead is so great.
11. Describe how lead poisoning could be reduced.
12. Identify the risks of skin cancer.
13. List the ABCD rule of melanoma.
14. Define *sun protection factor (SPF).*
15. Explain the relationship among Uranium-238, radon, and radon "daughters."
16. Describe the state of population growth in the world.
17. Interpret the relationship between population growth and human health.
18. Outline the solutions to population growth.
19. Define *natural disaster* and *disaster agent.*

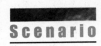

Pam and Gary were numb when their physician told them that the laboratory tests indicated that Gary had prostate cancer. Numb yes, shocked no, for Gary had served in Vietnam with the 151st Airborn Infantry Rangers in 1968–1969. During that time, his entire unit had been exposed to the herbicide Agent Orange, the defoliant used in Vietnam and Laos to eliminate enemy hiding places by destroying their crops. Agent Orange, comprised of an equal mixture of 2,4-D (2,4-dichlorophenoxyacetic acid) and 2,4 5-T (2,4 5-trichlorophenoxyacetic acid), was named for the bright orange stripes on the steel drums in which it was contained. Later it was found that the 2,4 5-T was contaminated with an extremely toxic compound known as *dioxin*. Gary was aware that a number of other men in his unit had been diagnosed with cancer in the past couple of years, but he thought that somehow maybe the dreaded disease might have passed him by. Prior to the diagnosis Gary had suffered from rashes, and his skin always seemed dry.

INTRODUCTION

In the previous chapter, we presented the concept of an environmental system and explained the interrelationships of its components. We also detailed the concerns associated with the wastes and pollutants created by human activities. In this chapter, we focus on how certain components of the environmental system can cause health problems in humans. No attempt is made to discuss all environmental hazards in this chapter; we have only selected a few to discuss. This is for one primary reason: the number of environmental hazards is overwhelming. In fact, to date, only a small fraction of the environmental substances with the potential to harm human health have been studied.[1] Also note that several other chapters in this book discuss the impact of the environment on human health. For example, Chapter 4 includes material on microorganisms that are biological hazards. Chapter 11 includes information on stress, a psychological hazard. Chapter 17 presents information about the sociological environmental hazard of violence. And Chapter 18 contains a discussion about the specific environmental hazards found in the workplace.

To begin the discussion of environmental health, we would like to present the definitions of two key terms. First, is the word *environment*. *Environment* is defined as all that affects an organism during its lifetime.[2] In turn, **environmental health** refers to characteristics of environmental conditions that affect the health and well-being of humans. It is a part of the larger concept of public health.[3]

There is no doubt that the hazards in the environment have produced ill health. For example, overexposure to ultraviolet light has produced both serious sunburns and skin cancer; lead poisoning has been shown to cause brain damage in the young; and it is known that photochemical smog irritates the eyes and lungs. However, it is close to impossible to determine the impact of many environmental conditions on health. For example, does acid rain con

---

environmental health Characteristics of environmental conditions that affect the health and well-being of humans.

tribute to respiratory disease, or do agricultural pesticides increase the risk of cancer among farmers? (See Figure 16.1.)[4]

One of the major obstacles to pinpointing the impact of environmental hazards on human health is the difficulty of controlling all the associated variables during the research process. For example, look at the difficulty in just trying to take a simple air sample. A sample taken in one part of a building may be quite different than one taken on another floor of the same building. Furthermore, the factors associated with air quality are constantly changing, and those who breath the air all have different levels of susceptibility because of such factors as age, gender, personal behavior, genetic makeup, present health status, and exposure to other substances. This does not even take into account that some environmental hazards interact with one another synergistically, like asbestos and cigarette smoke.[1]

No matter whether the environment contributes a little or a lot to disease, the tragedy is that all environmental-induced disease is highly preventable.[5] Communities influence their health by the ways in which they adopt and control technologies, permit the transport and storage of hazardous wastes through and in the community, and dispose of wastes. Individuals influence their health and the health of those around them via their behavior. Choices about what they eat and drink, whether

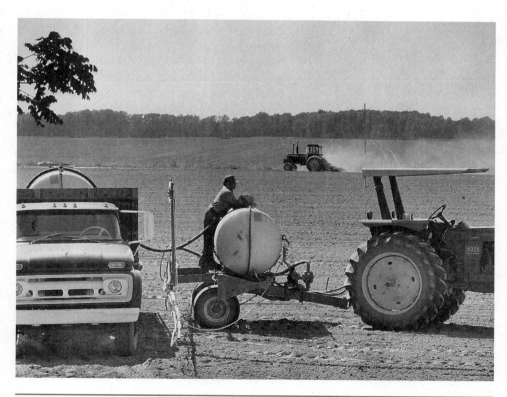

FIGURE 16.1

At what risk for cancer are farmers because of the pesticides they use?

they smoke, how they live and work can promote or jeopardize the health of those in the community.[1]

BIOLOGICAL HAZARDS AND HUMAN HEALTH

Biologically, the environment is a hazardous place. Life and death struggles between species for food, water, and shelter persist every hour and minute of every day. For each living species, there are natural enemies—predators, parasites, and disease agents, which can be considered biological hazards. Communities are just as much at risk as are individuals.

Biological hazards are living organisms (and viruses), or their products, that are harmful to humans. These may be animals or plants (such as poison ivy or poison oak), but are usually viruses or microbes such as bacteria.

In some community and public health texts, this topic can be found under the heading of **environmental sanitation,** the practice of effecting healthy or hygienic conditions in the environment. Since the immediate source of many biological hazards is humans themselves, the improper handling of human waste and waste water can jeopardize the health of the community.

The protection of communities from diseases that can result from the mismanagement of waste water or solid waste is the job of the **sanitary engineer.** This person is assisted by **sanitarians,** who inspect facilities and report breakdowns or violations of the public health code. Failure to maintain the integrity of the water supply can result in epidemics of **water-borne diseases;** those transmitted via fecal contamination of drinking water. Sanitarians also have a responsibility to inspect facilities to protect the food supply, which if improperly managed, can cause a number of **food-borne diseases.** Overflow of waste water into open fields and ditches or the mismanagement of solid waste near human habitation can result in epidemics of **vector-borne diseases**—diseases transmitted by insects.

Water-Borne Diseases

Water-borne agents continue to cause disease in the United States and around the world (see Figure 16.2). These diseases may be caused by viruses, bacteria, and protozoans (one-celled animals). Water-borne viral agents and the diseases they cause include poliomyelitis virus (polio) and Hepatitis A virus (hepatitis). Water-borne bacteria and the diseases they cause include *Salmonella typhi* (typhoid fever), *Shigella* spp. (shigellosis or bacillary dysentery), and *Vibrio cholerae* (cholera). Water-borne parasites include the protozoa *Entamoeba histolytica* (amebiasis or amoebic dysentery) and *Giardia lamblia* (giardiasis, lambliasis, or giardia enteritis). Each of these diseases can be serious (see Figure 16.3), and two in particular—typhoid fever and cholera—

---

biological hazards   Living organisms (and viruses), or their products, that are harmful to humans.

environmental sanitation   The practice of effecting healthy or hygienic conditions in the environment.

sanitary engineer   Environmental worker responsible for management of waste water and solid waste for a community.

sanitarians   Environmental workers responsible for inspection of facilities and investigation of complaints with regard to public health codes.

water-borne diseases   Diseases that are transmitted via fecal contamination of water.

food-borne diseases   Diseases that are transmitted via contaminated food.

vector-borne diseases   Diseases that are transmitted by insects.

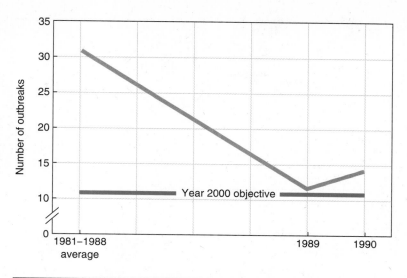

	1981–1988	1989	1990	Year 2000 Target
Outbreaks	31	12	14	11

FIGURE 16.2

Outbreaks of water-borne disease, United States, 1981–1988 average, 1989, 1990, and target for the year 2000.

From: U.S. Dept. of Health and Human Services, National Center for Health Statistics (1993). Healthy People 2000 Review 1992 *(DHHS pub. no. PHS-93-1232-1). Washington, D.C.: U.S. Government Printing Office.*

have killed thousands of people in single epidemics (see Table 16.1).

For the past ten years, the Number 1 agent in water-borne outbreaks in the United States has been the protozoal parasite *Giardia lamblia*.[6] Of the bacteria, *Shigella sonnei* was the most common pathogen reported. Another agent, *Cryptosporidium,* caused an outbreak of illness in 13,000 people in Georgia. Still another outbreak, a virus transported in commercial ice, caused illness in 5,000 people in several states. It is estimated that between 1971 and 1988, 136,833 cases of water-borne illness occurred; 43% of these outbreaks occurred via community water supply systems (see Box 16.1).

Public health laws that set standards for water and waste water treatment facilities and plumbing are a community's first line of defense against such epidemics. Chlorination of the water supply is a further safeguard. While epidemics of water-borne diseases do occur in the United States, they are more frequent in less-developed countries, where water is often not treated before being consumed. Wars and natural disasters such as floods and hurricanes, which disrupt normal water supplies, can result in epidemics of water-borne diseases.

Food-Borne Diseases

One way in which humans interact with their environment is by ingesting bits of it.

Table 16.1
Water-Borne Biological Hazards*

Hazard	Agent	Disease
Viruses	Poliomyelitis virus	Polio
	Hepatitis A virus	Infectious hepatitis
Bacteria	Vibrio cholerae	Cholera
	Salmonella typhi	Typhoid fever
	Shigella spp.	Bacillary dysentery
	Leptospira spp.	Leptospirosis
Protozoans (parasites)	Entamoeba histolitica	Amoebic dysentery
	Giardia lamblia	Giardiasis

*Generated from information derived from Benenson, A. S., ed (1990). *Control of Communicable Diseases in Man.* Washington, D.C.: American Public Health Assn.

BOX 16.1
Healthy People 2000— Objective

11.3 Reduce outbreaks of water-borne disease from infectious agents and chemical poisoning to no more than 11 per year. (Baseline: Average of 31 outbreaks per year during 1981–88)

Type-Specific Target

Average Annual Number of Water-Borne Disease Outbreaks	*1981–1988 Baseline*	*2000 Target*
11.3a People served by community water systems	13	6

Note: Community water systems are public- or investor-owned water systems that serve large or small communities, subdivisions, or trailer parks with at least 15 service connections or 25 yearround residents.

Baseline data source: Water-Borne Surveillance System, CDC.

For Further Thought

Do you know of anyone who has become ill from drinking water? If so, what were the circumstances, how ill was the person, and what was the causative agent?

The act of eating is, in effect, a way of bringing biological hazards into intimate contact with the tissues that line the intestinal tract. In these cases, food is the vehicle; and the agents can be viruses, bacteria, or parasites.

The Centers for Disease Control and Prevention defines a **food-borne outbreak** as an incident, confirmed by an epidemiological analysis, in which a commonly ingested food is the source of a similar illness in two or more people. Exceptions are that a single case of botulism or chemical poisoning is considered an outbreak.[7]

During the five-year period 1983–1987, 2,397 outbreaks of food-borne disease were reported, involving 91,678 cases; 139 more of these cases ended in death. The causative agent was not established in 62% of these outbreaks. In 66% of the outbreaks (92% of cases) in which the etiology was established, the agent was a bacterial pathogen. Viruses accounted for 5% of the outbreaks and 5% of the cases while parasites accounted for 4% of the outbreaks and less than 1% of the cases. Nonbiological agents accounted for the remainder, 26% of the outbreaks and 2% of the cases (see Figures 16.4 and 16.5).[7]

food-borne outbreak An incident, confirmed by an epidemiological analysis, in which a commonly ingested food is the source of a similar illness in two or more people.

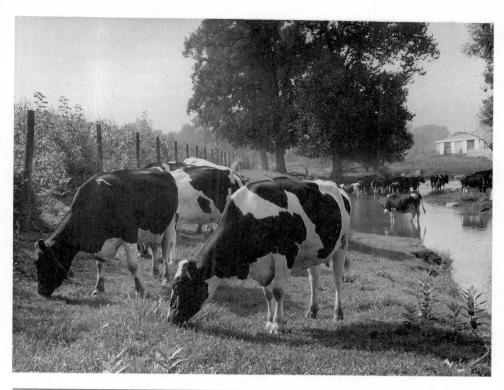

FIGURE 16.3

Outbreaks of water-borne diseases occur when drinking water becomes contaminated.

More than half (57%) of the bacterial disease outbreaks during 1983–1987 were traced to *Salmonella* (see Figure 16.6). Other bacteria to which multiple outbreaks were attributed were *Clostridium botulinum, Staphylococcus aureus, Clostridium perfringens,* and *Shigella.* Viruses implicated in food-borne disease outbreaks are Hepatitis A and Norwalk virus. Parasites identified were *Trichinella spiralis* and *Giardia.*

Almost any food can serve as a vehicle of transmission for a food-borne disease agent. The vehicle of infection for more than half of the cases was unknown. In another large proportion of cases, multiple foods were incriminated. Delicatessens, cafeterias, or restaurants were reported nearly twice as often as homes as places where the contaminated food was eaten. Also, more cases occur in the summer months than during any other season.[7]

The Number 1 contributing factor that preceded an outbreak of food-borne diseases was improper holding temperature for foods. This was followed by poor personal hygiene of preparers, inadequate cooking, contaminated equipment, and obtaining food from an unsafe source, such as shellfish from polluted waters.

To protect the public from food-borne diseases, sanitarians inspect restaurants and other food-serving establishments, such as churches and schools, to make sure that environmental conditions favorable to the

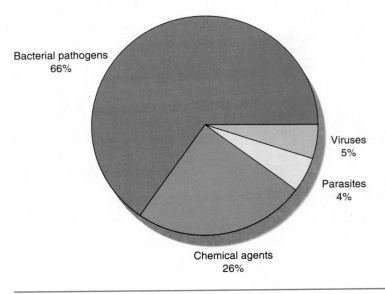

FIGURE 16.4

Outbreaks of food-borne disease by cause, United States, 1983–1987.

From: Centers for Disease Control (1990). "Food-borne Disease Outbreaks, 5-Year Summary, 1983–1987." In "CDC Surveillance Summaries, March, 1990," MMWR 1990; 34 (no. 55-1):15–57.

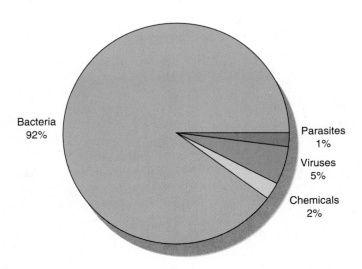

FIGURE 16.5

Cases of food-borne disease by cause, United States, 1983–1987.

From: Centers for Disease Control (1990). "Food-borne Disease Outbreaks, 5-Year Summary, 1983–1987." In "CDC Surveillance Summaries, March, 1990," MMWR 1990; 34 (no. 55-1):15–57.

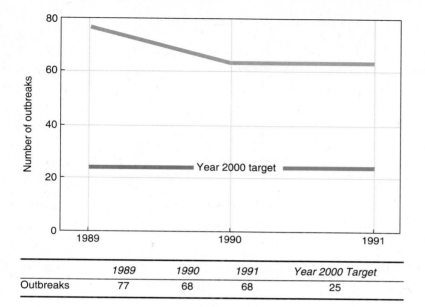

	1989	1990	1991	Year 2000 Target
Outbreaks	77	68	68	25

FIGURE 16.6

Food-borne disease outbreaks due to *Salmonella enteritidis,* United States, 1989–1991, and the target for the year 2000.

growth and development of pathogens do not exist. Sanitarians also inspect retail food outlets (grocery stores and supermarkets) to insure that foods are held at proper temperature to inhibit growth of biological hazards. By promulgating and enforcing food safety laws, public health officials protect the community.

Vector-Borne Diseases

Standing water, including runoff water from overflowing septic tanks or overloaded sewer systems, and improperly handled solid waste are more than unsavory sights. They provide habitat for and support the proliferation of disease vectors (see Figure 16.7). A vector is an invertebrate, usually an insect, that transmits microscopic disease agents to vertebrate hosts. Examples of vectors and the diseases they transmit include mosquitoes (St. Louis encephalitis), fleas (murine typhus, plague), lice (epidemic typhus), and ticks (Rocky Mountain spotted fever). (See Table 16.2.)

Mosquito larvae require standing water in which to complete their development. The improper handling of waste water or inadequate drainage of rainwater provides an ideal habitat for mosquitoes, particularly the northern house mosquito, *Culex pipiens. Culex pipiens* is the most important vector of St. Louis encephalitis (SLE) in the eastern United States. In California, the SLE virus is transmitted by another mosquito species, *Culex tarsalis,* which proliferates in mismanaged irrigation water. SLE is a disease to which the elderly are particularly susceptible. Those at greatest risk live in unscreened houses without air conditioning—usually in the poorer areas.

Another species of mosquito that thrives on environmental mismanagement is the eastern tree hole mosquito, *Aedes triseriatus.* While the natural habitat for this mosquito is tree holes, it flourishes in water held in discarded automobile and truck tires. It is estimated there are 2 billion used tires discarded in various places in the United States today, and 2 million more discarded tires are added to the environment each year. In the eastern United States, *Aedes triseriatus* is the vector for LaCrosse encephalitis, a serious and sometimes fatal disease of children.

Tires are also the favored habitat of the newly arrived asian tiger mosquito, *Aedes albopictus.* Since 1985, when this species was first discovered in Houston, Texas, it has been reported from 345 United States counties in 22 states.[8] The tiger mosquito arrived in the United States in used tires imported from Japan. Disease transmission experiments indicate that *Ae. albopictus* can transmit LaCrosse encephalitis, dengue fever, and Japanese B encephalitis. Larvae of the Asian tiger mosquito can develop in water held in almost any artificial container, including discarded cups and plastic wrap.

Improper management of solid waste—such as occurs at open dumps, ill-managed landfills, and urban slums—fosters the expansion of rat and mouse populations. These rodents are hosts for fleas, which transmit marine typhus, a rickettsial disease characterized by headache, fever, and rash. If the rodent population should decline rapidly because of disease or a successful rodent control program, these fleas could come into contact with humans and spread the disease directly to them. Diseases of animals that are transmissible to humans, such as murine typhus, are referred to as *zoonoses.*

Perhaps the most devastating zoonosis of all time is plague (see Chapter 1). The disease, caused by the bacterium *Yersinia pestis,* is often present in wild rodent populations such as rock squirrels in the southwest and ground squirrels in western forests. If the disease were to find its way into urban rodent populations and these populations were to become uncontrollably large, an epizoodemic could occur in which first rats, then humans, would be stricken with disease. As the rats die, their fleas, infected with the plague bacteria, jump on hu-

Table 16.2
Vector-Borne Biological Hazards[*]

Hazard	Agent	Vector	Disease
Virus	SLE virus	Mosquito	St. Louis encephalitis
	LaCrosse	Mosquito	LaCrosse encephalitis
Rickettsiae	*Rickettsia typhi*	Flea	Murine typhus
	Rickettsia rickettsii	Tick	Rocky Mountain spotted fever
Bacteria	*Yersinia pestis*	Flea	Bubonic plaque
	Borrelia burgdorferi	Tick	Lyme disease
Protozoa	*Plasmodium* spp.	Mosquito	Malaria
Nematodes	*Wuchereria bancrofti*	Mosquito	Filariasis (elephantiasis)

[*]Generated from data derived from Benenson, A. S., ed. (1990). *Control of Communicable Diseases in Man.* Washington, D.C.: American Public Health Association.

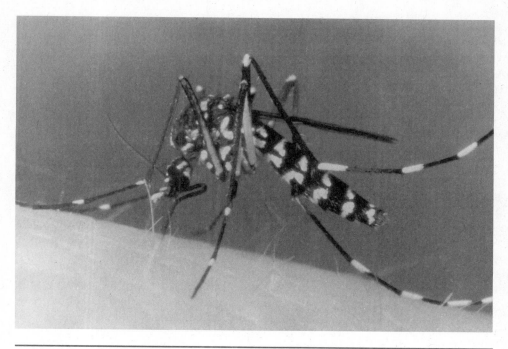

FIGURE 16.7

Asian tiger mosquitoes are the vectors that transmit two kinds of encephalitis and dengue fever.

mans. When they attempt to feed on the human, they transmit the disease agent. This is one reason why rodent control is an important community health service.

CHEMICAL HAZARDS AND HUMAN HEALTH

It is somewhat ironic to think that the very same chemical technology that permits us to modify the environment for our use, such as better insulated homes, crop protection, and more-effective medications, also poses a hazard to our health. Yet every day, the health of thousands is compromised by **chemical hazards,** which result from the mismanagement of the chemicals. Measure-

ment of these hazards is difficult because not all people exposed to chemical hazards react in the same way: some develop disease, others do not. For example, not all of the men of the 151st Airborn Infantry Unit who had been exposed to Agent Orange in Vietnam developed cancer. This phenomenon has been explained by the U.S. Department of Health and Human Services with the following statements:[1]

1. "There are variations among individuals in the concentration of the substance in their immediate environment and in the other kinds of toxins and chemicals to which they have been exposed."
2. "There is a variation among individuals in **pharmacokinetics** [rate of absorption, distribution, metabolism, excretion

---

chemical hazards Hazards caused by the mismanagement of chemicals.

pharmacokinetics Rate of absorption, distribution, metabolism, and excretion of substances from the body.

of substances from the body]: namely, those factors that govern the amount or concentration of the biologically active form of the toxic substance reaching target sites (places in the body where the substance is most active)."

3. "There is a variation among individuals in pharmacodynamics: namely, those factors that govern the reaction of active forms of the toxic substance with the body's target sites."

4. "There is a variation among individuals in factors that govern the progression of the successive chemical and biological reactions caused by the toxic substance within the body, reactions that ultimately may result in reversible or irreversible disease processes."

To examine the impact of chemicals on human health, we present information on pesticides, environmental tobacco smoke, and lead.

Pesticides

From a biological standpoint, there is no such thing as a "pest"; that is, mother nature has no favored species. The term **pest** is purely a human concept and refers to any organism (whether it is a multicelled animal or plant or a microbe) that has an adverse effect on human interests. Fortunately, the human species has the intelligence to moderate and counterbalance the actions of most pests. For example, by carefully managing the environment, the population of some pests, like the vectors discussed earlier in this chapter, is reduced. Humans also have the ability to create chemical solutions that eliminate some un-

wanted pests. Without chemical insecticides, it has been estimated that the agricultural production of the United States would decrease by 30% or more, food prices would soar, and there would be a distinct danger of starvation in this country. Developing countries would suffer even more from hunger and diseases without insecticides.[9] Though there are a number of ways of dealing with pests, such as mixing crops, crop rotation, and plant genetics to breed pest-resistant strains, many still rely on chemical pest control. However, it is this pest control strategy that causes the greatest potential for health problems.[10,11]

Pesticides are, for the most part, synthetic chemicals, developed and manufactured for the purpose of killing pests. While chemical companies market these chemicals to control a particular pest, most of them in fact kill a wide range of organisms. The pest organism against which the pesticide is applied is referred to as the **target pest** or **target organism** (see Table 16.3). All other organisms in the environment that may also be affected are called **nontarget organisms.** For example, most weed killers will not only kill the weeds, but also (nontarget) flowers and ornamental plant vegetation. Similarly, it is not uncommon for domestic animals to be poisoned and killed by rodenticides (rat poison). Some pesticides are also very toxic to humans. Overexposure to these chemicals can have adverse effects on their health.

The two most widely used pesticides are **herbicides** (pesticides to kill plants) and

---

pest Any organism—a multicelled animal or plant, or a microbe—that has an adverse effect on human interests.

pesticides Synthetic chemicals developed and manufactured for the purpose of killing pests.

target organism (target pest) The organism (or pest) for which a pesticide is applied.

nontarget organisms All other susceptible organisms in the environment, for which a pesticide was not intended.

herbicide Pesticide to kill plants.

Table 16.3
Types of Pesticides

Type of Agent	Target Pest to Be Destroyed
Acaricides/miticides	Mites
Bactericides	Bacteria
Fungicides	Fungi molds
Herbicides	Weeds
Insecticides	Insects
Larvicides/grubicides	Insect larvae
Molluscicides	Snails, slugs
Nematocides	Worms
Rodenticides	Rats, mice

insecticides (pesticides to kill insects). It is also from these two pesticides that most human pesticide poisonings occur. The two groups at highest risk for pesticide poisoning are young children and the workers who apply the pesticides. Many of these individuals are included in the 7.7 million persons living on farms or engaged in farm work in the United States.[12] Poisonings occur when the pesticides are consumed orally, inhaled, or when they come in contact with the skin. The majority of children poisoned by pesticides consume them orally. These are frequently unintentional poisonings that occur when pesticides are left within reach of children. Most adult poisonings occur because of careless practice. Examples include eating without washing hands after handling pesticides, mouth-siphoning to move pesticides from one container to another, applying pesticides while one's skin is exposed, or spilling the pesticide on one's body.

In agricultural settings, poisonings can occur when agricultural workers misuse pesticides. For example, illiterate workers or those who do not read English may enter sprayed fields too soon because of the inability to read product directions or posted warning signs. Their employers may even tell them to enter the field too soon, and the workers' children may be with them. In other cases, workers cannot follow the safety instructions printed on the labels.[11]

Exposures may be acute (one-time cases) or chronic (low-level exposure over an extended period of time). The effects of poisoning depend on many things, including the characteristics of the person exposed, the kind of pesticide, and the type and length of exposure. Some signals of poisoning are headaches, weakness, rashes, fatigue, and dizziness. More serious effects include cancer, mutations, birth defects, respiratory problems, convulsions, coma, and death.

Ideally, pesticide poisoning could be eliminated if a perfect pesticide could be produced and then used properly. Enger and Smith[3] stated that

> a perfect pesticide would have the following characteristics:
>
> 1. It would be inexpensive.
> 2. It would affect only the target organism.
> 3. It would have a short half-life.
> 4. It would break down into harmless materials.

Unfortunately, there is no such thing as a perfect pesticide. Developing a good pesticide is expensive because it requires years of research and testing. There are very good products available, which when used properly, are safe and effective.

An important characteristic of a pesticide is persistence. In the past, a majority of pesticides were very stable chemical compounds; that is, they had long half-lives. These pesticides are referred to as **hard pesticides.** This persistence was both good

---

insecticide   Pesticide to kill insects.

hard pesticide (persistent pesticide)   One that has a long-lasting effect.

and bad. It is good because one application can be counted on to have a long-lasting effect. Dichloro-diphenyl-trichloroethane (DDT) is the best example of a hard pesticide. While this chemical has saved more lives than any other through the killing of pest insects, its use was eventually banned because of its accumulation in the environment. Because persistent pesticides can become attached to the soil, they can also be transported—which means they will be carried to parts of the environment where they were not intended to go, thus exposing nonpests.

Beginning in the 1960s, a new generation of pesticides arrived on the market. These **soft pesticides** were less persistent, breaking down into harmless products within weeks. In the 1970s, even less-persistent chemicals were developed, with half-lives measured in days or hours. Many of these are still in use today. Many are not species-specific, and some are more toxic to humans and other animals than the hard pesticides.[2]

The immediate solutions to the problems of pesticide poisoning and environmental quality are better education about the safe use of pesticides, the government's ability to regulate safe products, and better compliance by the users to assure that the products are used in accordance with the instructions on the label. The long-term solution is to continue the research to develop better and better pesticides.

Environmental Tobacco Smoke

Approximately 25.5% (45.8 million) of adult Americans smoke cigarettes.[13] As a result, many nonsmokers are exposed to environmental tobacco smoke. As noted in

---

soft pesticide A less-persistent pesticide that breaks down into harmless products within weeks.

Chapter 15, environmental tobacco smoke (ETS), also known as *secondhand smoke,* includes both sidestream smoke and mainstream smoke. The process of inhaling ETS is referred to as passive smoking.

The association between ETS and adverse health effects has been demonstrated in a number of different epidemiological studies.[14, 15, 16] These studies provide evidence that adults exposed to ETS have an increased relative risk of lung cancer and possibly heart disease.[16] In addition, the studies show that about 50% of all American children five years of age and under have been exposed to ETS from prenatal maternal smoking and or sidestream smoke from household members after their birth (see Figure 16.8). Such exposure has been shown to increase the risk of adverse prenatal consequences and postnatal health conditions in infants. Specifically, this exposure may cause intrauterine growth retardation, low birth weight, preterm delivery, respiratory tract infections, and behavioral and cognitive abnormalities.[14]

Even though the research to date does not indicate a cause-effect relationship between ETS and ill health, a large body of evidence indicates that ETS is detrimental to human health. It is known that tobacco smoke contains about 4,000 substances, many of which have carcinogenic and mutagenic properties. The obvious solution to eliminate the increased health risks associated with ETS is to eliminate exposure to ETS. Though many people do their best to avoid ETS, it is not always possible. In fact, many individuals who report no exposure to ETS have low concentrations of cotinine (a metabolite of nicotine) in their urine, indicating they have indeed been exposed.[16] Such evidence led the EPA to issue a report on January 7, 1993, classifying ETS as a Group A carcinogen (known human carcinogen), like asbestos. In that report, the EPA stated that exposure to ETS is responsible for ap-

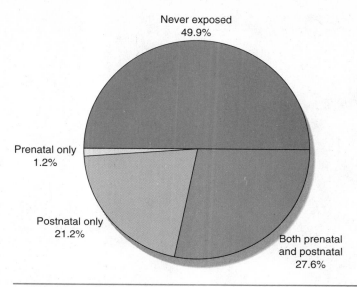

Never exposed
49.9%

Prenatal only
1.2%

Postnatal only
21.2%

Both prenatal
and postnatal
27.6%

FIGURE 16.8

Percentage of distribution of children five years of age and under by exposure to smoke before and after birth: United States, 1988.

From: Dept. of Health and Human Services, National Center for Health Statistics (1991). Pub no. (PHS) 91-1250. Hyattsville, Md.: U.S. Government Printing Office, p. 7.

proximately 3,000 lung cancer deaths per year in nonsmoking adults (see Figure 16.9).

Educational programs have been helpful in getting nonsmokers and smokers alike to understand the hazard of ETS. As a result, many nonsmokers attempt to avoid ETS, and many smokers have become more courteous about asking those around them for permission to smoke. At the same time, there are many smokers who believe that smoking whenever and wherever they wish is a right, not a privilege. It is these smokers who necessitate regulations against smoking in certain areas. Such regulation can originate at any level of government. For example, a federal regulation now prohibits smoking on all domestic air flights. Some states now have indoor clean air acts, which prohibit smoking in public places or restrict smoking to designated areas (see Box 16.2). Many communities throughout

the United States have adopted local ordinances, which regulate smoking in public places when state laws do not. It is anticipated that the EPA ruling on ETS as a carcinogen will have a ripple effect across the country and will increase the number of smoke-free public places.

In addition, many employers are now creating policies (administrative laws) that restrict or prohibit smoking in the workplace, on workplace grounds, and/or in company-owned vehicles. Many health agencies and health care facilities have led the way for smoke-free workplaces. Some of the smoking regulations are better than others. For example, many restaurants provide seating areas that are "no-smoking sections," but they are only an arm's length away from the smoking sections. Some employers prohibit smoking in common areas but allow it in individual offices.

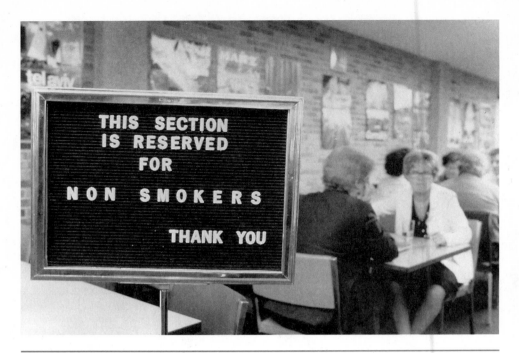

FIGURE 16.9
Environmental tobacco smoke is now considered a group A carcinogen.

Regulating smoking behavior, even though it makes perfectly good health sense, can cause hard feelings and much anger between smokers and nonsmokers. If regulation is going to be adopted, it should be jointly developed by representatives of all those impacted. The Association of Schools of Public Health has suggested the following procedure for developing smoking regulation in the workplace. Management and labor should work together to create appropriate policies, including some or all of the following:

- Prohibit smoking in the workplace and provide sufficient disincentives, such as fines, for those who do smoke.
- Provide information about health promotion and the adverse effects of smoking.
- Offer smoking cessation classes to all workers.

- Provide incentives (economic and otherwise) to encourage smokers to stop.[17]

Lead

Lead is a naturally occurring mineral element that is found throughout the environment and occurs in a variety of industrial products including electric batteries, pipe, solder, paint and plastic pigment, and leaded gasoline. (Note: Leaded gasoline has been outlawed in a number of states in the United States. Has it in yours?) Its industrial usefulness notwithstanding, lead can adversely affect human health. Lead poisoning is chronic in nature. The list of health problems that can occur is lengthy and in-

lead A naturally occurring mineral element that is found throughout the environment and which is produced in large quantities for industrial products.

cludes anemia, birth defects, bone damage, depression of neurological and psychological function, kidney damage, learning disabilities, miscarriages, and sterility[2,5,10,11,18,19] (see Table 16.4).

Humans are exposed to lead primarily by ingestion and inhalation. Those who are at greatest risk of lead poisoning are young children who may inadvertently ingest lead, adults whose jobs bring them in contact with lead, and people of all ages who live in homes with water pipes made of or soldered with lead. It has been estimated by the Centers for Disease Control and Prevention that 3–4 million American preschool children have elevated blood lead levels.[20] These young children consume lead by eating paint chips or dust in older dwellings that

---

BOX 16.2
Protect Indoor Air

On October 1, 1992, the state of Florida began to enforce its revised Clean Indoor Air Act in order to improve public health. Under the act, it is now illegal to smoke in health care and day care centers. The common areas of retirement homes, condominiums, and corridors, lobbies, stairways, and conference rooms of public places can no longer include smoking sections. Designated smoking areas in schools have also been outlawed. And restaurants that seat more than 50 people must reserve at least 35% of their seats for nonsmokers.

If smokers are caught violating this law, they can be fined $100 for the first offense and up to $500 for repeated offenses. When asked why she endorsed such legislation, State Representative Elaine Bloom, a prime sponsor of the measure, stated, "The high cost of health care is literally killing us, so anything we can do to minimize the burdens in the health care system is all to the good."

---

were painted with lead-base paint (see Figure 16.10). Lead paint has not been used indoors since 1940 and has been used only on a limited basis outdoors since 1971. But many older homes still have layers of old paint under newer coats. Children also consume lead by eating vegetation that has absorbed lead, primarily from auto emissions that have settled on its leaves, and by drinking water that contains lead. Such ingested lead poses a much greater health threat for small children than for adults. Whereas only 10% of the lead ingested by adults passes from the intestine into the bloodstream, 50% of the lead swallowed by preschoolers remains in their bodies. This makes these youngsters the highest risk group in the population.[11]

An example of the lead in the environment is illustrated by a study conducted in California. Because of great concern for exposing children to high concentrations of environmental lead, the California Department of Health Services conducted a study to measure the lead levels in: (1) children's blood (BLLs), (2) household paint, and (3) soil from three selected high-risk areas in California. The percentage of children with elevated BLLs (the "threshold of concern" for lead is 10 micrograms per deciliter [ugldL] of whole blood) ranged from 14%–67%. In addition, many of the dwellings in which the children lived and the soil in their respective yards contained high concentrations of lead[21] (see Table 16.5).

Occupational exposure to lead is the major source of lead intake for adults. Lead is produced for industrial use in larger quantities than any other heavy toxic metal. Though lead has many industrial uses, the most notable are in storage batteries and in gasoline. Inhaled lead poses a significant health threat because it enters the bloodstream rapidly.[11]

People of all age groups are exposed to lead if they consume water from lead pipes

Table 16.4
Summary of Lowest Observed Effect Levels
for Lead-Induced Health Effects in Adults and Children

BLL* (μg/dL)		Health Effect
>100	Adults:	Encephalopathic signs and symptoms
>80	Adults:	Anemia
	Children:	Encephalopathic signs and symptoms Chronic nephropathy (e.g., aminoaciduria)
>70	Adults:	Clinically evident peripheral neuropathy
	Children:	Colic and other gastrointestinal (GI) symptoms
>60	Adults:	Female reproductive effects Central nervous system symptoms (i.e., sleep disturbances, mood changes, memory and concentration problems, headaches)
>50	Adults:	Decreased hemoglobin production Decreased performance on neurobehavioral tests Altered testicular function GI symptoms (i.e., abdominal pain, constipation, diarrhea, nausea, anorexia)
	Children:	Peripheral neuropathy
>40	Adults:	Decreased peripheral nerve conduction Elevated blood pressure (white males aged 40–59 years) Chronic nephropathy
	Children:	Reduced hemoglobin synthesis
>25	Adults:	Elevated erythrocyte protoporphyrin levels in males
15–25	Adults:	Elevated erythrocyte protoporphyrin levels in females
	Children:	Decreased intelligence and growth
>10†	Fetus:	Preterm delivery Impaired learning Reduced birth weight Impaired mental ability

*Blood lead level.

†Safe BLLs have not been determined for fetuses.

From: Centers for Disease Control (1992). "Surveillance of Elevated Blood Lead Levels Among Adults—United States, 1992." *Morbidity and Mortality Weekly Report* 41(17): 288.

or pipes connected with lead solder. Lead pipes and solder can become corroded, and lead particles can be carried by the water. The EPA has estimated that about 40 million Americans who live in homes built before 1930 are drinking water containing more than the legally permissible level of lead (20 parts per billion). Around 1930, copper replaced lead as the metal of choice for water pipes. Federal laws now restrict the use of lead in pipe (no more than 8% lead) and solder (no more than 0.02% lead) in the installation and repair of public water systems. Some local governments have banned lead plumbing components altogether in drinking water systems.

It should also be noted that some well water used for drinking has been contaminated with lead by the inappropriate disposal of lead-containing materials such as old automobile batteries or solvents containing lead. Prior to passage of the laws governing disposal of toxic substances, it was very common for the toxic substance to end up in dumps or landfills where it could leak into the groundwater.

Yet another source of lead could be the community water supply. Traditionally, most water treatment facilities were designed to remove biological hazards such as pathogenic bacteria and protozoans and not lead and other heavy metals. As such, lead from gasoline and asbestos from brake linings that are carried into the streams by rainwater can enter the drinking water in communities that use surface water.

The solution to preventing lead poisoning includes several strategies: education, regulation, and prudent behavior. Educational efforts to inform people of the dangers of lead in paint have been in effect for a number of years; and for the most part, they seem to have been well received, even though there is still an unacceptable number of children being poisoned in this manner. The efforts to educate parents need to continue. National, state, and local laws have been useful in abating the lead poisoning problem. On the national level, the Lead-Based Paint Poisoning Prevention Act of 1971 initiated a national effort to identify children with lead poisoning and abate the sources in the environment. Passage of the Resource Conservation and Recovery Act (RCRA) in 1976 and the Comprehensive Environmental Response, Compensation, and

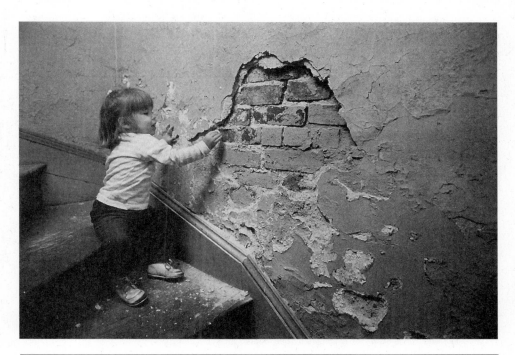

FIGURE 16.10

Lead poisoning from paint dust continues to be a problem in the United States.

Liability Act (CERCLA) in 1980 helped to regulate the disposal of lead-based products. Also at the federal level, the Lead Contamination Control Act of 1988 contributed to controlling lead poisoning. This act authorized the Centers for Disease Control and Prevention to provide grants to state and local agencies for comprehensive programs to: (1) screen infants and children for elevated blood lead levels, (2) ensure referral for medical and environmental intervention for infants and children who have been lead poisoned, and (3) provide educa-

tion to parents and children about childhood lead poisoning.[22]

An example of a state law to help abate lead poisoning was the enactment in January 1992 of a law to ban leaded gasoline in California. Similarly, a number of local governments have banned the use of lead materials in their water systems (see Box 16.3).

Both regulation and education are important in reducing lead poisoning; however, neither will be successful unless people heed safety advice and comply with

Table 16.5
Lead Concentrations in Paint from Survey Households in Selected High-Risk Areas—California, 1987–1990

Category	Oakland	Wilmington/ Compton	Sacramento
Number of households	358	350	232
Number with at least one interior paint sample	188	280	222
Geometric mean interior paint lead concentration (parts per million [ppm])	2,540	817	1,412
Range (ppm)	25–309,700	20–101,000	17–201,000
% with interior paint lead concentration ≥5000 ppm*	37%	13%	25%
Number with at least one exterior paint sample	215	268	218
Geometric mean exterior paint lead concentration (ppm)	13,545	3,100	8,430
Range (ppm)	9–347,900	9–216,200	57–320,000
% with exterior paint lead concentration ≥5000 ppm*	72%	45%	65%
Number with at least one soil sample	292	327	227
Geometric mean soil lead concentration (ppm)	897	188	236
Range (ppm)	50–88,000	30–2,000	26–2,700
% with soil lead concentration ≥1000 ppm†	46%	1%	5%

*According to U.S. Dept. of Housing and Urban Development guidelines, this is the level at which lead paint in public and Indian housing should be abated in comprehensive modernization programs (3).

†Threshold for hazardous waste under the California Dept. of Health Services' Toxic Substance Control Program.

From: Centers for Disease Control (1992). "Blood Lead Levels Among Children in High Risk Areas—California, 1987–1990." *Morbidity and Mortality Weekly Report* 41(17): 292.

BOX 16.3
Healthy People 2000—Objective

11.4 Reduce the prevalence of blood lead levels exceeding 15 µg/dL and 25 µg/dL among children aged six months through five years to no more than 500,000 and zero, respectively. (Baseline: An estimated 3 million children had levels exceeding 15 µg/dL, and 234,000 had levels exceeding 25 µg/dL, in 1984)

Special Population Target

Prevalence of Blood Lead Levels Exceeding 15 µg/dL & 25 µg/dL	1984 Baseline	2000 Target
11.4a Inner-city low-income black children (annual family income <$6,000 in 1984 dollars)	234,900 & 36,700	75,000 & 0

Baseline data sources: National Health and Nutrition Examination Survey, CDC; Agency for Toxic Substances and Disease Registry.

11.11 Perform testing for lead-based paint in at least 50% of homes built before 1950. (Baseline data not yet available)

11.16 Establish and monitor in at least 35 states plans to define and track sentinel environmental diseases. (Baseline: 0 states in 1990)

Note: Sentinel environmental diseases include lead poisoning, other heavy metal poisoning (e.g., cadmium, arsenic, and mercury), pesticide poisoning, carbon monoxide poisoning, heatstroke, hypothermia, acute chemical poisoning, methemoglobinemia, and respiratory diseases triggered by environmental factors (e.g., asthma).

Baseline data source: Center for Environmental Health and Injury Control, CDC.

For Further Thought

As can be seen above, there are several objectives associated with lead. If you were responsible for seeing that your community reduced the number of sentinel environmental diseases by the year 2000, what would be the first policy you would want to put in place? Explain the reasons for your choice.

---

regulations. Thus, modifying behavior is an important link in reducing the lead poison problem.

For example, a sizable number of dwellings in the United States have lead-contaminated water. The ideal solution would be to replace the entire water system. However, total replacement would be very expensive, as would be the second-best solution, an add-on filtration system. How-

ever, Nadakavakaren[11] has suggested two simple actions which, if taken by those at high risk, would help reduce their intake of lead. They are:

1. Avoid drinking water that has been in contact with pipes for more than six hours. (The longer water has been standing, the greater the amount of lead likely to be present. Before using such

water for drinking or cooking, flush out the pipes by allowing water to run for several minutes or until it is as cold as it will get. Water flushed from pipes need not be wasted; it can be used for washing, watering plants, etc.).

2. Don't consume or cook with hot tap water, since lead dissolves more readily in hot water than in cold. If you need hot water, draw it cold from the tap and use the stove to heat it.

PHYSICAL HAZARDS AND HUMAN HEALTH

There are a number of physical hazards in the environment that can negatively affect human health. They include dusts like silica and asbestos, humidity, equipment and environmental design, and radiation. We have selected two radiation physical hazards— radon and ultraviolet light—to discuss in relation to human health.

Ultraviolet (UV) Radiation

The health significance of any source of radiation is associated with the biological damage to cells due to ionization.[23] If Americans were told that they were regularly being overexposed to radiation because of the X-rays their dentists take or that their home was located on top of a known radiation waste site, they would be up in arms and would demand that some change take place. Ironically though, many Americans never think twice about overexposing themselves to radiation—solar radiation, that is—the radiation that we know as sunshine or **ultraviolet (UV) radiation.** Having a tan body is important to many.

---

ultraviolet (UV) radiation   Solar radiation.

UV radiation covers wavelengths between 0 and 400 nanometers (nm). The group of wavelengths between 290 and 330 nm are called *UV-B*. This is the group of wavelengths that reaches the earth's surface and causes most of the harm to humans. In recent years, with the destruction of the ozone layers, the quantity of UV-B radiation reaching the earth has been increasing.[24]

Epidemiological studies provide a link between the etiologic role of UV-B and skin cancer. The relationship has been shown in studies that have examined both geographic location (there is more skin cancer in those living closer to the equator if not protected by darker skin) and various anatomical sites (most skin cancer appears on the exposed body parts (i.e., arms, legs, head, neck).[25]

Each year over 700,000 new cases of skin cancer are reported in the United States. This is the most common form of cancer (see Figure 16.11). The vast majority of these cases are the highly curable **basal cell** and **squamous cell carcinomas**. The most serious and least common skin cancer is **malignant melanoma**. Approximately 32,000 new cases of this cancer are diagnosed every year in the United States, and each year about 6,800 patients die of melanoma. This type of skin cancer is the most dangerous because of its ability to grow and spread quickly. However, like the other skin cancers, melanoma is curable if discovered and treated early.[26]

Some solutions to dealing with this physical environmental hazard are simple. The first is for people to reduce their risk of exposure, and the second is to seek early treatment if cancer is suspected. Individuals who are at greatest risk include those who: (1) have excessive exposure to UV radiation, both natural-solar and artificial sources, such as sunlamps and tanning booths; (2) have fair complexions; and (3) are occupationally exposed to coal tar, pitch,

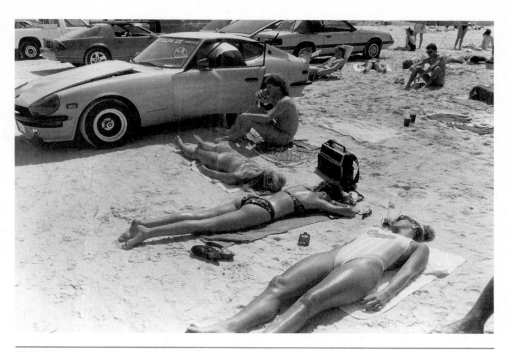

FIGURE 16.11

Skin cancer is the prevalent type of cancer in the United States.

creosote, and arsenic compounds or radium. These individuals should do their best to avoid excessive exposure to the sun, especially during midday (10 A.M. to 3 P.M.), when the sun's rays are the strongest. If they have to be out in the sun, they should cover exposed skin with either clothing (and hats) and/or sunscreens.[26,27] Sunscreens work by absorbing, reflecting, or scattering ultraviolet light, thereby reducing the amount that reaches the skin. Not all sunscreens are alike, and they vary in their protective quality. To help individuals select the sunscreen best suited for them, in 1978 the Food and Drug Administration (FDA) released a **sun protection factor (SPF)** rating scale ranging from 2–15. The higher the number, the greater the amount of protection. For example, an SPF of 10 allows a person who is likely to burn after half an hour's exposure to safely remain in the sun for five hours, or ten times as long as usual. Until 1986, the highest SPF endorsed by the FDA was 15. In 1993, the FDA endorsed SPFs of up to 30. However, today there are some products on the market that have SPFs as high as 50. There is some debate as to whether an SPF above 30 is necessary. One final note on sunscreens; recent developments in sunscreens include products that are greaseless, hypoallergenic, waterproof, and PABA-free (para-aminobenzoic acid). PABA is the protective agent in some sunscreens, but it can irritate skin and stain clothing.[28,29] (See Table 16.6 for suggested protection.)

The key to discovering whether treatment is warranted is to practice skin self-

---

sun protection factor (SPF) A scale used to indicate the protective quality of sunscreens.

Table 16.6
Sunscreen Guide

Skin Type	Pigmentation	Sunburn/Tanning History	Sun Protection Factor (SPF)
1.	Very fair skin; freckling; blond, red, or brown hair	Always burns easily; never tans	15–30
2.	Fair skin; blond, red, or brown hair	Always burns easily; tans minimally	15–20
3.	Brown hair and eyes, darker skin (light brown)	Burns moderately; tans gradually and uniformly	8–15
4.	Light brown skin; dark hair and eyes (moderate brown)	Burns minimally; always tans well	8–15
5.	Brown skin; dark hair and eyes	Rarely burns, tans profusely (dark brown)	Recommend same as Skin type 4
6.	Brown-black skin; dark hair and eyes	Never burns, deeply pigmented (black)	Recommend same as Skin Type 4

Note: As deterioration of the ozone layer continues, it may be necessary to use an even more protective sunscreen.

From: Payne, W. A., and D. B. Hahn (1992). *Understanding Your Health,* 3rd ed. St. Louis: Mosby Yearbook, p. 329.

examination once a month. Basal and squamous cell carcinomas often take the appearance of a pale, waxlike, peely nodule or a red, scaly, sharply outlined patch. Either of these abnormalities, or the sudden change in a mole's appearance, should be checked by a physician. Melanomas often start as small mole-like growths. T he simple ABCD rule from the American Cancer Society[26] outlines warning signs of melanoma.

A is for *asymmetry* (half of the mole does not match the other half).

B is for *border irregularity* (the edges are ragged, notched, or blurred).

C is for *color* (the pigmentation is not uniform).

D is for *diameter* greater than 6 millimeters (any sudden or progressive change in size should be of concern).

Radon Contamination

Radon is a colorless, tasteless, odorless gas that is formed during an intermediate step in the radioactive decay process of Uranium-238, a natural element that geologists estimate makes up about three parts per million of the earth's crust. Most soils and rocks contain varying amounts of uranium. It may also be found in well water. Radon gas has the ability to travel miles underground and rise to the earth's surface far away from any source of uranium. It enters buildings through cracks in the foundation walls and floors, joints, loose-fitting pipe penetrations, porous building materials, drain pipes, and dust floors. In some situations, radon can be released from the building itself if it is constructed with radon-bearing rocks, bricks, masonry or other components. Therefore, the magnitude of radon buildup indoors depends on the type of building materials, the quality of construction, and the concentration of radon in the underlying soil.[30,31]

Radon emanates from the earth into the air we breath. Outdoors, radon poses a very minimal health risk because it is diluted to low concentrations when mixed with large volumes of air. However, the primary danger from radon occurs from its production of a chain of radioactive isotopes called radon "daughters" (see Figure 16.12). The daughters can collect in high concentrations in buildings where there are inadequate air exchanges, and they can become attached to dust particles. The dust particles are then inhaled and may be deposited on lung tissues. This exposes the tissue to high-energy alpha particles and gamma radiation, thereby substantially increasing the risk of lung cancer.[30,31] In fact, long-term exposure to radon is estimated to be the second leading cause of lung cancer—second only to smoking—causing between 7,000 and 30,000 deaths annually.[13]

Radon has always existed, but it was not until the mid-1980s that dangerous levels of radon were found in homes across the United States. Prior to this time, the only major concern about radon exposure was among uranium miners. Epidemiological studies performed on the miners showed a

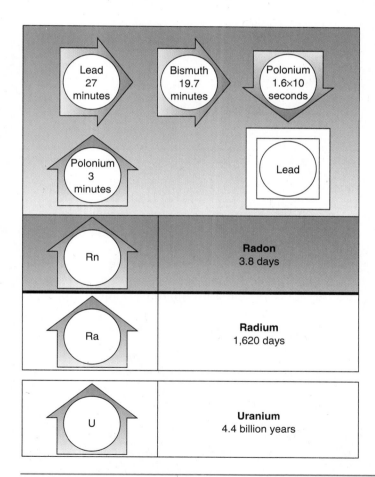

FIGURE 16.12

Uranium (the parent), its half-life, and its "daughters" and their half-lives.

From: Otton, J.K. (1992). The Geology of Radon. Washington, D.C.: U.S. Government Printing Office.

Table 16.7
Radon Risk Evaluation Chart

pCi/l	WL	Estimated Number of Lung Cancer Deaths due to Radon Exposure (out of 1,000)	Comparable Exposure Levels	Comparable Risk
200	1	440–770	1,000 times average outdoor level	More than 60 times
100	0.5	270–630	100 times average indoor level	4 pack-a-day smoker
40	0.2	120–380		20,000 chest x-rays per year
20	0.1	60–210	100 times average outdoor level	2 pack-a-day smoker
10	0.05	30–120	10 times average indoor level	1 pack-a-day smoker
4	0.02	13–50		5 times nonsmoker risk
2	0.01	7–30	10 times average outdoor level	200 chest X-rays per year
1	0.005	3–13	Average indoor level	Nonsmoker risk of dying from lung cancer
0.2	0.001	1–3	Average outdoor level	20 chest X-rays per year

From: Ganas, M. J., J. R. Schuring, and D. Raghu. "Radon Contamination in Dwellings." In J. Rose, ed. *Environmental Health* (pp. 103–116). New York: Gordon and Breach, p. 110.

correlation between radon and radon daughters and lung cancer. Based upon these studies, standards were set for the maximum permissible exposure of miners to radon. These standards are based on the concept of the "working level" unit (WL), which is equivalent to radiation exposure at a radon concentration of 200 pCi/L (picocurie per liter) of air.* Exposure at such a rate for 173 working hours is called a *working level month* or 1 *WLM*. In the studies of miners, it was found that excessive deaths due to lung cancer did not occur until miners were exposed to greater than 120 WLM. Thus, standards were set to make sure

*Radioactivity is measured in **picocuries (pCi)**. This unit of measurement is named for the French physicist Curie, who was a pioneer in the research on radioactive elements and their decay. One pCi is equal to the decay of about two radioactive atoms per minute.[32]

miners' exposure stayed below the 120 WLM level.[30]

In turn, based upon the studies on miners, predictions can be made on the cancer risks of radon exposure to the general population. It has been estimated that people who spend a lifetime in a home with a level of 1 pCi/L will have a 1 in 500 chance of dying from lung cancer due to exposure. However, the risk is directly proportional to the radon level. A concentration of 10pCi/L will increase the risk tenfold, to 1 in 50 (see Table 16.7).[30,33] In addition, there is also evidence that the combination of radon exposure and smoking may have a synergistic relationship. That is, exposure to both may exceed the effects of either alone.[31]

Like all other health problems related to environmental hazards, excessive exposure to radon can be prevented. The amount of

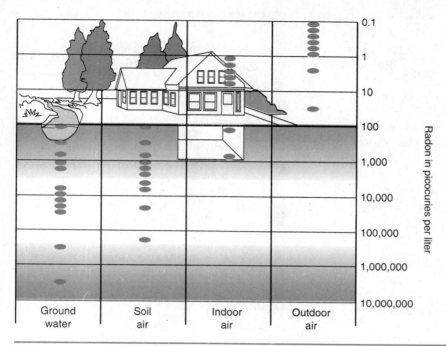

Radon in picocuries per liter

| Ground water | Soil air | Indoor air | Outdoor air |

FIGURE 16.13

Radon levels in ground water, soil, air, and indoor and outdoor air can vary dramatically.

radon in a home needs to be checked, and if levels are excessive, steps need to be taken to prevent the entry into the home. Radon levels can be tested by using an easy-to-use, relatively inexpensive (about $20) test kit. Kits are now available in most communities and are sometimes sold in hardware stores. Local health department personnel can usually help you locate one. Once the test has been administered, the kit is returned to the manufacturer for analysis. The average radon level in homes in the United States is 1.5 pCi/L (see Figure 16.13). If a home has a reading higher than 4pCi/L, steps should be taken to reduce the level. Such steps would include filling all cracks in the foundation and walls of a basement or crawl space; creating a barrier between the earth and home, by such means as pouring a concrete floor over a dust floor crawl space; and digging a new well if the radon is coming in with the water supply. Some of these steps can be expensive. Most homes with high radon levels can be fixed for $500 to $1,500 (in 1990 dollars). (See Box 16.4.)[31]

PSYCHOLOGICAL HAZARDS AND HUMAN HEALTH

Psychological hazards are not easy to define or measure. In fact, what may be a psychological hazard for one individual may be a variable that brings much pleasure to another. Research findings indicate that psychological hazards are just as important as biological, chemical, and physical hazards in the determination of human health. However, the precise effects of psychological hazards on humans is difficult to quantify.

There are a variety of mental states associated with psychological hazards, including but not limited to hypochondriasis, depression, hysteria, and stress. Because of the relationship of psychological hazards to mental health, we have chosen not to include an example of the impact of a psychological hazard on human health in this chapter. Instead, we refer the reader to Chapter 11, where stress is discussed in detail.

SOCIOLOGICAL HAZARDS AND HUMAN HEALTH

Living around other people can create a number of sociological hazards that can impact human health. It is known that noise, overcrowding, traffic jams, isolation, lack of privacy, and crowds can influence human health. As in the case of psychological hazards, the exact impact of these hazards to human health is unknown.

Although sociological hazards alone can create health problems, it is more likely for them to be found in combination with other environmental hazards. For example, the loud music created by a band could very well be harmless in a rural area but create a serious problem in a crowded housing project in the middle of a city. In order to demonstrate the impact of sociological problems on human health, we will discuss population growth.

Population Growth

A *population* is defined as a group of individuals of the same species that inhabits

---

BOX 16.4

Healthy People 2000— Objective

11.13   Increase to at least 30 the number of states requiring that prospective buyers be informed of the presence of lead-based paint and radon concentrations in all buildings offered for sale. (Baseline: 2 states required disclosure of lead-based paint in 1989; 1 state required disclosure of radon concentrations in 1989; 2 additional states required disclosure that radon has been found in the state and that testing is desirable in 1989)

Baseline data sources: Public Health Foundation; Environmental Law Institute.

For Further Thought

Is radon a problem in your part of the country? Has your residence ever been checked for radon? Should it be?

---

an area.[2] In this section, we focus on the human species and the area it inhabits, earth. Specifically, we will examine the growth of this population and the impact the growth has on health.

The Principles

The growth of a population can be attributed to three factors: its birth rate, its death rate, and migration. However, since we are discussing the human population on our entire planet, migration is not a factor. Population growth can be illustrated by an S-curve (see Figure 16.14). Such a curve consists of three phases: the **lag phase,** the

---

lag phase   Initial phase of the population growth S-curve, when growth is slow.

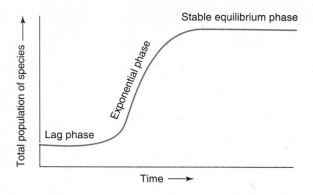

FIGURE 16.14

A theoretical population curve—S-curve

exponential phase, and the stable **equilibrium phase.** During the lag phase, the growth is slow because there are relatively few reproducing individuals and there is little difference between the death rate, and the birth rate. The exponential phase is characterized by a birth rate that is greater than the death rate, caused by more than one generation producing offspring. When the birth rate and death rate are equal, we have **zero population growth,** or the stable equilibrium phase. Prior to movement into the stable equilibrium phase, a J-curve is formed (see Figure 16.15). When a population grows in a J-curve pattern, the environment will eventually put it into an equilibrium phase, because the resources (food, water, shelter, etc.) to support such growth are limited and thus will not allow the population to grow any further. This is re-

ferred to as the **carrying capacity** of the environment.[2,11]

The Facts

In examining the population growth of the human species, one could say its growth has followed the J-curve pattern. Few facts and numbers exist about the population of the world prior to 1650 A.D., but educated guesses put the world population of 8000 B.C. at around 5 million people. By the year 1650, the population had grown to around 500 million. "It then doubled to one billion by 1850, to 2 billion by 1930, and to 4 billion by 1975; by the late 1980s, world population passed the 5 billion mark and continues to climb" today.[11] Not only does the world population continue to grow, but the larger it becomes, the faster it grows. This growth pattern is known as *exponential growth.* Table 16.8 provides a vivid example of the time it has taken for the world population to grow throughout history.

---

exponential phase Middle phase of the population growth S-curve, when the birth rate is greater than the death rate.

equilibrium phase Last phase of the population growth S-curve, when the birth and death rates are equal.

zero population growth (ZPG) When the birth and death rates for a given population are equal.

carrying capacity The amount of resources (air, water, shelter, etc.) of a given environment to support a certain-sized population.

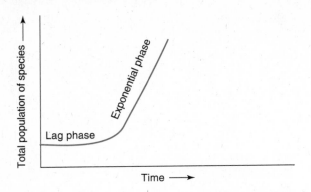

FIGURE 16.15

A population curve (growth phase)—J-curve

In 1992, the world population stood at 5.5 billion and it continues to grow at about 1.8% per year. At this rate, the United Nations projects that world population will reach 6.2 billion by the year 2000 and 8.5 bil- lion by 2025. More than three-fourths of the world's population lives in developing coun- tries, and 94% of the world's population in- crease between now and 2025 will occur in these countries.[34] For some underdeveloped

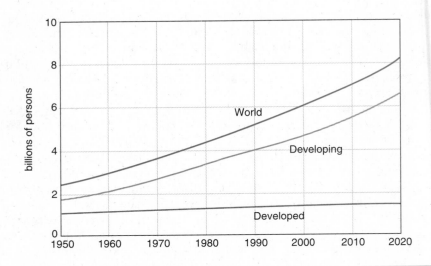

FIGURE 16.16

Developing regions account for most of the world's population growth.

From: U.S. Dept. of Commerce Economics and Statistics Administration (1992). "Our Increasingly Populated World." Bureau of the Census Statistical Brief (pub. no. SB/92-9). Washington, D.C.: U.S. Government Printing Office, p. 1.

Table 16.8
Doubling Time of World Population

Date	Estimated Human Population	Doubling Time (in years)
8000 B.C.	5 million	1,500
1650 A.D.	500 million	200
1850 A.D.	1 billion	80
1930 A.D.	2 billion	45
1975 A.D.	4 billion	36

From: Nadakavukaren, A. (1990). *Man and Environment: A Health Perspective,* 3rd ed. Prospect Heights, Ill.: Waveland Press, p. 47.

countries of the world, the growth rate is between 3% and 4%, while the U.S. rate is growing at about 1% per year (see Figures 16.16 and 16.17 and Table 16.9). Such low percentages seem insignificant until they are looked at in terms of population doubling time. Table 16.10 indicates the time it takes for a population to double based on the different percentage growth rates. Thus, a mere growth rate of 3%–4% means the population will double in 17–24 years. In human terms, that means that just to maintain the standard of living the population is enjoying today, the resources needed to sustain a population will also have to double. Such a task is difficult in a developed country and impossible in a underdeveloped country (see Figure 16.18). The world population cannot continue to grow exponentially; such growth raises many issues, not the least of which is the impact of the population's growth on human health (see Box 16.5).

The Issues

The health issues related to the exponential growth rate of the world population have already begun to surface. To date, few people have connected population growth with many health issues. While most are aware of the relationship of large populations and hunger, few associate larger popu-

---

BOX 16.5
Where in the World Do They Live?

Of every 100 people in the world in 1991:

21 lived in China (*mainland*)
16 lived in India
4 lived in Indonesia

2 lived in Japan, 2 in Pakistan, and 2 in Bangladesh
1 lived in Vietnam, 1 in the Philippines, 1 in Iran, and 1 in Thailand
5 lived in the United States

3 lived in Brazil
2 lived in Mexico
5 lived in the former Soviet Union

1 lived in Germany, 1 in Italy, 1 in the United Kingdom, and
1 in France
2 lived in Nigeria

1 lived in Ethiopia
1 lived in Turkey and 1 in Egypt.

Thus, 75 of each 100 persons lived in just 22 countries. The other 25 lived in the remaining 184 countries.

From: U.S. Dept. of Commerce, Bur. of the Census (Sept. 1992). *Statistical Brief: Our Increasingly Populated World* (pub. no. SB/92-9). Washington, D.C.: Author, p. 2.

lations with global warming, acid rain, bulging landfills, depletion of the ozone layer, crime, vulnerability to epidemics and pandemics, smog, exhaustion of soils and groundwater, and international tensions. All of these problems have an impact on human health, and, either in part or in whole, their problems are caused by increased population.

Listed below are some specific ways that population growth can impact human health. A larger world population:

Table 16.9

Total U.S. Population and Population Growth Rate, 1900–1991.

Year	Population (millions)	Growth Rate (%)	Year	Population (millions)	Growth Rate (%)	Year	Population (millions)	Growth Rate (%)
1900	76.09	na	1931	124.15	0.7	1962	186.54	1.5
1901	77.58	2.0	1932	124.95	0.6	1963	189.24	1.4
1902	79.16	2.0	1933	125.69	0.6	1964	191.89	1.3
1903	80.63	1.9	1934	126.49	0.7	1965	194.30	1.2
1904	82.17	1.9	1935	127.36	0.7	1966	196.56	1.1
1905	83.82	2.0	1936	128.18	0.6	1967	198.71	1.1
1906	85.45	1.9	1937	128.96	0.7	1968	200.71	1.0
1907	87.01	1.8	1938	129.97	0.8	1969	202.68	1.0
1908	88.71	2.0	1939	131.03	0.8	1970	205.05	1.3
1909	90.49	2.0	1940	132.59	0.9	1971	207.66	1.2
1910	92.41	2.1	1941	133.89	1.0	1972	209.90	1.0
1911	93.86	1.6	1942	135.36	1.3	1973	211.91	0.9
1912	95.34	1.6	1943	137.25	1.3	1974	213.85	0.9
1913	97.23	2.0	1944	138.92	1.2	1975	215.97	1.0
1914	99.11	1.9	1945	140.47	1.0	1976	218.04	1.0
1915	100.55	1.4	1946	141.94	1.5	1977	220.24	1.0
1916	101.96	1.4	1947	144.70	1.8	1978	222.59	1.1
1917	103.41	1.4	1948	147.21	1.7	1979	225.06	1.2
1918	104.55	1.1	1949	149.77	1.7	1980	227.72	1.1
1919	105.06	0.5	1950	152.27	1.7	1981	229.96	1.0
1920	106.46	1.3	1951	154.88	1.7	1982	232.19	1.0
1921	108.54	2.0	1952	157.55	1.7	1983	234.32	1.0
1922	110.05	1.4	1953	160.18	1.7	1984	236.37	0.9
1923	111.95	1.7	1954	163.03	1.8	1985	238.49	1.0
1924	114.11	1.9	1955	165.93	1.8	1986	240.68	1.0
1925	115.83	1.5	1956	168.90	1.8	1987	242.84	1.0
1926	117.40	1.4	1957	171.98	1.7	1988	245.06	1.0
1927	119.04	1.4	1958	174.88	1.7	1989	247.34	1.0
1928	120.51	1.2	1959	177.83	1.7	1990	249.98	1.0
1929	121.77	1.0	1960	180.67	1.6	1991	252.86	1.0
1930	123.19	0.9	1961	183.69	1.6			

Notes: The population estimates shown here are based on the April 1, 1990, population as enumerated in the 1990 census. Estimates for dates prior to April 1, 1990, have been revised. Except for 1991, annual population estimates are as of July 1 for the given year. Total population includes armed forces oversees.

Source: U.S. Dept. of Commerce, Bur. of the Census (1991). "Estimates of the Population of the United States to August 1, 1991." *Current Population Reports,* series P-25, no. 1078. Washington, D.C.: Author.

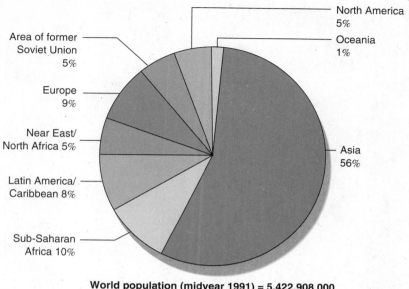

World population (midyear 1991) = 5,422,908,000

FIGURE 16.17

More people live in Asia than in the rest of the world combined (distribution of world population: 1991).

From: U.S. Dept. of Commerce Economics and Statistics Administration (1992). "Our Increasingly Populated World." Bureau of the Census Statistical Brief (pub. no. SB/92-9). Washington, D.C.: U.S. Government Printing Office, p. 1.

Note: "Asia" stretches from Iran to Indonesia and the Philippines; countries on the Asian continent west of Iran and the Arabian Sea are in the "Near East." Also, the Latin America/Caribbean region includes Mexico and Central America.

1. Will create more wastes, which in turn will increase the level of air and water pollution, resulting in a higher incidence of disease and premature death.
2. Will generate a greater demand for energy and increase utilization of fossil fuels, thus causing more pollution, depletion of the ozone layer, and global warming.
3. Will create a greater demand for food while reducing the amount of land available for cultivation; this in turn will lead to famine and malnutrition, which will result in more disease and premature deaths.

Table 16.10
Population Doubling Time by Growth Rate

Growth Rate	Doubling Time (in years)
0.5%	140
0.8	87
1.0	70
2.0	35
3.0	24
4.0	17

From: Nadakavukaren, A. (1990). Man and Environment: A Health Perspective, 3rd ed. Prospect Heights, Ill.: Waveland Press, p. 51.

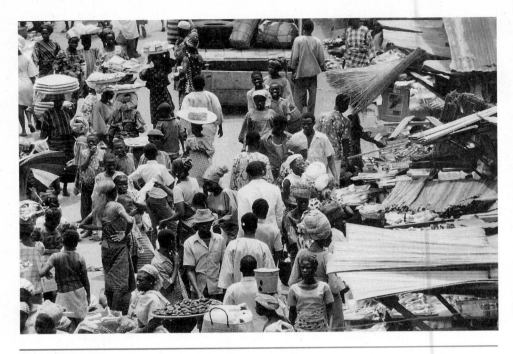

FIGURE 16.18

Three-fourths of the world's population lives in developing countries.

4. Will limit the amount of living space each person has, which means people will live closer together. Living closer together will make people more vulnerable to communicable diseases and stress.

5. Will create a greater demand on all necessary resources. Limited resources in the past have led to increases in crime and international tensions, including wars.

6. Will create a greater demand for health care in a world where current demands for health care are going unmet.

7. Will create a greater demand for housing in a world where many are already homeless.

The Solutions

Most experts agree that the world population is approaching the maximum sustainable limit. However, no one knows what the ultimate population size will be. Something different from what is presently being done must limit the growth. A stable population will occur either through (1) human action to conscientiously limit population growth or (2) actions taken by nature to limit population growth via survival of the fittest. Ehrlich and Ehrlich[35] have stated that "the population explosion will come to an end before very long. The only remaining question is whether it will be halted through the humane method of birth control, or by nature wiping out the surplus."

The so-called humane means of limiting population growth include: (1) various methods of conception control such as the oral contraceptive pill, cervical cap, diaphragm, sponges, Norplant (subdermal hormonal implant), condoms (both male and female), sterilization (tubal ligation and vasectomy), and spermicides; (2) birth control methods such as intrauterine devices, legalized abortion, and morning-after pills; and (3) social policies such as financial incentives and societal disincentives for having children, as is the practice in China's one-child family program. Each of these means has its good and bad points, and each has large groups of supporters and foes. However, all are proactive solutions to the mounting population problem. Nature's way of dealing with the problem would be through disease and famine, which would require reactive actions by humans to reduce the suffering. "Limiting human numbers will not alone end warfare, environmental deterioration, poverty, racism, religious prejudice, or sexism; it will just

buy us the opportunity to do so. As the old saying goes, whatever your cause, it is a lost cause without population control."[35] (see Box 16.6.)

Nature's methods of stabilizing the population are quite severe. They include wide-scale starvation, epidemics of acute and chronic communicable diseases, and wars. At times so many people die that the survivors are unable to bury them all.

SITE AND LOCATION HAZARDS AND HUMAN HEALTH

In Chapter 15, we outlined some natural and human-made site and location situations that can be hazardous to humans. To

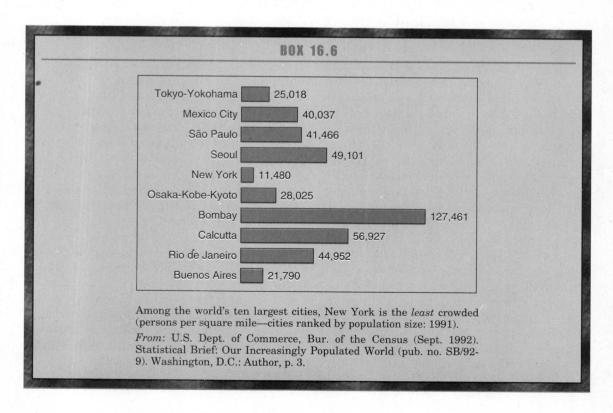

BOX 16.6

Tokyo-Yokohama	25,018
Mexico City	40,037
São Paulo	41,466
Seoul	49,101
New York	11,480
Osaka-Kobe-Kyoto	28,025
Bombay	127,461
Calcutta	56,927
Rio de Janeiro	44,952
Buenos Aires	21,790

Among the world's ten largest cities, New York is the *least* crowded (persons per square mile—cities ranked by population size: 1991).

From: U.S. Dept. of Commerce, Bur. of the Census (Sept. 1992). Statistical Brief: Our Increasingly Populated World (pub. no. SB/92-9). Washington, D.C.: Author, p. 3.

further explain the hazard to human health that site and location may bring, we have chosen to discuss natural disasters.

Natural Disasters

Natural disasters include those geophysical and meteorological events (disaster agents) that greatly exceed normal human expectations in terms of magnitude or frequency and which cause significant damage to individuals and/or their property.[36] From this definition, a few key points should be noted. First, disasters involve interactions of **disaster agents** such as cyclones, earthquakes, floods, hurricanes, tornadoes, typhoons, and volcanic eruptions, and people.[37] Take, for example, a hurricane. As long as it stays out at sea, it is just an event. As soon as it comes ashore in a populated area, it can create a disaster. Second, the concept of magnitude or overall loss to people and property are noted. Not only the density of a population is relevant, but also its size. For example, larger populations may be more affected than smaller populations in absolute terms, but less relatively. "The loss of tens of millions in China or India, though appalling, at least does not have an eliminating effect."[38]

Many times, human health is affected by natural disasters even prior to their occurrence because of impending dangers. Prior to the event, some disaster agents can be tracked or predicted (e.g., hurricanes, typhoons, floods, and volcanic eruptions). With such knowledge, oftentimes comes the psychological stress of an impending disaster. Such stress can cause serious health problems in those who are unable to control their reaction to the situation. During the event, health can again be affected because of the physical damage causing both injury and mortality casualties.

After a natural disaster because of the remaining biological, sociological, psychological, and physical conditions, a variety of needs may exist. The primary needs of people after a natural disaster usually include food, water, shelter, health care, and clothing. The availability and quality of these items can dictate the impact of the disaster on human health.

Hurricane Andrew, which came ashore during the summer of 1992, provides an example. Andrew made a swipe through the Bahamas before coming ashore on the southern tip of Florida and in southern Louisiana. The National Hurricane Center in Dade County, Florida, had been tracking the storm for almost a week, ever since it began as a tropical depression. Even with such close monitoring, the fury of the storm still caused 30 fatalities, left hundreds of thousands homeless, destroyed nearly 100,000 homes, left more than 3 million homes and businesses without power, and caused well over $20 billion in damage.[39] Hurricane Andrew was the most costly natural disaster in United States history.

In what ways was Hurricane Andrew a community health problem for the communities it struck? First, there were the injuries and deaths directly associated with the destructive force of the hurricane's wind and water. Second, many of those who survived uninjured found themselves without adequate food, water, shelter, or clothing. Much of the food in the area had become contaminated or ruined, so that grocery stores and restaurants were unable to meet the needs of the residents. Third, survivors were left in a community in which important health services such as water supply and sewage systems were inoperable. Thus, human waste and contaminated water posed serious public health problems. A source of pure water had to be supplied quickly. Fourth, many people were left without their medications. Finally, because of the destruction of homes, motels, and health care facilities (hospitals, nursing homes, etc.) and the lack of transportation out of the area, shelter also became a problem.

With all the above-mentioned problems, southern Florida was declared a Federal Disaster Area by President Bush. As such, the Federal Response Plan, which is included in the Robert T. Stafford Disaster Relief and Emergency Assistance Act (P.L. 93—288) was allowed to be put into action. This plan establishes the basis for federal assistance to a state and its affected local governments impacted by the disaster. The plan uses a functional approach to group the types of federal assistance that a state is most likely to need under 12 Emergency Support Functions (ESP).[40] (See Box 16.7.) Once the needs of an area are determined, appropriate assistance is rendered. As was the case with Hurricane Andrew, many of the primary needs of the people were met when the military supplied the area with portable toilets, food, water, tents, and hospital units. One might assume that people affected by such a disaster would pull together in a situation like this, and most do. But the affected areas also had to deal with the violence and crime of the looting that takes place after such disasters.

This scenario has been repeated several times since Hurricane Andrew. In the summer of 1993, massive flooding occurred in the American Midwest. (See Figure 16.19.) Though excessive rainfall was the natural disaster this time, the people of Iowa, Minnesota, and Missouri faced many of the same problems of those who dealt with Hurricane Andrew. Then in the early winter of 1994, the city of Los Angeles had to deal with an earthquake. Some experts indicated that the cost of the earthquake was greater

---

BOX 16.7

The 12 Emergency Support Functions (ESF) of the Federal Response Plan and the Lead Agency for Each ESF

1. Transportation—Department of Transportation

2. Communications—National Communications System

3. Construction management—Department of Defense

4. Firefighting—Department of Agriculture

5. Damage information—Federal Emergency Management Administration

6. Mass care—American Red Cross

7. Resources support—General Services Administration

8. Health and medical services—Department of Health and Human Services, Public Health Service*

9. Urban search and rescue—Department of Defense

10. Hazardous materials—Environmental Protection Agency

11. Food—Department of Agriculture

12. Energy—Department of Energy

*Supporting departments and agencies for this ESF are the Agency for International Development (Office of U.S. Foreign Disaster Assistance); American Red Cross; Departments of Agriculture, Defense (U.S. Army Corps of Engineers), Interior, Justice, Transportation, and Veterans Affairs; Environmental Protection Agency; Federal Emergency Management Agency; General Services Administration; U.S. Postal Service.

From: Ginzburg, H. M., R. J. Jevec, and T. Reutershan (1993). "The Public Health Service's Response to Hurricane Andrew." *Public Health Reports* 108(2):241–244.

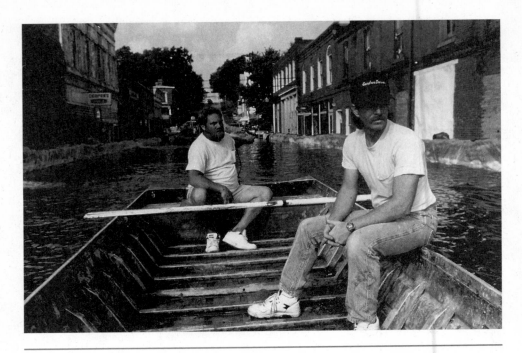

FIGURE 16.19

Natural disasters such as the floods that occurred in the midwestern United States in the summer of 1993 put an additional strain on a community's health resources.

than that of Hurricane Andrew.[41]

The seriousness of disasters seems to be directly related to the vulnerability of the people affected. The more vulnerable a group of people to a disaster, the more serious the outcomes. Mizutani and Nakano[41] have identified several factors that greatly affect human casualties from a natural disaster. These factors include the general preparedness for the event, previous disaster experience, time of day the disaster occurs, human behavior at the time of impact, and the locality of the event.

The key to recovery from any natural disaster lies with the ability of a community to mobilize to meet the needs of the people. In the United States, the American Red Cross has taken on the role of organizing such efforts.

CHAPTER SUMMARY

Chapter 15 presented information about the hazards found in the environmental system. This chapter focused on the way these environmental hazards affect human health. The environmental hazards that can affect human health are countless. In fact, there are probably a number of yet-unidentified hazards in the environment which will cause major problems in the future. For example, who could have predicted the pain and suffering that would result from the flooding in the midwestern United States during the summer of 1993? Or the Los Angeles earthquake in 1994?

Specifically, this chapter presents examples of hazards from six environmental hazard groups. Water-borne, food-borne, and vector-borne diseases are examples of biological hazards. Pesticides, environmental tobacco smoke, and lead are chemical hazards that affect many American lives. Ultraviolet radiation and radon are invisible physical hazards that have serious health consequences such as skin cancer and lung cancer. Worldwide population growth constitutes a potential sociological hazard for all. And finally, natural disasters, exemplified by Hurricane Andrew, are unpredictable site and location hazards that can profoundly disrupt community health services and put citizens at risk.

SCENARIO: ANALYSIS AND RESPONSE

1. At the present time, the U.S. government acknowledges that there is conclusive evidence that Agent Orange exposure is related to specific diseases, and compensates Vietnam veterans who are affected. Those diseases include three types of cancer (Hodgkin's disease, non-Hodgkin's lymphoma, and soft tissue sarcoma) and two other types of disorders (chloracne—a disfiguring skin disorder—and a metabolic disorder called porphyria cutanea tarda). The government does not compensate for prostate cancer. Even though science cannot prove it, do you believe Agent Orange caused Gary's cancer? Why?

2. Do you feel that the U.S. government owes Gary anything because of the exposure he had to the environmental hazard while serving his country? Would it make a difference whether he had enlisted or had been drafted?

3. Because of the adverse health conditions of many Vietnam veterans, a group of veterans filed suit against the seven United States chemical companies that produced Agent Orange. Before the case went to trial, the companies agreed to place $180 million into a fund that would be used to compensate victims and their families. The companies also denied any liability and stated they created the herbicide using the military's specifications. Do you feel these companies should be held responsible? Why or why not?

4. Do you feel that Gary was the victim of an environmental hazard (Agent Orange), or a sociological hazard (the war), or both? Explain your response.

REVIEW QUESTIONS

1. How are the following terms related: *environmental sanitation, sanitary engineer,* and *sanitarians?*

2. Explain the differences among water-borne, food-borne, and vector-borne diseases and give an example of each.

3. What is meant by the term *environmental health?*

4. What is so ironic about chemical hazards being detrimental to human health?

5. What is a pest? And what are pesticides?

6. What are the most common ways for pesticides to damage human health?

7. What is a perfect pesticide?

8. What is the difference between a hard pesticide and a soft one?

9. Explain the difference among environmental tobacco smoke, sidestream smoke, and mainstream smoke.

10. What is passive smoking?

11. To date, how has environmental tobacco smoke been regulated?

12. Who is at the highest risk for lead poisoning?

13. What are the most common ways to get lead poisoning?

14. What can be done to reduce the number of cases of lead poisoning?

15. Why is there such concern about ultraviolet radiation?

16. What carcinoma is the most dangerous type of skin cancer? Why?

17. Explain the ABCD rule of melanomas.

18. How is radon formed?

19. Why is radon such a concern?

20. Explain population growth using the S- and J-curves.

21. How fast is the population growing in the United States? In the world? What does such growth mean to all humans?

22. What are the solutions to population growth?

23. Explain the concept *disaster agent*.

ACTIVITIES

1. Make arrangements to "shadow" a sanitarian from a local health department for at least half a day. Record and summarize the tasks in which he/she is involved. Then write a two-page paper that answers the following:

   What professional training has the sanitarian completed to be qualified for this work?

   What role does this person play in protecting the community's health?

   What other tasks does the sanitarian routinely perform that he/she did not do on the day you visited?

   Would you like to be a sanitarian when you get out of school? Why or why not?

   Attach your notes of all the tasks that were performed when you were with the sanitarian.

2. Make arrangements to interview a director of environmental health in a local health department. Find answers to the following questions and summarize these answers in a paper.

   What are all the tasks your division of the health department carries out?

   What is the primary environmental health problem of your community? Why is it a problem? How is it being dealt with?

   If they inspect restaurants, find out which ones have the best sanitation practices.

   What is an average day like for a health department sanitarian?

3. Interview at least three different farm workers. Ask if they know anyone who has ever been poisoned by a pesticide. Find out how each poisoning happened, ask if it could have been prevented, and find out what happened to the person who was poisoned. Write the results of your findings in a two-page paper.

4. Visit three different restaurants in your community. Ask to speak with the manager or assistant manager about the smoking policy in the restaurants. Find out what the policy is, who determined the policy, why it was created, and what happens if someone violates it. Write the results of your findings in a two-page paper.

5. Call your local health department and find out what kind of efforts have been made to eliminate lead poisoning. Ask about education programs and possible state or local laws. Also, find out if the health department will test for lead in the water and paint. If they will, ask about the procedures they use to do so. Write the results of your findings in a two-page paper.

6. Survey five of your friends by asking them the following questions. Once the interviews are complete, write a two-page paper summarizing their responses.

   Do you lie out in the sun or go to tanning booths? If so, how often? Are you concerned about skin cancer?

   What are the risk factors for skin cancer?

   What is meant by the ABCD rule of melanoma?

   Is tan skin more important to you than not getting cancer? If so, why?

7. Is radon gas a problem in your area of the country? If so, find out to what extent it is a problem and what percentage of the dwellings are contaminated. Also, obtain a home test kit and use it in the place where you live. In a two-page paper, report: the extent of the problem in your community and the results of the test on your dwelling; then project what your risk of disease from radon would be. (Note: If you are not sure where to get a radon test kit, contact your local health department.)

8. Go to the student union on your campus to conduct a survey of those who use the building. Ask the questions below of at least 25 people (do not interview people in only one part of the building; get responses from people in the food service areas, the lounges, bookstore, etc. Also be sure to include students, faculty, and student union employees).

Are you a student, faculty member, or staff member?

Do you use tobacco in any form? If yes, what do you smoke or chew? How much?

Do you believe people should be allowed to smoke in this building? Why or why not?

Do you think smoking is a right or a privilege?

Are you in favor of a total ban on smoking on this campus? In all buildings? In offices? In residence halls?

After you have collected the data, summarize it in a written paper and report any trends you find. Be sure to compare the answers of students to faculty to staff.

9. Write a three-page position paper on one of the following questions. Make sure you cite references to support your position.

Should the United States be concerned with worldwide population growth?

Should the United States develop government policy to slow its population growth?

What is the best means for controlling population growth in any country?

10. Find an issue of a weekly news magazine (e.g., *Newsweek, Time,* etc.) that covers a recent natural disaster (Midwest flood in July 1993, Texas flood in January 1992, the Loma Prieta earthquake in San Francisco in October 1990, Hurricanes Hugo [in South Carolina], Bob [in New England], or Andrew [in Florida and Louisiana], or the Los Angeles earthquake in January 1994. Read all the stories covering the disaster, then write a two-page paper identifying what you believe to be the major community health concerns that resulted from the disaster and why.

REFERENCES

1. U.S. Dept. of Health and Human Services (1987). *Issues and Challenges in Environmental Health.* (NIH pub. no. 87-861) Washington, D.C.: U.S. Government Printing Office.

2. Enger, E. D., and B. F. Smith (1992). *Environmental Science: A Study of Interrelationships,* 4th ed. Dubuque, Ia.: Wm. C. Brown.

3. Purdom, P. W., ed. (1980). *Environmental Health,* 2nd ed. San Diego: Academic Press.

4. Doll, R. (1992). "Health and the Environment in the 1990s." *American Journal of Public Health* 82(7): 933–941.

5. Landrigan, P. J. (1992). "Commentary: Environmental Disease—A Preventable epidemic." *American Journal of Public Health* 82(7): 941–943.

6. Centers for Disease Control (1990). "Water-borne Disease Outbreaks, 1986–1988." In *CDC Surveillance Summaries, March 1990. MMWR* 39 (no. SS-1): 1–13.

7. Centers for Disease Control (1990). "Food-borne Disease Outbreaks, 5-Year Summary, 1983–1987. In *CDC Surveillance Summaries, March 1990. MMWR* 39 (No. SS-1): 15–57.

8. Moore, C. (1993). "Distribution of Aedes Ablopictus in the U.S.—September, 1992." *AMCA Newsletter* 19(2): 11. Lake Charles La.: American Mosquito Control Association.

9. Villee, C. A. (1985). "Consequences of World Population Growth on Natural Resources and Environment." In C. A. Villee, ed. *Fallout from the Population Explosion* (pp. 85–94). New York: Paragon House.

10. Benarde, M. A. (1989). *Our Precarious Habitat: Fifteen Years Later.* New York: John Wiley & Sons.

11. Nadakavukaren, A. (1990). *Man and Environment: A Health Perspective,* 3rd ed. Prospect Heights, Ill.: Waveland Press.

12. Blair, A., and S. H. Zabm (1992). "Agricultural Health: Pesticides and Cancer." *Health and Environment Digest* 6(5): 1–4.

13. Schultz, D. (1993). *Lung Disease Data 1993.* New York: American Lung Assn.

14. Overpeck, M. D., and A. J. Moss (1991). "Children's Exposure to Environmental Cigarette Smoke Before and After Birth." *Advance Data* no. 202 (DHHS pub. no. PHS-91-1250). Washington, D.C.: U.S. Government Printing Office.

15. U.S. Environmental Protection Agency (1993). *Respiratory Health Effects of Passive Smoking: Lung Cancer and Other Disorders* (EPA/600/6-90/006f). Washington, D.C.: U.S. Government Printing Office.

16. U.S. Dept. of Health and Human Services (1991). *Environmental Tobacco Smoke in the Workplace* (DHHS [NIOSH] pub. no. 91-108). Washington, D.C.: U.S. Government Printing Office.

17. National Inst. for Occupational Safety and Health (NIOSH) (1986). *Proposed National Strategy for the Prevention of Leading Work-related Diseases and Injuries: A Proposed National Strategy for the*

Prevention of Occupational Lung Disease (DHHS [NIOSH] pub. no. 89-128). Cincinnati: Author.

18. Goyer, R. A. (1990). "Lead Toxicity: From Overt to Subclinical to Subtle Health Effects." *Environmental Health Perspectives* 86(June): 171–181.

19. Centers for Disease Control (1992a). "Blood Lead Levels Among Children in High-Risk Areas—California, 1987–1990." *Morbidity and Mortality Weekly Report* 41(17): 291–294.

20. Centers for Disease Control (1991). *Preventing Lead Poisoning in Young Children.* Atlanta: Author.

21. Centers for Disease Control (1992c). "Surveillance of Elevated Blood Lead Levels Among Adults—United States, 1992." *Morbidity and Mortality Weekly Report* 41(17): 285–288.

22. Centers for Disease Control (1992b). "Implementation of the Lead Contamination Control Act of 1988." *Morbidity and Mortality Weekly Report* 41(17): 288–290.

23. Rogers, J. C. (1980). "Radiation: Ionizing and Nonionizing." In P. W. Purdom, ed. *Environmental Health,* 2nd ed. (pp. 393–433) San Diego, Calif.: Academic Press.

24. Bair, F. E., ed. (1990). *Cancer Sourcebook.* Detroit: Omnigraphics.

25. Dubin, N., M. Moseson, and B. S. Pasternack (1989). "Sun Exposure and Malignant Melanoma Among Susceptible Individuals." *Environmental Health Perspective* 81: 139–151.

26. American Cancer Society (1993). *Cancer Facts and Figures—1992.* Atlanta: Author.

27. American Cancer Society (1990). *Fry Now. Pay Later.* Atlanta: Author.

28. Sweet, C. A. (1989). "Healthy Tan—A Fast Fading Myth." *FDA Consumer* 23(5): 11–13.

29. Greeley, A. (1993). "Dodging the Rays," *FDA Consumer* 27(6): 30–33.

30. Ganas, M. J., J. R. Schuring, and D. Raghu (1990). "Radon Contamination in Dwellings." In J. Rose, ed. *Environmental Health* (pp. 103–116). New York: Gordon and Breach.

31. American Medical Assn. (1990). *"Radon, the Health Threat with a Simple Solution: A Physician's Guide."* Chicago: Author.

32. Otton, J. K. (1992). *The Geology of Radon.* Washington, D.C.: U.S. Government Printing Office.

33. Cohen, B. L. (1985). *Nuclear Energy, a Sensible Alternative.* New York: Plenum Press.

34. Associated Press (1992). "Planet Earth Could Get Awfully Crowded." *The Muncie Ind., Star.* July 11: 2D.

35. Ehrlich, P. R., and A. H. Ehrlich (1990). "The Population Explosion! Why Isn't Anyone as Scared as We Are?" *The Amicus Journal.* Winter: 22–29.

36. Heathcote, R. L. (1979). "The Threat from Natural Hazards in Australia. In R. L. Heathcote and B. G. Thom, eds. *Natural Hazards in Australia* (pp. 3–10). Canberra: Australian Academy of Sciences.

37. United Nations Disaster Relief Organization(1986). *Disaster Prevention and Mitigation: Social and Sociological Aspects,* vol. 12. New York: United Nations.

38. Clarke, J. I. (1989). "Conclusion." In J. I. Clarke, P. Curson, S. L. Kayastha, and P. Nag, eds. *Population and Disaster* (pp. 273–278). Cambridge, Mass.: Basil Blackwell.

39. Mathews, T., P. Katel, T. Barrett, D. Waller, C. Bingham, M. Liu, S. Waldman, and G. Carroll (1992). "Andrew's Wrath." *Newsweek* (Sept. 7): 16–27, 30–31.

40. Ginzburg, H. M., R. J. Jevec, and T. Reutershan (1993). "The Public Health Service's Response to Hurricane Andrew." *Public Health Reports* 108(2): 241–244.

41. Mizutani, T., and T. Nakano (1989). The Impact of Natural Disasters on the Population of Japan." In J. I. Clarke, P. Curson, S. L. Kayastha, and P. Nag, eds. *Population and Disaster* (pp. 24–33). Cambridge, Mass.: Basil Blackwell.

Chapter 17

INJURIES AS
A COMMUNITY
HEALTH PROBLEM

Chapter Outline

Chapter Objectives

After studying this chapter you will be able to:

1. Describe the importance of injuries as a community health problem.
2. Explain why the terms *accidents* and *safety* have been replaced by the currently more acceptable terms *unintentional injuries,* and *injury prevention* and *injury control* when dealing with such occurrences.
3. Briefly, explain the difference between intentional and unintentional injuries and provide examples of each.
4. List the four elements usually included in the definition of the term *unintentional injury.*
5. Summarize the epidemiology of unintentional injuries.
6. List strategies for the prevention and control of unintentional injuries.
7. Explain how education, regulation, automatic protection, and litigation can reduce the number and seriousness of unintentional injuries.
8. Define the term *intentional injuries* and provide examples of behavior that results in intentional injuries.
9. Describe the scope of intentional injuries as a community health problem in the United States.
10. List some contributing factors to domestic violence and some strategies for reducing it.
11. List some of the contributing factors to the increase in violence related to youth gangs and explain what communities can do to reduce the level of violence.
12. Discuss intervention approaches in preventing or controlling intentional injuries.

Peter decided to mow the lawn. He checked and filled the gas reservoir, started the mower and began mowing. He felt he should be finished in about 40 minutes, plenty of time to clean up before the ball game. In one corner of the yard, he found it easier to pull the lawnmower backward rather than to push it forward. Peter had done this many times before without incident; but this time, as he backed up, he tripped over a stump. To regain his balance, he automatically pulled harder on the mower, causing it to run over his foot. He felt an explosion of sharp pain and pulled his foot back, but it was too late; the mower blade had cut through Peter's shoe and big toe. Peter quickly turned off the mower and hobbled to the house. As he prepared to go to the emergency room at the local hospital, he thought only briefly about the ball game he would miss. The rest of the lawn would have to be mowed later.

INTRODUCTION

In this chapter, we first define and then examine the scope, causes, and effects on the community of both unintentional and intentional injuries. We also review approaches to the prevention and control of injuries and injury deaths.

Definitions

The word **injury** is derived from the Latin word for "not right."[1] It has been defined as "physical harm or damage to the body resulting from an exchange, usually acute, of mechanical, chemical, thermal or other environmental energy that exceeds the body's tolerance."[2] In this chapter we discuss both **unintentional injuries,** injuries judged to have occurred without anyone intending that harm be done, such as those that result from car crashes, falls, drownings and fires, and **intentional injuries,** injuries judged to have been purposely inflicted, either by the self or another, such as assaults, intentional shootings and stabbings, and suicides.

The term *accident* has fallen into disfavor and disuse with many public health officials, whose goal it is to reduce the number and seriousness of all injuries. The very word *accident* suggests a chance occurrence or an unpreventable mishap. Yet we know that many, if not most, accidents are preventable. The term *unintentional injury* is now used in its place. Similarly, the rather vague term *safety* has largely been replaced by **injury prevention** or **injury control.** These terms are inclusive of all measures to prevent injuries, both unintentional and intentional, or to minimize their severity.

Think for a moment about the term *unintentional injury,* which we have previ-

---

injury Physical damage to the body resulting from mechanical, chemical, thermal, or other environmental energy.
unintentional injury An injury that occurred without anyone intending that harm be done.

intentional injuries An injury that is purposely inflicted, either by the victim or by another.
injury prevention (control) An organized effort to prevent injuries or to minimize their severity.

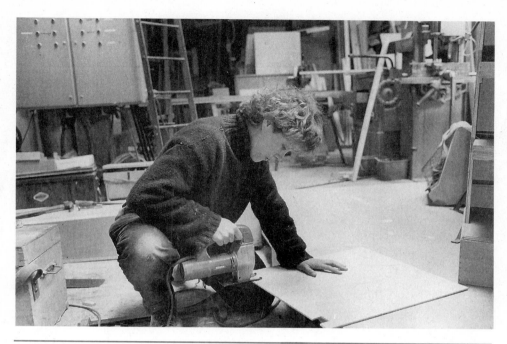

FIGURE 17.1

An unsafe act is a behavior that increases the probability of an injury. Should this person be wearing eye protection?

ously defined as an injury judged to have occurred without anyone intending that harm be done. If we examine it further, we can see that there are four characteristics of an *unintentional injury:* (1) it occurs following an unplanned event, (2) it is usually preceded by an *unsafe act* or *condition (hazard),* (3) it is often accompanied by economic loss or injury, and (4) it interrupts the efficient completion of a task.

An **unsafe act** is any behavior that would increase the probability of an unintentional injury. For example, driving an automobile while being impaired by alcohol or operating a power saw without eye protection creates a hazard (see Figure 17.1). An **unsafe condition** is any environmental factor (physical or social) that would increase the probability of an unintentional injury. Icy streets are an example of an unsafe condition. Note that these **hazards** do not *cause* unintentional injuries. (An alcohol-impaired person may reach home, even over icy streets.) Hazards do, however, *increase the probability* that an unintentional injury will occur.

Cost of Injuries to Society

Injuries are costly to society in terms of both human suffering and economic loss. Each year, more than 150,000 Americans

---

unsafe act Any behavior that would increase the probability of an injury occurring.

unsafe condition Any environmental factor or set of factors (physical or social) that would increase the probability of an injury occurring.
hazard An unsafe act or condition.

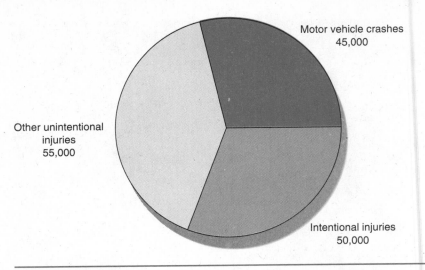

FIGURE 17.2

Injury deaths: 150,000 die annually from injuries in the United States.

Source: S. T. Brown, W. H. Folge, T. R. Bender, and N. Axnick (1990). "Injury Prevention Control: Prospects for the 1990s." Annual Review of Public Health *11:251–266.*

die from **fatal injuries,** injuries that result in one or more deaths.[3] Included in this staggering death toll are deaths that result from motor vehicle crashes, some 45,000; those that result from drownings, fires, falls, and other intentional injuries, another 55,000; and those that result from acts of violence such as homicide and suicide, about 50,000 (see Figure 17.2).[3]

Deaths are only a small part of the total cost of injuries. In 1985, 57 million Americans—one in four—was injured, and 2.3 million were hospitalized because of a **disabling injury,** an injury that causes restriction of normal activity beyond the day of the injury's occurrence.[4]

Not only are there unmeasurable social and psychological consequences for the victims and their families, there are also significant economic costs. It was estimated that the lifelong costs of the 1985 injuries cited above totaled $158 billion.[4]

In 1990, the cost of motor vehicle crashes and injuries alone was estimated at $137.5 billion.[5] Almost one-third of the cost of unintentional injuries can be attributed to the lost productivity of those who die prematurely. The other two-thirds of the cost is attributed to those who survive their injuries. This includes the costs of hospitalization, outpatient medical attention, and rehabilitation.[6]

Injury is the fifth leading cause of death in the United States,[7] but in terms of lost productivity, it ranks first. Each injury death represents an average of 36 *years of potential life lost (YPLL)* (refer to Chapter 4 to review YPLL) and a loss in productivity of $334,851. By way of comparison, only 12 years of life are lost for each death from cardiovascular disease (heart attack and stroke combined) and 16 years for each cancer death (see Figure 17.3). The comparable costs of lost productivity per death are

---

fatal injury   An injury that results in one or more deaths.
disabling injury   An injury causing any restriction of normal activity beyond the day of the injury's occurrence.

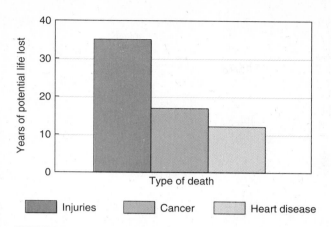

FIGURE 17.3

Average number of years of potential life lost (YPLL) per death from three causes in the United States: injuries, cancer, and heart disease.

Source: Rice, D. P., E. J. MacKenzie and Associates (1989). Cost of Injury in the United States: A report to Congress. San Francisco, Calif.: Inst. for Health and Aging, Univ. of California and Injury Prevention Center, the Johns Hopkins Univ.

$51,000 for cardiovascular diseases and $88,000 for cancer (see Figure 17.4).[4]

It is important to point out that federal funding for health research is not allocated on a cost-per-death basis. Expenditures for injury control in 1987 were only about 11% of those for the National Cancer Institute and 17% of those for the National Heart, Lung, and Blood Institute. Eighty-six dollars were spent on research for each heart

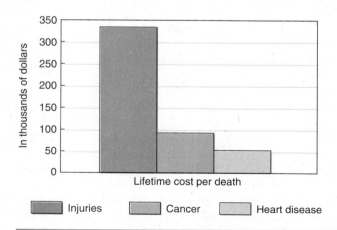

FIGURE 17.4

Cost per death for three causes of death in the United States: injuries, cancer, and heart disease.

Source: Rice, D. P., E. J. MacKenzie and Associates (1989). Cost of Injury in the United States: A report to Congress. San Francisco, Calif.: Inst. for Health and Aging, Univ. of California and Injury Prevention Center, the Johns Hopkins Univ.

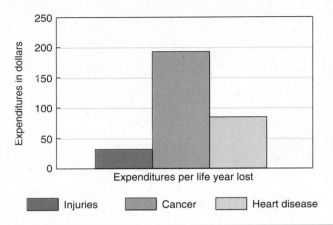

FIGURE 17.5

Research expenditures for three causes of death in the United States: injuries, cancer, and heart disease.

Source: Rice, D. P., E. J. MacKenzie and Associates (1989). Cost of Injury in the United States: A report to Congress. San Francisco, Calif.: Inst. for Health and Aging, Univ. of California and Injury Prevention Center, the Johns Hopkins Univ.

disease death and $195 for each cancer death, but only $31 for each injury death (see Figure 17.5).[4]

UNINTENTIONAL INJURIES

Even when intentional injury statistics are excluded, injuries remain the fifth leading cause of deaths in the United States (see Table 17.1).[7] In 1991, approximately 80,000 deaths resulting from unintentional injury were reported.[2] In addition, about 86 million disabling injuries were reported the same year. These deaths and injuries resulted in an economic loss to families and society of approximately $177.5 billion, when one considers lost wages, incurred medical expenses, property damage, insurance administration cost, and loss of productivity.[2] Clearly, unintentional injuries constitute a

major community health problem (see Boxes 17.1 and 17.2).

Types of Unintentional Injuries

There are many types of unintentional injuries. The majority occur as a result of motor vehicle crashes, falls, drownings, and fires.

Motor Vehicle Crashes

More people die from unintentional injuries associated with motor vehicle crashes than any other type of injury. In 1990, there were 44,531 fatalities, 5.4 million nonfatal injuries, and 28 million damaged vehicles.[5] There were also approximately 1.7 million disabling injuries as a result of car crashes that year.[8] Nearly 23 million Americans were involved in some type of motor vehicle crash that year—that is about one out of every ten people. To put the number of highway deaths each year in perspective, it is in-

Table 17.1
Estimated Deaths, Death Rates, and Percent of Total Deaths for the 15 Leading Causes of Death: United States, 1992

[Data are provisional, estimated from a 10-percent sample of deaths. Rate per 100,000 population. Figures may differ from those previously published. Due to rounding, figures may not add to totals. See table 10 for category numbers of causes of death.]

Rank	Cause of death (Ninth Revision, International Classification of Diseases, 1975)	Number	Death Rate	Percent of Total Deaths
	All causes	2,177,000	853.3	100.0
1	Diseases of heart	720,480	282.5	33.1
2	Malignant neoplasms, including neoplasms of lymphatic and hematopoietic tissues	521,090	204.3	23.9
3	Cerebrovascular diseases	143,640	56.3	6.6
4	Chronic obstructive pulmonary diseases and allied conditions	91,440	35.8	4.2
5	Accidents and adverse effects	86,310	33.8	4.0
	Motor vehicle accidents	41,710	16.4	1.9
	All other accidents and adverse effects	44,600	17.5	2.0
6	Pneumonia and influenza	76,120	29.8	3.5
7	Diabetes mellitus	50,180	19.7	2.3
8	Human immunodeficiency virus infection	33,590	13.2	1.5
9	Suicide	29,760	11.7	1.4
10	Homicide and legal intervention	26,570	10.4	1.2
11	Chronic liver disease and cirrhosis	24,830	9.7	1.1
12	Nephritis, nephrotic syndrome, and nephrosis	22,400	8.8	1.0
13	Septicemia	19,910	7.8	0.9
14	Atherosclerosis	16,100	6.3	0.7
15	Certain conditions originating in the perinatal period	15,790	6.2	0.7
	All other causes	298,430	117.0	13.7

Note: Rates have been recomputed based on revised population estimates; see Technical notes.

Source: National Center for Health Statistics. Annual summary of Births, Marriages, Divorces, and Deaths: United States, 1992. Monthly vital statistics report: vol. 41 no. 13. Hyattsville, Maryland: Public Health Services, 1993.

structive to note that in the ten years that the United States fought in Vietnam, a total of about 58,000 Americans lost their lives fighting. During that same period of time, between 500,000 and 600,000 Americans lost their lives on U.S. highways (see Boxes 17.3 and 17.4).

Other Types of Unintentional Injuries

Unintentional injuries also occur as a result of falls, fires, or the accidental discharge of firearms. Other injuries take place during swimming, boating, and hunting activities, or during natural disasters such as floods, tornados, earthquakes, or hurricanes. Deaths due to these types of injuries numbered about 19,000 in 1989. This total does not include deaths that occurred in the workplace. The Number 1 cause of nontransport, non-motor vehicle deaths is falls, followed by drownings, fires and burns, and firearms. Public transportation deaths (motor vehicles excluded) were led by air, then water, rail, and other types of transport such as street cars and bicycles.[2] An examination of the ranking of deaths resulting from unintentional injuries by number of potential years of life lost is as follows: motor vehicles, drowning, fires, poisonings, falls, firearms, and suffocation by ingestion (choking).

Epidemiology of Unintentional Injuries

As a community health problem, unintentional injuries constitute a major concern. As in the case of all injury deaths, unintentional injury deaths account for a disproportionately large number of early deaths in our society. For example, they claim more lives of people under 44 years of age than infectious or chronic diseases, and they account for more than 40% of the deaths of young people, ages 5–14 and 15–24 years.[7]

Again, it is important to remember that deaths are only a part of the human toll. Incapacitation by unintentional injuries is

---

BOX 17.1
Barriers to Unintentional Injury Control: Do You Have an Attitude?

One of the major reasons why unintentional injuries continue to be a community health problems is the general public attitude. Many people consider unintentional injuries as a part of life—something over which we have no control. Here is a list of common attitudes and an example of the consequences of each:

1. *It can happen to others, not me.* This is a common attitude taken by those who do not wear safety belts. People rationalize by saying, "I am a good defensive driver. Automobile accidents occur to those who are reckless and drunk. I am neither."

2. *It's faith—an act of God.* Those who play golf in the rain and those who do not take cover during a tornado warning believe that resulting injuries are acts of God—something over which they have no control.

3. *When it's your time to go, you go!* Again this is an attitude that reflects that hu-

man beings have no control over their destiny, no matter what they do or how they behave.

4. *He asked for it!* Some people feel if a person lives an evil life, then unintentional injuries are the payback.

5. *Law of averages.* If one engages in risky behavior often enough, sooner or later he or she is going to have an unintentional injury.

6. *It's the price we pay for progress.* People have come to accept the unintentional injuries that come with convenience and new ideas. People are not willing to change habits to reduce unintentional injuries. Little has been done by the average citizen to reduce automobile accidents. The majority of drivers in the United States still do not wear their safety belts, and many people continue to drive above the speed limits.

BOX 17.2
Healthy People 2000—Objective

9.1   Reduce deaths caused by unintentional injuries to no more than 29.3 per 100,000 people. (Age-adjusted baseline: 34.5 per 100,000 in 1987)

Special Population Targets

Deaths Caused by Unintentional Injuries (per 100,000)	1987 Baseline	2000 Target	Percent Increase
9.1a American Indians/Alaska Natives	82.6	66.1	
9.1b Black males	64.9	51.9	
9.1c White males	53.6	42.9	

Baseline data source: National Vital Statistics System, CDC.

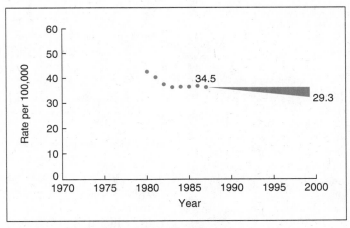

Age-adjusted unintentional injury death rate.

9.2   Reduce nonfatal unintentional injuries so that hospitalizations for this condition are no more than 754 per 100,000 people. (Baseline: 887 per 100,000 in 1988)

Baseline data source: National Hospital Discharge Survey, CDC.

For Further Thought

If unintentional injuries are such a problem in the United States, why do you think more emphasis is not placed on preventing them?

SPEED LIMITS ON
INTERSTATE HIGHWAYS

In 1973, as a result of the Arab oil embargo, the United States experienced a shortage of gasoline for automobiles. As a measure to encourage more efficient use of gasoline, a nationwide 55-mile-per-hour speed limit was put in force. As a result, traffic moved more slowly and traveled at a more uniform pace. Most importantly, deaths from motor vehicle crashes dropped 17%.*

In 1987, Congress enacted a law permitting states to raise the speed limits to 65 miles per hour on interstate highways passing through areas of less than 50,000 population. By 1988, 40 states had implemented the law on all or some of their interstate highways.

Studies of fatalities from vehicle crashes before and after the speed limit increase show an increase of 14%–27% on the affected highways.† There was an accompanying increase in fatalities on rural noninterstate highways, which researchers attributed to "speed spillover."

*National Safety Council (1975). *Accident Facts, 1975 Edition*. Chicago: Author, pp. 42–53.

†National Safety Council (1992). *Accident Facts, 1992 Edition*. Chicago: Author, p. 58.

Some of the factors that describe where, when, and to whom unintentional injuries occur are discussed in the sections that follow. In addition to describing the occurrence of injuries by person, place, and time, we include a discussion of alcohol and other drugs as risk factors in unintentional injuries.

Person

Unintentional injuries resulting in death and disability occur in all age groups, sexes, races, and socioeconomic groupings. However, certain groups are at greater risk for injury than others.

Age

After the first few months of life, unintentional injuries become the leading cause of death in children. Children under the age of 15 make nearly 10 million emergency visits due to injuries each year.[9] It is often not their fault, but rather the fault of their parents, or in some cases, of the community. Box 17.5 lists 12 measures that could reduce childhood deaths from unintentional injuries by 29%.[9] Unintentional injuries constitute the leading cause of death not only in children but in all age groups from 1 to 44 years.[7] For youths, 15–24 years old, unintentional injuries claim more than twice as many lives as the next leading cause of death, homicide.[7]

Children and teenagers, particularly, are at risk of dying as a result of unintentional firearm injury. While this cause was the eighth leading cause of death in all age groups in 1988, it was the third leading cause of death among teenagers, ages 10–19. From 1982–1988, 3,607 children and teenagers died from unintentional firearm-related injuries.[10] Since it has been estimated that there are at least 100 nonfatal gunshot wounds for each fatal one, unintentional firearm injuries constitute an impor-

another significant aspect of the problem. One in six hospital days can be attributed to unintentional injuries. These injuries cost Americans $45.8 billion in lost wages, $29.6 billion in medical expenses, $35.4 billion in insurance costs, and $29.0 billion in motor vehicle damage in 1991.[2] Many of these injuries, such as head and spinal cord injuries, result in long-term or permanent disabilities that affect individuals and their families for years.

BOX 17.4
Healthy People 2000—Objective

9.3 Reduce deaths caused by motor vehicle crashes to no more than 1.9 per 100 million vehicle miles traveled and 16.8 per 100,000 people. (Baseline: 2.4 per 100 million vehicle miles traveled (VMT) and 18.8 per 100,000 people [age adjusted] in 1987)

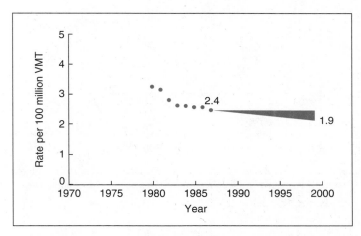

Motor vehicle crash death rate per 100 million vehicle miles traveled.

Special Population Targets

Deaths Caused by Motor Vehicle Crashes (per 100,000)	1987 Baseline	2000 Target	Percent Change
9.3a Children aged 14 and younger	6.2	5.5	
9.3a Youth aged 15–24	36.9	33	
9.3c People aged 70 and older	22.6	20	
9.3d American Indians/Alaska Natives	46.8	39.2	

Type-Specific Targets

Deaths Caused by Motor VehicleCrashes	1987 Baseline	2000 Target
9.3e Motorcyclists	40.9/100 million VMT & 1.7/100,000	33/100 million VMT & 1.5/100,000
9.3f Pedestrians	3.1/100,000	2.7/100,000

Baseline data sources: Fatal Accident Reporting System (FARS), U.S. Dept. of Transportation; for American Indians/Alaska Natives, National Vital Statistics System, CDC.

(continued)

BOX 17.4 (continued)

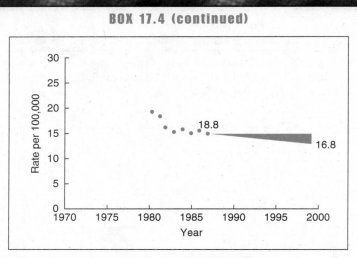

Age-adjusted vehicle crash death rate per 100,000 people.

9.12 Increase use of occupant protection systems, such as safety belts, inflatable safety restraints, and child safety seats, to at least 85% of motor vehicle occupants. (Baseline: 42% in 1988)

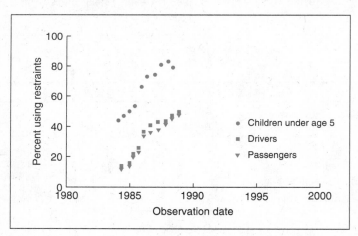

Occupant restraint use by drivers, passengers, and children aged four and younger.

(continued)

tant public health problem. Two states, California and Florida, have enacted legislation making adults legally responsible for inappropriate storage of firearms.

Motor vehicle crashes are the leading cause of unintentional injury deaths for all age groups except for persons 75 years of age and older. Fatal injury involvement rates per 100,000 are highest for drivers 19 years of age and under.[2] Falls are the Number 1 cause of unintentional injury deaths for those 75 years of age and older.

BOX 17.4 (continued)

Special Population Target

Use of Occupant Protection Systems	1988 Baseline	2000 Target
9.12a Children aged 4 and younger	84%	95%

Baseline data sources: National Highway Traffic Safety Admin. and Fatal Accident Reporting System (FARS), U.S. Dept. of Transportation.

9.13 Increase use of helmets to at least 80% of motorcyclists and at least 50% of bicyclists. (Baseline: 60% of motorcyclists in 1988 and an estimated 8% of bicyclists in 1984)

Baseline data sources: For motorcyclists, National Highway Traffic Safety Administration 19 Cities Survey, U.S. Department of Transportation; for bicyclists, R. C. Wasserman, et al. (1988).

For Further Thought

Several of the year 2000 objectives are related to motor vehicle crashes. Of the three objectives presented above, which one do you think has the best chance of being met by the year 2000? Explain your reasoning.

Gender

Statistics indicate that males at every age level are much more likely to become involved in a fatal unintentional injury than females. Overall, the ratio of male deaths to female deaths is 2:1. Males in the 15–24- and 25–64-year age groups, however, die from unintentional injuries at greater than three times the rate of their female counterparts. Differences in unintentional injury death rates between the sexes decline with age, but men retain a marginally higher rate even in the over-75-year age group. The type of unintentional fatality with the widest disparity is firearm injuries (88% males); the type with the narrowest is falls (52% males).[2]

Race

Deaths caused by unintentional injuries occur at different rates depending upon race. In 1987, white males suffered 54 deaths per 100,000 population, while the unintentional injury death rate for black males was 65 per 100,000. During the same period, Native Americans had the highest rate, 83/100,000.[11] Such differences in unintentional injury death rates reflect differences in living conditions, life-styles, and types of employment rather than any inherited tendencies toward unintentional injuries. (See Chapter 9 for other differences in community health problems associated with race.)

Place

Unintentional injuries occur wherever people are: at home, at work, or on the road. While more injuries occur at home, more injury deaths occur on the road.

BOX 17.5
Reducing Childhood Deaths Due to Injuries

These 12 currently known or available preventive interventions could, if universally applied, reduce childhood deaths due to injuries by 29%.*

- Infant seat restraints in automobiles.
- Air bags for front-seat motor vehicle occupants.
- Helmets for motorcyclists.
- Helmets for bicyclists.
- Expansion and enforcement of the Poison Prevention Packaging Act.
- Barriers around swimming pools.
- Self-extinguishing cigarettes.
- Smoke detectors.
- Elimination of handguns.
- Knowledge of the Heimlich maneuver.
- Adherence to Consumer Product Safety Commission regulations.
- Window bars on windows above the first floor.

*U.S. Congress, Office of Technology Assessment (1988). *Healthy Children: Investing in the Future* (pub. no. OTA-H-345). Washington, D.C.: U.S. Government Printing Office.

Home

People spend more time at home than any other place, so it is not surprising that most accidents and unintentional injuries occur in the home. Unintentional injuries in the home result from falls, burns, poisonings, accidental shootings and stabbings, and suffocation. Specifically, unintentional injuries in the home can be classified by the rooms or places in the house where they occur. The presence of appliances (including stoves, toasters, mixers, and so on) and sharp knives in the kitchen makes this room one of the more dangerous ones in the house. Another location where many unintentional injuries occur, particularly to the very young and old, is on stairways. For children, the bathroom, garage, and basement are hazardous areas because of the drugs, cleaning agents, and other poisonous materials that are often stored in these areas. In the home, more people die in bedrooms, where they may be sleeping during a fire, than in any other room.

Residential Institutions

After homes, residential institutions are the most common site of unintentional injuries. Residential institutions include nursing homes and other long-term care facilities.

Workplace

Industry ranks third as a location where injuries frequently occur, primarily because of the machinery that workers use. As one might imagine, there is a wide range of levels of injury between one occupation and another. Three of the most dangerous occupations are mining, farming (including logging), and construction. More is said about injuries in the workplace in Chapter 18.

Highway

Although more unintentional injuries happen in the home, more unintentional injury deaths occur on highways. Approximately 50% of all unintentional injury deaths are motor vehicle deaths (see Figure 17.6). In spite of significant progress in reducing highway deaths during the 1980s, the mortality rate is still about 19/100,000 population,[2] which amounted to 44,531 deaths in 1990.[5]

Time

There are seasonal variations in the incidence of some types of unintentional injuries, but these depend upon the types of accident. For example, 62% of all drownings occur in four months: May, June, July, and August, when people take part in water sports. Conversely, 65% of all deaths due to fires and burns are recorded during the six months from October through March, when furnaces, fireplaces, wood-burning stoves, and electric and kerosene space heaters are most often in use.

Death rates from motor vehicle crashes can be calculated for every 100 million miles traveled. When this is done, the lowest death rates occur during January to April, while the highest rates occur in the late summer and early fall. In 1989, the overall annual rate of 2.01 deaths/100 million miles traveled was the lowest rate on record.[2]

Motor vehicle related deaths increase markedly at night. While mileage death rates average 1.21 (per 100 million miles) in the daytime, they average 4.41 at night. Fatalities also occur at a higher rate on weekends (Friday through Sunday), with Saturday being the most dangerous day to travel.[2]

Much publicity surrounds motor vehicle deaths that occur during the following six major holiday periods: Memorial Day, Fourth of July, Labor Day, Thanksgiving, Christmas, and New Year. However, recent data show that, taken together, these holidays have slightly lower death rates than they would if they were nonholiday periods. Interestingly, the three winter holidays have enjoyed a 7% drop in fatalities while the summer holidays have showed an 8% increase over previous years.[8]

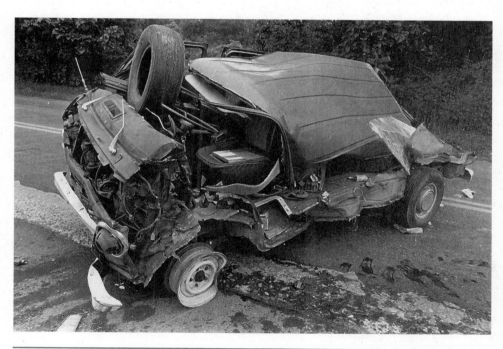

FIGURE 17.6

Approximately 50% of highway fatalities involve the use of alcohol.

Alcohol and Other Drugs as Risk Factors

An examination of the factors that contribute to intentional and unintentional injuries reveals that alcohol may be the single most important factor. This has proven to be the case in fatal motor vehicle crashes. While there has been a decrease from 57% in 1982 to 49% in 1990, alcohol is still involved in about half of all fatalities.[2] Recently, some progress has been noted in the percentage of fatal traffic crashes involving legally intoxicated drivers, drivers whose blood alcohol concentration exceeds .10% (BAC > .10%). The percentage dropped from 46% in 1982 to 39% in 1988. Unfortunately, the number of drivers with BACs between 0.01 and 0.09% remained around 10%. The highest rates of intoxication occur in drivers in their early twenties (see Figure 17.7).

Alcohol use often contributes to motor vehicle injuries and deaths in another way. Safety-belt use by drinking drivers is lower than for their nondrinking counterparts, increasing the likelihood of a fatal outcome if there is a crash. During the period 1982–1989, safety belt use increased from 6.3% to 53.6% among nondrinking drivers involved in fatal crashes, but from only 2.0% to 19.6% among drinking drivers. During each of the years in this period, safety-belt use was lower for drinking drivers.[12]

Alcohol has been determined also to be an important factor in other types of unintentional injuries and deaths. For example, a study of aquatic-related deaths revealed that 47% of adults who drowned had evidence of alcohol in their blood.[13]

There is mounting evidence that alcohol is a major risk factor for boating fatalities. In one study, 60% of those dying in boating

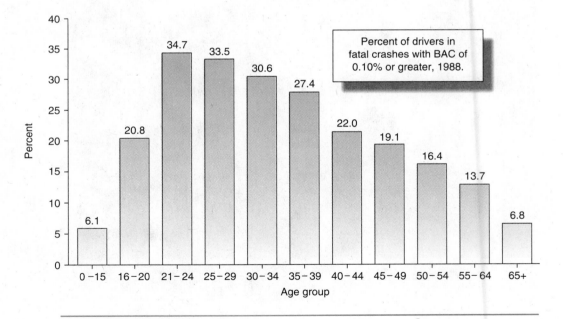

FIGURE 17.7

Alcohol involvement in fatal crashes by age, United States, 1988.

From: National Safety Council (1990). Accident Facts, 1990 Edition. Chicago: Author, p. 56.

fatalities had elevated BACs, and 30% were above 0.10%. In another study, it was found that nearly half of all boating fatalities occurred when vessels were *not* underway. The point is, that while it is dangerous when the person who is operating the boat is drinking, it is also dangerous when passengers have been drinking. Lastly, alcohol consumption lowers your chance of survival should you end up in the water. Clearly, and in contrast to beer companies' messages, alcohol consumption and aquatic recreation are a dangerous combination.[14]

Alcohol is also a factor in bicycle injuries. An investigation of brain injuries sustained by bicyclists in San Diego County, California, revealed that 15 (65%) of 23 brain-injured bicyclists over the age of 14 who were blood-tested for alcohol within four hours of their crash were positive and 12 (52%) were legally intoxicated.[15]

Prevention Through Epidemiology

It is human nature to wait until after a tragedy before correcting an existing hazard or dangerous situation. Most advances in the prevention of unintentional injuries occurred only after costly disasters.

Early Contributors to Injury Prevention and Control

In spite of the extent of the problem, relatively little effort was made to prevent and control injuries until this century. Three of the most important contributors to early efforts at injury control were Hugh DeHaven, John E. Gordon, and William Haddon, Jr. Hugh DeHaven was a World War I combat pilot, who, after surviving a plane crash, dedicated his professional life to studying victims of falls in an effort to design ways to reduce the force of impact on a body. Many of his ideas have led to better design concepts, including structural adaptations to protect drivers and other occupants of moving vehicles. For example, today we enjoy the protection of safety belts, air bags, collapsible steering assemblies, and padded dashboards.[16]

John E. Gordon proposed in 1949 that the tools of epidemiology be used to analyze injuries. Because of Gordon's work, a great deal was learned about risk factors, susceptible populations, and the distribution of injuries in populations.

William Haddon, Jr., was both an engineer and a physician and is often considered the founding father of modern injury-prevention research.[16] He was an unrelenting proponent of the epidemiologic approach to injury control and insisted that the results of this work be used in the development of public policy. He was the foremost expert on highway safety in the 1960s and developed many successful countermeasures to reduce the number of unintentional highway injuries.

A Model for Unintentional Injuries

Until the middle of this century, little progress occurred in the reduction of unintentional injuries and deaths. One reason for this was the failure to identify the causative agent associated with unintentional injuries. In Chapter 4, we discussed the public health model that describes communicable diseases in terms of the host, agent, and environment, arranged in a triangle. A similar **model for unintentional injuries** has been proposed. In this model, the injury-producing agent is *energy* (see Figure. 17.8).

Examples of injury-producing energy are plentiful. A moving car, a falling object (or person), and a speeding bullet all have kinetic energy. When one of these moving objects strikes another object, energy is released, often resulting in injury or trauma.

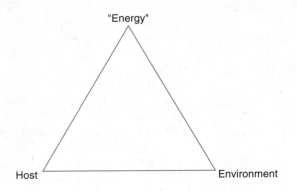

FIGURE 17.8

The public health model for unintentional injuries.

Similarly, a hot stove or pan contains energy in the form of heat. Contact with one of these objects results in the rapid transfer of heat. If the skin is unprotected, tissue damage (a burn) occurs. Electrical energy is all around us and represents a potential source of unintentional injuries. Even accidental poisonings fit nicely into our model. Cleansers, drugs, and medicines represent stored chemical energy which, when released inappropriately, can cause serious injury or death.

Prevention and Control Tactics Based Upon the Model

Based upon the epidemiological model described above, there are four types of actions that can be taken to prevent or reduce the number and seriousness of unintentional injuries and deaths.[17] These four tactics are modified from those of Haddon.[18] The first is to prevent the accumulation of

---

model for unintentional injuries The public health triangle (host, agent, and environment) modified to indicate energy as the causative agent of injuries.

the injury-producing agent, energy. Examples of implementing this principle include reducing speed limits to decrease motor vehicle injuries, lowering the height of children's high chairs and diving boards to reduce fall injuries and lowering the settings on hot water heaters to reduce the number and seriousness of burns. In our electrical example, circuit breakers in the home prevent the accumulation of excess electrical energy.

The second type of action is to prevent the inappropriate release of excess energy or to modify its release in some way. Flame retardant fabric that will not ignite is an example of such a prevention. Currently, there is a law that requires that such a fabric be used in the manufacture of children's pajamas. The use of automobile safety belts is another example. In this case, excess energy (movement of a human body) is released into the safety belt instead of into the car's windshield (see Figure 17.9). In the prevention of fall injuries, handrails, walkers, and nonslip surfaces in bathtubs prevent the inappro-

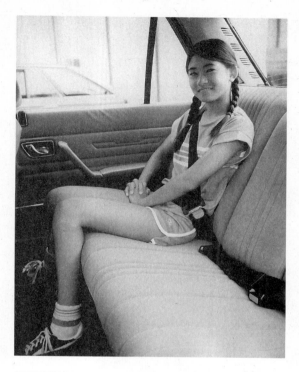

FIGURE 17.9

Safety belts prevent the inappropriate release of excess energy.

priate release of kinetic energy resulting from falls.

The third tactic involves placing a barrier between the host and agent. The insulation around electrical wires and the use of potholders and nonheat-transferring handles on cookware are examples of this preventive strategy. The use of sunscreen lotion and the wearing of a hat in the summer place a barrier between the sun's energy and you.

Finally, it is sometimes necessary or useful to completely separate the host from potentially dangerous sources of energy. Examples include the locked gates and high fences around electrical substations and swimming pools. At home, locking up guns and poisons provides protection against the likelihood of unintentional injury of young children.

Other Tactics

By viewing energy as the cause of unintentional injuries and deaths, it is possible to take positive steps in their prevention and control. Still there are other actions that a community can take. First, injury-control education in the schools and in other public forums can be helpful. Second, improvements in the community's ability to respond to emergencies, such as encouraging the public to enroll in first aid and cardiopulmonary resuscitation (CPR) classes and expanding 911 telephone services, can limit disability and save lives. During the last decade, significant strides have been made in this direction. Third, communities can insure that they have superior emergency and paramedic personnel by instituting the best possible training programs. The result will be improved emergency medical care and rehabilitation for the injured. Finally, communities can strengthen ordinances against high-risk behaviors, such as driving while impaired by alcohol, and then support their enforcement.

Approaches to the Prevention of Unintentional Injuries

There are four broad strategies for the prevention of unintentional injuries: education, regulation, automatic protection, and litigation.

Education

Injury prevention education is the process of changing people's health-directed

---

injury prevention education The process of changing people's health-directed behavior so as to reduce unintentional injuries.

behavior in such a way as to reduce unintentional injuries. Education certainly has a place in injury prevention. Many of us remember the school fire drill, lessons on bicycle safety, and the school crossing guard. Undoubtedly, millions of injuries were prevented in these ways. However, injury prevention education has limitations. For example, Figure 17.10 illustrates both the inefficiency of public education and the difficulties of measuring a successful outcome.

Regulation

For years, motorists were advised to drive more slowly. Some of us can still remember public service announcements in the 1960s and 1970s that reminded us that "speed kills," and not to "drink and drive." Yet the highway death toll continued to mount until 1974, when then president Gerald Ford issued the national 55-mile-per-hour speed limit. Although the slower speed limit was ordered to help conserve gasoline, more than 9,000 lives were saved as the number of motor vehicle deaths dropped from 55,511 in 1973 to 46,200 in 1974.[2] The 55-mile-per-hour speed limit is an example of the power of **regulation,** the enactment and enforcement of laws to control conduct, as a means of reducing the number and seriousness of unintentional injuries (see Figure 17.11). State laws requiring safety belts and motorcycle helmet use are another example of regulation to reduce injuries.

In another example of the power of legislation, Honolulu reports a fatality rate of 0.9/100,000 for swimming pool drownings while Brisbane, Australia, reports a rate of 2.6/100,000. Honolulu requires all public and private pools to be surrounded with protective fencing.[17]

---

regulation The enactment and enforcement of laws to control conduct.

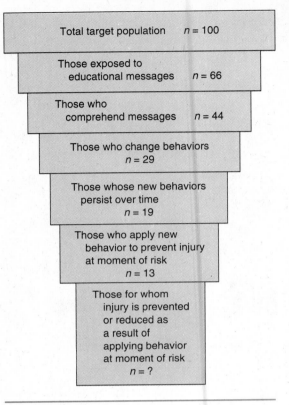

FIGURE 17.10

Attenuation of the effect of a public health education program.

From: E. McLoughlin, C. J. Vince, A. M. Lee, et al., "Project Burn Prevention: Outcome and Implications," *American Journal of Public Health 72(3): 241-247, 1982. As presented in U.S. Congress, Office of Technology Assessment (Feb. 1988). Healthy Children: Investing in the Future, pub. no. OTA-H-345. Washington, D.C.: U.S. Government Printing Office.*

In a "free society," such as the one in which Americans live, there is a limit to how much can be accomplished through legislation. For example, it has been very difficult to reduce the number of firearm injuries in the United States through legislation, because the National Rifle Association has been able to lobby successfully against firearm legislation.

Regulation is not always successful in reducing injuries. Between 1976 and 1980, state laws requiring the use of helmets for

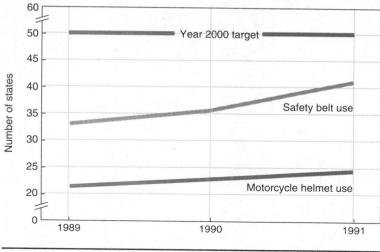

	1989	1990	1991	Year 2000 Target
Safety belt laws	33	36	41	50
Motorcycle helmet laws	22	23	24	50

FIGURE 17.11

Number of states with laws requiring safety belt and motorcycle helmet use for all ages: United States, 1989–1991, and the target for the year 2000.

From: U.S. Dept. of Health and Human Services, National Center for Health Statistics (1993). Healthy People 2000 Review 1992 (DHHS pub. no. PHS-93-1232-1). Washington, D.C.: U.S. Government Printing Office.

motorcyclists were repealed in 28 states. In those states, fatalities due to motorcycle crashes increased 56% while motorcycle registration increased only 1%.[11]

The strategy of prevention through regulation is indeed a complicated move to implement. The idea of regulating health behavior grates against the individual freedom that Americans have come to expect. Why should someone be forced to wear a safety belt? The answer to that is, for the good of the total public; to protect the resources, including human life, of the greater public. Others say, "It's my life, and if I choose to take the risk of dying by not wearing a safety belt, who should care?" That response is all well and good; but when life is lost, it affects many others, such as family members, friends, and co-workers, not just the deceased. This scenario would become worse if the person not wearing a safety belt does not die but becomes a paraplegic and a ward of the state. Many public resources would have to be used.

At what point is some legislation enough? It is known that safety belts and air bags are good and effective, but so are helmets—at least they think so at the Indianapolis 500-mile auto race. So should people now work to pass a law that requires all automobile and truck drivers to wear helmets? How much legislated health behavior is enough?

Automatic Protection

When engineered changes are combined with regulatory efforts, remarkable results are sometimes achieved. The technique of improving product or environmental design to reduce unintentional injuries is termed **automatic (or passive) protection.**[17] Examples include child-proof safety caps and automatic safety belts (see Figure 17.12). Child-proof safety caps on aspirin and other medicine were introduced in 1972. Deaths attributed to ingestion of analgesics and antipyretics had decreased 41% by 1977. Beginning in 1973, free, easily installed window guards were provided to New York City families living in high-risk areas. By 1975, there was a 50% reduction in falls of young children from windows and a 35% decrease in deaths from such falls.

In recent years, automobile safety belt and child restraint legislation has spread in the United States. By 1988, 33 states and the District of Columbia had legislation requiring the use of safety belts. Beginning with the 1990 models, car makers were required to equip all passenger cars with *automatic* crash protection, either automatic safety belts or air bags.[11] Since there are still millions of cars without these automatic devices, it is important that the 17 remaining states enact laws requiring the use of such devices and support vigorous enforcement if the United States is to achieve its national goals of vehicle occupant-protection-system use of 85% of vehicle occupants and 95% of children under five.[11]

Litigation

When other methods fail, behavioral changes can sometimes come about through the courts. Lawsuits filed by injured victims or their families have been successful in removing dangerous products from store

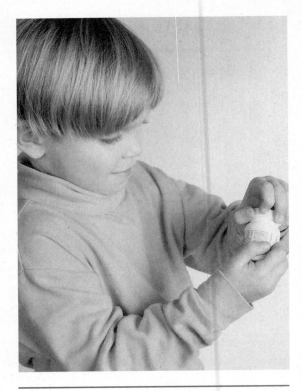

FIGURE 17.12

Child safety caps are an example of automatic or passive protection.

shelves or otherwise influencing changes in dangerous behavior. Lawsuits against bartenders and bar owners for serving alcohol to a drunken customer who has later injured another person have produced more responsible behavior at public bars. Alcohol-related deaths and injuries on college campuses have caused insurance companies to reexamine their liability insurance policies with fraternities and sororities. This has forced some of these organizations and the universities themselves to restrict the way alcohol is used. The outcome may be a drop in unintentional injuries on these campuses.

---

automatic (passive) protection The modification of a product or environment so as to reduce unintentional injuries.

It is important to remember, however, that **litigation,** the process of seeking justice for injury through the courts, is a "double-edged sword." The threat of lawsuits can result in the delay or failure to introduce potentially beneficial products on the market. For example, it has been suggested that the tobacco industry has been slow to introduce cigarettes that self-extinguish when unattended because this might imply that their previous liability for fire injuries caused by current products.[3]

INTENTIONAL INJURIES

Intentional injuries, the outcome of self-directed and interpersonal violence, are a staggering community health problem in the United States. Approximately 50,000 people die and another 2.2 million receive nonfatal injuries each year as a result of interpersonal violence.[19,20,21]

The spectrum of violence includes assaults, abuse (child, spouse, elder), rape, robbery, suicide, and homicide. An estimated 35 million violent crimes and attempted crimes (excluding homicide) occurred in 1991. Stated another way, there were 31 attempted or committed violent crimes per 1,000 people in the United States. This rate is higher than that reported in 1990 but below the record rate of 35 per 1,000 reported in 1981.

In 1992, homicide ranked as the tenth leading cause of death in the United States, accounting for 26,570 deaths.[7] The homicide rate in the United States is significantly higher than in other industrialized nations.

During that same year (1992), suicide ranked as the ninth leading cause of death,

accounting for 29,760 deaths.[7] Suicides account for 20% of all injury deaths.[20] Suicide rates among youth (15–24-year age group) and the elderly have been increasing in recent years.

Interpersonal violence is a costly community health problem not only because of the loss of life and productivity but also because of the economic cost to the community. Consider the community resources expended for each violent act. There are those of the police, the legal system, the penal system, emergency health care services, medical services, social workers, and many others. Clearly, this is a problem for which prevention is the most economic approach.

Epidemiology of Intentional Injuries

To better understand the problem of intentional injuries, there is a need to look more closely at those involved. Interpersonal violence disproportionately affects those who are frustrated and hopeless, those who are jobless and live in poverty, and those with low self-esteem. More violent acts are committed by males. Firearms or other weapons are often involved, as are drugs, especially alcohol. Perpetrators of violent acts are more likely to have been abused as children or exposed to violence and aggression earlier in their lives.

Homicide, Assault, Rape

Most assaults and homicides were committed among minorities, black Americans, Hispanic Americans, and Native Americans (see Box 17.6). "In 1989, an African American male had a lifetime probability of being a murder victim of 1 in 27, compared to a white male's probability of 1 in 205."[22] To put this in perspective, black males are more likely to die on the streets of a major American city today than an American

---

litigation The process of seeking justice for injury through courts.

BOX 17.6
Healthy People 2000—Objective

7.1 Reduce homicides to no more than 7.2 per 100,000 people. (Age-adjusted baseline: 8.5 per 100,000 in 1987)

Special Population Targets

Homicide Rate (per 100,000)	1987 Baseline	2000 Target	Percent Decrease
7.1a Children aged 3 and younger	3.9	3.1	
7.1b Spouses aged 15–34	1.7	1.4	
7.1c Black men aged 15–34	90.5	72.4	
7.1d Hispanic men aged 15–34	53.1	42.5	
7.1e Black women aged 15–34	20.0	16.0	
7.1f American Indians/Alaska Natives in Reservation States	14.1	11.3	

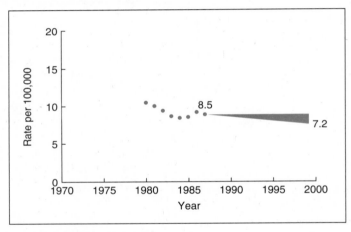

Baseline data source: National Vital Statistics System, CDC.

Age-adjusted homicide rate.

For Further Thought

Why do you think the homicide rates are so much higher in minorities than the general population?

soldier was to die in Vietnam. In 1990, the homicide rates for black males (aged 15–34) was 130/100,000, nearly twice that target goal for the year 2000 (72.4). (See Figure 17.13.)

Most victims of assault are between the ages of 12–34 years. Many, perhaps 2 million, victims of assault are women battered by husbands, former husbands, boyfriends, and lovers.[3]

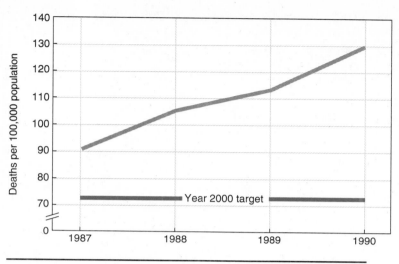

	1987	1988	1989	1990	Year 2000 Target
Black males 15–34 years	91.1	104.9	113.2	130.5	72.4

Note: Death rates are age adjusted. ICD codes differ from similar categories published in *Health, United States* and elsewhere. Related tables in *Health, United States, 1992,* are 28, 30, and 43.

FIGURE 17.13

Death rates for homicide among African-American males 15–34 years of age: United States, 1987–1990, and the target for the year 2000.

From: U.S. Dept. of Health and Human Services, National Center for Health Statistics (1993). Healthy People 2000 Review 1992 *(DHHS pub. no. PHS-93-1232-1). Washington, D.C.: U.S. Government Printing Office.*

Only about half of all rape victims contact law enforcement officials to report the crime, making the acquisition of accurate statistics on rape and attempted rape difficult. Nonetheless, the estimated rates for rape and attempted rape in 1985 were 120/100,000 for women over 12 years of age and 250/100,000 for women aged 12–34. Although reported offenders are usually strangers, this may reflect a reluctance of victims to report acquaintance and date rapes to authorities (see Box 17.7).

Suicide and Attempted Suicide

As indicated above, nearly 30,000 suicides are reported each year in the United States. Provisional data for 1992 indicate that there were a total of 29,760 suicide deaths for that year.[7] Men are about three and one-half times more likely to commit suicide than women.[2] The rates of suicide in young people (15–24 years of age) have tripled since 1950 and those for the elderly have been increasing since 1979.[20]

Firearm Injuries

Firearm injuries and injury death statistics include reports from both unintentional and intentional injuries. For example, if one considers all firearm deaths, those that result from violent and unintentional acts, firearms are the sec-

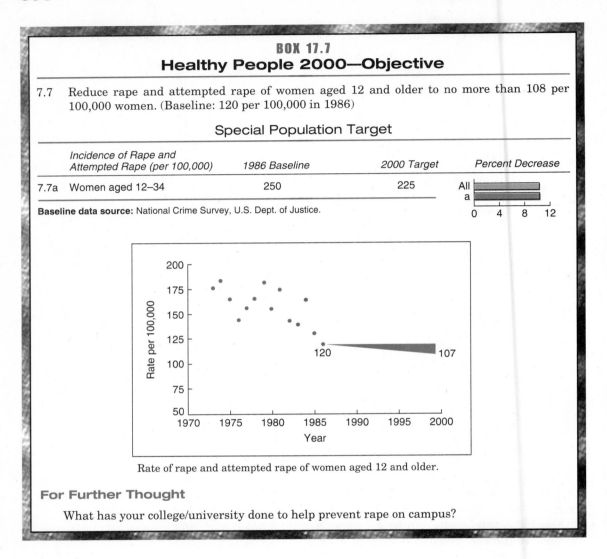

BOX 17.7
Healthy People 2000—Objective

7.7 Reduce rape and attempted rape of women aged 12 and older to no more than 108 per 100,000 women. (Baseline: 120 per 100,000 in 1986)

Special Population Target

Incidence of Rape and Attempted Rape (per 100,000)	1986 Baseline	2000 Target	Percent Decrease
7.7a Women aged 12–34	250	225	All a

Baseline data source: National Crime Survey, U.S. Dept. of Justice.

Rate of rape and attempted rape of women aged 12 and older.

For Further Thought

What has your college/university done to help prevent rape on campus?

ond leading cause of injury deaths after motor vehicles; firearms were the weapons used in 31,566 deaths in 1985.[11] More than 60% of the homicides and 55% of the suicides committed each year involve the use of firearms. At highest risk for homicide and suicide involving firearms, are teenage boys and young men (ages 15–34 years).

Violence in our Society

A Japanese foreign exchange student is shot by a homeowner, a young man is killed for "cutting" in line, and a child dies from punishment for breaking a rule at home. These are signs of the violent society in which Americans now find themselves living. Over the past few years, violence in America has increased. Many young people do not have the interest or skills to work out a solution to a conflict through verbal negotiation, and they resort to physical violence to resolve it. Some of these confrontations are gang-related, while others are simply individual actions. The availability of firearms in America makes violence all the more deadly, both for those in conflict and for innocent bystanders. In the next sections, we will discuss individual, family, and gang violence.

Individuals and Violence

A significant number of violent acts committed in the United States each year are committed by individuals who lack basic communication and problem-solving skills.[23] Many of these people are not interested in resolving an argument through discussion or compromise. Instead, they are intent on "winning" their argument, by physical force if necessary. (After all, isn't that the way arguments are won in the movies?)

The availability and proliferation of firearms makes this approach particularly deadly. In some black American communities, murder is the Number 1 cause of death for black American males and females, aged 15–34.[24] Unfortunately, violent confrontations often result in injuries and deaths to others who are not directly involved in the confrontation.

Because of the escalating violence, conflict resolution programs are now being offered by schools and other community organizations. One of these courses, "Dealing with Anger. Givin' It, Takin' It, and Workin' It Out," includes a videotape program to teach conflict resolution skills to black American youth. Among the skills taught are how to determine which battles are worth fighting and which are not, that controlling one's own behavior is more important than controlling another's, and that life is more valuable than winning an argument.[25]

Family Violence and Abuse

One in every six homicides is the result of family violence. **Family violence** includes the abuse of children, spouses, and older persons; sibling violence; and violence between intimates and separated or divorced partners. Because being abused or neglected as a child increases one's risk for violent behavior as an adult, it is of paramount importance that society increase its efforts to intervene in cases of family violence, particularly child abuse and child neglect.

Child Abuse

Child abuse can be physical, emotional, verbal, or sexual. Physical abuse is the intentional (nonaccidental) inflicting of injury on another person by shaking, throwing, beating, burning, or other means. Emotional abuse can take many forms including showing no emotion; failure to provide warmth, attention, supervision, or normal living experiences. Verbal abuse is the demeaning or teasing of another verbally. Sexual abuse includes the physical acts of fondling or intercourse, nonphysical acts such as indecent exposure or obscene phone calls, or violent physical acts such as rape and battery.

An estimated 1.6 million children experienced some type of abuse or neglect in 1986.[11] Physical abuse was the most common form of reported abuse, followed by emotional and then sexual abuse.

Child Neglect

Child neglect is the failure of a parent or guardian to care for or otherwise to pro-

---

family violence The use of physical force by one family member against another, with the intent to hurt, injure, or cause death.

child abuse The intentional physical, emotional, verbal, or sexual mistreatment of a minor.

child neglect The failure of a parent or guardian to care for or otherwise provide the necessary subsistence for a child.

vide the necessary subsistence for a child (see Figure 17.14). Neglect may be physical, such as the failure to provide food, clothing, medical care, shelter, or cleanliness. It may be emotional, such as failure to provide attention, supervision, or other support necessary for well-being. Or it may by educational, such as failure to ensure that a child attends school regularly.

Educational neglect is the most common category of neglect, followed by physical, and then emotional neglect.[11] Signs of neglect are apparent to the trained professional, such as a teacher, school nurse, or other community health professional. Such signs include extremes in behavior, an uncared for appearance, evidence of a lack of supervision at home, or an untended need for medical care.

Children are neglected for several different reasons. The parent or parents may have emotional problems, financial difficulties, limited parenting skills, or substance abuse problems. Sometimes, the parents themselves were victims of abuse or neglect as children. Another contributing factor is that there may not be an extended family (grandparents, aunts and uncles) nearby to lend a helping hand or to provide relief for parenting problems (see Box 17.8).

Spouse Abuse

Between 2 million and 4 million spouses are physically battered each year. The violence is often severe, involving such acts as "kicking, biting, punching, hitting with an object, beating up, threatening with a knife or gun, or using a knife or

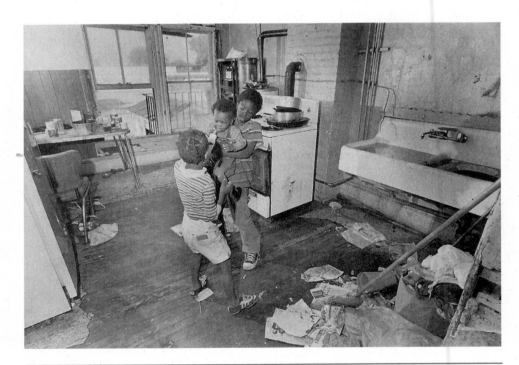

FIGURE 17.14
Child neglect is the failure to provide care or other necessary subsistence for a child.

What Do You Know About Child Abuse and Neglect?

Which of These Statements Are Correct?

1. In many states, certain professionals such as physicians, dentists, police, and teachers are legally required to report cases of neglect and abuse.
2. Common signs of neglect are extreme behavior (aggressive or passive), uncared for appearance, lack of supervision, need for medical care.
3. Child abuse and neglect are rare occurrences.
4. Many abused or neglected children grow up to be abusive or neglectful parents.
5. Emotional abuse can be just as damaging as physical abuse.
6. Oftentimes, child abuse is only directed at one child in the family.
7. Most abusive parents suffer from severe mental illness.
8. The difference between neglect and abuse is that neglect represents a lack of action for a child while abuse represents an action against the child.
9. The incidence of abuse is higher than that of neglect.
10. Many cases of neglect and abuse go unreported.

Answers

1. T; 2. T; 3. F; 4. T; 5. T; 6. T; 7. F; 8. T; 9. F; 10. T.

women in this country have been beaten by a partner at least once. Data show that once abuse has occurred in a family, it is likely to recur.[11]

A Model for Abuse

A **model for abuse** of a family member has been developed. It is a triangle similar to the vector-host-environment model for communicable diseases presented in Chapter 4. In this case, however, the apices are labeled *abuser, abused,* and *crisis* (see Figure 17.15). The crisis may result from the loss of a job, a divorce, illness, death of a family member, or misbehavior (actual or perceived) of children. The likelihood that abuse will occur is greatly increased if alcohol has been consumed. While selected interventions aimed at one factor, for example the abuser, might mitigate against family violence, community efforts to reduce violence should be both comprehensive, involving a variety of approaches, and coordinated among all agencies involved in order to be effective.

Gangs and Violence

While many young women and men in the United States grow up subscribing to such American ideals as democracy, individualism, equality, and education, others do not. Many of these, who are often among the economically poor, have lost faith in society's capacity to work on their behalf. Some of these seek refuge and reward in organized subculture groups of youngsters who feel similarly disenfranchised.[26]

One popular subculture structure is the **youth gang,** a self-formed association of

gun."[11] Abuse can also be emotional or sexual.

More than 1 million women seek medical attention for injuries received from domestic violence each year. Only half of the women who are abused are married; the rest are single, separated or divorced. It is estimated that between 21%–30% of all

model for abuse The public health triangle (host, agent, and environment) modified to indicate the abused (host), the abuser (agent), and a crisis (the environment).
youth gang An association of peers, bound by mutual interests and identifiable lines of authority, whose acts generally include illegal activity and control over a territory or an enterprise.

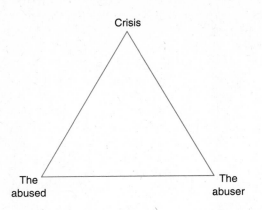

FIGURE 17.15

The public health model for child or spouse abuse.

peers, bound together by mutual interests, with identifiable leadership and well-defined lines of authority. Youth gangs act in concert to achieve a specific purpose, and their acts generally include illegal activities and the control over a particular territory or enterprise.[27]

While youth gangs and gang violence have been around for centuries, the frequency and level of gang violence have increased in the United States in recent years. This increase has resulted in a corresponding increase in the number of intentional and unintentional injuries and deaths.

In Los Angeles County, the number of gang-related homicides rose from 271 in 1979 to 771 in 1991. There has been a corresponding increase in the number of nonfatal injuries. It has been estimated that for every homicide, there are approximately 100 nonfatal intentional injuries.[28] Thus, the number of nonfatal intentional injuries during the same period (1979–1991) rose by some 50,000 (27,100–77,100).

Two factors have contributed to these increases: the epidemic of illicit drug trafficking and abuse, and the availability of firearms, particularly semi-automatic assault weapons. Involvement in the lucrative illegal drug trade has enabled gangs and gang members to purchase and stockpile large inventories of such weapons. For example, it was estimated that the cocaine trade alone was worth more than $1 million per week to four gangs in Los Angeles. It is little wonder then, that one L.A. gun dealer reported sales of 1,000 AK semi-automatic military assault weapons in a one-month period.[28]

While many of the injuries and deaths from gang-related violence occur among the gang members themselves because of intergang rivalries and vendettas, the violence also affects the rest of the community. First of all, many of the gang members still belong to families in the community. Second, other family members and innocent bystanders are often injured or killed in acts of violence such as drive-by shootings or bombings.

Other Costs to the Community

Gangs and gang-related violence present an enormous drain on the law enforcement resources of a community. Pressured to "do something," field officers may be pulled from other duties and not replaced. If additional police are hired, it can cost the community $50,000 per year per officer.[29] There is the additional need to strengthen the prosecutor's office if the operation is to be effective. In short, the suppression of gangs by law enforcement is costly for the communities, often depleting resources for other needed community improvements.

Another problem is the defacing of public and private buildings by gang-related graffiti. One school district in California spends about $1,700 per month removing such graffiti. This money could hire another teacher or otherwise support educational activities.

Community Response

Communities must respond to the increase in violence resulting from gang-related activity. Perhaps the best approach would be a multifaceted effort that would include: law enforcement, education, diversion activities, and social services support.

Suppression of gang activity by law enforcement is justified because many gang-related activities—such as selling illicit drugs, carrying and discharging weapons, and defacing property—are illegal. In many communities, special units with names like SMASH (San Bernadino County Movement Against Street Hoodlums) or CRASH (Community Resources Against Street Hoodlums) have been formed. These groups are made up of representatives from different law enforcement agencies that gather and share information about street gangs and coordinate efforts to combat the problem.[29]

Diversion activities that involve youths in positive activities have evolved in some

communities, as have efforts to resolve disputes between rival gangs. Recently, leaders of two rival gangs in Los Angeles joined hands to work toward community improvement and even attended President Clinton's inauguration.

Education of children, teachers, parents, and community leaders is another facet of gang-related violence prevention. Just as there are antidrug curricula in schools, there are now antigang awareness programs. In one school, the gang awareness program begins in the second grade.[29]

Approaches to the Prevention of Intentional Injuries

Examples of approaches to the reduction of intentional injuries include education, providing better opportunities for employment and recreation, regulation and enforcement, and improving social services such as counseling and treatment.

Education

The most useful education programs for adults have been those which improve parenting skills and nonviolent conflict resolution skills. For youth, the most meaningful programs have been those that develop nonviolent, interpersonal problem-solving skills and social skills, and those that demonstrate and promote appropriate norms of nonviolent behavior. Because young people with low self-esteem are at risk for engaging in violent behavior, programs that develop an increased level of self-esteem are also meaningful.

Opportunities for Employment and Recreation

Many of those involved in the violence in Los Angeles in the summer of 1992 have suggested that a key factor contributing to that violence was the failure of the community to provide greater opportunities for employment, education, and healthful free-time activities for inner-city populations. Similar situations exist in other American cities. Experimental data on violent behavior indicate that participants are usually the uneducated or undereducated and the unemployed segments of the population. Violent behavior not only provides a release of the frustrations of chronic unemployment but, in the case of looting and stealing, fulfills a need for money, food, and shelter, denied by normal means (see Figure 17.16).

Sports and recreational activities have long been touted as a healthy outlet for pent-up physical energy. It seems logical to assume that young persons who participate in such activities would be less likely to become involved in destructive, violent behav-

ior. Yet many communities fail to provide their youth with such opportunities as organized sports programs or other recreational activities (see Figure 17.17).

Regulation and Enforcement

In America, where personal freedoms are regarded as inalienable rights, regulation and enforcement are viewed by many as actions of the last resort. Yet most would agree that these approaches are an important facet of a community's protection against violent acts.

Hence, virtually all state and local governments have laws aimed at reducing injuries and deaths resulting from both intentional and unintentional acts of violence. Examples of such statutes include laws against the carrying of concealed weapons, laws prohibiting the sale of alcohol to mi-

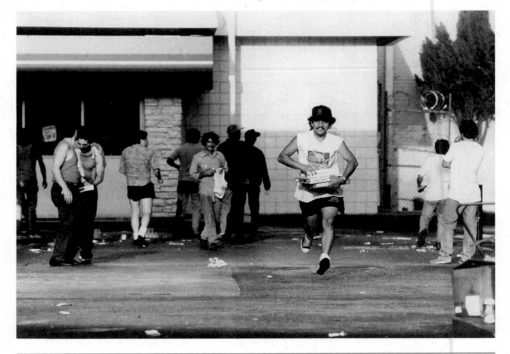

FIGURE 17.16
Rioting and looting are in part a result of the anger and frustration from chronic unemployment.

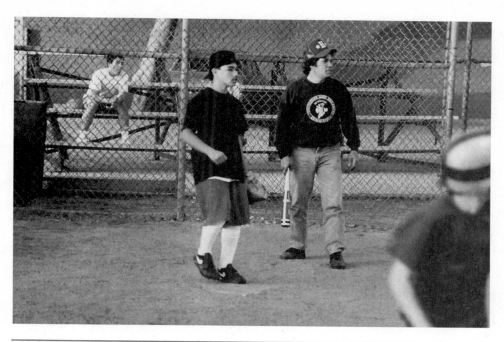

FIGURE 17.17

Adequate recreational opportunities for youth can reduce violence in a community.

nors, and most recently, a federal law that requires a five-day waiting period for the purchase of handguns.

On November 30, 1993, President Clinton signed into law the "Brady Bill" stating, "Americans are finally fed up with violence that cuts down another citizen with gunfire every 20 minutes" (see Figure 17.18). This new law was named after James Brady, the White House press secretary who suffered a disabling injury in a 1981 assassination attempt against then president Ronald Reagan and who, along with his wife, Sarah, lobbied seven years for its passage. The new law will require a five-day waiting period and a background check on all handgun buyers.[30]

Enforcement is often aided by advances in technology. One example is the metal detectors and X-ray units that are used in airports to screen passengers and their luggage. This technology has now spread to inner-city high schools, where it is used to detect concealed weapons. Technology, in the form of computers and communications networks, has also enabled law enforcement agencies to maintain, access, and exchange information electronically. Photographs and fingerprints can now be sent digitally from coast to coast in seconds.

Examples of uses of technology in the prevention of unintentional injuries include the use of the radar gun to apprehend speeders and the use of the Breathalyzer to measure blood alcohol concentrations of drivers. Although there is little doubt that the use of these technologies has prevented injuries and fatalities, they are not useful without citizen support and cooperation.

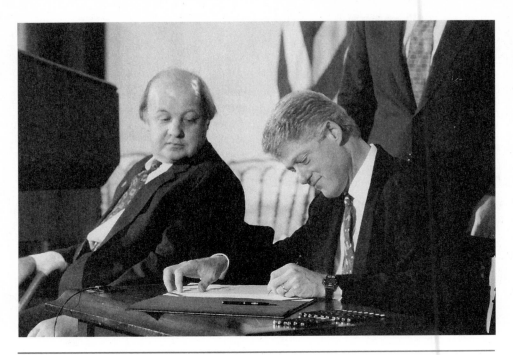

FIGURE 17.18
On November 30, 1993, President Clinton signed into law the "Brady Bill."

While regulations such as these can provide communities with better control over some of the factors that contribute to intentional and unintentional injuries, such regulations may also jeopardize or otherwise interfere with legal activities of certain business groups. When this occurs, proposals for such regulations are likely to be met with resistance. An example of such conflict is provided by the state of Indiana, which has been unable to pass an "open container law," a law that would forbid the consumption of alcohol in the passenger compartment of a moving motor vehicle. The legislation has been successfully defeated in the state legislature each time it has been proposed. To overcome this opposition, concerned citizens have approached individual city and county governments to enact local ordinances to prohibit such behavior. Such local efforts often meet with resistance from the tavern owners and some organized labor groups who sometimes succeed in defeating or "watering down" (weakening) the final version of these ordinances. Hence, there is a limit to what can be accomplished in violent-injury reduction through legislation and enforcement.

Counseling and Treatment

In addition to preventing violent acts by first-time offenders, it is essential that efforts be made to identify and treat past and current offenders as well as those at high risk for perpetrating violent acts. It is important that communities provide outreach counseling and treatment services to those who need it.

A Comprehensive Approach to Prevention of Intentional Injuries

A **comprehensive approach to violence prevention** was outlined in a position paper from the Third National Injury Control Conference.[20] It includes targeting resources "to improve surveillance, to empower communities to develop their own violence prevention programs, to broaden training for violence prevention, and to evaluate rigorously promising prevention programs." The panel who issued this position paper made the following priority recommendations:

- Develop culturally appropriate violence prevention and intervention programs for communities with high rates of violent injury in order to address the specific needs, characteristics, and circumstances of these communities.

- Improve recognition, referral, and treatment of people at high risk for violence or violent injury (e.g., battered spouses, suicidal persons, and victims of child abuse or neglect).

- Set up a system for E-codes (codes to identify the external causes of injury (e.g., attempted suicide or child abuse) to be included with the usual nature-of-injury data in all hospital-discharge data.

- Develop and disseminate at the community level guidelines for preventing violent injuries.

- Develop new financial and other resources for the development and long-term support of community-based violence prevention programs.

- Establish fellowship training programs in violence prevention, with special efforts to recruit minorities and women.

The panel further noted four specific areas of emphasis: (1) injuries from firearm violence, (2) alcohol and other drug use, (3) early childhood experiences that affect the risk of future violent behavior or victimization, and (4) treatable mental disorders associated with an increased risk of suicide.

Firearms

Strategies for the reduction of injuries resulting from firearm violence were designed to minimize ready access to handguns and other firearms. They include educational and behavioral change, technological and environmental efforts, enhanced enforcement of existing laws, and new legislative and regulatory efforts.

Alcohol and Other Drugs

Recommendations target decreasing chronic use of alcohol and other drugs by persons at high risk of violent behavior, by properly identifying such persons and providing them with adequate treatment. Other recommendations are aimed at preventing the initiation of substance use by those already at high risk of interpersonal or self-directed violence. The committee also suggested research to explore alternatives to current drug laws.

Childhood Experiences

Recommendations to reduce instances of child abuse and neglect, witnessing violence in the home, and viewing media violence include: (1) home visitation programs involving nurses; (2) educational intervention programs for children, such as nonviolent interpersonal problem solving; (3) timely crisis intervention for families at risk; and (4) the development of media programs that foster nonviolent behavior.

Mental Disorders

The panel recommends the expansion of efforts to identify and treat those suffering from treatable disorders (such as depression) that are associated with suicide. Secondly, they recommend expanded training for those professionals who are potential gatekeepers for treatment services. Finally, the panel recommends that both public health and insurance funding be increased for outpatient treatment of patients with mental disorders.

CHAPTER SUMMARY

Injuries are the fifth leading cause of death in the United States. Unintentional and intentional injuries represent a major community health problem, not only because of the loss of life but also because of the lost productivity and the increase in the number of disabled Americans.

Unintentional injuries are those resulting from unplanned events that are usually preceded by an unsafe act or condition. They are often accompanied by economic loss or injury, and they interrupt the efficient completion of a task. Most unintentional injuries occur in the home; most fatal unintentional injuries occur on the highway. Although unintentional injuries occur across all age groups, they are the leading cause of death for ages 1–44. Motor vehicle accidents are the leading cause of unintentional injury deaths. Males and minority groups suffer proportionately more unintentional injuries.

Prevention and control of unintentional injuries and fatalities can be instituted based upon a model in which energy is the causative agent for injuries. There are also four broad strategies that can prevent unintentional injuries: education, regulation, automatic protection, and litigation. Together, these strategies may be used to reduce the numbers and seriousness of unintentional injuries in the community.

Intentional injuries are the outcome of self-directed and interpersonal violence. The spectrum of violence includes assaults, abuse (child, spouse, elder), rape, robbery, suicide, and homicide. Suicide and homicide are the ninth and tenth leading causes of death in the United States. Minorities and youths are at highest risk for injury or death from an intentional violent act. Family violence, including spouse, child, and elder abuse and neglect, are serious and pervasive community health problems. Prevention and intervention approaches aimed at reducing intentional injuries and injury deaths must be comprehensive and coordinated in order to be effective.

SCENARIO: ANALYSIS AND RESPONSE

1. Reread the scenario at the beginning of the chapter (about Peter mowing the lawn). How does the description of the unintentional injury fit the definition provided in the chapter? Can you identify each element of the definition as it pertains to this particular scenario?

2. Think about the four approaches to the prevention of unintentional injuries (education, regulation, automatic protection, and litigation). Provide an example of how each of these four approaches could prevent another, similar injury from occurring.

REVIEW QUESTIONS

1. List the ways injuries are costly to society and quantify the costs in terms of the United States.

2. Identify the leading types of unintentional injury deaths and the risk factors associated with each type of death.

3. Why have the terms *accident* and *safety* lost favor with injury prevention professionals?

4. What is a hazard? Do hazards cause accidents? Explain your answer.

5. What types of injuries are most likely to occur in the home, and in which rooms are they most likely to occur?

6. Characterize injuries from the following activities by time: motor vehicle driving, swimming, heating the home.

7. How does alcohol consumption contribute to unintentional injuries?

8. Summarize the contribution of Hugh DeHaven, John E. Gordon, and William Hadden, Jr., to injury prevention and control.

9. Describe the epidemiological model for injuries, and provide three examples of how energy causes injuries.

10. For each of your examples, explain how the injury could have been prevented using prevention and control tactics.

11. List four broad strategies for the reduction of unintentional injuries and give an example of each.

12. Identify the different types of violent behavior that result in intentional injuries.

13. Describe the cost of intentional injuries to society.

14. Define *family violence* and give some examples.

15. Explain the difference between child abuse and child neglect. List some contributing factors to these phenomena.

16. Identify two factors that have contributed to the increase in youth gang violence.

17. Explain what may be the best response communities can make to youth gang violence.

18. Outline four approaches for the prevention of intentional injuries.

19. List and explain four specific areas that experts believe should be emphasized in a coordinated program of prevention of intentional injuries.

ACTIVITIES

1. Obtain a copy of a local newspaper and find three stories dealing with unintentional injuries. Provide a two- or three-sentence summary of each article and then provide your best guess of: (a) what the unsafe act or condition that preceded the event is, (b) what the resulting economic loss or injury was, and (c) what task was not completed.

2. Make an appointment and interview the director of safety on your campus. Find out what the most prevalent unintentional injuries are on campus, what strategies have been used to deal with them, and what could be done to eliminate them.

3. With guidance from your course instructor, conduct a random survey of safety belt use at your campus. Collect the data in such a manner that you can compare the results between school employees and students. Then analyze your results and draw some conclusions.

4. Survey your home, apartment, or residence hall and create a room-by-room list of the unsafe conditions that may exist. Then create a strategy for changing each condition.

5. Using a local newspaper, locate three articles that deal with violence. For each article: (a) provide a two-sentence summary, (b) identify and describe the victim and the perpetrator, (c) identify what you feel was the underlying cause of the violence, and (d) offer a suggestion as to how the violence could have been avoided or prevented.

6. Make an appointment with an officer of the local police department to interview him or her about violent crime in your hometown. Write a two-page summary of your interview and include answers to the following questions: (a) What is the Number 1 violent crime? (b) What is the law enforcement department doing to control violent crime? (c) Does the city have a comprehensive program against crime? (d) What can the typical citizen do to help reduce violence?

7. Write a two-page paper on what the typical citizen can do about violence.

8. Think about the public health triangle model of disease (agent, host, and environment) and gang violence. Describe in writing who or what represents each of these factors. What steps can be taken to reduce gang-related violence using this public health model? List the steps and explain each.

REFERENCES

1. Baker, S. P. (1989). "Injury Science Comes of Age." *JAMA* 262(16): 2284–2285.

2. National Safety Council (1992). *Accident Facts, 1992 Edition.* Chicago: Author, p. 105.

3. Brown, S. T., W. H. Foege, T. R. Bender, and N. Axnick (1990). "Injury Prevention and Control:

Prospects for the 1990s." *Annual Review of Public Health* 11: 251–266.

4. Rice, D. P., E. J. MacKenzie, and Associates (1989). *Cost of Injury in the United States:* A Report to Congress. San Francisco: Inst. for Health and Aging, Univ. of California; and Injury Prevention Center, The Johns Hopkins Univ.

5. National Highway Traffic Safety Administration (1992). *The Economic Cost of Motor Vehicle Crashes, 1990.* (pub. no. DOT HS 807876) Washington, D.C.: U.S. Dept. of Transportation, p. I-1.

6. Max, W., D. P. Rice, and E. J. MacKenzie (1990). "The Lifetime Cost of Injury." *Inquiry* 27: 332–343.

7. National Center for Health Statistics (1993). "Annual Summary of Births, Marriages, Divorces, and Deaths: United States, 1992." *Monthly Vital Statistics Report* 41 (13)1-33. Hyattsville, MD.

8. National Safety Council (1991). *Accident Facts 1991 Edition.* Chicago: Author, p. 51.

9. U.S. Congress, Office of Technology Assessment (1988). *Healthy Children: Investing in the Future* (pub. no. OTA-H-345). Washington D.C.: U.S. Government Printing Office.

10. Centers for Disease Control and Prevention (1992). "Unintentional Firearm-related Fatalities Among Children and Teenagers—United States, 1982–1988." *Morbidity and Mortality Weekly Reports* 41(25): 442–451.

11. U.S. Dept. of Health and Human Services, U.S. Public Health Service (1991). *Healthy People 2000. National Health Promotion and Disease Prevention Objectives* (pub. no. PHS-91-50212). Washington, D.C.: U.S. Government Printing Office.

12. Centers for Disease Control (1991). "Safety-Belt Use Among Drivers Involved in Alcohol-related Fatal Motor-Vehicle Crashes—United States, 1982–1989." *Morbidity and Mortality Weekly Report* 40(24): 397–400.

13. Centers for Disease Control (1982). "Aquatic Deaths and Injuries—United States." *Morbidity and Mortality Weekly Report* 31(31): 417–419.

14. Howland, J., G.S. Smith, T. Mangione, R. Hingson, W. DeJong, and N. Bell (July 7 1993). "Missing the Boat on Drinking and Boating." *JAMA* 270(1): 91–92.

15. Kraus, J. F., D. Fife, and C. Conray (1987). "Incidence, Severity and Outcomes of Brain Injuries Involving Bicycles." *American Journal of Public Health* 77(1): 76–78.

16. Lescohier, I., S. S. Gallagher, and B. Guyer (1990). "Not by Accident." *Issues in Science and Technology* 6: 35–42.

17. Centers for Disease Control (1982). "Unintentional and Intentional Injuries—United States." *Morbidity and Mortality Weekly Report* 31(18): 240–248.

18. Haddon, W. (1980). "Advances in the Epidemiology of Injuries as a Basis for Public Policy." *Public Health Reports* 95(5): 411–421.

19. Centers for Disease Control (1986). "Homicide Surveillance: High-Risk Racial and Ethnic Groups—Blacks and Hispanics, 1970–1983." Atlanta: Author.

20. Centers for Disease Control (1992). "Position Papers from the Third National Injury Control Conference: Setting the National Agenda for Injury Control in the 1990s—Executive Summary." *Morbidity and Mortality Weekly Report* 41(6): 1–38.

21. Bur. of Justice Statistics (1989). "Injuries from Crime: Special Report." Washington, D.C.: U.S. Dept. of Justice.

22. Houk, V. N., and R. C. Warren (1991). "Background of the Forum—The Necessity of Social Change in Preventing Violence." *Public Health Reports* 106(3): 225–228.

23. Rice, K. E. (1993). "Conflict-Resolution Curriculum Teaches Adolescents to 'win' without Violence." *Prevention Newsline* 6(3): 4–5. Indiana Prevention Resource Center.

24. Will, G. F. (Nov. 29, 1992). "The Disease of Violence." *The Washington Post*, p. 26.

25. Baxley, N., and Associates (1991). *Dealing with Anger. Givin' It, Takin' It and Workin' It Out.* Champaign, Ill.: Research Press.

26. Padilla, F. M. *The Gang as an American Enterprise* (1992). New Brunswick, N.J.: Rutgers Univ. Press, pp. 1–2.

27. Covey, H. C., S. Menard, and R. J. Franzese *Juvenile Gangs* (1992). Springfield, Ill.: Charles C. Thomas, p. 5.

28. U.S. Dept. of Justice (Sept 1988). "Juvenile Gangs: Crime and Drug Trafficking." *Juvenile Justice Bulletin.* Washington D.C.: Office of Juvenile Justice and Delinquency Prevention.

29. Martinez, F. B. (1992). "The Impact of Gangs and Drugs in the Community." In R. C. Cervantes, ed. *Substance Abuse and Gang Violence.* Beverly Hills, Calif.: Sage Publications, pp. 60–73.

30. Hunt, T. (1993). "Brady Bill Becomes Law." *The Muncie Star.* Muncie, Ind., p. 1.

Chapter 18

SAFETY AND HEALTH
IN THE WORKPLACE

Chapter Outline

Chapter Objectives

After studying this chapter, you will be able to:

1. Describe the scope of the occupational safety and health problem in the United States and its importance to the community.
2. Identify some of the pioneers in the prevention of occupational injuries and disease.
3. Provide a short history of state and federal legislation on occupational safety and health.
4. Explain the difference between occupational injuries and occupational diseases and give several examples of each.
5. Discuss the types of injuries that frequently occur in the workplace and describe their occurrence with regard to person, place, and time.
6. Briefly describe broad strategies for preventing injuries in the workplace.
7. Identify the different types of occupational diseases and some of the causative agents and general strategies for controlling these diseases.
8. List several occupational safety and health professions and describe what the professionals in each of these do.
9. List and briefly describe several occupational safety and health programs for the workplace.

"I was reading a book and ran across something on the symptoms of chronic lead poisoning. What it will do to you is restrict the blood vessels to the kidneys so that the kidneys absorb more salt to raise their blood pressure. At the same time they raise the blood pressure over the whole body. I read that and thought to myself, '. . . you know, S. had high blood pressure and he's been painting since 1950 when they used lead paint.' Then I thought, 'Gee, P.'s got high blood pressure too and he's been painting since the forties.' The cases just started multiplying. The more I thought about it, the more painters I knew with high blood pressure. There's got to be some relation. Out of 15 painters in our crew maybe 10 of them are old enough to have spent a lot of time with lead paints, and out of that 10, 6 or 7 have high blood pressure and nobody ever connected it. But you can't prove it. How are you going prove that it's a job-related disease? It's impossible. You go to the doctor and he'll tell you, 'Well, you're 10 pounds overweight and smoke too much, that's why you've got high blood pressure.' They don't connect it with the lead."[1]

INTRODUCTION

The work force in America numbers approximately 112 million.[2] After home, Americans spend the next largest portion of their time at work, sometimes in unsafe or unhealthy environments. Although it is not always easy to distinguish between the terms *occupational injury* and *occupational illness* or *disease,* it is generally accepted that an **occupational disease** is any abnormal condition or disorder, other than one resulting from an occupational injury, caused by factors associated with employment. Included are acute or chronic diseases that result from cumulative or repetitive exposures to workplace hazards. **Occupational injuries** are injuries that

result from "a work accident or from exposure involving a single incident in the work environment."[3]

Scope of the Problem

Estimates of the annual cost of occupational injuries, illnesses, and deaths in the United States range from $83 billion[4] to $136 billion.[5] The average cost per injury is $13,000. Data suggest that the occupational fatality rate is higher in the United States than in Sweden, Germany, or Japan[4] and that improvements in workplace safety could reduce health-related fringe benefit costs and medical costs without reducing benefits offered by employers, thereby making U.S. firms more competitive.[5] (The cost categories for the employer are listed in Box 18.1.)

Workplace safety and health can be measured by numbers of deaths resulting from occupational injuries and diseases,

---

occupational disease An abnormal condition, other than an occupational injury, caused by an exposure to environmental factors associated with employment.
occupational injury An injury that results from exposure to a single incident in the work environment.

BOX 18.1
Cost Categories

Injury-related costs to employers include:

- Medical payments.
- Wage replacement.
- Incident investigation and litigation.
- Other administrative expenses.
- Workplace disruption and lost productivity.
- Property damage.
- Tax payments that support emergency services and other government aid to the injured.
- Third-party payments when the employer or its agent is liable for damages to nonemployees.
- Wage risk premiums—extra wages that compensate workers for taking the risks involved in their jobs.

---

numbers of injuries, numbers of workers who become permanently disabled, number of those who become ill, and the dollar cost of these occurrences. For example, it is estimated that 7,000–11,000 men and women die each year from workplace injuries, and 47,377–95,479 people die from occupationally related diseases.[4] Each year, there are approximately 2.5 million serious injuries and 70,000 workers who become permanently disabled.[4]

Importance of Occupational Safety and Health to the Community

Beyond the grim statistics stated above, it is important to recognize how occupational and community health problems are linked. The population of those working in industry is a subset of the population of the larger community in which the industry is located. Workers, usually the healthiest people in the community, are exposed in the course of their jobs to specific hazardous materials at the highest concentrations. It is in the factory that the most accurate exposure and health data are available for extrapolation to the general community. Most pollutants for which exposure levels have been calculated are workplace materials for which occupational exposures were studied first.

Hazardous agents in the workplace affect not only workers but those outside the worksite. This can occur through soil and groundwater contamination with solids and liquids, or air pollution with industrial gases and dusts. It can also occur through clothing and vehicle contamination, as in the case of asbestos workers whose wives and children became exposed to asbestos from these sources.[6] It is important to note that the general population, which includes children, elderly, and pregnant women, is more sensitive to exposure to pollutants than the work force, who usually represent the fittest members of the population.

Another way that industries and their communities share health problems is in the instance of an industrial disaster. Examples include the Bhopal tragedy in India, the Three Mile Island nuclear reactor meltdown in the United States, and the Chernobyl catastrophe in Ukraine.

Finally, it is important to recognize the workers themselves as a community, with common social problems and environmental risks. The failure to recognize the community nature of occupational groups and to monitor chronic conditions such as dermatitis, headaches, blood pressure, or blood chemistries has been a major weakness in our conventional approach to occupational health problems.[6]

HISTORY OF OCCUPATIONAL SAFETY AND HEALTH PROBLEMS

Occupational risks undoubtedly occurred even in prehistoric times, not only during hunting and warfare but also in more peaceful activities such as the preparation of flint by knapping. The discovery of flint heaps suggests that even these earliest of workers may have been at risk for silicosis (dust on the lungs).

An extensive historical review of occupational safety and health problems, from early Egyptian times to the present day, has been published.[7] In this chapter, we will concentrate only on recent events in the United States and make only brief reference to earlier milestones.

Origins of the Occupational Safety and Health Movement

The first of these milestones occurred in 1561, with George Agricola's treatise on mining, *De Re Metallica,* which emphasized the need for ventilation of mines. In 1567, the work of Philippus Aureolus Theophrastus Bombastus von Hohenheim, also known as Paracelsus, was published under the title *On the Miners' Sickness and Other Miners' Diseases.* These were the first significant works describing specific occupational diseases. The first work on occupational diseases in general was Ramazzini's *Discourse on the Diseases of Workers,* which appeared in 1700.[7,8]

Occupational Safety and Health in the United States

The Industrial Revolution, which began in Britain in the eighteenth century, soon spread to continental Europe and to the United States. Factors creating and driving the Industrial Revolution were the substitution of steam and coal for animal power, the substitution of machines for human skills, and other advances in industrial technology.[7] These changes resulted in the rise of mass manufacturing, the organization of large work units such as mills and factories, and eventually, the exposure of masses of workers to new hazards. Although mining remained the most dangerous form of work, there were soon other unsafe occupations such as iron smelting and working in cotton mills and textile factories (see Figure 18.1).

The recognition of the need to reduce workplace injuries began long before any attention was paid to workplace diseases. The earliest efforts of those responsible for inspecting workplaces were aimed primarily at the sanitation and cleanliness of workplaces. They soon became concerned with equipment safeguards and tending to those who had become injured or ill at work.[9] These efforts, while much needed and appreciated, did little to improve the overall health of the work force.

State Legislation

The first official responses to new hazards in the workplace did not occur until 1835, when Massachusetts passed the first Child Labor Law and later in 1867, when it created a Department of Factory Inspection to enforce it (see Figure 18.2). Under this law, factories were prohibited from hiring children under ten years of age.[10] At this time the federal government was concerned only with working conditions of federal employees. In 1877, Massachusetts passed the first worker safety law aimed at protecting textile workers from hazardous spinning machinery.[11]

The first state to pass any kind of workers' compensation legislation was Maryland in 1902. In 1908, Congress, at the insis-

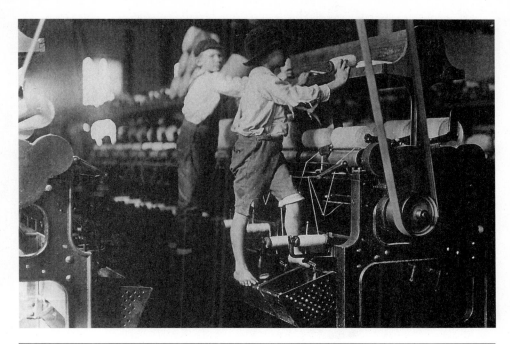

FIGURE 18.1

Cotton mills in the late nineteenth century offered little protection from injuries.

tence of President Theodore Roosevelt, finally enacted the first of several **workers' compensation laws;** this one covered certain federal employees. Over the next 40 years, all states and territories eventually enacted some type of workers' compensation legislation, beginning with New York in 1910 and ending with Mississippi in 1948.[7] So ended the first wave of reform in occupational safety and health. With the exception of several legislative efforts, little further progress was achieved during the first half of the century in protecting workers from injuries in the workplace, and almost nothing was done about occupational illnesses.

There was one exception. Alice Hamilton (1869–1970) was a strong proponent of occupational health and a true pioneer in this field (see Figure 18.3). Over her 40-year career in occupational health, she led crusades to reduce poisonings from heavy metals such as lead and mercury. She investigated silicosis in Arizona copper mines, disulphide poisoning in the viscose rayon industry, and many other industrial health problems.[10]

In spite of Hamilton's efforts, progress in occupational health legislation was slow in the first half of the twentieth century. Occupational diseases were by and large ignored. There was some safety legislation, such as the Coal Mine Safety Act of 1952. Beginning in the 1960s, some people began to take a closer look at the various state worker safety and workers' compensation laws. It was discovered that in most states,

---

workers' compensation laws A set of federal laws designed to compensate those workers and their families who suffer injuries, disease, or death from workplace exposure.

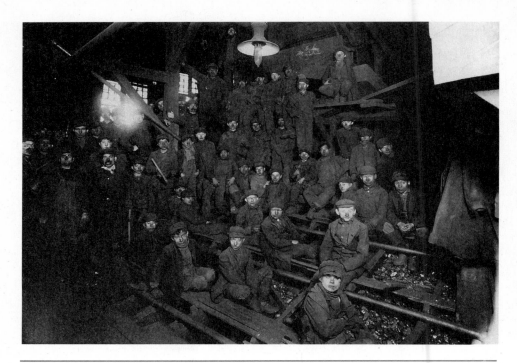

FIGURE 18.2

Before child labor laws were passed, many children worked long hours at dangerous jobs such as mining.

legislation was a patchwork of fragmentary laws; some states had good laws, but many had inadequate legislation. Many of the laws had kept up with neither new technology nor inflation. Some groups of workers, including agricultural workers, were not covered at all by legislation. Other problems were the division of authority among various departments within state governments, fragmented record keeping, and inadequate administrative personnel.[12]

Federal Legislation

In 1884, the federal government created a Bureau of Labor, in 1910, the Federal Bureau of Mines; and in 1914, the Office of Industrial Hygiene and Sanitation in the Public Health Service. In 1916, Congress passed the Federal Employees' Compensation Act, which provided federal employees compensation if injured while on the job.[11] There have been some important laws passed since 1916 (see Table 18.1), but the two most comprehensive laws were the Coal Mine Health and Safety Act of 1969 and the **Occupational Safety and Health Act of 1970 (OSHAct)**. The Occupational Safety and Health Act, now about 25 years old, served to raise the consciousness of both management and labor to the problems of health and safety in the workplace.

Occupational Safety and Health Act of 1970 (OSHAct)
Comprehensive federal legislation aimed at assuring safe and healthful working conditions for working men and women.

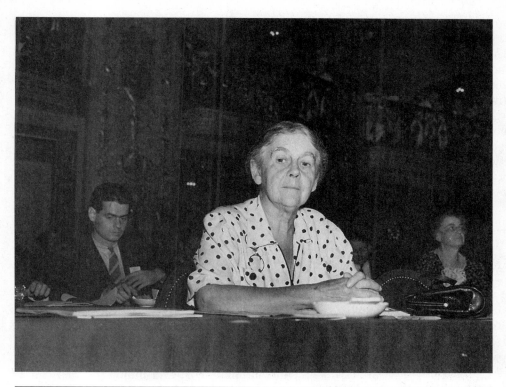

FIGURE 18.3

Alice Hamilton (1869–1970) was a pioneer in occupational safety and health in America.

Occupational Safety and Health Act of 1970

The purpose of the Occupational Safety and Health Act of 1970 (OSHAct) is to assure that employers in the private sector furnish each employee "employment and a place of employment which are free from recognized hazards that are causing or likely to cause death or serious physical harm."[11] Furthermore, employers were henceforth required to comply with all occupational safety and health standards promulgated and enforced under the act by the **Occupational Safety and Health Administration (OSHA),** which was also established by the act.

Also established by the OSHAct was the **National Institute for Occupational Safety and Health (NIOSH),** a research body, now located in the Centers for Disease Control and Prevention of the Department of Health and Human Services. NIOSH is responsible for recommending occupational

Occupational Safety and Health Administration (OSHA) The federal agency located within the Department of Labor and created by the OSHAct that is charged with the responsibility of administering the provisions of the OSHAct.

National Institute for Occupational Safety and Health (NIOSH) A research body within the Department of Health and Human Services that is responsible for developing and recommending occupational safety and health standards.

saftey and health standards to OSHA, which is located in the Department of Labor.

The OSHAct contains several noteworthy provisions. Perhaps the most important is the employee's right to request an OSHA inspection. Under this right, any employee or any employee representative may notify OSHA of violations of standards or of the general duty obligation (to provide a safe and healthy workplace) by the employer. Under the act, the employee's name must be withheld if desired and the employee or a representative may accompany the OSHA inspectors in their inspection. For another provision of the OSHAct, individual states can regain local authority over occupational health and safety by submitting state laws that are and will continue to be as effective as the federal programs.[11]

EPIDEMIOLOGY OF OCCUPATIONAL INJURIES AND DISEASES

The following paragraphs present an epidemiological description of workplace injuries followed by workplace diseases.

Injuries in the Workplace

Injuries in the workplace include minor injuries, such as bruises, cuts, abrasions, and minor burns; and major injuries, such as amputations, fractures, severe lacerations, eye losses, acute poisonings, and severe burns. Statistics on injuries and injury deaths are available from several sources, including the National Center for Health Statistics (NCHS), the National Safety Council (NSC), the Bureau of Labor Statistics (BLS), and the National Institute for Occupational Safety and Health (NIOSH). For this reason, estimates of the number of occupational injuries and injury deaths vary considerably. For example, the estimated number of annual work-related deaths is 3,000 (BLS), 6,000 (NIOSH), and 10,000 (NSC).[13]

It is estimated that for the 20–64-year-old age group, one-third of all injuries and one-sixth of all injury deaths occur on the job.[13] According to NIOSH data, prepared from the National Traumatic Occupational Fatality (NTOF) file, 36,210 fatal occupa-

Table 18.1
Highlights of Federal Occupational Safety and Health Legislation

Year	Legislation
1908	Federal Workmen's Compensation Act—limited coverage
1916	Federal Highway Aid Act
1926	Federal Workmen's Compensation Act amended to include all workers
1927	Federal Longshoremen's and Harbor Workers' Compensation Act
1936	Walsh-Healey Public Contracts Act
1952	Coal Mine Safety Act
1958	Federal Longshoremen's and Harbor Workers Compensation Act amended to include rigid safety precautions
1959	Radiation Standards Act
1960	Federal Hazardous Substances Labeling Act
1966	National Traffic and Motor Vehicle Safety Act
1966	Child Protection Act—banned hazardous household substances
1967	National Commission on Product Safety created
1968	Natural Gas Pipeline Safety Act
1969	Construction Safety Act
1969	Child Protection Act amended to broaden the coverage
1969	Coal Mine Health and Safety Act
1970	Occupational Safety and Health Act
1970	Poison Prevention Packaging Act

BOX 18.2
Healthy People 2000—Objective

10.2 Reduce work-related injuries resulting in medical treatment, lost time from work, or restricted work activity to no more than six cases per 100 full-time workers. (Baseline: 7.7 per 100 in 1987)

Special Population Targets

	Work-Related Injuries (per 100)	1983–87 Average	2000 Target	Percent Decrease
10.2a	Construction workers	14.9	10	
10.2b	Nursing and personal care workers	12.7	9	
10.2c	Farm workers	12.4	8	
10.2d	Transportation workers	8.3	6	
10.2e	Mine workers	8.3	6	

Baseline data source: Annual Survey of Occupational Injuries and Illnesses, U.S. Dept. of Labor.

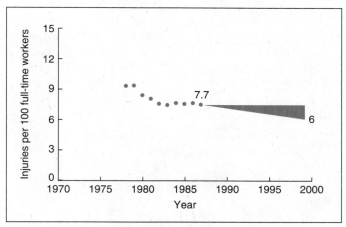

Work-related injuries resulting in medical treatment, lost time from work, or restricted work activity.

For Further Thought

Think back to a job you held in the past. Was there anything dangerous about the work? Did your employer see to it that you were trained properly for the work? Did you wear or have to use safety equipment? Were you ever injured? If so, could it have been prevented?

tional injuries occurred during the six-year period, 1980–1985—this amounts to about 6,000 deaths per year[13] (see Box 18.2).

Types of Injuries

The leading cause of occupational injury deaths by any agency's estimate is motor-vehicle crashes, but these estimates vary.

According to the National Safety Council, 36% of work-related injury deaths are the result of motor vehicle crashes.[14] According to the U.S. Department of Transportation, this figure is only 27.4%.[5] Other leading causes of work related injury deaths are machinery, homicide, falls, and electricity (see Figure 18.4).

The leading cause of nonfatal injury, and the one that accounts for the greatest cost from workers' compensation funds, is back injuries (see Figure 18.5), which affect about 1 in 50 workers per year.[13] These injuries are often caused by overexertion, stooped posture, or other postural stress. Legs, fingers, arms, and hands are also leading injury sites, followed by head and eyes, and feet and toes.

Person

Differences in injury and injury death rates are often related to the age and gender of the worker. Injury death rate differences also occur between those of different income levels and races.

Age and Gender

Injuries are highest for the younger workers of each gender, but males sustain more injuries at each age level than females (see Figure 18.6). While injury rates are higher for younger workers, death rates are highest for workers 65 years of age and older. This group makes up only 3% of the work force but suffers 7% of the fatal accidents. The rate of fatal injuries for workers aged 65 years and older is 14.75/100,000, twice the rate for the next younger age group, 55–64 years, 7.24/100,000 (see Figure 18.7).

One group of workers that has been increasingly exploited in recent years is children. In a recent study, it was determined that the annual number of child labor violations increased from 9,679 in 1983 to 42,696 in 1990 (Figure 18.8).[15] The Government Accounting Office estimates that 18% of all

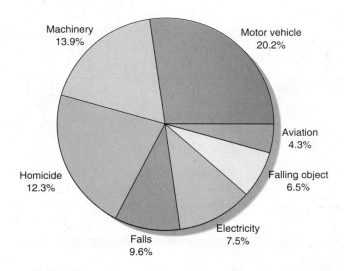

FIGURE 18.4

Occupational injury deaths, United States, 1980–1985.

From: National Institute for Occupational Safety and Health.

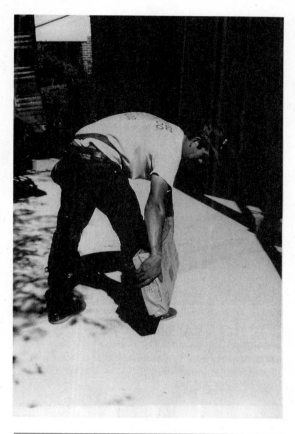

FIGURE 18.5

Back injuries are the leading cause of nonfatal injuries on the job.

working 15-years-olds are illegally employed; that is, they are employed in occupations prohibited to them because of age, or there are standard-hour violations.

During the same 1983–1990 period, serious injuries in illegally employed children increased 100%.[15] It has been estimated that 100,000 children are injured on the job each year. Lastly, a study in Massachusetts found that nearly one-quarter of all emergency room visits by adolescents for treatment of injuries were job-related injuries.[15] One of the most serious situations for children is the agricultural setting, where an estimated 24,000 children are injured each

year, and one in every five deaths is a child under the age of 16.[16] Sixty-five percent of farm boys drive tractors before the age of 12 (see Figure 18.9). It is not difficult to understand why boys are much more likely to be involved in a fatal injury event than girls. The most dangerous ages for fatal injuries for children living on farms are under 2 and over 13.[17]

Only 6% of those killed in the general work force are women; but when figures are adjusted for the numbers of each sex in the work force, the overall occupational death rate for men is 12 times higher than for women (9.9 versus 0.8 per 100,000 workers).[13] A significant portion of the difference results from men being employed in more dangerous jobs.

Poverty and Race

Studies show that those living in counties were income is lower have significantly higher occupational death rates than those living in higher-income counties. In general, death rates for nonwhites are about 12% higher than for whites. However, machinery injury death rates for whites are twice those of blacks. Native Americans are at highest risk for death from explosions and falling objects. Asians have very low death rates for occupational injuries.[13] Occupational injury rates may reflect the types of employment in which workers find themselves.

Place

Occupational injury death rates per 100,000 workers are highest from the mountain states and Alaska and lowest from the northeastern states. Deaths from nonfarm machinery are higher in the mountain states, but deaths from farm machinery are higher in the north central states. Work-related death rates from machinery, falling objects, electric current, and explosion are all higher in rural states. Within states,

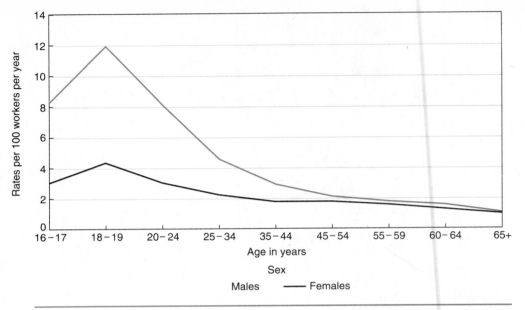

FIGURE 18.6
Occupational injuries by age and sex.
From: MMWR *32(2855).*

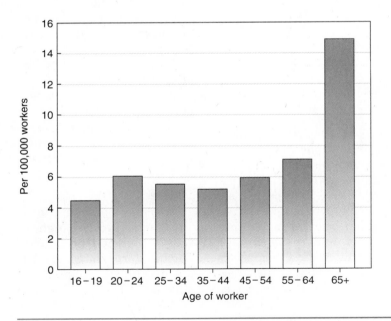

FIGURE 18.7
Death rates from occupational injuries by age, 1980–1985.
From: National Institute for Occupational Safety and Health.

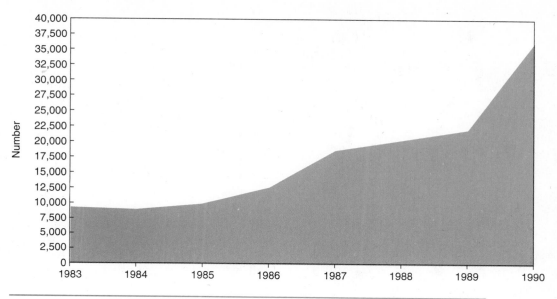

FIGURE 18.8

Federally detected illegally employed minors, United States, 1983–1990.

From: Committee on Labor and Human Resources (1992). Childhood Labor Amendments Report no. 102–380, to accompany Senate Bill 600, Aug. 12, 1992, p. 3.

work-related deaths are higher in rural areas than in more urban areas.

Time

It is important to note that between 1912 and 1989, injury death rates per 100,000 workers have declined 81%, from 21 to 4 while the amount of goods and services produced has increased eleven-fold.[14] There is a seasonality to work-related deaths. Injury death rates from machinery, falling objects, electric current, and explosions are highest in the summer, when farming and construction work increase. Deaths from these causes are also more often reported during weekdays than on weekends, when, in general, more injury deaths occur.

Industry and Occupation

Injury death rates by type of industry and occupation vary depending upon the source of one's statistics. Industry fatality rates are highest for mining, construction,

transportation, and agriculture (see Figure 18.10). When these data are separated into more specific job categories, the highest job-related death rates are found among timber cutters/loggers and pilots (see Table 18.2 and Figure 18.11).[13]

One particularly hazardous occupation is farming. With more than 1,400 deaths and 140,000 disabling nonfatal injuries in 1991,[14] farming ranks fourth among major U.S. industries for work-related fatalities (see Figure 18.10). A major contribution to farm-related fatalities is farm machinery, particularly farm tractors. Deaths occur during rollover incidents in which the tractor tips sideways or backwards, crushing the operator. While all tractors manufactured since 1985 are fitted with seat belts and **rollover protective structures (ROPS),**

rollover protective structures (ROPS) Factory-installed or retrofitted reinforced framework on a cab to protect the operator of a tractor in case of a rollover.

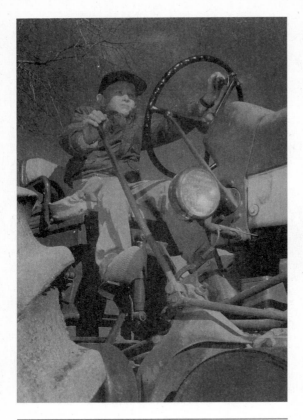

FIGURE 18.9

Sixty-five percent of all farm boys drive a tractor before the age of 12.

more than half of the approximately 4.6 million tractors in use in the United States lack this equipment.[18] The effectiveness of ROPS in protecting the tractor operator has been demonstrated in Nebraska, where only 1 (2%) of 61 persons operating ROPS-equipped tractors that rolled over died. This data compares favorably with a 40% death rate for the 250 persons involved in unprotected tractor rollover incidents. The single fatality in the ROPS-equipped tractor was not wearing a seatbelt and was ejected from the ROPS-protected area.[18]

    Tractor rollover incidents reflect injuries that occur on family farms, and while the statistics seem gruesome, they

underestimate the actual injury rate in all agricultural settings. The highest injury rates probably occur in the migrant work force, where children as young as 12, 10, 8, and even 4 years of age can be found working in the fields. Testimony before the U.S. Senate Committee on Labor and Human Resources by Fernando Cuevas, Jr., paints a grim picture for migrant children (see Box 18.3).[15]

    Of our 50 states, 48 rely heavily on migrant workers during the peak harvest season. These migrant workers have poor access to health care facilities; infant mortality is about 50 per 1,000. In many cases, working conditions are hazardous and water shortages require workers to drink water from irrigation ditches. Not

Table 18.2

Occupations with Highest Job-Related Death Rates, 11 States, 1977–1980

Occupation	Estimated Deaths Annually per 100,000 Workers
Timber cutters/loggers	129
Pilots	98
Asbestos/insulation workers	79
Structural metal workers	72
Electric line installers/repairers	51
Firefighters	49
Garbage collectors	40
Truck drivers	40
Bulldozer operators	39
Earth drillers	39
Specified craft apprentices	38
Mine operatives	38
Boilermakers	35
Taxi drivers/chauffeurs	34
Construction laborers	34

Source: Leigh, J.P. (1987). "Estimates of the Probability of Job-Related Death in 347 Occupations. *Journal of Occupational Medicine* 29: 510–519.

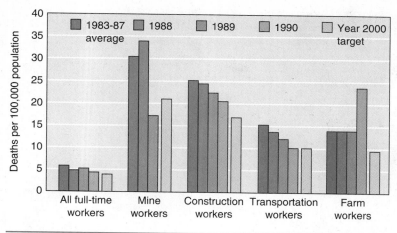

	1983–1987	1988	1989	1990	Year 2000 Target
All full-time workers	5.9	5.0	5.4	4.3	4.0
Mine workers	30.3	33.8	17.3	—	21.0
Construction workers	25.0	24.5	22.4	20.6	17.0
Transportation workers	15.2	13.5	12.2	10.0	10.0
Farm workers	14.0	13.8	13.9	23.8	9.5

Note: Death rates are crude rates. Related tables in *Health, United States, 1992,* are 46, 47, and 75. The data in tables 46, 47, and 75 are age-adjusted.

Source: Bur. of Labor Statistics, *Annual Summary of Occupational Injuries and Illnesses.*

FIGURE 18.10

Death rates for work-related injuries among full-time workers, according to selected occupations: United States, 1983–1990, and the target for the year 2000.

From: U.S. Dept. of Health and Human Services, National Center for Health Statistics (1993). Healthy People 2000 Review 1992. *(DHHS pub. no. PHS-93-1232-1). Washington, D.C.: U.S. Government Printing Office.*

only is such water unpurified, it is usually laden with agricultural chemicals and biological wastes. Migrant workers are also exposed to long hours in the sun, other unsanitary conditions, and numerous harmful pesticides from crop-dusting airplanes.[19]

Controlling Injuries in the Workplace

There are several principles that can point in the direction of controlling workplace injuries. These stem from the theory presented in Chapter 17, that injuries are the result of unintended exposure to energy in amounts that injure the body. As such, injuries on the job can be reduced by: (1) modifying the job to make it safer, (2) changing the work environment, physically or psychosocially, to make it less hazardous, (3) making machinery (including vehicles) safer, and (4) improving the selection, training, and education of the workers.[20,21] It is important to recognize that these strategies are listed in descending order of effectiveness. That is, eliminating or modifying a dangerous task is preferable to changing the work environment, safeguarding the machinery, or im-

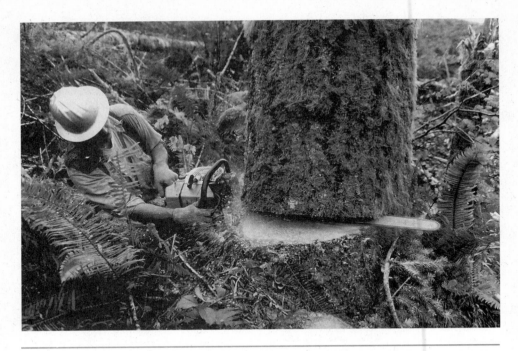

FIGURE 18.11

The highest job-related death rates can be found among loggers and pilots.

proving the selection and training of the worker.

Occupational Diseases

More than 330,000 cases of occupational illness were reported in 1990.[13] The leading types of disorders were those caused by repeated trauma (185,400 cases), skin diseases (60,900), and respiratory conditions due to toxic agents (20,500). In another estimate, deaths from occupational diseases in the United States ranged from 47,377 to 95,479 in 1987 (see Table 18.3).[4]

Types of Diseases

Occupational diseases can be categorized by cause and by organ or system affected. For example, repetitive motion is the cause of injury, but musculoskeletal disor-

Table 18.3
Estimates of U.S. Occupational Disease Deaths, 1987

Cause of Death (ICD Code)	Total Deaths	Proportion Related to Work Exposure	Proportional Ranges (low–high)
Cancer (140–239)	483,497	5–10%	24,175–48,350
Neurologic disease (330–337, 340–359)	34,100	3–5	1,023–1,705
Cardiovascular disease (390–448)	963,611	1–3	9,636–28,908
Pneumoconioses (500–508)	8,670	100	8,670–8,670
Other pulmonary disease (460–499,509–519)	164,164	2–4	3,283–6,567
Renal disease (580–589)	22,052	1–3	220–662
Congenital anomalies (740–759)	12,333	3–5	370–617
Total deaths	**1,688,427**	**47,377–95,479**	
Midpoint:	71,428		

ICD Code: International Classification of Diseases.

Source: National Safe Workplace Institute.

der is the result. Exposure to asbestos is a cause; cancer of the respiratory system, especially the lung, is the result. In this discussion, the categories proposed by NIOSH in the series of booklets *Proposed National Strategies for the Prevention of Leading Work-Related Diseases and Injuries* will be followed.[20–27] Included are musculoskeletal injuries, dermatological conditions, lung diseases, psychological disorders, neurotoxic disorders, disorders of reproduction, occupational cardiovascular diseases, and occupational cancers.

Musculoskeletal Conditions

Musculoskeletal injuries include both acute and chronic injury to muscles, tendons, ligaments, nerves, joints, bones, and supporting vasculature. The leading type of musculoskeletal injury is back injury. Taken together, acute and chronic musculoskeletal injuries are the leading cause of disability in the work force. When one considers both the loss of earnings and the workers' compensation payments, the cost of musculoskeletal injuries exceeds that of any other single health disorder.[21]

In this category of conditions, our concern lies with injury resulting from exposure to continued trauma (see Figure 18.12), in which structures are often described as "inflamed, irritated, or strained, for example, tendonitis, synovitis, bursitis, nerve entrapment, and lumbar pain." These conditions are often referred to as *cumulative trauma disorders* to distinguish them from acute, single exposure injuries. The manufacturing industry reports the highest rate of such injuries. The incidence of musculoskeletal injuries is likely to increase as the work force ages.

Dermatological Conditions

Occupational skin disorders are one of the ten leading causes of morbidity and disability in the workplace. The skin may serve as the target organ for disease, or it may be the route through which toxic chemicals enter the worker's body. Because the integument is the largest organ of the body, and because it is often directly exposed to the environment, it is particularly vulnerable to occupational diseases. In one Bureau of Labor Statistics (BLS) survey, dermatological disease accounted for 34% of all identified occupational diseases (see Figure 18.13).

The greatest number of cases of skin disorders occurs in manufacturing. However, an examination of incidence rates reveals that the rates of occupational skin diseases in agriculture are more than twice as high as those in manufacturing.[25]

Some common types of skin diseases include contact dermatitis, skin cancer, infections (such as erysipeloid, anthrax, mycobacteria, herpes simplex virus, and grain-mite), and other miscellaneous skin diseases. Common chemicals that can enter the body by absorption through the skin (and the diseases they cause) include: aniline (methemoglobinemia, bladder cancer), benzene (aplastic anemia, leukemia), cyanide salts (acute cellular asphyxia and death), and mercury (central nervous system intoxication, kidney failure). Dermal toxicity data are available on about only 1,600 of the 85,000 chemical substances currently listed in the *Registry of Toxic Effects of Chemical Substances*.[25]

Lung Diseases

Occupational lung disease is the result of the inhalation of toxic substances present in the workplace. The lungs, like the skin, can be both the target organ of disease and a portal of entry for toxic substances. Characteristic of occupational lung disease is the difficulty in early recognition (the latent period for such diseases may be 15–30 years) and the problem of multiple or mixed exposures—home and the workplace. Examples of occupational lung diseases include asbestosis, byssinosis, silicosis, and coal workers' pneumoconiosis.

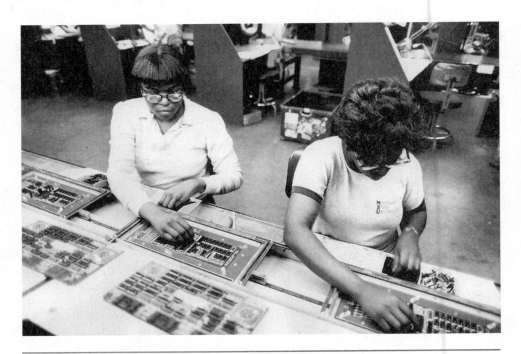

FIGURE 18.12

Exposure to repetitive strain can result in cumulative trauma disorder.

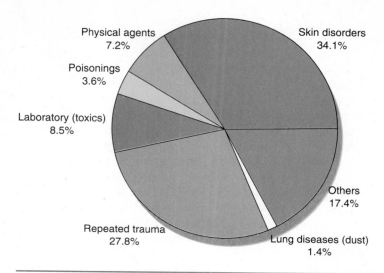

Physical agents
7.2%

Poisonings
3.6%

Laboratory (toxics)
8.5%

Repeated trauma
27.8%

Skin disorders
34.1%

Others
17.4%

Lung diseases (dust)
1.4%

FIGURE 18.13

Occupational illnesses by type, United States, 1984.

From: U.S. Dept. of Health and Human Services (1988). Proposed National Strategies for the Prevention of Leading Work-related Diseases and Injury: Dermatological Conditions. Cincinnati: NIOSH Publications, p. 3.

Asbestos workers suffer from diseases that include **asbestosis**—an acute or chronic lung disease, lung cancer, and mesothelioma (cancer of the epithelial linings of the heart and other internal organs). Textile factory workers who inhale dusts from cotton, flax, or hemp often acquire **byssinosis** (sometimes called *brown lung disease*), an acute or chronic lung disease. Workers in mines, stone quarries, sand and gravel operations, foundries, abrasive blasting operations, and glass manufacturing run the risk of **silicosis** (sometimes referred to as *dust on the lungs*) from inhaling crystalline silica. Coal miners often suffer from **coal workers' pneumoconiosis** (also called *black lung disease*), an acute or chronic lung disease, caused by inhaling coal dust (see Figure 18.14).

Other agents that can affect the lungs include metallic dusts, gases and fumes, and aerosols of biological agents (viruses, bacteria, and fungi). Health conditions that can result from exposure to these agents include occupational asthma, asphyxiation, pulmonary edema, histoplasmosis, and lung cancer (see Table 18.4).[22]

Other Occupational Diseases

Among the other types of occupational disorders are neurotoxic disorders, reproductive disorders, occupational cardiovascular diseases, occupational cancers, and psychological disorders. Neurological disorders

asbestosis Acute or chronic lung disease caused by the deposit of asbestos fibers on lungs.

byssinosis Acute or chronic lung disease caused by the inhalation of cotton, flax, or hemp dusts (brown lung disease).

silicosis Acute or chronic lung disease caused by the inhalation of free crystalline silica.

coal workers' pneumoconiosis Acute and chronic lung disease caused by the inhalation of coal dust (black lung disease).

are one of the ten leading causes of work-related diseases. There are more than 750 potentially neurotoxic chemicals, and an estimated 8 million workers may be exposed
full-time to one or more of these neurotoxic
agents.[26] Both the peripheral and central
nervous systems can be affected. Effects on
the peripheral nervous system include motor neuropathy and mixed sensorimotor
neuropathy. Affects on the central nervous
system include cranial neuropathy, vision
problems, Parkinsonism, seizures, memory
impairment, impaired psychomotor function, and psychosis.[26]

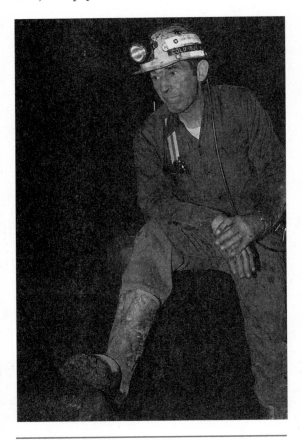

FIGURE 18.14

Mining is a dangerous occupation because of exposure
to both injuries and disease.

"Disorders of reproduction include infertility, impotence, menstrual disorders,
spontaneous abortion, low birth weight,
birth defects, congenital mental retardation, and various genetic diseases."[27] About
20% (17,000) of the 85,000 chemicals listed
in the NIOSH *Registry of Toxic Effects of
Chemical Substances* cite data on reproductive effects. However, the data on many of
these effects have been incompletely evaluated. Only about 30–40 physical, chemical,
or biological agents are generally recognized as causing teratogenic effects (birth
defects) in humans. Proving that an agent
at the workplace is the cause of a reproductive problem is very difficult. People have
nonoccupational exposures resulting from
personal habits or hobbies that make analysis of data difficult. Nonetheless, interest in
agents that are hazardous to reproductive
health will remain high. Legal precedents
are "established almost daily" as the rights
of the embryo or fetus, the rights of the
woman bearing the embryo (or fetus), and
society's interests come into moral and legal conflict.[27]

Cardiovascular diseases (CVDs) include
ischemic heart disease, hypertension,
stroke, and peripheral vascular diseases.
While it is recognized that the greatest opportunity for progress against CVDs lies in
decreasing alterable personal risk factors
such as cigarette smoking, dietary intake,
and hypertension, the workplace can have a
deleterious effect on cardiovascular health.
Specific chemical and physical agents that
are known to contribute to CVDs are carbon
disulfide, carbon monoxide, halogenated hydrocarbons, nitroglycerin, heat stress, and
noise.[23] Prevention of CVDs should include
efforts to reduce both work-related and personal risk factors.

Estimates for the number of cancer
deaths that are attributable each year to
workplace exposures range from a low of

Table 18.4
Examples of Occupational Lung Diseases

Agent	Examples of Agent	Disease/Response
Inorganic dusts	Crystalline silica	Silicosis*
	Asbestos	Asbestosis,* lung cancer, mesothelioma
	Coal dust	Coal workers' pneumoconiosis*
Organic and metallic dusts	Cotton, flax, hemp	Byssinosis*
	Proteins, metallic salts, antibiotics, chemicals (TDI, TMA)	Occupational asthma
	Moldy hay, grain, sugar cane, contaminated humidifiers	Hypersensitivity pneumonitis
Gases and fumes	Nitrogen, CO_2, CO, methane, H_2S, NH_3, SO_2, phosgene, ozone	Asphyxiation, irritation, pulmonary edema
Viable aerosols	Bacteria, viruses	Brucellosis, psitticosis, anthrax, mycobacterioses
	Fungi	Histoplasmosis, aspergillosis, cocidioidomycosis
Respiratory carcinogens	Arsenic, asbestos, chromium, radon daughters, nickel, coke oven emissions	Lung cancer*

*Identified in PHS 1990 Objectives

Source: U.S. Dept. of Health and Human Services (1986). *Proposed National Strategies for the Prevention of Leading Work-Related Diseases and Injuries: Occupational Lung Diseases.* Cincinnati: NIOSH Publications.

$17,000^{24}$ to a higher range of 24,175–48,350.[4] Using any of these estimates, occupational cancer deaths are a leading cause of occupational disease fatalities. It is estimated that more than a million workers are potentially exposed to agents that can produce cancer. Examples of industrial agents and the types of cancers they cause is presented in Table 18.5.

Controlling Occupational Diseases

Preventing and controlling occupational diseases requires the vigilance of employer and employee alike and the assistance of governmental agencies. The agent-host-environment disease model discussed earlier in this book is applicable to preventive strategies outlined here. Specific activities that should be employed to control occupational diseases include: identification and evaluation of agents, standard setting for handling and exposure to causative agents, elimination or substitution of causative factors, engineering controls to provide for a safer work area, environmental monitoring, medical screening, personal protective devices, health promotion, disease surveillance, therapeutic medical care and rehabilitation, and compliance activities.[24] Coordinated programs to monitor and reduce occupational hazards require professionally trained personnel. In a well-functioning program, these professionals work together as members of the occupational health and safety team.

Table 18.5
Industrial Agents Associated with Cancer*

Agent	Target Organ	Relative Risk†
Asbestos	Lung, pleura, peritoneum, (mesothelioma)	1.5–12.0 100.0
2-Naphthylamine	Bladder	87.0
Benzidine	Bladder	14.0
Coke oven emissions	Lung, kidney	2.7
Benzene	Blood (leukemia)	2.5
Wood dust	Nasal cavity	500.0
Arsenic	Lung, skin	2.3–8.0
Chromium and chromates	Lung, nasal sinuses	4.0–20.0
Vinyl chloride	Angiosarcoma of the liver	Marked
Bis(chloro-methyl) ether	Lung	100.0

*Abstracted from Schottenfeld and Haas (1979), CA: *A Cancer Journal for Clinicians* 29:144–168.

†Estimated relative risk for workers exposed to agent.

Source: U.S. Dept. of Health and Human Services (1986). *Proposed Strategies for the Prevention of Leading Work-Related Diseases and Injuries: Occupational Cancers.* Cincinnati: NIOSH Publications.

RESOURCES FOR THE PREVENTION OF OCCUPATIONAL INJURIES AND DISEASES

Community resources for the prevention of injuries and diseases attributable to the workplace include a variety of professional personnel and programs.

Occupational Safety and Health Professionals

The need for health professionals in the workplace is substantial. It was estimated that more than 2,100 students trained in occupational health and safety would graduate in 1990, and that this would constitute a 50% increase from 1980.[28] Among those with specialized training in their fields are safety engineers, certified safety professionals, health physicists, industrial hygienists, occupational health nurses, and medical doctors with a specialization in occupational medicine.

Safety Engineers and Certified Safety Professionals

Approximately 400 academic institutions offer accredited programs that train occupational safety professionals.[28] Many of these will join the professional organization, the American Society of Safety Engineers. In spite of the name of this society, not all members are engineers. The background of this group is varied and includes a number of health educators.

Another recognized group of trained professionals in this field is the **Certified Safety Professionals (CSPs)**. This group is somewhat smaller; there are about 6,000

certified safety professional (CSP) A health and safety professional, trained in industrial and workplace safety, who has met specific requirements for board certification.

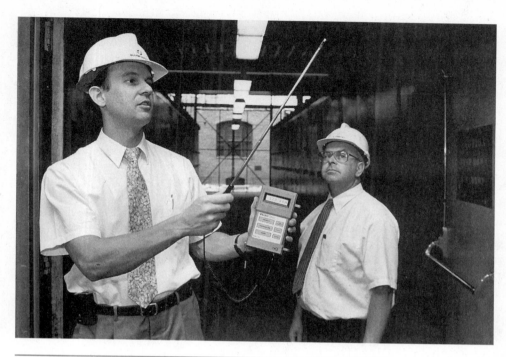

FIGURE 18.15

Safety engineers prevent workplace injuries by detecting hazards.

CSPs. Certification usually requires a bachelor's degree in engineering or another scientific curriculum and the passing of two examinations.

Safety engineers and CSPs design safety education programs, detect hazards in the workplace, and try to correct them (see Figure 18.15). Increased federal regulations have made the work load heavier for these occupational health professionals.

Health Physicists

Health physicists are concerned with radiation safety in the workplace. They mon-itor radiation within the work environment and develop plans for decontamination and coping with accidents involving radiation. It is estimated that there are approximately 11,000 health physicists in the United States. Many of these belong to the Health Physicist Society. Probably less than 10% of health physicists are board certified.[28]

Industrial Hygienists

Whereas the safety engineer or certified safety professional is primarily concerned with hazards in the workplace and injury control, the **industrial hygienist** is con-

---

safety engineer A safety professional employed by a company for the purpose of reducing unintentional injuries in the workplace.

health physicist A safety professional with responsibility for developing plans for coping with radiation accidents.

industrial hygienist A health professional concerned with health hazards in the workplace and with recommending plans for improving the healthiness of workplace environments.

cerned with environmental factors that might cause illness. Examples for such factors might include poor ventilation, excessive noise, poor lighting, and the presence of hazardous substances.

It is estimated that there are 7,600 industrial hygienists practicing in the United States. Perhaps a third of them hold the title of Certified Industrial Hygienist (CIH), and many belong to the American Industrial Hygiene Association. To be certified requires a two-part written examination; the first part is given following one year of post-baccalaureate experience. The second is given after five years of professional activity.

Occupational Physicians

The **occupational physician (OP) (Occupational Medical Practioner)** is a medical practitioner whose primary concern is preventive medicine in the workplace. The only official certification the OP is likely to have is that of the American Board of Preventative Medicine. Since there is little formal training in occupational medicine in most medical schools, OPs must acquire most of their knowledge on the job.

With physicians being highly skilled and highly paid occupational health professionals, only the largest companies maintain full-time OPs. In other cases, they are hired on a part-time basis or as consultants. Approximately 4,000 physicians belong to the American Occupational Medical Associates. Only a small percentage of them, 700–1,000, are actually board certified.

Occupational Health Nurses

The role of the **occupational health nurse (OHN)** has changed over the years from running the industry's medical department and first aid station to one of greater emphasis in health promotion and illness prevention. Because in smaller plants the OHN may be the only health professional employed, it is clear that if injury prevention and health promotion programs are to be offered, the job will fall to this individual.

The OHN must be a registered nurse (RN) in the state in which he or she practices. It is unlikely that these persons will have had much formal training in occupational health nursing prior to receiving their baccalaureate degrees because most nursing curricula do not provide much training in this area. However, the American Board of Occupational Health Nurses, Inc., established in 1972, now offers certifications. Requirements include many hours of continuing-education credits and five years' experience in the field of occupational health nursing. Many OHNs belong to the American Association of Occupational Health Nurses (AAOHN), which includes about 12,000 members.

Occupational Safety and Health Programs

There are a number of programs that can be put in place in occupational settings to reduce injuries and diseases. These include preplacement examinations, health maintenance programs, safety awareness programs, health promotion programs, investigation of accidents, stress management programs, employee assistance programs, and rehabilitation programs.

Preplacement Examinations

The purpose of **preplacement examinations** is to make sure that the worker fits

---

occupational physician (OP) or **(occupational medical practitioner)** A physician whose primary concern is preventive medicine in the workplace.
occupational health nurse (OHN) A registered nurse whose primary responsibilities include prevention of illness and promotion of health in the workplace.

---

preplacement examination A physical examination of a newly hired or transferred worker to determine medical suitability for placement in a specific position.

the job. By selecting the employee best physically and mentally qualified for a specific job, probabilities of job-related injuries or illnesses are minimized. Periodic evaluations are necessary to assure that the individual selected continues to be physically and mentally qualified to carry out the job assignment. Examinations are also recommended for transferred and return-to-work employees. Sometimes a phasing in of these employees is desirable.[29]

Health Maintenance Programs

The purpose of **health maintenance programs** is to monitor employees for the onset of chronic health problems and intervene with appropriate care to prevent the worsening of such problems. The early detection and treatment of such diseases as hypertension, diabetes, obesity, and heart disease can keep employees healthier and on the job longer. Health maintenance programs might include health promotion programs and safety programs.

Health Promotion Programs

The inclusion of workplace **health promotion programs** in the United States is driven by three major factors. The first is to promote the health of the employee. A healthy employee is a more productive employee. Such an employee also is less likely to use health care dollars—the most rapidly growing cost of doing business today. The second major factor is the personal concern employers have for their employees. Corporations who provide health promotion programs for their employees show a personal concern for the employees and their

families. This in turn increases employee morale. And third, workplace health promotion programs offer the potential of not only affecting the health of the workers and their families, but also the health of the corporation and the community.

A national survey conducted on worksites with 50 or more employees by the U.S. Department of Health and Human Services in 1992 indicated that approximately 81% of all worksites had one or more areas of health promotion activity. These data represented a 25% increase since the first survey in 1985. Included in those activities were smoking control, health risk abatement, back care, stress management, exercise/fitness, off-the-job accident prevention, nutrition education, high-blood-pressure control, cholesterol reduction, and weight control. In addition, the percentage of worksites with formal policies that prohibit or severely restrict smoking more than doubled from the 1985 study, increasing from 27% to 59%.[30,31] (See Figure 18.16.)

All indications are that workplace health promotion programs will continue to grow. Corporations not only see them as a means to control health care costs and show a concern for the employees, but also as a means by which to recruit new employees and to retain the ones currently in the organization. (See Chapter 5 for more information on health promotion programs.)

Safety Programs

Safety programs are those portions of the workplace health and safety program aimed at reducing the number and seriousness of unintentional injuries on the job. A successful safety program requires that senior management lead, that middle management be involved, that supervisors serve

---

health maintenance programs Worksite programs that monitor employees for the onset of chronic health problems and intervene with treatment.
health promotion program That part of a worksite health maintenance program aimed at improving employee health through changes in behavior and lifestyle.

---

safety program That part of the workplace health and safety program aimed at reducing unintentional injuries on the job.

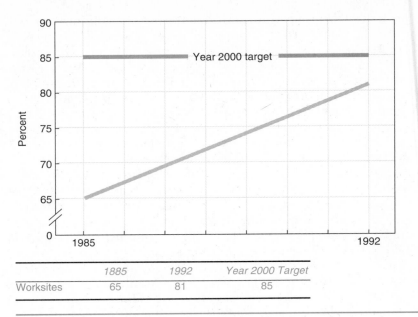

FIGURE 18.16

Percent of worksites offering health promotion activities, United States, 1985, 1992, and the target for the year 2000.

From: U.S. Dept. of Health and Human Services, National Center for Health Statistics (1993). Healthy People 2000 Review 1992. *(DHHS pub. no. PHS-93-1232-1). Washington, D.C.: U.S. Government Printing Office.*

as key coordinators, and that employees participate.[32] Each company needs to have a policy statement, safe operating procedures, a disaster plan, policies for hazard control, and policies for the investigation of injuries in the workplace. Provision must be made for regular safety inspections of the workplace and for the maintenance of accurate records for each injury and for analysis of such records. Each safety program should include safety orientation and training programs and programs on first aid and cardiopulmonary resuscitation.

Employee Assistance Programs

Employee assistance programs (EAPs) are programs that assist employees who have substance abuse, domestic, psychological, or social problems that interfere with the performance of their work. These programs have as their goal the rehabilitation of employees who need help.

CHAPTER SUMMARY

The work force in America now numbers approximately 112 million. Occupational injuries and illnesses cost our society $83 billion each year. Occupational health issues affect the quality of life economically as well as medically in communities in which workers live.

Although the awareness of occupational injuries and diseases is longstanding, only relatively recently has progress been made in reducing the number and seriousness of certain types of injuries and illnesses. An example of progress is the Occupational Safety and Health Act of 1970, which established the Occupational Safety and Health Administration and the

National Institute of Occupational Safety and Health.

The number and type of workplace injuries vary by person, place, time, and type of industry. Workplace injuries can be controlled by applying strategies based on the control of excess energy, the agent that causes injuries.

Occupational diseases kill thousands of workers each year. The types of diseases that can be attributed to workplace exposure are many, including musculoskeletal conditions, dermatological conditions, lung diseases, cancers, and reproductive disorders.

There are numerous resources to aid in the prevention of occupational injuries and diseases. These include occupational health professionals, such as safety engineers and industrial hygienists; and workplace health maintenance, health promotion, and safety programs.

SCENARIO: ANALYSIS AND RESPONSE

1. In the scenario, the exposure of painters to the toxic agent, lead, is an example of situations that occur daily in the workplace. Suppose you suspected that you were being exposed to a toxic agent where you worked. What would you do? Who would you contact? How could OSHA be of assistance?

2. Think about some of the jobs held by your fellow students. Do any of those jobs expose them to hazardous substances? Do any of the jobs students have put them at risk for injuries?

REVIEW QUESTIONS

1. Provide definitions of the terms *occupational injury* and *occupational disease* and give three examples of each.

2. In what ways are health problems in the workplace related to health problems in the general community?

3. How did the Industrial Revolution contribute to an increase in occupational health problems?

4. Who was Alice Hamilton?

5. What were the deficiencies in state occupational safety and health laws in the early 1960s?

6. Discuss briefly the purpose of the Occupational Safety and Health Act of 1970 and outline its provisions.

7. What does the National Institute of Occupational Safety and Health do?

8. What are some of the most frequently reported workplace injuries? Which are the leading causes of workplace injury deaths?

9. Which age group and gender of workers suffer the most occupational injuries? Which have the most fatal injuries?

10. During which days of the week and seasons do more occupational injuries occur?

11. Outline some general control strategies that can reduce the number and seriousness of workplace injuries.

12. What are some of the most frequently reported occupational diseases?

13. What determines whether a musculoskeletal condition or skin condition should be considered an injury or a disease?

14. List four well-documented lung conditions that are related to occupational exposure. Name the occupations whose workers are at high risk for each of these conditions.

15. Why is it often difficult to prove that a disease or condition resulted from workplace exposure?

16. Outline some features of a workplace program to prevent or control occupational diseases. For each activity, indicate whether it is aimed at the agent, host, or environment aspect of the disease model.

17. List five health occupations that deal with worker safety and health. Describe their training and job assignments.

18. Name and describe four occupational safety and health programs.

19. What are some of the more common worksite health promotion activities offered today in the United States?

ACTIVITIES

1. Examine your local newspaper every day for a week, looking for articles dealing with occupational injury or disease. Find three articles and, after reading them, provide the following: a brief summary, the resulting injury or disease, the cause of the injury or disease, and a brief plan for how the organization could eliminate the cause.

2. Interview an individual who works in the profession you wish to enter after graduation. Ask him or her to describe what he or she feels are the most prevalent injuries and illnesses connected with the job. Also ask about specific preservice and in-service education the interviewee has had to protect against these problems. Finally, ask him or her to propose measures to limit future problems. Summarize your interview on paper in no more than two pages.

3. If you have ever become injured or ill as a result of a job, explain what happened to you. In a two-page paper, identify the causative agent, how the injury could have been prevented, and what kind of training you had to prepare you for a safe working environment.

4. Go to the school library and research the injuries and diseases connected with your future profession. In a two-page paper, identify the major problems and what employers and employees should do about them, and express concerns you have about working in the profession because of the problems.

5. Visit any jobsite related to your future profession. At that site, find ten things that employers and employees are doing to make it a safe work environment. List the ten briefly and explain the benefit of each one.

REFERENCES

1. Nelkin, D., and M. S. Brown (1984). *Workers at Risk: Voices from the Workplace*. Chicago: Univ. of Chicago Press, p. 32.

2. U.S. Bur. of the Census (1989). *Statistical Abstract of the United States*. Washington, D.C.: U.S. Government Printing Office.

3. Persmick, M. E., and K. Taylor-Shirley (May 1992). "Profiles in Safety and Health: Occupational Hazards of Meat Packing." *Monthly Labor Review,* pp. 1–28

4. National Safe Workplace Institute (1992). *Basic Information on Workplace Safety and Health in the United States*. Chicago: Author.

5. National Highway Traffic Safety Admin. (1993). *The Cost of Injuries to Employees. A Traffic Safety Compendium.* (pub. no. HS 807 970). Washington, D.C.: U.S. Dept. of Transportation, p. 39

6. Goldsmith, J. R., ed. (1986). *Environmental Epidemiology*. Boca Raton, Fl.: CRC Press.

7. Felton, J. S. (1986). "History of Occupational Health and Safety." In *Introduction to Occupational Health and Safety,* J. LaDou, ed. Chicago: National Safety Council.

8. Rosen, G. (1958). *A History of Public Health*. New York: M.D. Publications.

9. LaDou, J., J. Olishifski, and C. Zenz (1986). "Occupational Health and Safety Today." In *Introduction to Occupational Health and Safety,* J. LaDou, ed. Chicago: National Safety Council.

10. Waldron, H. A. (1989). *Occupational Health Practice*. Boston: Butterworths & Co.

11. Ashford, N. A. (1976). *Crisis in the Workplace: Occupational Disease and Injury, a Report to the Ford Foundation*. Cambridge, Mass.: MIT Press.

12. Page, J. A., and M. W. O'Brien (1973). *Bitter Wages*. New York: Grossman.

13. Baker, S. P., B. O'Neill, M. J. Ginsburg, and G. Li (1992). *The Injury Fact Book*. New York: Oxford Univ. Press.

14. National Safety Council (1992). *Accident Facts*. Chicago: Author.

15. Committee on Labor and Human Resources (Aug. 12, 1992). *Childhood Labor Amendments* (report no. 102-380, to accompany Senate Bill 600).

16. Novello, A. C. (1991). "A Charge to the Conference." *Papers and Proceedings from the Surgeon General's Conference on Agricultural Safety and Health: Farm Safe 2000*. Des Moines, Ia., April 30–May 3, 1991, pp. 48–54.

17. Lee, B. C., and P. D. Gunderson, eds. (1992). "Epidemiology Public Health Perspective." *Proceedings from the Childhood Agricultural Injury Prevention*

Symposium. Marshfield, Wis. April 1–3, 1992, pp. 17–18.

18. Centers for Disease Control (1993). "Public Health Focus: Effectiveness of Rollover Protective Structures for Preventing Injuries Associated with Agricultural Tractors." *Morbidity and Mortality Weekly Report* 42(3): 57–59.

19. Novello, A. C. (1991). "Surgeon General Conferences: A Model for the Future." *Papers and Proceedings from the Surgeon General's Conference on Agricultural Safety and Health: Farm Safe 2000.* Des Moines, Ia. April 30–May 3, 1991, pp. 30–34.

20. U.S. Dept. of Health and Human Services (1986a). *Proposed National Strategies for the Prevention of Leading Work-Related Diseases and Injury: Severe Occupational Traumatic Injuries.* Cincinnati: NIOSH Publications.

21. U.S. Dept. of Health and Human Services (1986b). *Proposed National Strategies for the Prevention of Leading Work-Related Diseases and Injury: Musculoskeletal Injuries.* Cincinnati: NIOSH Publications.

22. U.S. Dept. of Health and Human Services (1986c). *Proposed National Strategies for the Prevention of Leading Work-Related Diseases and Injury: Occupational Lung Diseases.* Cincinnati: NIOSH Publications.

23. U.S. Dept. of Health and Human Services (1986d). *Proposed National Strategies for the Prevention of Leading Work-Related Diseases and Injury: Occupational Cardiovascular Diseases.* Cincinnati: NIOSH Publications.

24. U.S. Dept. of Health and Human Services (1986e). *Proposed National Strategies for the Prevention of Leading Work-Related Diseases and Injury: Occupational Cancers.* Cincinnati: NIOSH Publications.

25. U.S. Dept. of Health and Human Services (1988a). *Proposed National Strategies for the Prevention of Leading Work-Related Diseases and Injury: Dermatological Conditions.* Cincinnati: NIOSH Publications.

26. U.S. Dept. of Health and Human Services (1988b). *Proposed National Strategies for the Prevention of Leading Work-Related Diseases and Injury: Neurotoxic Disorders.* Cincinnati: NIOSH Publications.

27. U.S. Dept. of Health and Human Services (1988c). *Proposed National Strategies for the Prevention of Leading Work-Related Diseases and Injury: Disorders of Reproduction.* Cincinnati: NIOSH Publications.

28. Olishifski, J. B., J. E. Parker, R. J. Vernon, and C. Zenz (1986). "The Occupational Health and Safety Team." In *An Introduction to Occupational Health and Safety,* J. LaDou, ed. Chicago: National Safety Council.

29. Cowles, S. R. (1986). "Occupational Health." In *An Introduction to Occupational Health and Safety,* J. LaDou, ed. Chicago: National Safety Council.

30. No Author (1993). "Worksite Health Promotion Increases by 25 Percent." *Public Health Reports* 108(4): 523–524.

31. Fielding, J. E., and P. V. Piserchia (1989). "Frequency of Worksite Health Promotion Activities." *American Journal of Public Health,* 79: 16–20.

32. Peterson, D. (1986). "Safety Programs." In *An Introduction to Occupational Health and Safety,* J. LaDou, ed. Chicago: National Safety Council.

Appendix 1

State and Territorial Health Departments

States

Alabama
Public Health Dept.
434 Monroe Street
Montgomery, AL 36130-1701

Alaska
Div. of Public Health
P.O. Box H
Juneau, AK 99811-0610

Arizona
Dept. of Health Services
1740 West Adams St.
Phoenix, AZ 85007

Arkansas
Dept. of Health
4815 W. Markham St.
Little Rock, AR 72205

California
Dept. of Health Services
714 P St., Rm. 1253
Sacramento, CA 95814

Colorado
State Health Dept.
4300 Cherry Creek Dr. South
Denver, CO 80222-1530

Connecticut
State Dept. of Health
150 Washington St.
Hartford, CT 06106

Delaware
Div. of Public Health
P.O. Box 637
Dover, DE 19901

District of Columbia
Dept. of Public Health
1660 L St., NW, 12th Floor
Washington, DC 20036

Florida
Dept. of Health and Rehab.
Services
1323 Winewood Blvd., #115
Tallahassee, FL 32399-0700

Georgia
DHR/Public Health, Suite 201
878 Peachtree St., NE
Atlanta, GA 30309

Hawaii
Dept. of Health
Kiau Hale, P.O. Box 3378
Honolulu, HI 96801

Idaho
Dept. of Health and Welfare
450 W. State St.
Boise, ID 83720

Illinois
IL Dept. of Public Health
535 W. Jefferson St.
Springfield, IL 62761

Indiana
State Dept. of Health
1330 W. Michigan St.
P.O. Box 1964
Indianapolis, IN 46206-1964

Iowa
Iowa Dept. of Public Health
Lucas State Office Bldg.
Des Moines, IA 50319

Kansas
Dept. of Health
900 SW Jackson, Rm. 901
Topeka, KS 66612

Kentucky
Dept. for Health Services
275 E. Main St.
Frankfort, KY 40621

Louisiana
Dept. of Health
Two United Plaza, Suite 300
8550 United Plaza Blvd.
Baton Rouge, LA 70801

Maine
Bur. of Health
State House Station #11
Augusta, ME 04333

Maryland
Dept. of Health
201 W. Preston Street
Baltimore, MD 21201

Massachusetts
Dept. of Public Health
150 Tremont St., 10th Flr.
Boston, MA 02111

Michigan
Dept. of Public Health
3423 N. Logan St., Box 30035
Lansing, MI 48909

Minnesota
Dept. of Health
717 Delaware St, SE
Minneapolis, MN 55440

Mississippi
State Health Dept.
2423 N. State St., Box 1700
Jackson, MS 39215

Missouri
Dept. of Health
P.O. Box 570
Jefferson City, MO 65102

Montana
Dept. of Health and Environment
Cogswell Bldg.
Helena, MT 59620

Nebraska
State Dept. of Health
301 Centennial Mall South
Lincoln, NE 68509

Nevada
Dept. of Health
Capitol Complex
505 E. King St.
Carson City, NV 89710

New Hampshire
Dept. of Health
H&W Building, 6 Hazen Dr.
Concord, NH 03301-6527

New Jersey
Dept. of Health
CN 360
Trenton, NJ 08625

New Mexico
Dept. of Health
1190 St. Francis Dr.
Santa Fe, NM 87503

New York
NY State Health Dept.
ESP—Corning Tower
Albany, NY 12237

North Carolina
Dept. of Environment, Health,
and Natural Resources
P.O. Box 27687
Raleigh, NC 27611-7687

North Dakota
Dept. of Health
600 E. Boulevard Ave.
Bismarck, ND 58505-0200

Ohio
Dept. of Health
246 N. High St.
Columbus, OH 43266-0588

Oklahoma
Dept. of Health
1000 N.E. 10th St.
Oklahoma City, OK 73117

Oregon
Oregon Health Div.
950 State Office Bldg.
P.O. Box 14450
Portland, OR 97214-0405

Pennsylvania
Dept. of Health
P.O. Box 90, Rm. 802
Harrisburg, PA 17108

Rhode Island
Dept. of Health
Cannon Bldg., Rm. 401
3 Capitol Hill
Providence, RI 02908-5097

South Carolina
Dept. of Health and Environment
2600 Bull St.
Columbia, SC 29201

South Dakota
State Dept. of Health
445 East Capitol
Pierre, SD 57501-3185

Tennessee
Dept. of Public Health
344 Cordell Hull Bldg.
Nashville, TN 37247-0101

Texas
Texas Dept. of Health
1100 W. 49th St.
Austin, TX 78756

Utah
Utah Dept. of Health
288 N. 1460 West
Salt Lake City, UT 84116-0700

Vermont
State Health Dept.
108 Cherry St.
Burlington, VT 05402

Virginia
State Health Dept.
P.O. Box 2448
Richmond, VA 23218

Washington
Dept. of Health
1112 S.E. Quince St.
P.O. Box 47890
Olympia, WA 98504-7890

West Virginia
Dept. of Health
Bldg. 3, Rm. 519
State Capitol Complex
Charleston, WV 25305-0501

Wisconsin
Div. of Health
1 W. Wilson St., Box 309
Madison, WI 53701-0309

Wyoming
Dept. of Health
117 Hathaway Bldg.
Cheyenne, WY 82002

Territories

American Samoa
Dept. of Health
Govt. of American Samoa
Pago Pago, A. Samoa 96799

Micronesia
Dept. of Human Resources
P.O. Box PS70
Palikir, Pohnpei FM 96941

Guam
Dept. of Public Health
P.O. Box 2816
Agana, Guam 96901

Puerto Rico
Dept. of Health
Bldg. A, Call Box 70184
San Juan, PR 00936

Mariana Islands
Dept. of Public Health
P.O. Box 409CK
Saipan, CM 96950

Virgin Islands
Dept. of Health
P.O. Box 7309
Charlotte Amalie
St. Thomas, VI 00801

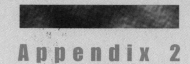

Appendix 2

Selected List of Voluntary Health Agencies

Alcoholics Anonymous
P.O. Box 459
Grand Central Station
New York, NY 10017

American Cancer Society
1599 Clifton Rd., N.E.
Atlanta, GA 30329

American Diabetes Association
2 Park Ave.
New York, NY 10016

American Heart Association
7320 Greenville Ave.
Dallas, TX 75231-4596

American Lung Association
1740 Broadway
New York, NY 10019-8700

American Parkinson's Disease Association
116 John St.
New York, NY 10038

Anorexia Nervosa and Associated Disorders
Box 271
Highland Park, IL 60035

Arthritis Foundation
1314 Spring St., N.W.
Atlanta, GA 30309

Cystic Fibrosis Foundation
6000 Executive Blvd.
Suite 510
Rockville, MD 20852

Juvenile Diabetes Foundation
23 E. 26th St.
New York, NY 10010

Leukemia Society of America
800 Second Ave.
New York, NY 10017

March of Dimes, Birth Defects Foundation
1275 Mamaroneck Ave.
White Plains, NY 10605

National Kidney Foundation
2 Park Ave.
New York, NY 10016

National Multiple Sclerosis Society
205 E. 42nd St.
New York, NY 10017

Planned Parenthood Federation of America
810 Seventh Ave.
New York, NY 10019

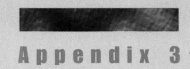

Appendix 3

Retrospective Studies:
How to Calculate an Odds Ratio

Let us assume that you selected 100 lung cancer cases and 1,000 controls of the same age, sex, and socioeconomic status as the cases. Suppose 80 of 100 cases of lung cancer had been regular smokers, but only 270 of 1,000 controls smoked, an odds ratio could be calculated by the formula $(A \times D) \div (B \times C)$ where cases and controls are designated as follows:

		Disease Present	
		Yes	No
Risk Factor Present	Yes	A	B
	No	C	D

In our example:

		Disease Present	
		Yes	No
Risk Factor Present	Yes	80	730
	No	270	20

Substituting our data into the formula:

$[(80 \times 730) \div (270 \times 20)] = 58400 \div 5400 = 10.8$. Thus, lung cancer victims have 10.8 times greater probability of having been a smoker.

Prospective Studies: How to Calculate
Relative and Attributable Risk

Let us assume that in a cohort of 4,000 there were 1,000 smokers and 3,000 nonsmokers. If, after 20 years, cancer develops in 22 smokers (22 per 1,000) and in 6 nonsmokers (6 per 3,000 or 2 per 1,000), *relative risk* is the ratio of the incidence rates, 22 per thousand: 2 per thousand or 22:2 or **11 to 1.**

Further, one can calculate an *attributable risk* by subtracting the deaths in the nonsmoking group (2 deaths) from the number of lung cancer deaths in the smoking group (22 deaths). Thus, 20 deaths attributable to smoking; the attributable risk is 20 per 1,000.

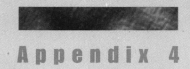

Appendix 4

Answers to Questions about the Picnic Lunch

1. The first cases of illness had onsets between 7 and 8 hours after the picnic. The last cases had onsets beginning 12 hours after the picnic. Therefore, the incubation period for this outbreak was 7–12 hours.

2. The epidemic curve in Figure A4.1 suggests a single (point) exposure; all the reported cases were exposed at the same time, to the same source.

3. It seems almost certain that the cause of this outbreak is one of the foods served at the picnic. Food can serve as a vehicle for a wide variety of pathologic and toxic agents, including chemicals; *Staphylococcus, Salmonella,* and *Clostridium* bacteria; and a number of parasites.

4. The attack rates can be calculated for each food and then compared against the illnes rates of those not eating the foods (Table A4.1). Seventy-six percent of those eating turkey became ill while only 6% (one person) became ill who did not eat turkey. Thus, the chances of becoming ill for those eating turkey was 12–13 times greater than for those who did not eat turkey. While people who ate potato salad were 3 times more

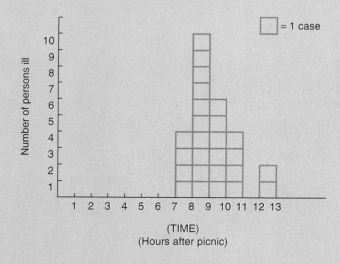

FIGURE A4.1

Epidemic curve for a disease outbreak following a picnic lunch.

Table A4.1

Attack Rate Worksheet for Foods Served at Picnic

Food	Persons Eating Food				Persons Not Eating Food			
	Total	Ill	Well	Attack Rate	Total	Ill	Well	Attack Rate
Bread	31	16	15	52%	18	10	8	56%
Butter	27	16	11	59%	22	10	12	45%
Turkey	33	25	8	76%	16	1	15	6%
Potato Salad	35	22	13	63%	14	4	10	29%
Milk	45	26	19	58%	4	0	4	0%
Jell-O	34	18	16	53%	15	8	7	53%

likely to become ill than those who did not, all those who ate potato salad and became ill also ate turkey. Therefore, turkey was almost certainly the vehicle for this food-borne outbreak.

5. The Centers for Disease Control and Prevention defines a food-borne disease outbreak as:

> . . . an incident in which (1) 2 or more persons experience a similar illness, usually gastrointestinal, after ingestion of a common food, and (2) epidemiologic analysis implicates the food as the source of the illness.[1]

In outbreaks in which epidemologic evidence implicates a food source, but adequate laboratory confirmation is not obtained, CDC subdivides outbreaks into 4 categories by incubation period of illness:

> . . . less than 1 hour (probable chemical poisoning), 1–7 hours (probable *Staphylococcus* food poisoning), 8–14 hours (probable *Clostridium perfringens* food poisoning), and greater than 14 hours (infectious or toxic agents).*

In our example, the picnic lunch, in which we determined the incubation period to be 7–12 hours, it seems likely that the causative agent was *Clostridium perfringens*. This bacterium is often found in beef and beef products, in turkey, and in chicken, and is a not infrequent cause of food-bourne disease outbreaks in the United States. A report of one such outbreak in a Meals on Wheels program can be found in *Morbidity and Mortality Weekly Report*, Vol 30, No. 14, p. 171 (1981).

---

*Centers for Disease Control (1990). Foodbourne Disease Outbreaks, 5-Year Summary, 1983–1987. *Morbidity and Mortality Weekly Report*, CDC Surveillance Summaries, 39SS-1): 15–23.

Appendix 5

Operational Definitions for the 1990 Census

American Indian, Eskimo, or Aleut Includes persons who classified themselves as such in one of the specific race categories identified below.

American Indian Includes persons who indicated their race as "American Indian," entered the name of an Indian tribe, or reported such entries as Canadian Indian, French-American Indian, or Spanish-American Indian.

Eskimo Includes persons who indicated their race as "Eskimo" or reported entries such as Arctic Slope, Inupiat, and Yupik.

Aleut Includes persons who indicated their race as "Aleut" or reported entries such as Alutiiq, Egegik, and Pribilovian.

Asian or Pacific Islander Includes persons who reported in one of the Asian or Pacific Islander groups listed on the questionnaire or who provided write-in responses such as Thai, Nepaili, or Tongan.

Asian Includes "Chinese", "Filipino," "Japanese," "Asian Indian," "Korean," "Vietnamese," and "Other Asian."

Chinese Includes persons who indicated their race as "Chinese" or who identified themselves as Cantonese, Tibetan, or Chinese American. In standard census reports, persons who reported as "Taiwanese" or "Formosan" are included here with Chinese. In special reports on the Asian or Pacific Islander population, information on persons who identified themselves as Taiwanese are shown separately.

Note: These definitions were taken directly from U.S. Dept. of Commerce. *1990 Census of Population and Housing, Summary Population and Housing, Characteristics, United States.* Washington, D.C.: U.S. Government Printing Office.

Filipino Includes persons who indicated their race as "Filipino" or reported entries such as Philipino, Philipine, or Filipino American.

Japanese Includes persons who indicated their race as "Japanese" and persons who identified themselves as Nipponese or Japanese American.

Asian Indian Includes persons who indicated their race as "Asian Indian" and persons who identified themselves as Bengalese, Bharat, Dravidian, East Indian, or Goanese.

Korean Includes persons who indicated their race as "Korean" and persons who identified themselves as Korean American.

Vietnamese Includes persons who indicated their race as "Vietnamese" and persons who identified themselves as Vietnamese American.

Cambodian Includes persons who provided a write-in response such as Cambodian or Cambodia.

Hmong Includes persons who provided a write-in response such as Hmong, Laohmong, or Mong.

Laotian Includes persons who provided a write-in response such as Laotian, Laos, or Lao.

Thai Includes persons who provided a write-in response such as Thai, Thailand, or Siamese.

Other Asian Includes persons who provided a write-in response of Bangladeshi, Burmese, Indonesian, Pakistani, Sri Lankan, Amerasian, or Eurasian. See Table 9.2 for other groups comprising "Other Asian."

Pacific Islander Includes persons who indicated their race as "Pacific Islander" by classifying themselves into one of the following race categories or identifying themselves as one of the Pacific Islander cultural groups of Polynesian, Micronesian, or Melanesian.

Hawaiian Includes persons who indicated their race as "Hawaiian" as well as persons who identified themselves as Part Hawaiian or Native Hawaiian.

Samoan Includes persons who indicated their race as "Samoan" or persons who identified themselves as American Samoan or Western Samoan.

Guamanian Includes persons who indicated their race as "Guamanian" or persons who identified themselves as Chamorro or Guam.

Other Pacific Islander Includes persons who provided a write-in response of a Pacific Islander group such as Tahitian, Northern Mariana Islander, Palauan, Fijiian, or a cultural group such as Polynesian, Micronesian, or Melanesian. See Table 9.2 for other groups comprising "Other Pacific Islander."

Black Includes persons who indicated their race as "black or Negro" or reported entries such as African American, Afro-American, black Puerto Rican, Jamaican, Nigerian, West Indian, or Haitian.

White Includes persons who indicated their race as "white" or reported entries such as Canadian, German, Italian, Lebanese, Near Easterner, Arab, or Polish.

Other race Includes all other persons not included in "white," "black," "American Indian, Eskimo, or Aleut," and "Asian or Pacific Islander" race categories described above. Persons reporting in the "Other race" category and providing write-in entries such as multiracial, multiethnic, mixed, interracial, Wesort, or a Spanish/Hispanic origin group (such Mexican, Cuban, or Puerto Rican) are included here.

Hispanic origin Of Hispanic origin are those who classified themselves in one of the specific Hispanic origin categories listed on the questionnaire: "Mexican," "Puerto Rican," or "Cuban"; as well as those who indicated that they were of "other Spanish/Hispanic" origin. Persons of "Other Spanish/Hispanic" origin are those whose origins are from Spain, the Spanish-speaking countries of Central or South America, or the Dominican Republic; or they are persons of Hispanic origin identifying themselves generally as Spanish, Spanish-American, Hispanic, Hispano, Latino, and so on.

Glossary Terms

absorption field The element of a septic system in which the liquid portion of waste is distributed.

acid rain Both wet and dry acidic deposits, which occur both within and downwind of areas that produce emissions containing sulfur dioxide and oxides of nitrogen (also called *acid deposition*).

Activities of Daily Living (ADLs) Eating, toileting, dressing, bathing, walking, getting in and out of a bed or chair, and getting outside.

acute disease A disease in which the peak severity of symptoms occurs and subsides within three months of onset, usually within days or weeks.

Administration for Children and Families A division of DHHS that coordinates programs to enhance the functioning of the family.

adolescents and young adults Individuals between the ages of 15 and 24 years.

adult day care programs Daytime care provided to seniors who are unable to be left alone.

aeroallergens Biological organisms or products that float in the air and invoke an immune response in humans.

affective disorder Mental disorder characterized by a disturbance of mood, either depression or elation (mania); for example, bipolar disorder, major depression.

age pyramid A conceptual model that illustrates the age distribution of a population.

aged The state of being old.

ageism Prejudice and discrimination against the aged.

Agency for Toxic Substances and Disease Registry (ATSDR) An agency created by Superfund legislation to prevent or mitigate adverse health effects and diminished quality of life resulting from exposure to hazardous substances in the environment.

agent (pathogenic agent) The cause of the disease or health problem, the factor that must be present in order for the disease to occur.

aging The physiological changes that occur normally in plants and animals as they grow older.

Aid to Families with Dependent Children (AFDC) Program of the Social Security Administration that pays benefits to single mothers and their children who find themselves with minimal resources.

Aid to the Permanently and Totally Disabled (APTD) 1962 amendments to the Social Security Act aimed at providing federal funds for social services to the mentally ill.

air pollution The contamination of the air by gases, liquids, or solids that interfere with the comfort, safety, or health of living organisms.

air-borne disease A communicable disease that is transmitted through the air (e.g., influenza).

Alcoholics Anonymous (AA) A fellowship of recovering alcoholics who offer support to anyone who desires to stop drinking.

alcoholism A disease characterized by impaired control over drinking, preoccupation with drinking, and continued use of alcohol despite adverse consequences.

alien A person born in and owing allegiance to a country other than the one in which he or she lives.

allied health care professionals Health care workers who provide services that assist, facilitate, and complement the work of physicians and other health care specialists.

allopathic providers Independent health care providers whose remedies for illnesses produce effects different from those of the disease. These people are doctors of medicine (MDs).

American Cancer Society A voluntary health agency dedicated to fighting cancer and educating the public about cancer.

amotivational syndrome A pattern of behavior characterized by apathy, loss of effectiveness, and a more passive, introverted personality.

amphetamines A group of synthetic drugs that act as stimulants.

amplitude The intensity of sound measured in decibels.

anabolic drugs Compounds, structurally similar to the male hormone testosterone, that increase protein synthesis.

analytical study A type of epidemiological study aimed at testing hypotheses (e.g., case/control study, cohort study).

anthroponosis A disease that infects only humans.

aquifers Underground water reservoirs.

asbestos A naturally occurring mineral fiber that has been identified as a class A carcinogen by the Environmental Protection Agency.

asbestosis Acute or chronic lung disease caused by the deposit of asbestos fibers on lungs.

attack rate A special incidence rate calculated for a particular population for a single disease outbreak and expressed as a percent.

automatic (passive) protection The modification of a product or the environment in such a way as to reduce unintentional injuries.

bacteriological period The period in public health history from 1875 to 1900.

barbiturates Depressant drugs based on the structure of barbituric acid; for example, phenobarbital.

basal cell carcinoma A common, highly curable type of skin cancer.

Beers, Clifford (1876–1943) A leader in the mental hygiene movement, Beers suffered from bipolar disorder and underwent repeated hospitalizations; he wrote a book entitled *A Mind That Found Itself* and founded the forerunner of the National Mental Health Association.

behavioral therapy A treatment methodology, based on learning theory, aimed at encouraging desired behavior and extinguishing undesirable behavior.

benzodiazapines Nonbarbiturate depressant drugs; examples: Librium, Valium.

biological hazards Living organisms (and viruses), or their products, that are harmful to humans.

biological system All living organisms and their interactions.

biological transmission A type of vector-borne disease transmission in which there is multiplication and or development of the disease agent in the vector.

biomedical therapy A treatment methodology based on the theory that mental disorders result from a physical or biochemical lesion that can be treated with drugs or electric shock.

biosphere Sum total of all life forms on earth.

bipolar disorder An affective mental disorder characterized by distinct periods of elevated mood alternating with periods of depression.

birth defects Deleterious medical conditions present at birth.

birth rate See **natality rate.**

blood-alcohol concentration (BAC) The percentage of concentration of alcohol in the blood; a BAC of 0.1% or greater is regarded as the legal level of intoxication in most states.

bottle bills Laws that require consumers to pay refundable deposits on beer and soft drink containers.

bottom-up community organization Organization efforts that begin with those who live within the community affected.

built environment The portion of the environment that is built by humans.

Bureau of Indian Affairs (BIA) The original federal government agency charged with the responsibility for the welfare of Native Americans.

byssinosis Acute or chronic lung disease caused by the inhalation of cotton, flax, or hemp dusts; those affected include workers in cotton textile plants (sometimes called *brown lung disease).*

carcinogens Agents that are known to cause cancer.

care-manager One who helps identify the health care needs of an individual but does not actually provide the health care services.

care-provider One who helps identify the health care needs of an individual and also personally performs the caregiving service.

carrier A person or animal that harbors a specific communicable disease agent in the absence of discernible clinical disease and serves as a potential source of infection to others.

carrying capacity The amount of resources (air, water, shelter, etc.) of a given environment to support a certain-sized population.

case fatality rate (CFR) The percentage of cases of a particular disease that result in death.

case/control study (retrospective study) An epidemiological study that seeks to compare those diagnosed with a disease (cases) with those who do not have the disease (controls) for prior exposure to specific risk factors.

cases People afflicted with a disease.

categorical programs Those programs available only to people who can be categorized into a specific group based on disease, age, family means, geography, or other variables.

cause-specific mortality rate (CSMR) An expression of the death rate due to a particular disease; the CSMR is calculated by dividing the number of deaths due to a particular disease by the total population and multiplying by 100,000.

Centers for Disease Control and Prevention (CDC) One of the seven divisions of the Public Health Service; charged with the responsibility for surveillance and control of diseases and other health problems in the United States.

cerebrovascular disease (stroke) A disease in which the blood supply to the brain is interrupted.

certified safety professional (CSP) A health and safety professional, trained in industrial and workplace safety, who has met specific requirements for board certification.

chain of infection A model to conceptualize the transmission of a communicable disease from its source to a susceptible host.

chemical hazards Hazards caused by the mismanagement of chemicals.

chemical straitjacket The concept of a mental patient's behavior being restrained or subdued by a drug (chemical) such as Thorazine instead of by a physical straitjacket.

child abuse The intentional physical, emotional, verbal, or sexual mistreatment of a minor.

child neglect The failure of a parent or guardian to care for or otherwise provide the necessary subsistence for a child.

childhood diseases Infectious diseases that normally affect people in their childhood (e.g., are measles, mumps, rubella, and pertussis).

children Persons between 1 and 14 years of age.

chiropractor A nonallopathic, independent health care provider who treats health problems by adjusting the spinal column.

chlorofluorocarbons (CFCs) A family of chemical agents used in industry for such items as propellants, refrigeration, solvent cleaning, and insulation.

chlorpromazine The first and most famous antipsychotic drug introduced in 1954 under the brand name Thorazine.

chronic disease A disease or health condition that lasts longer than three months, sometimes for the remainder of one's life.

citizen initiated community organization See **bottom-up community organization.**

Clean Air Act (CAA) (P.L. 88-206) A 1963 law that provided the federal government with authority to address interstate air pollution problems.

Clean Water Act (CWA) (P.L. 92-500) A 1972 law that provided the federal government with authority to ensure water quality by controlling water pollution; first known as Federal Water Pollution Control Act Amendments.

coal workers' pneumoconiosis Acute and chronic lung disease caused by the inhalation of coal dust (sometimes called *black lung disease*).

cocaine The psychoactive ingredient in the leaves of the coca plant, *Erythoxolyn coca*.

cohort A group of people who share some important demographic characteristic—year of birth, for example.

cohort study (prospective study) An epidemiological study in which a cohort is selected, classified on the basis of exposure to one or more specific risk factors, and observed into the future to determine the rates at which disease develops in each class.

coinsurance Portion or percentage of insurance company's approved amounts for covered services that the beneficiary is responsible for paying.

combustion by-products Gases and other particles generated by controlled or uncontrolled burning.

comminutor A large grinder; part of a waste water treatment system.

common law Legal principles and rules based on past legal decisions; judge-made law.

communicable disease (infectious disease) An illness due to a specific communicable agent or its toxic products, which arises through transmission of that agent or its products from an infected person, animal, or inanimate reservoir to a susceptible host.

communicable disease model A visual representation of the interrelationships of agent, host, and environment—the three entities necessary for communicable disease transmission.

community A group of people with a shared location, shared environment, and shared fate.

community analysis A process by which community needs are identified.

community development A process by which community members work to create conditions of economic and social progress for the whole community.

community diagnosis See **community analysis.**

community health Both private and public efforts of individuals, groups, and organizations to promote, protect, and preserve the health of those in the community.

community mental health centers Local agencies, initially built with federal funding, that provide the community members with mental health services.

community organization The process by which individuals, groups, and organizations engage in planned action to influence social problems.

Community Support Program A federal program that offers financial incentives to communities to develop a social support system for the mentally ill.

composting The natural, aerobic biodegradation of organic plant and animal matter to compost.

comprehensive approach to violence prevention An organized effort to apply all methods to prevent intentional injuries.

Comprehensive Environmental Response, Compensation, and Liability Act (CERCLA) (Superfund) A 1980 law created by the federal government primarily to clean up abandoned hazardous waste sites.

comprehensive school health program "An organized set of policies, procedures, and activities designed to protect and promote the health and well-being of students and staff which has traditionally included health services, healthful school environment, and health education. It should also include, but not be limited to guidance and counseling, physical education, food service, social work, psychological services, and employee health promotion."*

congregate meal programs Community-sponsored nutrition programs that provide meals at a central site, such as a senior center.

continuing care Long-term care for chronic health problems, usually including personal care.

continuing-care retirement communities (CCRCs) Planned communities for seniors that guarantee a lifelong residence and health care.

control The containment of a disease by prevention and/or intervention measures.

copayment See **coinsurance.**

coronary heart (artery) disease A noncommunicable disease characterized by damage to the coronary arteries which supply blood to the heart.

correlated instruction Pattern of instruction in which the subject matter is taught in many other subjects and not as its own subject.

cosmic radiation That radiation which comes from outer space and the sun.

criteria pollutants The six most pervasive air pollutants in the United States.

crude birth rate An expression of the number of live births per unit of population in a given period of time. For example, the crude birth rate in the United States in 1992 was 16.0 births per 1,000 population.

crude death rate (CDR) An expression of the total number of deaths (from all causes) per unit of population in a given period of time. For example, the crude death rate in the United States in 1990 was 8.5 per 1,000 population.

*From: Joint Committee on Health Education Terminology (1991). "Report of the 1990 Joint Committee on Health Education Terminology." *Journal of School Health* 22(2): 105–106.

crude rate A rate in which the denominator includes the total population.

culturally sensitive Having respect for cultures other than one's own.

curriculum Written plan for instruction.

cycles per second (cps) A measure of sound frequency.

dangerous drugs A term used by the Drug Enforcement Agency to denote any controlled substances other than cocaine, opiates (narcotics), and *cannabis* products (such as marijuana); for example, LSD.

death rate The number of deaths per unit of resident population.

decibels (dB) A measure of sound amplitude.

deductible The amount of expense that the beneficiary must incur before the insurance company begins to pay for covered services.

deinstitutionalization The process of discharging, on a large scale, patients from state mental hospitals to less restrictive community settings.

demography (demographers) The study of a population and those variables bringing about change in that population.

Department of Health and Human Services (DHHS) The largest federal department in the United States government, formed in 1980 and headed by the secretary who is a member of the president's cabinet.

dependency (support) ratio A ratio that compares the number of individuals whom society considers economically productive (the working population) to the number of those it considers economically unproductive (the nonworking or dependent population).

desalinization The process used to remove salt from salt water.

descriptive study An epidemiological study that describes an epidemic with respect to person, place, and time.

designer drugs Mind-altering drugs, synthesized in clandestine laboratories, that are similar to but structurally different from known controlled substances.

diagnosis-related groups (DRGs) A procedure used to classify the health problems of all Medicare patients when they are admitted to a hospital.

direct instruction Pattern of instruction in which subject matter is identified as a separate subject and is allocated a specific amount of teaching time in the school day.

direct transmission The immediate transfer of an infectious agent by direct contact between infected and susceptible individuals.

directly observed therapy (DOT) Visual verification of an individual taking prescribed therapy.

disability-adjusted life years (DALYs) A measure for the burden of disease that takes into account premature death and loss of healthy life resulting from disability.

disabling injury An injury causing any restriction of normal activity beyond the day of the injury's occurrence.

disaster agents Occurrences such as cyclones, earthquakes, floods, hurricanes, tornadoes, typhoons, and volcanic eruptions.

diseases of adaptation Diseases that result from chronic exposure to excess levels of stressors which elicit GAS.

Dix, Dorothea (1802–1897) Nineteenth century leader in the cause of public care for the mentally ill, personally involved in founding of many state mental hospitals.

dose rate The rate at which a dose of radiation is received.

drug A substance other than food or vitamins, that upon entering the body in small amounts, alters one's physical, mental, or emotional state.

drug abuse Use of a drug despite the knowledge that continued use is detrimental to one's health or well-being.

drug (chemical) dependence A psychological and sometimes physical state characterized by a craving for a drug.

drug misuse Inappropriate use of prescription or nonprescription drugs.

drug use Any drug-taking behavior.

DSM-III-R *Diagnostic and Statistical Manual of Mental Disorders,* third ed., revised, published by the American Psychiatric Association.

dump Open pits in which solid waste is placed.

Earth Day Annual public observance for concerns about the environment; the first was held April 22, 1970.

ecology Interrelationship of organisms and their environments.

elder hostel Education programs specifically for seniors, held on college campuses.

elderly (or elder) Individuals over 60 years of age.

elderly dependency (support) ratio The dependency ratio that includes only the elderly.

employee assistance program (EAP) That aspect of a workplace drug program devoted to assisting employees in recovering from their alcohol or other drug problems.

empower To give power or authority; to enable, to permit.

endemic disease A disease that occurs regularly in a population as a matter of course.

environment The physical, biological, and social surroundings.

environmental hazards Conditions that threaten the well-being of the environment.

environmental health Characteristics of environmental conditions that affect the health and well-being of humans.

Environmental Protection Agency (EPA) The federal agency primarily responsible for setting, maintaining, and enforcing environmental standards.

environmental sanitation The practice of effecting healthy or hygienic conditions in the environment.

environmental system The place where humans interact with their environment and vice versa.

environmental tobacco smoke (ETS) Tobacco smoke in the ambient air.

epidemic An unexpectedly large number of cases of disease in a particular population for a particular time period.

epidemic curve A graphic display of the cases of disease according to the time or date of onset of symptoms.

epidemiologist One who practices epidemiology.

epidemiology The study of the distribution and determinants of diseases and injuries in human populations.

equilibrium phase Last phase of the population growth S-curve, when the birth and death rates are equal.

eradication The complete elimination or uprooting of a disease (e.g., smallpox eradication).

etiology The cause of a disease (e.g., the etiology of mumps is the mumps virus).

evaluation The process in which the value or worth of the objective of interest is compared to a standard of acceptability.

exclusion A health condition that is written into the health insurance policy indicating what is not covered by the policy.

exclusive provider organization Similar to a preferred provider organization but with fewer providers and greater discounts. See **preferred provides organization (PPO).**

experimental study An epidemiological study carried out under controlled conditions, usually to determine the effectiveness of a vaccine, therapeutic drug, or surgical technique.

exponential phase Middle phase of the population growth S-curve, when the birth rate is greater than the death rate.

Family and Medical Leave Act Federal legislation that provides up to a 12-week unpaid leave to men and women after the birth of a child, an adoption, or an event of illness in the immediate family.

family planning Determining the preferred number and spacing of children and choosing the appropriate means to achieve this preference.

family violence The use of physical force by one family member against another, with the intent to hurt, injure, or cause death.

fatal injury An injury that results in one or more deaths.

fatality rate See **mortality rate.**

Federal Water Pollution Control Act Amendments See **Clean Water Act.**

Fee-for-service A method of paying for health care in which after the care (service) is rendered, a bill (fee) is paid.

fertility rate The number of live births per 1,000 women of childbearing age (15–44 years).

fetal alcohol syndrome (FAS) A characteristic group of defects in babies born to mothers who have consumed large amounts of alcohol during their pregnancies.

fetal deaths Deaths in utero with a gestational age of at least 20 weeks.

fight or flight reaction An alarm reaction that prepares one physiologically for sudden action (heart rate, blood pressure, and respiration increase).

fixed indemnity The maximum amount an insurer will pay for a certain service.

Food and Drug Administration (FDA) A regulatory agency of the DHHS that sets safety standards for all food, drugs, and cosmetics.

food-borne diseases Diseases that are transmitted via contaminated food.

food-borne outbreak An incident, confirmed by an epidemiological analysis, in which a commonly ingested food is the source of a similar illness in two or more people.

formaldehyde (CH_2O) A water-soluble gas used in aqueous solutions in hundreds of consumer products.

formative evaluation The evaluation that is conducted during the planning and implementing processes to improve or refine a community health program.

frequency The rate of vibrations created by the transmission of energy. In the case of sound, it is measured in cycles per second, hertz, or vibrations per second.

full-service hospitals Hospitals that offer services in all or most of the six levels of care defined by the spectrum of health care.

functional limitations Difficulty in performing personal care and home management tasks.

gag rule Regulations that barred physicians and nurses in clinics receiving federal funds from counseling clients about abortions.

gatekeepers Those who control, both formally and informally, the political climate of the community.

General Adaptation Syndrome (GAS) The complex physiological responses resulting from exposure to stressors that can in time result in health deficits.

geophysical system The earth, its water, and its atmosphere.

geriatrics The branch of medicine that deals with the structural changes, physiology, diseases, and hygiene of old age.

gerontology The study of aging, from the broadest perspective.

global warming The gradual increase in the earth's surface temperature.

government hospital One that is partially or fully funded by tax dollars.

governmental health agency (or official health agencies) A local, state, national, or international agency funded primarily by tax dollars.

grass-roots community organization See **bottom-up community organization.**

greenhouse effect The trapping of heat in the atmosphere by greenhouse gases.

greenhouse gases Atmosphere gases, principally carbon dioxide, the CFCs, methane, and nitrous oxide, that are transparent to visible light but absorb infrared radiation (heat).

groundwater Water that sinks into the soil.

group model HMO An HMO that contracts with a physicians' group practice to provide care for a specific number of HMO enrollees.

"Growing Healthy" A health education curriculum for grades K–6, distributed by the National Center for Health Education.

hallucinogens Drugs that produce profound distortions of the senses.

hard pesticide A chemical substance used for pest control that persists unchanged in the environment for months or years.

hard-to-reach population Those in a target population that are not easily reached by normal programming efforts.

hazard An unsafe act or condition.

hazardous waste A solid waste or combination of solid wastes which—because of its quantity, concentration, or physical, chemical, or infectious characteristics—may: (A) cause or significantly contribute to an increase in mortality or an increase in serious irreversible, or incapacitating reversible, illness; or (B) pose a substantial present or potential hazard to human health or the environment when improperly treated, stored, transported, or disposed of, or otherwise managed.*

health The blending of physical, emotional, social, intellectual, and spiritual resources as they assist one in mastering the developmental tasks necessary to enjoy a satisfying and protective life.

Health Care Financing Administration (HCFA) A division of the DHHS that oversees the expenditure of all federal monies appropriated for health care services.

health education "A continuum of learning which enables people, as individuals and as members of social structures, to voluntarily

---

*Note: This definition was taken from the Resource Conservation and Recovery Act of 1976 (RCRA).

make decisions, modify behaviors, and change social conditions in ways which are health enhancing."*

health instruction "The development, delivery, and evaluation of a planned curriculum, preschool through [grade] 12, with goals, objectives, content sequence, and specific classroom lessons which include, but are not limited to the following major content areas: community health, consumer health, environmental health, family life, mental emotional health, injury prevention and safety, nutrition, personal health, prevention and control of disease, substance use and abuse."*

health maintenance organization (HMOs) Groups that supply prepaid comprehensive health care with an emphasis on prevention.

health maintenance programs Worksite programs that monitor employees for the onset of chronic health problems and intervene with treatment to correct or prevent the worsening of such problems.

health physicist A safety professional with responsibility for monitoring radiation within the plant environment, developing instrumentation for the purpose, and developing plans for coping with radiation accidents.

health promotion and disease prevention "The aggregate of all purposeful activities designed to improve personal and public health through a combination of strategies, including the competent implementation of behavioral change strategies, health education, health protection measures, risk factor detection, health enhancement, and health maintenance."*

health promotion program That part of a worksite health maintenance program aimed at improving employee health through changes in behavior and life-style.

Health Resources and Service Administration (HRSA) An agency of DHHS established in 1982 to improve the nation's health resources and services and their distribution to underserved populations.

health resources development period The period in public health history from 1900 to 1960; a time of great growth in health care facilities.

healthful school environment "The promotion, maintenance, and utilization of safe and wholesome surroundings, organization of day-by-day experiences and planned learning procedures to influence favorable emotional, physical and social health."†

herbicide A pesticide designed specifically to kill plants.

herd immunity The overall immunity of a population against a particular disease.

hertz (HZ) A measure of sound frequency.

home health care services Health care services provided in the patient's place of residence (home or apartment).

home health care Care that is provided in the patient's residence for the purpose of promoting, maintaining, or restoring health.

homebound A person unable to leave home for normal activities such as shopping, meals, or other activities.

Hospital Survey and Construction Act of 1946 (Hill-Burton Act) Federal legislation that provided substantial funds for hospital construction.

host A person or other living animal that affords subsistence or lodgment to a communicable agent under natural conditions.

human activities All activities of human beings.

---

*From: Joint Committee on Health Education Terminology (1991). "Report of the 1990 Joint Committee on Health Education Terminology." *Journal of School Health* 22(2): 103–106.

†From: Joint Committee on Health Education Terminology. (1974). "New Definitions: Report of the 1972–73 Joint Committee on Health Education terminology." *Journal of School Health* 44 (1): 33–37.

hydrologic cycle The endless movement of water from the earth's surface to the atmosphere and back to the earth's surface.

hypertension A chronic condition characterized by a resting blood pressure reading of 140/90mm of mercury or higher.

illegal alien An individual who entered this country without permission.

illicit (illegal) drugs Drugs that cannot be legally manufactured, distributed, bought, or sold, and that lack recognized medical value.

immigrant Individuals who migrate to this country from another country for the purpose of seeking permanent residence.

impairments Defects in the functioning of one's sense organs or limitations in one's mobility or range of motion.

incidence rate The number of *new* cases of a disease in a population-at-risk during a particular period of time, divided by the total number in that same population.

incineration The burning of wastes.

incubation period The period of time between exposure to an infectious agent and the onset of symptoms.

Independent practice association (IPA) model HMO An HMO in which individual physicians contract with the HMO to provide care for a certain number of enrollees.

independent providers Health care professionals with the education and legal authority to treat any health problem.

Indian Health Service (IHS) An agency whose goal is to raise the health status of the American Indian and Alaskan Native to the highest possible level by providing a comprehensive health services delivery system.

indirect transmission Communicable disease transmission involving an intermediate step; for example, air-borne, vehicle-borne, or vector-borne transmission.

indoor air pollution The buildup of undesirable gases and particles in the air inside a building.

industrial hygienist A health professional concerned with health hazards in the workplace, including such things as problems with ventilation, noise and lighting; also responsible for measuring air quality and with recommending plans for improving the healthiness of work environments.

infant death (infant mortality) Death of a child under one year of age.

infant mortality rate The number of deaths of children under one year of age per 1,000 live births.

infection The lodgment and growth of a virus or microorganism in a host organism.

infectious disease (See **communicable disease.**)

informal caregiver One who provides unpaid care or assistance to one who has some physical, mental, emotional, or financial need that limits his or her independence.

inhalants Breathable substances that produce mind-altering effects; for example, glue.

injury prevention (control) An organized effort to prevent injuries or to minimize their severity.

injury Physical harm or damage to the body resulting from an exchange, usually acute, of mechanical, chemical, thermal, or other environmental energy that exceeds the body's tolerance.

injury prevention education The process of changing people's health-directed behavior in such a way as to reduce unintentional injuries.

insecticides Pesticides designed specifically to kill insects.

integrated instruction Pattern of instruction in which a certain subject matter is the vehicle used to teach other subjects.

integrated waste management approach An approach to disposing of solid waste that includes sanitary landfills, incineration, recycling, and source reduction.

intensity Cardiovascular work load measured by heart rate.

intentional injury An injury that is judged to have been purposely inflicted, either by the victim or another.

intern Title given to a physician who, after passing a licensing examination, joins the staff of a hospital for practical experience.

internal radiation Radiation in the human body that occurs as a result of ingesting food or inhaling air.

intervention Efforts to control a disease in progress.

involuntary outpatient commitment Court-ordered outpatient treatment.

labor-force dependency ratio A ratio of the number of those individuals who are working (regardless of age) to the number of those who are not.

lag phase Initial phase of the population growth S-curve, when growth is slow.

leachates Liquids created when water mixes with wastes and removes soluble constituents from them by percolation.

lead A naturally occurring mineral element that is found throughout the environment and is produced in large quantities for industrial products.

legal intervention deaths Deaths attributable to police action or legal execution.

licensed practical nurse (LPN)/ licensed vocational nurse (LVN) Those prepared in one- to two-year programs to provide nontechnical bedside nursing care under the supervision of physicians or registered nurses.

life expectancy The average number of years a person from a specific cohort is projected to live from a given point in time.

life support systems Those elements in the environment that provide the basis for life.

limited care providers Health care providers who provide care for a specific part of the body; for example, dentists.

limited-service hospitals Hospitals that offer only the specific services needed by the population served.

litigation The process of seeking justice for injury through courts.

low-birth-weight infant An infant that weighs less than 2,500 grams, or 5.5 pounds, at birth.

macro intervention activities Activities aimed at groups of people.

mainstream tobacco smoke The smoke of burning tobacco inhaled and exhaled by the smoker.

major depression An affective mental disorder characterized by a dysphoric mood, usually depression, or loss of interest or pleasure in almost all usual activities or pastimes.

majority Those with characteristics that are found in over 50% of a population.

malignant melanoma Most serious and least common skin cancer.

malignant neoplasm Uncontrolled new tissue growth resulting from cells that have lost control over their growth and division.

marijuana Dried plant parts of *Cannabis sativa.*

maternal mortality rate Number of mothers dying per 100,000 live births in a given year.

maternal, infant, and child health The health of women of childbearing age: from prepregnancy through pregnancy, labor and delivery, and the postpartum period. Also includes the health of the child prior to birth through adolescence.

Meals-on-Wheels program A community supported nutrition program in which prepared meals are delivered to seniors in their homes, usually by volunteers.

mechanical transmission Communicable disease transmission that occurs without incubation, growth, or multiplication of the infectious agent.

median age The age at which half of the population is older and half is younger.

medigap Private health insurance to supplement Medicare benefits—that is, to fill in the gaps of Medicare.

mental disorder Deficiency in one's psychological resources for dealing with everyday life, usually characterized by distress or impairment of one or more areas of functioning.

mental health Emotional and social well-being, including one's psychological resources for dealing with the day-to-day problems of life.

mental hygiene movement A movement by those who believed that mental illness could be cured if identified and treated at an early stage; proponents were Adolph Meyer and Clifford Beers.

Mental Retardation Facilities and Community Mental Health Centers (CMHC) Act of 1963 (Community Mental Health Act of 1963) A law that provided federal funds directly to communities to assist in the building and funding of community mental health centers.

metastasis The spread of a disease, such as cancer, by the transfer of cells by means of the blood or lymphatics.

methaqualone A depressant drug that has no recognized medical use but is sometimes subject to abuse; also known as quaaludes ("ludes").

methcathinone ("cat") An illicit, synthetic drug, similar to the amphetamines, that first appeared in the United States in 1991.

Meyer, Adolf (1866–1950) A Swiss-born psychiatrist, prominent at the turn of the century, who was influential in establishing psychiatric hospitals for mentally ill.

micro intervention activities Intervention activities aimed at individuals.

migration Movement of people from one country to another.

minority groups Subgroups of the population that make up less than 50% of the total population.

model for abuse The public health triangle (host, agent, and environment) modified to indicate the abused (host), the abuser (agent), and a crisis (the environment).

model for unintentional injuries The public health triangle (host, agent, and environment) modified to indicate energy as the causative agent of injuries.

modern era of public health The era of American public health that began in 1850 and continues today.

modifiable risk factor Factors contributing to the development of a noncommunicable disease that can be altered by modifying one's behavior or environment; for example, cigarette smoking is a modifiable risk factor for coronary heart disease.

moral treatment Treatment for mental illness in eighteenth and nineteenth centuries, based on belief that mental illness was caused by moral deterioration.

morbidity rate The rate of illness in a population.

mortality (fatality) rate The rate of deaths in a population.

Mothers Against Drunk Driving (MADD) A voluntary organization that encourages removal of drunk drivers from the nation's highways.

multicausation disease model A visual representation of the host, together with various internal and external factors that promote and protect against disease.

municipal waste Waste generated by individual households, businesses, and institutions located within municipalities.

narcotics Durgs similar to morphine that reduce pain and induce a stuporous state.

Narcotics Anonymous A fellowship of recovering narcotics users who offer support to anyone who desires to remain free of drugs.

natality (birth) rate The rate of births in a population.

National Alliance for the Mentally Ill (NAMI) A national voluntary health agency that advocates for the mentally ill.

National Ambient Air Quality Standards (NAAQSs) Standards created by the EPA for allowable concentration levels of the six criteria pollutants and nine others in outdoor air.

National Diffusion Network (NDN) An organization that reviews and rates curricula.

National Electronic Telecommunications System (NETS) The electronic reporting system by which state health departments send health records to the Centers for Disease Control and Prevention (CDC).

National Institute for Occupational Safety and Health (NIOSH) A research body within the Centers for Disease Control and Prevention, Department of Health and Human Services, that is responsible for developing and recommending occupational safety and health standards.

National Institute of Mental Health (NIMH) The primary federal agency for mental health research.

National Institutes of Health (NIH) The research division of the Public Health Service.

National Mental Health Act of 1946 Landmark federal legislation which established the National Institute of Mental Health and grants in aid to states to provide mental health services.

National Mental Health Association (NMHA) A national voluntary health association that advocates for mental health and for those with mental illnesses; it has 600 affiliates in 43 states.

National Mental Health Foundation (NMHF) A national organization (1946–1950) formed by mental health attendants who were appalled at conditions in mental hospitals.

nativity Birthplace.

natural disasters Geophysical and meteorological events that frequently exceed normal human expectation in terms of magnitude or frequency and which cause significant damage; example, flood.

needs assessment A process by which needs of individuals, groups, organizations, or communities are identified.

neonatal deaths (neonatal mortality) Deaths occurring during the first 28 days after birth.

neonatologist A medical doctor who specializes in the care of newborns from birth to two months of age.

net migration The population gain or loss resulting from migration.

network model HMO An HMO in which the HMO contracts with several physicians' group practices to provide care for a specified number of HMO enrollees.

neuroleptic drug A drug that reduces nervous activity; another term for *antipsychotic drug.*

noise Unwanted sound.

Noise Control Act (NCA) (P.L. 92-574) A federal law aimed at regulating the noise emissions from new consumer products. Amended to include the Quiet Communities Act.

noise pollution Excessive sound.

nonallopathic providers Independent providers who provide nontraditional forms of health care.

noncommunicable disease (noninfectious disease) A disease not caused by a communicable agent, and that thus cannot be transmitted from infected host to susceptible host.

noninfectious disease (See **noncommunicable disease.**)

nonnutritive energy Energy sources that provide shelter, fiber, heat, and transportation (e.g., oil, electricity, gas, solar, etc.).

nonpoint source pollution All pollution that occurs through the runoff, seepage, or falling of pollutants into the water.

nontarget organisms All other susceptible organisms in the environment, for which a pesticide was not intended.

notifiable diseases Infectious diseases for which health officials request or require reporting for public health reasons.

nutritive energy Food.

occupational disease Any abnormal condition or disorder, other than one resulting from an occupational injury, caused by an exposure to environmental factors associated with employment.

occupational health nurse (OHN) A registered nurse whose primary responsibilities include prevention of illness and promotion of health in the workplace.

occupational injury An injury that results from exposure to a single incident in the work environment (e.g., cut, fracture, sprain, amputation).

occupational physician (OP) or **(occupational medical practitioner)** A medical practiner (doctor) whose primary concern is preventive medicine in the workplace.

Occupational Safety and Health Act of 1970 (OSHAct) Comprehensive federal legislation aimed at assuring safe and healthful working conditions for working men and women.

Occupational Safety and Health Administration (OSHA) The federal agency located within the Department of Labor and created by the OSHAct that is charged with the responsibility of administering the provisions of the OSHAct.

odds ratio A probability statement about the association between a particular disease and a specific risk factor, often the outcome of a retrospective (case/control) study.

official health agency See governmental health agency.

old Those 65 years of age and older.

old old Those 75 years of age and older.

Older Americans Act of 1965 Federal legislation to improve the lives of seniors.

oldest old Those 85 years of age and older.

operationalize (operational definition) Provide working definitions.

osteopathic providers Independent health care providers whose remedies are based on a philosophy that emphasizes the interrelationships of the body's systems in the prevention, diagnosis, and treatment of illness, disease, and injury.

outside community organization Organization efforts that begin with individuals from outside the affected community.

over-the-counter (OTC) drugs (nonprescription drugs) Drugs (except tobacco and alcohol) that can be legally purchased without a physician's prescription; example, aspirin.

ownership A feeling that one has a stake in or "owns" the object of interest.

ozone layer Ozone gas (O_3) found in the stratosphere.

pandemic An outbreak of disease over a wide geographical area, such as a continent.

passive smoking The inhalation of environmental tobacco smoke by nonsmokers.

pathogenicity The capability of a communicable agent to cause disease in a susceptible host.

peer counseling programs School-based drug education programs in which students discuss alcohol and other drug-related problems with other students.

perceived or felt needs Needs that those in the target population believe must be met in order to resolve a problem.

persistent pesticide See **hard pesticide.**

pest Any organism—multicelled animal or plant, or microbe—that has an adverse effect on human health or well-being.

pesticides Synthetic chemicals developed and manufactured for the purpose of killing pests.

pharmacokinetics Rate of absorption, distribution, metabolism, and excretion of substances from the body.

phasing in Implementation of an intervention with small groups prior to the entire population.

philanthropic foundation An endowed institution that donates money for the good of mankind.

photochemical smog A secondary air pollutant created when primary pollutants react with oxygen and sunlight.

physical dependence Drug dependence in which discontinued use results in the onset of physical illness.

picocurie (pCi) A means of expressing the rate of radioactive disintegration. One pCi equals the decay of about two radioactive atoms per minute.

pilot test Presentation of the intervention to just a few individuals, who are either from the intended target population or from a very similar population.

placebo A blank treatment (e.g., a sugar pill).

point source epidemic curve An epidemic curve depicting a distribution of cases that can all be traced to a single source of exposure.

point source pollution Pollution that can be traced to a single identifiable source.

Pollutant Standard Index (PSI) A scale developed by the EPA which relates air pollutant concentrations to health effects.

polydrug use Concurrent use of multiple drugs.

population-at-risk Those in the population who are susceptible to a particular disease or condition.

portal of entry The route by which a communicable agent invades a susceptible host.

portal of exit The route by which a communicable agent leaves an infected host.

postneonatal deaths (postneonatal mortality) Deaths that occur between 28 days and 365 days after birth.

preexisting condition A medical condition that places the insured and insurer at a higher risk for having to make medical payments.

preferred provider organization (PPO) An organization that buys fixed-rate (discount) health services from providers and sells them (via premiums) to consumers.

premature infant One born following a gestation period of 38 weeks or less, or one born at a low birth weight.

prenatal health care (prenatal care) Medical care provided to a pregnant woman from the time of conception until the birth process occurs, including counseling about appropriate and inappropriate health behavior.

preplacement examination A physical examination of a newly hired or transferred worker to determine medical suitability for placement in a specific position.

prevalence rate The number of *new and old* cases of a disease in a population in a given period of time, divided by the total number of that population.

prevention The planning for and taking of action to forestall the onset of a disease or other health problem before the occurrence of undesirable health events.

preventive care Care given to healthy people to keep them healthy.

primary care Regular and routine front-line health care.

primary prevention Preventive measures that forestall the onset of illness or injury during the prepathogenesis period.

private (proprietary) hospitals For-profit hospitals.

pro-choice A medical/ethical position that holds that women have a right to reproductive freedom.

pro-life A medical/ethical position that holds that performing an abortion is an act of murder.

problem drinker One for whom alcohol consumption results in personal, economic, medical, social, or any other type of problem.

professional nurse (BSN) A registered nurse holding a bachelor of science degree in nursing.

program planning A process by which an intervention is planned to help meet the needs of a target population.

propagated epidemic curve An epidemic curve depicting a distribution of cases traceable to multiple sources of exposure over time.

proportionate mortality ratio (PMR) The percentage of overall mortality in a population that can be assigned to a particular cause or disease.

prospective pricing system One in which providers are paid predetermined amounts of money per procedure for services provided.

prospective study An epidemiological study that begins in the present and continues into the future for the purpose of observing the development of disease (e.g., cohort study).

providers of health care Those individuals educated to provide health services, such as physicians, dentists, nurses, etc.

psychoactive drugs Mind-altering drugs; drugs that affect the central nervous system.

psychological dependence A psychological state characterized by an overwhelming desire to continue use of a drug.

psychotherapy A treatment methodology based on the Freudian concept of emotional (catharsis) release, sexual conflict resolution, and subconscious drives.

public health The sum of all official or government efforts to promote, protect, and preserve the people's health.

public health professional A health care worker who works at a public health clinic or in another public health organization.

Public Health Service (PHS) A major division of the Department of Health and Human Services and the one most directly responsible for the community health of Americans.

quasi-governmental health organizations Organizations that have some responsibilities assigned by the government but operate more like voluntary agencies; example, the American Red Cross.

radiation Energy released when an atom is split during the process of fission.

radon A naturally occurring radioactive gas that cannot be seen, smelled, or tasted.

rate The number of events (cases of disease) that occur in a given period of time.

recycling The collection and reprocessing of a resource after use so it can be reused for the same or another purpose.

reform phase of public health The period of public health from 1900 to 1920, characterized by social movements to improve health conditions in cities and in the workplace.

refugee A person who flees one area or country to seek shelter or protection from danger in another.

registered nurse (RN) An associate or baccalaureate degree–prepared nurse who has passed the state licensing examination.

regulation The enactment and enforcement of laws to control conduct.

rehabilitation center A facility in which restorative care is provided following injury, disease, or surgery.

relative risk A statement of the relationship between the risk of acquiring a disease when a specific risk factor is present and the risk of acquiring that same disease when the risk factor is not present.

rems (roentgen equivalent man) A measure of the biological damage of radiation to human tissues.

reservoir Any person, animal, arthropod, plant, soil, or substance in which a communicable agent normally lives and multiplies and which can serve as a source of infection to a susceptible host.

resident A physician who is training in a specialty.

residues and wastes By-products of human activities.

Resource Conservation and Recovery Act (RCRA) A federal law that regulates solid and hazardous wastes.

respite care Planned short-term care, usually for the purpose of relieving a full-time informal caregiver.

restorative care Care provided to patients after a successful treatment or when the progress of a incurable disease has been arrested.

retirement communities Residential communities that have been specifically developed for those in their retirement years.

retrospective study An epidemiological study that looks into the past for clues to explain the present distribution of disease.

risk factors Factors that increase the probability of disease, injury, or death.

Roe vs. Wade A 1973 Supreme Court decision that made it unconstitutional for state laws to prohibit abortions.

rollover protective structures (ROPS) Factory-installed or retrofitted reinforced framework on a cab to protect the operator of a tractor in case of a rollover.

Safe Drinking Water Act (SDWA) A 1974 federal law that instructed the EPA to set maximum contaminant levels for specific pollutants in drinking water.

safety engineer A health and safety professional, sometimes with an engineering background, employed by a company for the purpose of reducing unintentional injuries in the workplace.

safety program That part of the workplace health and safety program aimed at reducing unintentional injuries on the job.

sanitarians Environmental workers responsible for inspection of facilities and investigation of complaints with regard to public health codes.

sanitary engineer Environmental worker responsible for management of waste water and solid waste for a community.

sanitary landfill A site judged suitable for in-ground disposal of solid waste.

school health coordinator Person who coordinates the school health program for a school district.

School Health Education Study (SHES) A study that began in 1960 to determine the status of health education in U.S. schools.

school health policies Written statements that describe the nature and procedures of a school health program.

school health services Health services "provided by physicians, nurses, dentists, health educators, other allied health personnel, social workers, teachers, and others to appraise, protect and promote the health of students and school personnel."*

school health team Those individuals who work together to plan and implement the school health program.

scope Part of the curriculum that outlines what will be taught.

secondary (acute) care That which includes intense and elaborate diagnosis and treatment.

secondary prevention Preventive measures that lead to early diagnosis and prompt treatment of a disease or injury to limit disability and prevent more severe pathogenesis.

secondhand smoke Environmental tobacco smoke (ETS), tobacco smoke in the ambient air.

secured landfill A double-lined landfill located above flood plain and away from a fault zone, equipped with monitoring pipes for seepage, used primarily for hazardous waste.

self-insured organization One that pays the health care costs of its employees with the premiums collected from the employees and the contributions made by the employer.

seniors Those 65 years of age or older.

senior centers Facilities where seniors can congregate for fellowship, meals, education, and recreation.

septic tank A watertight concrete or fiberglass tank that holds sewage; one of two main parts of a septic system.

sequence Part of the curriculum that states in what order the content will be taught.

---

*From: Joint Committee on Health Education Terminology (1991). "Report of the 1990 Joint Committee on Health Education Terminology." *Journal of School Health* 22(2): 105–106.

service demands or wants See **perceived or felt needs.**

service needs or real needs Needs that health professionals believe the target population must have met in order to resolve a problem.

sexually transmitted diseases (STDs) Diseases that are spread primarily through unprotected sexual activity.

sick building syndrome A term to describe a situation in which the air quality in a building produces signs and symptoms of ill health in the building's occupants.

sickle cell disease A genetic disease of the red blood cells characterized by atypical hemoglobin; most common in black Americans and those of Mediterranean, Caribbean, South and Central American, Arabian, and East Indian ancestry.

sidestream tobacco smoke The smoke that comes off the end of burning tobacco products.

silicosis Acute or chronic lung disease caused by the inhalation of free crystalline silica; those affected include workers in mines, stone quarries, sand and gravel operations, and abrasive blasting operations.

sludge A gooey mixture of solid waste that includes bacteria, viruses, organic matter, toxic metals, synthetic organic chemicals, and solid chemicals.

smokeless tobacco Snuff and chewing tobacco.

social interaction Interaction between human beings.

Social Security Administration (SSA) An agency of DHHS that administers programs that provide financial support to special groups of Americans. (See note on p. 35.)

soft pesticide A chemical substance used for controlling pests that breaks down into harmless products within weeks.

solid waste Refuse from households, agriculture, and businesses, including garbage, yard waste, paper products, manure, excess stone generated from mining, and building material scraps.

sound-level meter Instrument used to measure sound.

source reduction A waste management approach entailing the reduction or elimination of use of materials that result in the accumulation of solid waste.

specific rate A rate of a specific disease in a population or the rate of events in a specific population (e.g., cause-specific death rate, age-specific death rate).

spectrum of health care delivery The array of types of care—from preventive to continuing, or long-term, care. It comprises six levels of care.

spiritual era of public health A time during the Middle Ages when the physical and biological environment in the causation of communicable disease were ignored.

squamous cell carcinoma A common, highly curable type of skin cancer.

staff model HMO A health maintenance organization that hires its own staff of physicians.

standard of acceptability A comparative mandate, value, norm, or group.

State Implementation Plans (SIPS) Documents submitted by each state to the EPA outlining their plan for achieving and maintaining air-quality standards.

statutory law Law passed by state or federal legislatures or other governing body, as opposed to common law.

stimulant A drug that increases the activity of the central nervous system; for example, methamphetamine.

stress One's psychological and physiological response to stressors.

stressors Stimuli in one's physical and social environment that produce feelings of tension and strain.

Student Assistance Programs (SAPs) School-based drug education programs to assist students who have alcohol or other drug problems.

Students Against Driving Drunk (SADD) A national organization, composed primarily of high school students, whose goal it is to reduce drinking and driving deaths of teenagers.

Substance Abuse and Mental Health Services Administration (SAMHSA) Federal agency in DHHS established in 1992 to superceed Alcohol, Drug Abuse, and Mental Health Association (ADAMHA), whose stated mission is the reduction of the incidence and prevalence of alcohol and other drug abuse and mental disorders, the improvement of treatment outcomes, and the curtailment of the consequences of mental health problems for families and communities.

sudden infant death syndrome (SIDS) Sudden unanticipated death of an infant in whom, after examination, there is no recognized cause of death.

summative evaluation The evaluation that determines the impact of a program on the target population.

sun protection factor (SPF) A scale used to indicate the protective quality of sunscreens.

Superfund Amendments Reauthorization Act (SARA) 1986 reauthorization of Comprehensive Environmental Response, Compensation, and Liability Act (CERCLA).

Supplemental Security Program of the Social Security Administration that provides cash benefits to elderly, blind, and disabled Americans with minimal resources.

surface water Water that is found on the earth's surface (e.g., oceans, rivers, streams, ponds, lakes, etc.).

synesthesia Impairment of mind (by hallucinogens), characterized by a sensation that senses are mixed (e.g., seeing sounds and hearing images).

tardive dyskinesia Irreversible, involuntary, and abnormal movements of the tongue, mouth, arms, and legs which can result from long-term use of certain antipsychotic drugs such as chlorpromazine.

target organism The organism for which a pesticide is applied.

target pest See **target organism.**

target population Those whom a planned program is intended to serve.

technical nurse An associate degree–prepared registered nurse.

"Teenage Health Teaching Modules" (THTM) A health education curriculum developed by the Education Development Center for the secondary level.

terrestrial radiation Radiation that comes from radioactive minerals within the earth, as opposed to celestial radiation.

tertiary (special) care Advanced care that often requires highly technical services for patients; example, heart by-pass surgery.

tertiary prevention Measures aimed at rehabilitation following significant pathogenesis.

thermal inversion Condition that occurs when warm air traps cooler air at the surface of the earth.

thermal pollution The contamination of surface water at ambient temperatures with excessively heated water.

Third World country A country with meager economic resources.

third-party payment system A health insurance term indicating that bills will be paid by the insurer (the government or private insurance company) and not the patient (first party) or the health care provider (the second party).

Thorazine (See *chlorpromazine*).

Title X A portion of the Public Health Service Act of 1970 that provides funds for family planning services for low-income people.

tolerance Physiological and enzymatic adjustments that occur in response to the chronic presence of drugs, reflected in the need for ever-increasing doses to achieve a previous level of effect.

top-down community organization See **outside community organization.**

top-down funding Money that comes from either the federal or state government to the local level.

total dependency (support) ratio The dependency ratio that includes both youth and elderly.

transinstitutionalization The process by which patients from one type of public institution, a mental hospital for example, end up in a different institution, such as a nursing home or jail, because of changes in federal policy.

transitional care facilities Residential housing that enables a mental patient to live in a community by providing some social support.

transmission (of communicable agents) Any mechanism by which a communicable agent is spread from a source or reservoir to a host.

treatment An activity or activities designed to create change in people.

turfism The protectionism of the subgroups within the larger group.

U.S. Census The enumeration of the population of the United States that is conducted every ten years.

ultraviolet radiation Solar radiation.

unintentional injury An injury judged to have occurred w8ithout anyone intending that harm be done.

universal precautions Disease prevention guidelines for health workers and others who may come into contact with human body fluids, which involve the use of appropriate barriers to reduce or eliminate exposure to these fluids.

unsafe act Any behavior that would increase the probability of an injury occurring.

unsafe condition Any environmental factor or set of factors (physical or social) that would increase the probability of an injury occurring.

urbanization The process by which people come together to live in cities.

vector A living organism, usually an arthropod, that can transmit a communicable disease agent to susceptible hosts (e.g., mosquitoes, ticks, lice, fleas).

vector-borne disease A communicable disease transmitted by vectors; for example, Lyme disease is transmitted by ticks.

vehicle Inanimate materials or objects, such as clothes, bedding, toys, hypodermic needles; or nonliving biological materials such as food, milk, water, blood, serum or plasma, tissues or organs, that can serve as a source of infection.

vehicle-borne disease A communicable disease transmitted by nonliving objects; for example, typhoid fever can be transmitted by water.

vibrations per second (vps) A measurement of sound frequency.

visitor services A community social service involving one individual taking time to visit with another who is unable to leave his/her residence.

vital statistics Statistical summaries of vital records—records of major life events, such as births, deaths, marriages, divorces, and infant deaths.

volatile organic compounds (VOCs) Compounds that exist as vapors over the normal range of air pressures and temperatures.

voluntary (independent) hospital A nonprofit hospital administered by religious, fraternal, and other charitable community organizations.

voluntary health agency An organization created by concerned citizens to deal with health needs not met by governmental health agencies.

waste exchanges Managed exchanges in which a contract is written between those who want to dispose of hazardous wastes and those who can use them as raw materials.

waste-to-energy (WTE) plants Incinerators that are able to convert some heat generated from the burning of trash into steam and electricity.

waste water The aqueous mixture that remains after water has been used or consumed by humans.

water pollution Any physical or chemical change in water that can harm living organisms or make the water unfit for other uses.

water-borne diseases Diseases that are transmitted via fecal contamination of water.

WIC program A special supplemental food program for women, infants, and children, sponsored by the United States Department of Agriculture.

workers' compensation laws A set of federal laws designed to compensate those workers and their families who suffer injuries, disease, or death from workplace exposure.

World Health Assembly Body of delegates of the member nations of the World Health Organization.

World Health Organization (WHO) Most widely recognized international governmental health organization today. Created in 1948 by representatives of United Nations countries.

years of potential life lost The number of years lost when death occurs before the age of 65.

young old Those 65–74 years of age.

youth dependency (support) ratio The dependency ratio that includes only youth.

youth gang A self-formed association of peers, bound together by mutual interests, with identifiable leadership and well-defined lines of authority, who act in concert to achieve a specific purpose and whose acts generally include illegal activity and control over a territory or an enterprise.

zero population growth (ZPG) A state in which the birth and death rates for a given population are equal.

zoonosis A communicable disease transmissible under natural conditions from vertebrate animals to man.

Acknowledgments

Unless otherwise acknowledged, all photographs are the property of Scott, Foresman and Company.

1: Bob Daemmrich; **6:** Mike Mazzaschi/Stock Boston; **8:** Margaret Thompson/The Picture Cube; **16:** © American Public Health Assoc.; **17:** Robert Harding Picture Library Ltd., London; **19:** Library of Congress; **23:** Courtesy Center for Attitudinal Healing; **32 left:** Courtesy World Health Organization; **32 right:** Courtesy Pan American Sanitary Bureau; **46:** Courtesy The American Red Cross; **53:** Milt & Joan Mann/Cameramann International, Ltd.; **61:** The National Archives; **68:** Ellis Herwig/The Picture Cube; **75:** Griffin/The Image Works; **85:** Teresa Delgadillo-Bevington; **89:** Bernard Furnival/Fran Heyl Assoc.; **102:** Doug Plummer/Photo Researchers; **103:** Jim Pickerell/Stock Boston; **109:** Jean-Claude LeJeune; **111:** Courtesy Peace Corps; **115:** Peter Simon/Stock Boston; **123:** Michael Hayman/Stock Boston; **129:** David Sams/Stock Boston; **138:** Bob Daemmrich; **148:** Mary Kate Denny/Photo Edit; **150:** Rick Friedman/The Picture Cube; **151:** Richard Hutchings/Photo Researchers; **161:** Courtesy The School Based Adolescent Health Care Program, Washington, DC; **167:** Paul Conklin; **170:** Cynthia W. Sterling/The Picture Cube; **189:** Robert Brenner/Photo Edit; **190:** Richard Frear/Photo Researchers; **199:** Courtesy, American Cancer Society; **203:** Joel Gordon Photography; **204:** Therese Frare/The Picture Cube; **214:** Beryl Goldberg; **216:** Robert Brenner/Photo Edit; **221:** Mel Rosenthal/The Image Works; **235:** Paul Fusco/Magnum Photos; **238:** Beryl Goldberg; **245:** Rhoda Sidney/Photo Edit; **251:** Paul Conklin; **256:** Beryl Goldberg; **283:** Joel Gordon Photography; **288:** Susan Greenwood/Gamma-Liaison; **299:** Ulrike Welsch/Photo Edit; **300:** AP/Wide World; **301:** Okoniewski/The Image Works; **312:** Preuss/The Image Works; **313:** Ulrike Welsch/Photo Edit; **321:** Milt & Joan Mann/Cameramann International, Ltd.; **328, 332:** Paul Fusco/Magnum Photos; **338:** Judy Gelles/Stock Boston; **340:** Robert Brenner/Photo Edit; **346:** National Library of Medicine, Bethesda, MD; **347:** Historical Pictures/Stock Montage, Inc.; **348:** UPI/Bettmann; **349:** The National Committee for Mental Hygiene, NY; **351:** Jerry Cooke; **355:** Beryl Goldberg; **361:** P.Beringer/Dratch/The Image Works; **373:** Robert Brenner/Photo Edit; **375:** Richard Hutchings/Photo Edit; **376:** Michael Newman/Photo Edit; **382:** Pierre Marie/Gamma-Liaison; **384:** Hap Stewart/Jeroboam Inc.; **394:** Lynne Sladky/AP/Wide World; **397:** Joel Gordon Photography; **398:** Gale Zucker/Stock Boston; **405:** Wally McNamee/Sygma; **408:** Eduardo Contreras/Copyrighted, Chicago Tribune Company, all rights reserved; **411:** David Jennings/The Image Works; **417:** Tim Barnwell/Stock Boston; **421:** J.P.Laffont/Sygma; **423:** Watson/The Image Works; **428:** Wells/The Image Works; **430:** Bob Daemmrich/The Image Works; **436:** N.R.Rowan/Stock Boston; **443:** Mark Antman/The Image Works; **445:** H.Dratch/The Image Works; **456,457:** Martin Benjamin/The Image Works; **458:** Ron Edmonds/AP/Wide World; **462:** Courtesy Ministry of Health,Ontario; **469:** Courtesy *Successful Farming;* **476:** AP/Wide World; **478:** David Wells/The Image Works; **481:** J.Fossett/The Image Works; **489:** Liliana Nieto DelRio/NYT Pictures; **491:** Jesse Mobley/The Image Works; **494:** Shoemaker ©1970 Chicago Today; **498:** AP/Wide World; **509:** Okoniewski/The Image Works; **531,535:** Grant Heilman Photography; **539:** Dr. Leonard E. Munstermann/Fran Heyl Associates; **547:** Jeff Albertson/Stock Boston; **551:** Dion Ogust/The Image Works; **562:** Owen Franken/Stock Boston; **566:** Brooks Kraft/Sygma; **573:** Peter Menzel/Stock Boston; **585:** Alan Carey/The Image Works; **598:** Spencer Grant/Stock Boston; **602:** Allan Tannenbaum/Sygma; **603:** Michael Newman/Photo Edit; **604:** AP/Wide World; **613,614:** George Eastman House; **615:** AP/Wide World; **619:** Milt & Joan Mann/Cameramann International, Ltd.; **622:** Courtesy *Successful Farming;* **624,626:** Milt & Joan Mann/Cameramann International, Ltd.; **628:** Jon Chase/Stock Boston; **631:** John Coletti/Stock Boston.

Index